Healthy Ageing and Aged Care

EDITED BY

Maree Bernoth and
Denise Winkler

DEDICATION

Dedicated to:

Our husbands: Maxwell Bernoth and John Winkler who have contributed to the content, sustained us and provided learning opportunities for both us and the readers.

Our parents: Mary Blackford OAM, and John and Darlene Cantrell, who demonstrate how to live well despite the challenges ageing provides.

Healthy Ageing and Aged Care

EDITED BY

Maree Bernoth and Denise Winkler

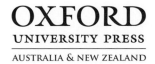

OXFORD
UNIVERSITY PRESS
AUSTRALIA & NEW ZEALAND

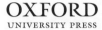

OXFORD
UNIVERSITY PRESS

Oxford University Press is a department of the University of Oxford.
It furthers the University's objective of excellence in research,
scholarship, and education by publishing worldwide. Oxford is a registered
trademark of Oxford University Press in the UK and in certain other countries.

Published in Australia by
Oxford University Press
Level 8, 737 Bourke Street, Docklands, Victoria 3008, Australia.

A catalogue record for this
book is available from the
National Library of Australia

ISBN 9780190326234

Edited by Sandra Balonyi
Typeset by Integra Software Services Pvt. Ltd
Proofread by Peter Cruttenden
Indexed by Mary Russell
Printed in Singapore by Markono Print Media Pte Ltd.

Disclaimer

Aboriginal and Torres Strait Islander peoples are advised that this publication may include
images or names of people now deceased.

*Links to third party websites are provided by Oxford in good faith and for information only.
Oxford disclaims any responsibility for the materials contained in any third party website referenced in this
work.*

Brief Contents

PART 1 » The Context of Ageing   1

PART 2 » The Social Aspects of Ageing   91

PART 3 » The Clinical Aspects of Ageing and Aged Care 189

OXFORD UNIVERSITY PRESS

OXFORD UNIVERSITY PRESS

Contents

PART 1 » The Context of Ageing   1

Chapter 1: The Opportunities and Challenges of Ageing in Australia

Clarissa Hughes, Christine Stirling and Robin Harvey

Chapter 2: Policies Influencing Aged Care in Australia: Past, Present and Future

J. Michael Wynne, Lynda Saltarelli and Denise Winkler

Chapter 3: Healthy Ageing and Aged Care of First Nations Australians

Jayne Lawrence

Chapter 4: The Personal Perspective of Ageing in a Complex World   75
Denise Winkler

PART 2 » The Social Aspects of Ageing   91

Chapter 5: Family Relationships and Informal Care   92
Belinda Cash

Chapter 6: Ageing in Rural Areas: Embracing Diversity   109
Karen Bell and Sabine Wardle

PART 3 » The Clinical Aspects of Ageing and Aged Care 189

Chapter 18: Managing Multiple Chronic Conditions (Multimorbidity)

Alison Devitt

Jenny McKenzie and Melissa Brodie

GUIDED TOUR

This book comes equipped with a range of carefully designed learning features, both in the text and online. These will help you gain a deeper understanding of ageing and aged care, and to develop the essential knowledge and skills you'll need for your future career.

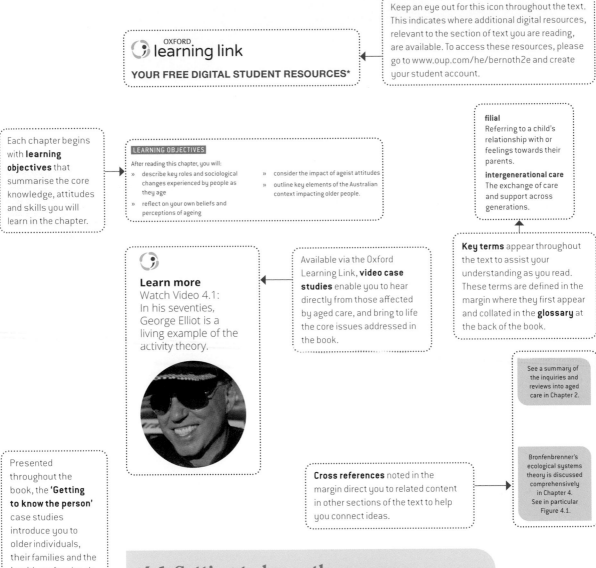

OXFORD learning link

YOUR FREE DIGITAL STUDENT RESOURCES*

Keep an eye out for this icon throughout the text. This indicates where additional digital resources, relevant to the section of text you are reading, are available. To access these resources, please go to www.oup.com/he/bernoth2e and create your student account.

Each chapter begins with **learning objectives** that summarise the core knowledge, attitudes and skills you will learn in the chapter.

LEARNING OBJECTIVES

After reading this chapter, you will:
» describe key roles and sociological changes experienced by people as they age
» reflect on your own beliefs and perceptions of ageing
» consider the impact of ageist attitudes
» outline key elements of the Australian context impacting older people.

filial
Referring to a child's relationship with or feelings towards their parents.
intergenerational care
The exchange of care and support across generations.

Key terms appear throughout the text to assist your understanding as you read. These terms are defined in the margin where they first appear and collated in the **glossary** at the back of the book.

Learn more
Watch Video 4.1: In his seventies, George Elliot is a living example of the activity theory.

Available via the Oxford Learning Link, **video case studies** enable you to hear directly from those affected by aged care, and bring to life the core issues addressed in the book.

See a summary of the inquiries and reviews into aged care in Chapter 2.

Bronfenbrenner's ecological systems theory is discussed comprehensively in Chapter 4. See in particular Figure 4.1.

Presented throughout the book, the **'Getting to know the person'** case studies introduce you to older individuals, their families and the health professionals involved in their care. These stories reveal the complex and individual nature of ageing, and provide context to the issues discussed in each chapter.

Cross references noted in the margin direct you to related content in other sections of the text to help you connect ideas.

4.1 Getting to know the person: Darlene's story

During January 2020, Darlene was anticipating her eightieth birthday. Her four children were planning a big party at the local RSL club; the Chinese food there was her favourite meal. Three of her children, her grandchildren and great grandchildren would be travelling interstate and staying at the bed and breakfast on the street of the country village where she now lived.

- Is there validity in Darlene's perspective of her current situation? Which of her life experiences support your answer?
- Is Darlene ageing successfully?
- To what extent do activity, continuity and disassociation theories explain Darlene's experience of ageing?
- What are the implications for clinical practice if health professionals hold to the disassociation theory?

FOCUS QUESTIONS

You will find several sets of **focus questions** in each chapter inviting you to reflect on the content and encouraging independent thinking and reasoning. These questions often refer to the case studies.

Implications for practice

These are some useful reflections for you as a health professional to consider in relation to the impact of family diversity on care:

- Health professionals should hold a stance of curiosity and awareness about diversity in all assessment and practice contexts to encourage asking questions without making assumptions about how an individual or family might understand and approach ageing and caregiving.
- All health professionals should continue reflecting on their own cultural and family experiences to understand how these can influence assumptions and expectations of care in practice.
- The richness of an individual's family and social background enables health professionals to respectfully identify potential risks while enhancing and utilising existing strengths.

Implications for practice features interpret the information contained in the chapter and show how it can impact current nursing and health-care practices.

Box 3.2

Robyn's experience

Robyn's cultural connection is to the Kamilaroi Nation on her mother's side. She has been on the Cancer Council committee for five years and a board member of Dubbo Health Service and Lourdes Hospital. She shares with you what she has heard from older First Nations peoples.

I have spoken to a number of Elders about their ageing process. Some said it is a part of the life cycle. Some don't like it as they say it comes with many aches and pains and more visits to the 'white' doctor. When they visit the doctor, they don't listen to them as they are always at the computer. Most of the Elders I spoke with said they would like to go back to Country but can't as they have no money. They also commented that they would be buried in the town where they have lived for many years.

They don't like going to hospital as they say that their culture and age is not respected, and they would rather have Aboriginal nurses looking after them. For me, my own experience in the local hospital was not a pleasant one and I was left in a ward without a drink of water for over 24 hours. My friend made a complaint about my treatment and I received an apology. One thing, as a health professional, you must remember is that the current generation of older Aboriginal people may have never learnt to read as they were raised on Aboriginal missions and reserves.

Throughout the book, **Boxes** are used to highlight key material. Chapter 3, specifically uses these to present invaluable insights from First Nations Elders and health-care professionals.

EXAMPLE DIALOGUE

Conversation starters you can use to display acceptance may include:

- How can we best help you?
- What do I need to know to provide the best care for you and your family?
- What would you like us to call you?
- What is your preferred pronoun: he, she or they?
- Who is your best support person or persons? (This might not be a blood relative.)
- Is there anything I can read, or person I can talk to, to assist us to care for you?

Allow time and privacy for these conversations, understanding that there can be fear of judgment, persecution and distrust of health-care providers, which can make rapport-building difficult.

The **example dialogues** featured in Chapters 12 (Mental health) and 19 (End-of-life care) contain constructive conversations and communication points for you as a health professional to use.

Conclusion

In this chapter we encouraged you to understand the holistic perspectives of First Nations peoples, which include the health of the community and the environment. Both the statistics and the lived experiences shared provide unique details of healthy ageing and aged care for First Nations peoples. Critically reflecting on this information over the course of your professional career will allow you to provide culturally safe care to older First Nations peoples. In your role as a nurse or other health-care professional in First Nations aged care, you must have strategies for assessment and communication to create culturally safe experiences. We hope you will benefit from the techniques to build culturally safe communication such as building a rapport, non-verbal communication and respecting silence.

Each chapter ends with a **conclusion** which draws together important ideas. It links back to the chapter's learning objectives to reinforce the information presented in the chapter

Learn more
Access additional resources – such as weblinks, further readings and podcasts – to broaden your understanding of this chapter. See the Guided Tour for access details.

1 Consider the impact that changing family dynamics has on older adults and informal caregivers. How do cultural and social diversity influence expectations of familial care?

2 How does the complex and diverse nature of family relationships impact an individual's experience of ageing?

3 List both the opportunities and barriers to healthy ageing caused by social determinants of health.

4 Identify the significant risks to the health and well-being of families and caregivers of older adults, including spousal caregiving and co-dependence in older couples.

5 Explain why assessment and practice with older adults should take place within a family and social context.

REVISION QUESTIONS

Available via the Oxford Learning Link and arranged by chapter, annotated **additional resources and weblinks** identify key further readings and useful online resources available to support the material presented in the chapter. **Podcasts** are also available to broaden your understanding of chapter topics.

Revision questions at the end of each chapter encourage you to reflect on what you have learnt in the chapter and to consider how you would use this knowledge in your role as a health professional.

LISTS OF TABLES AND FIGURES

List of Tables

List of Figures

LIST OF VIDEO CASE STUDIES

Accompanying this book are 10 bespoke award-winning video case studies created to enable you to hear directly from those affected by aged care. The videos come from the authors, older Australians, carers and volunteers, and directly relate to material covered in this book. Access your digital student resources for the video case studies by creating a student account at www.oup.com/he/bernoth2e

Keep an eye out for this icon throughout the text. This indicates where additional digital resources are available.

1.1   Ray

Ray talks about the importance of Men's Sheds.

4.1   George

George Elliot, the race car driver, talks about his ageing experience.

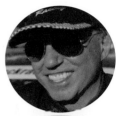

4.2   George

We revisit George five years later to discuss his life experience as he navigated Erikson's eight stages.

6.1   Preet

Preet talks about the challenges of living in rural Australia.

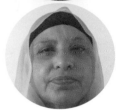

7.1   Mardi

Mardi discusses the abuse and neglect of her grandmother in residential aged care.

8.1   Mary

Mary discusses what volunteering means to her.

8.2   Wallsend Area Community Care volunteers

Wallsend Area Community Care volunteers discuss their experiences.

11.1   Max

Max discusses the delirium he experienced in hospital.

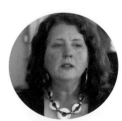

11.2   Denise

Denise talks about the importance of communication during palliative care.

13.1   David

David and his wife Ronita talk leisure and recreation while living with dementia.

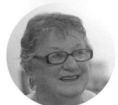

ACKNOWLEDGMENTS

We would like to thank all the individuals who generously allowed us to share their stories and to video them.

We would like to give appreciation to the people who supported us during our editing. A huge shout-out to Vince, Marni, Tennison and Jaxson Cantrell who gave me time, space and energy to pursue my passion. To Heather Arnold, who came to the rescue when I needed you most. Thank you dear friend.

DENISE WINKLER

To Max Bernoth, Rebecca, Simone, their partners and my precious grandsons, I appreciate your love and support through the writing and editing phases of this second edition. I also want to acknowledge the students who are the motivating factor for the book and who continue to challenge me as a teacher.

MAREE BERNOTH

We would like to give a special thanks to Debra James and Sarah Fay, who got us started on the second edition. To Helen Carter, who got us through to the end with her insightful comments: a huge thanks!

We would also like to acknowledge the following people:

- for his expertise with a camera and for his contribution in providing rich stories through the videos and podcasts: Matthew Olsen
- for her masterful skill at editing and referencing: Carmel Davies
- for their contribution to the first edition: Jane Anderson-Wurf, Stephen Neville, Pam Foster, Susan Mlcck, Robyn and Faye McMillan, Travis Ingersoll, Andeia Schineanu, Fredrik Velander, Gary Forrest, Susan Baldawi, Tanya Atkinson, Helen Small, Robyn Bryant, Margaret Roberts, Belinda Scott, Kay Shannon, Carmel Davies and Megan Daniel
- for their contribution to chapter content: Robert Salt, Robyne Payne and Harkiran Kaur.

The author and the publisher wish to thank the following copyright holders for reproduction of their material.

World Health Organization Publication for fig 1.1 from Model of disability, the basis for ICF Source: ICF -Towards a Common Language for Functioning, Disability and Health, WHO, Geneva 2002, p. 9.
https://www.who.int/classifications/icf/icfbeginnersguide.pdf WHO Reference Number WHO/EIP/GPE/CAS/01.3; World Health Organization Publication for box 1.1 The WHO Age Friendly Cities and Communities framework https://extranet.who.int/agefriendlyworld/age-friendly-practices/; Dr. Brian Walker for fig 2.1A, fig 2.1B, fig 2.2; Australian Bureau of Statistics (ABS) for fig 3.1 © Commonwealth of Australia, Creative Commons Attribution 4.0 International licence; University of Minneapolis for Fig 4.1 McEathron, Mary & Beuhring, Trisha. (2011). Postsecondary Education for Students with Intellectual and Developmental Disabilities: A Critical Review of the State of Knowledge and a Taxonomy to Guide Future

Research. Policy Research Brief, 21(1). [Minneapolis: University of Minnesota, Research and Training Centre on Community Living, Institute on Community Integration].(fig based on Bronfenbrenner (1998, 2006); Australian Bureau of Statistics (ABS) for fig 5.1 © Commonwealth of Australia, Creative Commons Attribution 4.0 International licence; Age Action Ireland for extracts from O'Brien et al. (2011) A Total Indifference to Our Dignity: Older people's understandings of elder abuse. pp. 37 and p.43; Elder Abuse Action Australia for fig 7.1; Senior Rights Victoria for fig 7.2; SAGE Publications for fig 9.1, Reprinted from Moving beyond patient and client approaches: Mobilizing 'authentic partnerships' in dementia care, support and services; Sherry L. Dupuis, Jennifer Gillies, Jennifer Carson, et al; Publication: Dementia Copyright © 2012 SAGE Publications; Taylor and Francis for fig 9.2 from Lopez, K. J. & Dupuis, S. L. (2014). Exploring meanings and experiences of wellness from residents living in long- term care homes. World Leisure Journal, 56(2), 141–150, reprinted by permission of the publisher (Taylor & Francis Ltd, http://www.tandfonline.com); Commonwealth of Australia, 2019b. Royal Commission into Aged Care Quality and Safety for extract from Aged care program redesign: Services for the future. Consultation paper 1, p. 3 © Commonwealth of Australia. Released under CC BY 4.0 licence www.creativecommons.org/licenses; World Health Organization Publication for fig 10.1 WHO: Number of people over 60 years set to double by 2050; major societal changes required https://www.who.int/ageing/events/world-report-2015-launch/healthy-ageing-infographic.jpg; Springer Nature for fig 10.2 Reprinted by permission from Springer Nature: Nature, Fig. 2: The concept of geroscience and its approach to age-related disease from Discoveries in ageing research to therapeutics for healthy ageing, Campisi, J., Kapahi, P., Lithgow, G. J., Melov, S., Newman, J. C., & Verdin, E. Nature, 571(7764), 183-192. (2019); RCN Publishing Co for fig 11.1. Republished with permission of RCN Publishing Co, from A short mnemonic to support the comprehensive geriatric assessment model by Brenda Han and Cristin Grant; Emergency Nurse, 24(6), 18-22.2016; permission conveyed through Copyright Clearance Center, Inc.; Elsevier for fig 11.2. Reprinted from Behavioral Emergencies: Special Considerations in the Geriatric Psychiatric Patient. Psychiatric Clinics of North America, 40(3), 449-462. with permission from Elsevier; Alzheimer's Association for fig 13.1, Terese Winslow for fig 16.3 © 2012 Terese Winslow LLC, U.S. Govt. has certain rights; Dementia Australia for fig 13.3 from Dementia Practice Guidelines; Dr Sue-Ching Yeoh for table 16.3, table 16.4; Extract from Cameron, I. D., Dyer, S. M., Panagoda, C. E., Murray, G. R., Hill, K. D., Cumming, R. G., & Kerse, N. (2018). Interventions for preventing falls in older people in care facilities and hospitals. Cochrane Database of Systematic Reviews, (9). https://doi.org/10.1002/14651858.CD005465.pub4 Copyright © 2020 The Authors. Cochrane Database of Systematic Reviews published by John Wiley & Sons, Ltd. on behalf of The Cochrane Collaboration.

Images: Ippei Naoi/Getty Images: Cover; World Image Archive / Alamy Stock Photo, p.33; Dr Soseh Yekanians: p.301, p.302; Shutterstock: p.1, p.2, p.24, p.54, p.75, p.91, p.92, p.109, p.130, p.151, p.172, p.189, p.190, p.216, p.258, p.275, p.307, p.326, p.349, p.355 (fig 16.2), p.368, p.394, p.415

PREFACE

This is a book about life – the continuum of life, the impact of choices made throughout life, changes that happen during our lives and a celebration of lives lived! Even as the world changes around us, our lives go on. Australians have experienced uniquely different aspects of life since our first edition in 2017. We all have aged too. This second edition of *Healthy Ageing and Aged Care* reflects the changes brought about by global pandemics, immigration, and the Royal Commission into Aged Care Quality and Safety. Changes in the world, specifically in Australia and the need to provide readers with contemporary information about the issues impacting ageing, are the reasons and motivations for writing a new edition.

As with the first edition, at the very heart of the book is the people who are living, who have lived their lives and are generously and courageously sharing their personal experiences with you – people who are ageing, people who make up families and communities and people who are health professionals, especially registered nurses, who work with and provide support for individuals, families and communities to ensure the best possible outcomes. Our goal, in making this book about people, their stories and experiences, is to make learning real and engaging, to capture your hearts as well as your minds, and teach you about how best to work with older people and support them.

The significance of storytelling in teaching and learning is recognised by First Nations peoples, so our use of stories reflects our willingness to learn from this ancient culture.

In the stories and the interviews, wellness continues to be a strong theme. Even though older people may have multiple chronic conditions, they consider themselves well, and remain active and involved. Registered nurses have a significant role in working with older people to enhance their wellness, and support them to be as active as they wish to be and to remain engaged with the community of their choice. The registered nurse will encounter the well older person and our role, in collaboration with the older person, is to optimise their functionality. After astute assessment, interventions can be instigated to maintain health and wellness rather than wait for an illness or disability to become evident. This is one of the rewarding aspects of working with older people – assessing accurately and collaboratively putting in place strategies that can maintain the person's quality of life. Our goal is for you to be able to develop those skills by engaging with the material in this book.

In this second edition, we address the impact COVID-19 has had on our health care system, health professionals, and older people. From the small things, such as the communication barriers that wearing masks creates, to the mental health impacts of isolation, and nutritional information for boosting our immune systems. We use the global pandemic in stories of older people to facilitate your understanding of the complexity of working with older people.

The increasing diversity of Australia is also highlighted in this edition to continue to challenge your attitudes and possible stereotypes. The photos and stories in this book represent all of the people in our country, no matter when and how they arrived. As our population ages, the need for sensitive, respectful care increases. Strategies, communication examples, and videos are included so that you may adapt your professional practice to the people you will be working with.

Learn more
Watch the Video preface: Maree and Denise introduce the approach taken by this book.

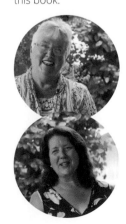

There is a wonderful reciprocity in working with older people. As you work with them and support them, you are learning about life from them. A skilled, informed health professional can ensure wonderful outcomes for the individual and their family and be part of a team that enhances quality of life for an older person, eventually ensuring the delivery of appropriate palliative care. Our authors, many of whom are practising clinicians, have enjoyed these rewards and we want to share with you how to do the same.

Although the recommendations of the Royal Commission into Aged Care Quality and Safety are predominantly yet to be implemented, we offer a timeline of history leading up to them. Poised in a time that holds great hope and potential in aged care, we know that inevitably the information in this edition and its presentation will empower and equip you to face the future. We hope this edition shows you practical, hopeful ways to engage with people who have survived the changes in the world and can continue to live healthy, happy lives with your support.

CONTRIBUTORS

Simone Alexander has extensive experience as an oral hygienist in private practice and has held an academic position at Charles Sturt University. Her work with Murrumbidgee Medicare Local involved visiting residential aged care facilities to provide assessments of the oral health of residents and education for the care staff. Currently she works in private practice, is supporting undergraduate oral therapy students with their clinical skills and works at Wagga Wagga Base Hospital providing outpatient support for older patients and patients with disability. She is also an Australian junior and master's cycling champion.

Karen Bell is an associate professor and a social work academic and co-leader of the Environmental and Social Justice Research Group at Charles Sturt University. Karen's record of research and publication reflects her interest in the philosophy of social work, post-conventional theory, gender and eco-social work. Many of Karen's publications explore the potential of post-conventional theory in relation to social work, qualitative research, gender and climate change. Karen's current research collaborations include projects on healthy ageing, disaster resilience, professional identity, international education, research capacity-building, gender and inter-professional practice.

Maree Bernoth is an associate professor in the School of Nursing, Paramedicine and Healthcare Sciences at Charles Sturt University, based in Wagga Wagga. Since 1985, Maree has worked with and supported older people and those who care for them. Her roles have included registered nurse, educator and researcher in regional and rural areas of New South Wales, and in residential facilities and the community. Maree is a member of the Australasian Association of Gerontology and the NSWNA Aged Care Reference Group, and she chairs the Murrumbidgee Primary Health Network Aged Care Consortium. Maree was a recipient of an Australian Government Office of Learning and Teaching Award for her teaching of ageing. The desire to improve the support of older people and carers is the driving force in her writing and co-editing this text.

Marguerite Bramble is an associate professor with national and international recognition for her contribution to evidence-based knowledge of neurological conditions affecting our older population, such as dementia and Parkinson's disease. As a registered nurse, educator and researcher she has implemented innovative, evidence-based models and clinical trial interventions, working collaboratively on projects with industry stakeholders, managers, health professionals, clients and families. Marguerite is currently President of the Australian Association of Gerontology.

Bianca Brijnath is an associate professor and the Divisional Director of Social Gerontology at the National Ageing Research Institute (NARI). A medical anthropologist and public health practitioner by training, her research explores elder abuse prevalence, primary prevention, screening tool development, management in the context of dementia and big-data analysis of service responses.

Melissa Brodie is a project coordinator for the national End of Life Directions for Aged Care (ELDAC) project and is based at the Queensland University of Technology in Brisbane. Melissa has worked across acute, aged care and community sectors, providing the highest quality care in roles that span clinical, management and education settings. Melissa is committed to leading change through collaboration, and to the integration of practical and sustainable practices to optimise models of care.

Belinda Cash has clinical and academic expertise in ageing, disability and mental health. Before her move to academia, Belinda practised as a social worker in clinical mental health and disability service settings in rural and regional areas. Her teaching and research interests include mental health and psychosocial well-being for older adults and informal caregivers, social policy, service provision in rural areas and social determinants of health in later life. She works full time at Charles Sturt University, teaching, researching and supervising students in the social work and gerontology programs.

Ruth Crawford is an accredited practising dietitian who has worked in a variety of settings including food service, education and institutional care (aged care, disability homes and correctional facilities). Ruth started teaching the Bachelor of Health Science (Nutrition and Dietetics) degree at Charles Sturt University in 2011.

Megan Daniel has extensive experience in caring for older people in residential aged care, acute care and palliative care settings and in teaching undergraduate nurses. Megan is a former lecturer in the School of Nursing, Midwifery and Indigenous Health at Charles Sturt University.

Alison Devitt is a lecturer at Charles Sturt University and a Clinical Nurse Consultant in a specialised intellectual disability health team. Her clinical background in primary healthcare, disability and chronic disease management combined with her post-graduate studies in education, fuels her passion to help nursing students to understand the complex and holistic needs of people living with chronic health issues. She has a research interest in using technology in chronic disease management, including nurse-led in-home telemonitoring and virtual assessment of people with intellectual disability. She has been part of clinical teams pioneering the way in these areas in Australia.

Rylee A. Dionigi is a professor in the School of Allied Health, Exercise & Sports Science at Charles Sturt University, New South Wales. Rylee has expertise in qualitative methodologies and knowledge on the personal and cultural meanings of sport, leisure and exercise participation in later life. Overall, Rylee calls for an acceptance of diversity and difference in ageing. She expects governments and stakeholders to provide the systems, policies and conditions that enable people to make choices affecting their lifelong health.

John Dobrohotoff is a specialist psychiatrist working with older people since 2000. He is a clinical adviser at the Older People's Mental Health Policy Unit at the NSW Ministry of Health and clinical director of the Older People's Mental Health Service of the Central Coast LHD.

Briony Dow is the director of the National Ageing Research Institute (NARI), Honorary Professor at the School of Population and Global Health at the University of Melbourne, and Honorary Professor at the School of Nursing and Midwifery at Deakin University. As NARI director, she leads a range of studies that incorporate her research expertise in elder abuse and carer mental health.

Phillip Ebbs is a paramedic, university lecturer and researcher who has extensive experience in the field of clinical governance. He commenced his paramedicine career in 2001 and has since been involved in clinical, educational, managerial, research and advisory roles across New South Wales and internationally within this profession. He is a member of the Paramedicine Council of New South Wales, was a paramedic advisor to the New South Wales Clinical Excellence Commission, and served as Deputy Chair of the CEC Clinical Council from 2012 to 2015. A key area of his research explores the complex factors that can contribute to mistakes, misunderstandings and 'blind-spots' in clinical practice settings, and the types of strategies needed to help address these complexities.

Gael Evans-Barr is a communications and engagement director with the Victorian State Government and a health service board. For more than 15 years, Gael has worked in positions that require significant and geographically dispersed volunteer management, primarily in state and national not-for-profit organisations. An active volunteer herself, Gael's volunteer experience spans various sectors including health, education, early childhood, community and emergency services. Gael is currently completing doctoral research into the health and organisational effects of older people ceasing volunteering.

Elyce Green is the rural health education lead at the University Department of Rural Health at Charles Sturt University. She has worked as a registered nurse across the areas of aged care, palliative care and intensive care and has conducted clinical research in these specialty areas.

Robin Harvey is a Course Director and lecturer in the inter-disciplinary Master of Ageing and Health program at Charles Sturt University. She has extensive clinical experience as a social worker with older adults in mental health and health promotion fields. Robin is a founding Co-Convenor of the national Ageing, Workforce and Education Special Interest Group of the Australian Association of Gerontology and has a commitment to increasing opportunities for specialist education in ageing for professionals working across health, human services and aged care. She created the 'Understanding Ageing' free online course for CSU in 2020.

Bridget Honan is an emergency physician with a special interest in pre-hospital and retrieval medicine. She is involved in interprofessional research and education on delivering high-quality care of older people in emergency departments and pre-hospital settings, particularly in rural and remote areas.

Clarissa Hughes spent the first two decades of her post-PhD career in teaching and research roles at the University of Tasmania and Charles Sturt University, before qualifying as a Speech Pathologist in 2021. Her new clinical role complements her background in Sociology, and encompasses her passions for health, education, social care, qualitative research and social justice. Clarissa's most recent teaching responsibilities included coordinating undergraduate and postgraduate subjects in nursing, paramedicine and health sciences, and supervising PhD projects on such diverse topics such as cancer care, rural health, consumer participation, health policy, and child protection. Clarissa has authored and co-authored over thirty peer-reviewed articles, book chapters and commissioned reports, and has presented at conferences in Australia, New Zealand, and the United States. She first worked with Maree Bernoth and Denise Winkler on the Opteach project (www.opteach.com.au) in 2017–18, and she continues to get a buzz from multidisciplinary collaboration and applying theoretical knowledge to real-world problems.

Jayne Lawrence has been a registered nurse for 35 years and a registered midwife for 20 years, with the majority of her experience in rural New South Wales. She has a passion for achieving better health outcomes in regional and rural areas and is blessed to have the opportunity in her current role with Charles Sturt University to establish and provide curriculum, support and mentoring to clinicians and health professional students to advance their education and practice. Her strengths lie in communication and engagement in a diverse variety of health-care contexts with clinicians, students and stakeholders. She is committed to improving health outcomes for First Nations communities and growing the rural health workforce.

Kathryn Little has 30-plus years' nursing experience and continues in both a clinical and educational role across several health sectors. In her role as Clinical Educator she delivers educational sessions to staff in aged care and acute care. Kathryn also teaches and lectures enrolled nurses and registered nurses at TAFE and Charles Sturt University respectively where clinical education necessitates clear and current application of clinical education principles.

Jenny McKenzie is a palliative care nurse practitioner located in regional New South Wales. She is passionate about promoting evidence-based, high-quality, equitable palliative care services to people living in rural and remote areas. Jenny enjoys mentoring clinicians new to palliative care.

Jed Montayre is a senior lecturer in the School of Nursing and Midwifery at Western Sydney University. He teaches and coordinates the Masters of Ageing, Wellbeing and Sustainability course. Jed has a strong clinical background in gerontology and medical-surgical nursing. Jed's research areas include age-friendly communities, social gerontology, aged care nursing and nursing workforce development in the aged care sector. Jed led an international team for a project commissioned and funded by the World Health Organization to conduct a review of the community-based, age-friendly interventions and programs as part of the WHO and UN Decade of Healthy Ageing 2020–2030 initiative. Jed also serves as an associate editor of *Australasian Journal on Ageing*.

Kate O'Halloran is a research fellow in social gerontology in the Division of Social Gerontology at the National Ageing Research Institute (NARI). Her research focuses on the primary prevention of intergenerational elder abuse, and on elder abuse and disaster (including COVID-19). She serves on the Senior Rights Victoria elder abuse roundtable, and the Compass content committee.

Kristy Robson is an experienced allied health professional with more than 25 years' experience working in rural and regional Australia. Through clinical experience and research interests, Kristy has extensive knowledge in enhancing mobility, particularly in older populations, to maintain quality of life. Her PhD focused on exploring falls risks in older people living within the community and she has considerable experience in undertaking collaborative research in improving mobility and preventing falls in both the community and hospital settings. Kristy has published her research in peer-reviewed journals and has been an invited speaker both nationally and internationally presenting on a range of topics that focus on mobility and falls prevention.

Lynda Saltarelli has a background in application and website development. A personal experience led her to found independent voluntary advocacy group Aged Care Crisis. She has used her technical skills to collect data, and to develop an advocacy and information website where feedback and discussion is encouraged for family members and staff. She uses social media to challenge fake news and mobilise the community to engage in aged care issues. Aged Care Crisis has, along with its supporters, written approximately 100 submissions to aged care–related inquiries. It presses for management and oversight to be conducted through and in cooperation with empowered regional and local bodies, so enabling greater accountability to, and involvement of, communities.

Marissa Samuelson is an accredited practising dietitian who has worked in a variety of settings including community health, private practice and acute care. Marissa started teaching nutrition and dietetics at Charles Sturt University in 2003. Her PhD topic combined her interest in the education and practice development of health practitioners, working in rural and regional environments and patient-centred communication. Her current research interests include healthy ageing and weight stigma in the health professions.

Peter Santangelo is a credentialled mental health nurse with the Australian College of Mental Health Nurses, a fellow and a past president. He has worked as a registered mental health nurse for more than 40 years. Peter's substantive clinical background has been in community mental health nursing in Sydney and the Central Coast of New South Wales. He has held senior management positions and holds conjoint and adjunct positions with a number of universities in Australia.

Christine Stirling is a Professor of Nursing with the University of Tasmania and leads the Transforming Research in Ageing research group. Christine has more than two decades of experience in working with industry, research and government in the area of ageing, culminating in a strong national policy presence in her role as immediate past president for the Australian Association of Gerontology (AAG). She has improved experiences for older Australians through pioneering person-centred research to promote voice and improve access.

Sabine Wardle is a lecturer in social work and human services at Charles Sturt University. Her research interests include aged care, culturally and linguistically diverse populations, grief and loss, rehabilitation, and community development. Sabine grew knowing various cultures and religions. She has maintained an interest in spiritual and religious aspects of the culturally and linguistically diverse population within an Australian context, particularly in palliative and end-of-life care. Sabine's PhD thesis concerned lived experiences of a culturally and linguistically diverse population group (the Punjabi Indians) with palliative care services at residential aged care facilities in regional New South Wales.

Denise Winkler is a writer, editor and research assistant. Her primary focus is qualitative research with older people and their experience of ageing.

J. Michael Wynne is a surgeon who has worked in private, public and academic surgery in three countries. He has had a long interest in the impact of ideological beliefs and policies on healthcare. Over the past 30 years he has focused on the impact of free-market policies on health and aged care in the United States and Australia. He has been a whistleblower and supplied information to several state probity investigations when large medical and aged care megacorps with poor track records attempted to buy into Australia during the 1990s. During the past 20 years he has focused on the impact on aged care. He is a member of Aged Care Crisis, where he contributes to data analysis and the writing of submissions.

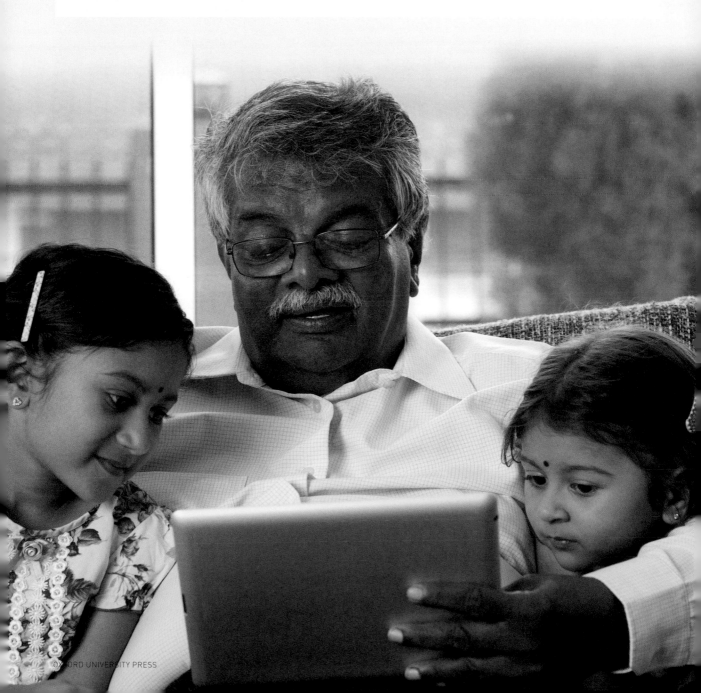

PART 1

THE CONTEXT OF AGEING

1

The Opportunities and Challenges of Ageing in Australia

CLARISSA HUGHES, CHRISTINE STIRLING AND ROBIN HARVEY

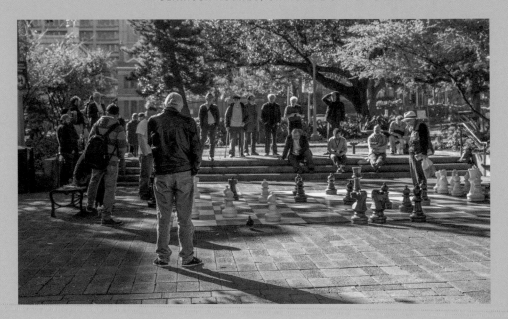

LEARNING OBJECTIVES

After reading this chapter, you will:

» describe key roles and sociological changes experienced by people as they age

» reflect on your own beliefs and perceptions of ageing

» consider the impact of ageist attitudes

» outline key elements of the Australian context impacting older people.

Introduction

People lie at the heart of this book. While many textbooks are filled with facts and figures, in *Healthy Ageing and Aged Care* we hope our readers never lose sight of the fact that the statistics relate to *real people* – each with their own histories, experiences, personalities, skills, challenges and aspirations. Of course, the facts and figures remain important for appreciating the patterns and shared experiences of older people in Australia – but we will aim to balance those commonalities against an understanding of individuality and diversity.

As a future health professional, you will learn how to apply your knowledge and skills to the care of each individual patient or client. You will come to the role of health professional with certain beliefs or expectations about what 'old people' are like and what is involved in the ageing process. Part of this will have come from your experiences throughout your life and the cultural influences to which you have been exposed. These beliefs will inevitably influence how you think about, and relate to, older people – and can affect the care you provide in either positive or negative ways.

One of the most important roles of this book is to help the reader 'peel back the layers' of their underlying beliefs and stereotypes about ageing and older people. At times, this will be an uncomfortable process. At this point you may be thinking that this does not apply to you, since you pride yourself on being non-judgmental and open-minded. However, we are very confident that when reading and thinking about the following chapters, you will discover some subconscious and unquestioned assumptions and biases. Some introspection, honesty and emotional maturity will be required as you confront the less palatable aspects of how your world view relates to older people and their place in society.

If you found you were going to meet a fashion designer, or a musician, or someone who runs marathons, would you have any assumptions about the likely age of those people? If you had to guess, would you expect them to be in their twenties, thirties or forties – or older? What does your mental image of them look like? What if you found out that the fashion designer has grey hair, the musician collects stamps and the marathon runner lives alone in a caravan. Would this change your age estimates?

Without even realising it, most of us have assumptions or biases about what older and younger people do and are interested in. These assumptions often extend to mental or physical capacities. Of course, many of these assumptions are accurate and are reflected in the data on older people, some of which you'll encounter in this chapter and elsewhere in this book. However, as a clinician providing person-centred care, it is your responsibility to be aware of your stereotypes, and to not let them get in the way of treating each of your patients as a unique individual with their own particular combination of interests, history, culture, impairments and capabilities.

In the spirit of recognising both diversity and commonality, let's meet some of the people whose stories and experiences will be woven through this chapter:

- **Helen**, a former fashion model, moved back to Australia to work on planning committees for elite fashion shows. Prior to the COVID-19 pandemic, she regularly travelled to New York and Paris. During the lockdowns in Melbourne, Helen used the time to focus on barre workouts to keep her body toned and fit and to create an Instagram channel. Although her finances were never a worry, she was surprised at the passive income stream the social media platform provided. The channel attracted thousands of subscribers, who followed her posts and videos.

- **Binyan (Ben)** lives in Darwin with his wife Jill. He is heavily involved in music camps for at-risk children. He loves volunteering his time and talents to watch the children grow during the camp. Ben becomes very concerned about being able to continue his involvement with music because he needs hearing aids.
- **Paul** lives in a cottage in a small town on the Central Coast of New South Wales. He breeds and hand-raises budgerigars, and also enjoys surfing and whale-watching along the coast. Paul served a short sentence in a low-security prison. He is currently a carer for his brother, who has spina bifida and requires help with his activities of daily living.
- **Chakrii** is a retired engineer who lives in inner-city Sydney with his wife and her mother. Since retiring, he has become heavily involved in the local cricket team. Over the years, he has sustained many injuries while playing cricket: he has had knee replacements, a shoulder reconstruction and other surgeries. Chakrii was diagnosed with Parkinson's disease, which is debilitating, and requires help from his wife.
- **Fran** lives on a large property in rural Victoria. She lives in a caravan with her small dog, who is her only companion. Fran's frugal lifestyle allows her to pursue her interests of rock-climbing and marathon running. She supplements her pension by doing gardening jobs in the rural community.

Helen, Binyan, Paul, Chakrii and Fran have one important thing in common: they are all aged fifty-five or over. Beyond that commonality, you can see that there is great diversity. Two live in large cities, while the others live in small towns or villages. Some live with a partner – and, in Chakrii's case, one other person – while three live alone (albeit that Fran has a dog). Some are unpaid carers, while others are themselves cared for (or are likely to be in the future). Some are 'financially comfortable', while others struggle to meet their basic living costs. Some are dealing with one or more chronic or degenerative conditions, while others are fit and active. These older people have a wide variety of life experiences and interests. Over the course of this chapter (and the rest of this book) you will learn more about these people and be introduced to others. You will be asked to focus on people as individuals, but also consider the ways in which the experience of ageing is inevitably influenced by factors *beyond the individual*.

The experience of ageing: change and transitions

Getting older is inevitably accompanied by change. Some of these changes (like reduced mobility and changes to vision) are anticipated, while others (like a sudden illness or an accident) may be completely unexpected and come as a shock. Likewise, as we get older, we will be confronted with a range of changes affecting ourselves, our family and friends, our communities, our country and even our planet. Our ability to cope and adjust with anticipated and unanticipated changes will be at least partly influenced by our personality, expectations, personal 'life narratives', support networks and a range of other factors. Other significant factors are socio-economic status, proximity to medical services and whether we live in rural, remote, regional or metropolitan communities.

Think back to a time when you needed to adjust to change. Perhaps when you were a young child you had to go to a new school, or your best friend moved interstate or your parents started living in separate houses. How well do you think you adjusted to this 'new reality'? What helped you to come to terms with the change? Now that you are older, do you think you would respond differently? What changes were associated with young adulthood? Maybe you made the transition from school to university or lost your job as a result of the COVID-19 pandemic, started or ended a relationship or became a parent. Do you think of yourself as someone who readily adapts to change, or do you struggle with it?

When we think of the changes associated with ageing, it is easy to assume that they will be unwelcome and negative. Take a moment to consider whether your first thoughts about change and ageing relate to *loss* – such as the loss of a youthful appearance, independence, hearing or social status. However, just like earlier in our lives, some changes are positive – and some that seemed unpleasant or negative at the start may even turn out to be good in the longer term, or with the benefit of hindsight.

Although it may seem counter-intuitive, some of the changes associated with ageing may actually be welcome! Some people experience a sense of liberation as they begin to experience freedom from the societal expectations attached to being a 'younger' person. Older people may enjoy finally having the time to spend doing things they enjoy, such as travelling, taking up a hobby or learning a new skill. They can potentially invest more fully in relationships that matter to them, such as with family members (particularly children and grandchildren), friends, neighbours and the wider community.

Freed from the expectation of being 'productive' in a financial or employment sense, older people may have more capacity to redefine productivity and balance it with a desire for meaning. Older age may be a time of having fewer debts and less interest in purchasing items. It is common for older people to 'declutter' their homes and lives and to report having less attachment to material things. It can also be liberating to be less concerned about, and restricted by, what others think of you: your appearance, life choices and behaviour. In her TEDx Talk 'How to live passionately – no matter your age' (2014), South American author Isabel Allende insists that as she has aged, she has gained freedom since she is no longer 'stuck in the idea of who I was, who I want to be or what other people expect me to be'.

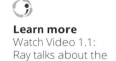

Learn more
Watch Video 1.1: Ray talks about the importance of Men's Sheds.

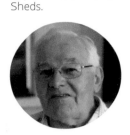

Milestones and mindsets

Ageing is commonly associated with changes in how others see you as well as how you see yourself. Particular life experiences and milestones can mark salient points in the ageing journey, such as stopping paid work or becoming a grandparent. They can be influenced by factors beyond the individual person. For example, stopping paid work may be related to a person having reached retirement age; or it may be due to a person's position being made redundant in the context of company closure or industry collapse; or the person may have an acute or chronic illness that makes continuing in a paid work role problematic or impossible. Similarly, how that 'milestone' is experienced will be affected by many factors, such as how important paid work is to that person's identity and whether their post-retirement income will allow (or necessitate) moving home or other changes to lifestyle or daily routine.

Another 'milestone' associated with ageing is becoming a grandparent. Many older people report thoroughly enjoying being grandparents because it entails having 'all of the joy, but none of the responsibility' of having children. Again, how this is experienced will depend on various factors beyond the individuals involved. Some people relish this transition, whereas others struggle with it because it denotes a social marker of being 'an older person'. Some grandparents are heavily involved in the lives of their grandchildren, and some need to take on parenting roles. Others may rarely, or never, see their grandchildren due to relationship issues, physical distance or other restrictions. Our very ideas of the role of grandparents in the family (and society more generally) are strongly influenced by the culture and society we live in.

Adjustment and adaptation to change

As noted at the start of this chapter, ageing is inevitably associated with change. In this section, we will start to consider a range of changes that individuals may encounter as they get older. Our aim is to prompt you to start thinking about ageing as a complex and nuanced process that does not just happen 'to other people'. We also want you to become aware of your prejudices and assumptions so you can acknowledge them and consider how they could affect your interactions and decisions. These are both important steps in the journey of becoming a health-care professional who places 'the person' at the centre of every episode of care.

CHANGES TO APPEARANCE

When somebody mentions 'ageing', changes to appearance come to mind. Older people look different from younger people in terms of their skin, hair, style of dress, physique and posture, for example. In cultures where youth is idealised and beauty is defined in terms of youthfulness, many of the changes associated with ageing may be unwelcome – or even actively resisted. A Google search of the term 'anti-ageing' (or 'anti-aging') is likely to produce thousands of results including skin products and treatments, diets, supplements and more. Many of these target women, but if you repeat the search, you'll see that looking younger is not solely a female concern. As noted earlier, people differ in the extent to which they accept and adapt to age-related changes. The discovery of your first grey hairs may be a 'non-event', or it may trigger feelings of disgust or panic! Let's meet one of our case-study individuals, Helen, and read how she has adapted to physical changes as she has grown older.

1.1 Getting to know the person: Helen's story

Helen was a fashion model in Australia during her late teens and early twenties. Looking back, she can see that she and other young women in the industry were under great pressure to maintain a certain image. This image involved staying extremely slim and avoiding sun exposure. After a few years in the industry, she started to resent being valued only for her appearance, as well as the restrictions on her lifestyle. With the support and encouragement of her family, Helen studied fashion design. Her existing links to the industry helped her secure mentoring and work overseas. She worked as a fashion designer for several decades before moving back to Australia with the intention of working on planning committees for elite fashion shows. She enjoyed this because she could continue her involvement in the industry in a way that seemed appropriate for 'an older woman' and that was less demanding of her energy. The work saw her regularly travelling to New York and Paris – until the COVID-19 pandemic hit. Since then, Helen has devoted time to her Instagram channel, where thousands of subscribers follow her posts and videos on the latest fashion trends.

CHANGES TO FUNCTIONING

The myriad physical changes associated with ageing can bring about many changes to functioning. Ageing is presumed to involve the loss of many functions, including hearing, vision and memory. Some people experience significant reductions in their cardiovascular fitness or physical strength. Other, less obvious issues include changes to libido and trouble eating and/or drinking. Some of these changes to functioning can be 'corrected' (e.g. through glasses or surgery for vision impairment, hearing aids for hearing impairment, or dentures or dental implants for tooth loss), while others require that the person (and perhaps also those around them) draw on strategies to cope with, compensate for or minimise the impact of the issue. It is also important that communities and organisations play their part in assisting older people to live engaged and enjoyable lives – for example, by ensuring that their patient handouts are printed in a large, readable font – and that there are ramps, lifts and well-formed footpaths available for those with mobility challenges. We'll learn more about those and other 'age-friendly' considerations in later chapters. But first, let's read about how Binyan coped with a specific age-related change.

Read more about the impact of physiological changes on older people in Chapter 10.

1.2 Getting to know the person: Binyan's story

Binyan (who also calls himself Ben) was born in Borroloola, a remote community about seven hours' drive south-east of Katherine. He is in his mid-fifties and volunteers at music camps for at-risk children. He and his wife Jill are currently living in Darwin, but when they get the chance, they travel to the Gulf of Carpentaria, where Ben's brother is setting up an ecotourism business. Like many First Nations children, Ben suffered recurrent ear infections during infancy and early childhood. These infections affected his hearing, which in turn affected his ability to learn language. Throughout much of his adult life, Ben did not really notice that his hearing was impaired unless he was trying to follow a conversation with lots of background noise. More recently, however, Jill has noticed that he often does not hear her call out to him, and he does not respond to some sounds (such as their small dog barking) like he used to. After initially resisting, Ben had a hearing test, which revealed significant hearing loss in one ear and mild loss in the other. He is now worried about how they will afford hearing aids – and if his hearing continues to worsen, whether he will be able to continue his role at the music camps.

 CLARISSA HUGHES, CHRISTINE STIRLING AND ROBIN HARVEY

CHANGES TO EMPLOYMENT

At some time as we grow older, most of us will experience changes to paid employment, either through retirement due to personal choice, or perhaps due to external issues such as economic trends, ageist expectations of older workers or government workforce policies and incentives associated with the ageing population.

Taylor and Earl (2016) pointed out the existence of two competing stories affecting older workers: a 'victim' narrative associated with the incidence of ageism in workplaces and the denial of opportunities for work that this creates; and a 'productivity' narrative that promotes older workers as having desirable traits such as experience and reliability. Both these disparate trends may be present in reality, with the differences being associated with factors such as the type of work/industry, availability of flexible employment options, employment history, health, retraining and upskilling opportunities available to older workers and availability of younger workers, as well as economic conditions that generate or limit growth in employment more generally. Some older people may have opportunities to work longer and/or retire by choice. Others may be forced to continue working due to a lack of financial security, or forced to retire via redundancies or because they have difficulty finding employment as their skills are no longer considered current or in demand.

Paid work

Macro-economic and policy trends affect the paid employment and retirement plans of older adults in Australia. Working longer has been seen as a public and individual 'good' to the extent that those whose health, skills or choice leads them to retire, and those who face unemployment at a later age with the consequent likelihood of remaining so for a considerable period, may be stigmatised as 'non-productive'. Research indicates that being able to choose to voluntarily leave work leads to better health and well-being outcomes in retirement (Tavares & Cohen, 2019). However, there are substantial numbers of older adults whose retirement is involuntary. These people are therefore more likely to find adaptation to retirement more difficult and will have a higher risk of economic, health and well-being problems.

There is also a substantial number of older adults who cannot afford to retire prior to being able to access the age pension. This is particularly the case for all low-income workers and for women whose workforce participation has been interrupted by periods of (child/parental) care. Women whose remuneration during their working lives was below that of their male counterparts retire with low levels of superannuation. Older women in these circumstances are unable to exercise choice in their decision making on employment and may either be forced by economic necessity to continue working or may find themselves in poverty, if they are unable to remain employed or regain employment prior to reaching pension age. Single older women are at greatest risk of poverty and homelessness due to these factors.

Chronological age is clearly of importance in determining an individual's prospects of employment, as is gender. However, of itself, chronological age is relatively unimportant as a determinant of the potential and capabilities of workers. It has been suggested by Taylor and Smith (2017) that policies that aim to address the difficulties that face some older and younger workers should seek to be 'age neutral'. In addition, the dependency ratio used as an economic planning tool should be adapted to include a broader range of voluntary and social participation as contributions, rather than only paid work, and recognise the diversity of age and participation to more accurately reflect the productive activity of older adults (Taylor & Smith, 2017), such as volunteering, care of grandchildren, and creative or social support pursuits.

Volunteering

Volunteering is mostly a reciprocal arrangement where services benefit from volunteers' free labour and volunteers gain a range of personal benefits such as feeling valued, better health or improved social connection. This is evidenced in Binyan's story. As you read this section, consider the potential loss Binyan will experience as his hearing deteriorates and he can no longer contribute in the way he did previously to music camps.

Volunteers can be classed as formal volunteers (who volunteer for an organisation) or informal volunteers (who help out in the community). According to the Australian census (ABS, 2020), formal volunteering has declined over the past decade in both the number of people (less than one-third of Australian adults) and the hours volunteered (a 20% decline). While older people have often been viewed as a source of volunteers, given their likely retirement from the workplace and assumed spare time, formal volunteering actually drops off from age 55 years. Older people, though, are more likely to volunteer in the health, welfare and community settings and have sustained organisations such as Meals on Wheels for decades.

The benefits of volunteering, particularly when focused on helping others, include better mental and physical health, and better life satisfaction and social well-being (Yeung et al., 2018). Volunteering, then, could be a way for older people to increase social interaction and prevent isolation. However, some may need additional help to access volunteering opportunities if they have barriers to participation – for example, financial barriers (e.g. the cost of travelling to volunteer) or physical barriers (e.g. difficulty climbing stairs). Volunteering can provide mutual benefits and is worthy of further exploration.

> Read more about volunteering in Chapter 8.

Learn more
Watch Video 1.2: Mary talks about the benefits of volunteering.

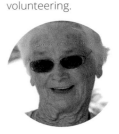

CHANGES TO RELATIONSHIPS: CAREGIVING

Like volunteers, informal carers receive no payment for the work they do and are critical in providing care for older people. Most research focuses on the primary carer (the person providing the majority of care), who is most likely a family member, though they may be a neighbour or a friend. Carers reduce the need for formal care, supplement the care provided by aged care services, and maintain critical social and community connections. In Australia, around seven in 10 (69%) of informal carers and those they care for are over the age of 45 (ABS, 2019). Like volunteering, being an informal carer has some benefits and many couples operate as dyads, supporting each other to continue ageing in place. However, informal care also places a burden on carers and this can have negative consequences. Measures of carer burden and interventions to support carers have proliferated over the past decade, particularly for carers of people with dementia, with respite care and in-home support being two key mechanisms. If the care recipient is admitted to a residential aged care facility, the informal carer role usually continues, but in a changed form. This ongoing involvement is often central to the life satisfaction of the carer and care recipient, and engaging carers in decisions and care activities can be an important aspect of the health professional's role.

1.3 Getting to know the person: Paul's story

Paul, whom we met at the start of this chapter, is an informal carer for his brother Tyson. Tyson was born with spina bifida and uses a wheelchair. Until recently, Tyson was cared for by their elderly mother, April. While Paul was in prison, April was diagnosed with Alzheimer's disease. Unfortunately, the disease progressed rapidly, and shortly after Paul's release from prison, she was admitted to residential aged care. Paul took over as Tyson's carer. While this went well initially, as Paul is getting older, he is struggling with the physical demands of caring for his brother. The lack of wheelchair-friendly paths in their area make outdoor activities and socialising difficult. Paul's stress levels are increasing, and he tends to smoke more when he is stressed. He has noticed he becomes breathless when pushing Tyson's wheelchair, and he is worried that his long history as a smoker has damaged his lungs – or worse.

FOCUS QUESTIONS

- What would Paul perceive as imposing carer burdens? Are there any conditions influencing his feelings?
- What are the costs and benefits of this relationship for Paul and for Tyson?
- How can Paul advocate for Tyson and others with impaired mobility?

CHANGES TO PRIORITIES

Like many others, Paul is noticing that his priorities are changing as he ages. As a younger person, Paul was very focused on his career and possessions. He moved house many times and lived in different states and countries. He always maintained contact with his family, even during his time in prison. He was deeply affected by his mother's diagnosis with Alzheimer's and is determined to not 'take anyone for granted'. His priorities are now having the best relationship he can with his brother, taking good care of him and making the most of whatever time they have together. Paul is an example of changing priorities being psychological evidence of ageing.

Swiss psychiatrist Carl Jung was one of the forerunners of modern gerontological thinking. His writings during the 1920s and 1930s have had a longstanding influence (see, for example Jung, 1933) on psychology and other disciplines. Jung saw the so-called 'afternoon of life' as a time when people undergo 'a process of psychological turning inward' (Martin et al., 2015, p. 16). Another influential theorist, Erik Erikson, argued that people pass through eight developmental stages as they grow and mature. He considered that those over the age of 65 are in the eighth stage of 'integrity versus despair'. This is the stage of reflection, during which people look back over their lives and make sense of their experiences (Martin et al., 2015). According to Erikson's theory, achieving 'wisdom' in later life involves 'revisiting previous crises and reviewing psychosocial accomplishments' (Perry et al., 2015, p. 253).

More recently, social researchers have expanded on these ideas in their theories on ageing. For example, according to Socioemotional Selectivity Theory (Carstensen, 2006), as people grow older, they perceive that they have 'limited time left'. This awareness motivates them to prioritise deriving emotional meaning from life (Fung, 2013), which includes pursuing meaningful experiences and connections, but also reviewing their past. This 'life review' process consists of remembering and emotionally processing the full range of life experiences involving happiness, pleasure and success as well as disappointment, loss and trauma (Westerhof, 2015). In your future work with older people (particularly if you are caring for those with dementia), you may be involved in 'reminiscence interventions' in which cultural artefacts such as music or photographs from a person's youth are used to stimulate the recollection of memories (Subramaniam & Woods, 2012).

Socioemotional Selectivity Theory also argues that as people age, they gain knowledge about how to regulate their emotions, and may successfully avoid negative experiences by applying this knowledge (Charles & Carstensen, 2010). Of course, not all negative experiences can be avoided! For example, an unavoidable aspect of ageing is death – both our own and that of those around us. When reading the newspaper, some older people observe a daily ritual of reading through the death notices. Over time, as a person's partner, relatives, friends and associates pass away, their social circle reduces in size and their sources of social support may be diminished. If their social network becomes too small, they may be placed at risk of isolation. However, research has shown that for many older people, the 'quality' (closeness and importance) of their relationships is more important than the 'quantity' of people in the social network (Charles & Carstensen, 2010). Having meaningful connections with others may even contribute to longevity (Pressman & Cohen, 2007).

Read more about the theories of ageing in Chapter 4.

Social attitudes towards ageing and older people

If we are lucky enough, we are all going to grow old; the alternative is certainly a less desirable option. Despite an anti-ageing industry and a field of scientific research aimed at slowing or reversing the ageing process (Kane & Sinclair, 2019a, 2019b; Bertoldo et al., 2020), ageing is currently still a physiological imperative and something that starts as soon as we begin life. As ageing is an experience that everybody still alive is undergoing, we should all be very familiar with the shape, colour and flavour – that is, the terms and conditions of growing old.

So, what do we know about ageing and older adults? What are some of the commonly held beliefs in our society about being old? We will consider these questions shortly. First, how do we define 'older'? Who are referred to as 'elderly' in our community? Depending on the age of the speaker and their purpose in defining it, 'elderly' can mean anyone in their fifties (as is the parameter for First Nations peoples), sixties, seventies, eighties, nineties, or even in our fastest growing age-group, that of centenarians.

A category that potentially stretches across five decades is clearly not a very useful one for understanding or predicting much about the people in it. And, in fact, chronological age (although significantly associated with increasing health risks) is not actually a very precise predictor of an individual's health or functional capacity. People's biological, physical or social age and functional ability change at different rates and according to different trajectories (Hooyman & Kiyak, 2018, p. 3).

Back to some of the commonly held beliefs about ageing. Does getting older mean a steady process of decline and frailty until a merciful release? Or a period of relaxation and retirement after a busy life? An opportunity to try something new, or to focus on interests and adventures? A time of poverty, hardship and illness? A time of reconciling how life has been lived and finding meaning from this reflection? Or a time to be satisfied with the accumulation of wealth from a long life (perhaps guarding this accumulation at the expense of other generations as per the 'boomer' memes)?

Ageing and becoming old could, of course, mean any of these things or none of them, or perhaps something completely different. In contrast to widely held ideas that there is a category of people called 'the elderly' who share a set of homogenous characteristics to be entered at a certain age (65?, 70?), the reality is that we actually grow more different from each other as we age.

FOCUS QUESTIONS

Think for a moment about how you will be as an older version of yourself.

- What physical attributes, state of health, values, attitudes and interests do you imagine yourself to have? What will you be doing? What will your hopes and dreams be?
- Why do you expect these things to be your future?
- What other opportunities might there be?

AGEISM

gerontologist
A scientist who focuses on supporting education about and understanding of ageing.

Ageism is a term that was first coined in 1969 by American **gerontologist** Robert N. Butler, the founding director of the National Institute on Aging in the United States (Butler, 1969). It is defined as systematic stereotyping of (usually) older people and discrimination against them due to chronological age.

There are three commonly accepted types of ageism:

1 stereotyped attitudes and beliefs (e.g. 'All old people are frail/are forgetful/need help/are wise')

2 behavioural discrimination (e.g. treating older people differently because of unfounded beliefs such as those described above)

3 structural ageism (e.g. policies and practices of governments, businesses, organisations, health services etc.).

There is significant evidence that ageism causes harm to the health of those people affected. In a recently reported global systematic review of studies of ageism at the individual and structural levels, the authors reported a link between ageism and poor health outcomes (E-Shien et al., 2020).

At the individual level, feeling yourself subjected to negative stereotyped beliefs is psychologically and emotionally damaging. One of the most serious consequences occurs when an older person accepts the ageist stereotypes. This acceptance of negativity about their age may reduce their expectations of their capacity and future plans and may contribute to anxiety and depression. They may then make choices to limit their activities and aspirations due to underrating their capabilities. 'I'm too old' can be a harmful state of mind if, in the absence of a reasoned assessment of the chances of success, it prevents someone from trying to achieve something they desire or need. Internalised ageist expectations can prevent someone seeking medical care if they believe that the symptoms they are noticing are 'just getting old' rather than signs of being unwell.

Ageism can also be viewed positively (e.g. 'I love old people because they are so wise and kind'). Yes, older people may have developed wisdom from the experiences of their lives, and many may be kind. However, not all people of a certain age share the same characteristics. Examples of ageism such as these may be based on a foundation of respect for older people, but are just as much an untested assumption as the more negative framings of 'what all older people are like'.

Language can also reveal an unconscious ageism. For example, when we use the term 'elderly' we turn a group of diverse older individuals into a category, a noun. They are the elderly. Terms such as 'older adults' or 'older people' maintain the emphasis on the generic noun (adult/people) and simply add the qualifying information that these particular adults are older than some others. We acknowledge the person first and add 'older' as a secondary characteristic, a description among many that we could use to describe that person. Do you see the difference this change of language makes? Another use of language that devalues older people is the use of 'baby talk' – for example, 'What do we want for dinner today, love?' Using the third person 'we' infantilises the person as not being a full individual in their own right. Many people find the familiarity of terms such as 'love' and 'darling' disrespectful if used outside of an intimate relationship with that person, irrespective of their wishes, or as a standard way of addressing an older person.

Structural ageism can be found in policies of all levels of government that impact on the health, well-being and opportunities of older people and also within health services. Health services are not free of ageism; neither are those who work within health systems and services for older people. To illustrate this, you may have heard stories such as that of the doctor who told a patient that the pain experienced in his knee was to be expected 'at your age'. The patient's response was, 'So what about my other knee? It's the same age and it doesn't hurt!'

When you think about growing older, what are your first thoughts and feelings? Happy expectation or dread? Visualise an 'older person' in your mind. Do you visualise someone who is active or frail? It is important to be reflective as a health professional and maintain awareness about how you may be stereotyping older people so that you can counter the influence of any bias. Any unrecognised bias could negatively impact the care you provide. For example, a normally fit older person may not receive as rapid a response to a deteriorating condition post-operatively if health professionals assume they are usually frail and confused. It is therefore important to understand, and be able to assess, gerontological conditions so that appropriate care is given.

Read more about this topic in Chapters 10 and 11.

'THEY'RE NOT ALL THE SAME!': STEREOTYPING AND DIVERSITY

 If you've seen one older adult, you've seen ONE older adult. The complexity and variability [of older people] is profound and should be respected. (Robertson, 2020)

Mariah Robertson, a clinical educator in geriatric medicine and **gerontology** at Johns Hopkins University, provides this guidance for all trainee health practitioners and gerontic specialists: Don't expect that the next older person you meet will be like the last. Each one is different, even if some superficial characteristics might seem to be the same.

It makes sense that older people are diverse. Even within a fairly homogenous population we all start out with different genetic characteristics and we grow up via different parenting, educational, cultural and social experiences, and work in different jobs and roles. As we

gerontology
The study of all aspects of ageing: social, spiritual, psychological, physical, cultural and cognitive.

grow older, we accumulate different experiences, make different choices, and are exposed to different environmental and societal challenges or benefits. We experience different health and medical conditions, have differential access to socio-economic security, healthy lifestyles and medical care, and experience different family and friendship networks and interests.

The intersection of age with the experiences of older people of diverse backgrounds – such as the First Nations peoples of Australia, people of CALD (culturally and linguistically diverse) backgrounds, lesbian, gay, bisexual, transgender, gender diverse, intersex, queer, asexual and questioning (LGBTIQ+) Australians, and people living with disability – creates substantial diversity not only in the way ageing is experienced, but also in the need for specific service options and attention to cultural safety requirements for health and social support services. It is important for health professionals to understand that an older adult may have experienced discrimination due to one or more of these intersecting factors at some time during their life and be able to recognise and address any personal biases or lack of cultural awareness in order to provide appropriate treatment, care and support.

Read more about stereotyping and diversity in Chapters 3, 10 and 11.

 If you're going to keep on living, you've got to keep on growing! (Anon. male aged 80)

Ageing, like any other stage of life, involves challenges and joys, losses and opportunities, sadness, frustration and achievements. It can be a time of personal growth as we adapt to changes and exercise our agency in choosing how we participate in life. It is never too late (and never too early!) to start and maintain appropriate physical activity to build muscle tone, strength and flexibility to improve mobility. Physical activity also has important health benefits to reduce risks of many age-related medical conditions and supports cognitive health and emotional well-being (Hooyman & Kiyak, 2018). Attitudes to ageing, social connections, meaningful activity and the absence of ageist expectations support personal growth, but so too do external factors. Opportunities for growth as we age are significantly enhanced or limited depending on a range of external factors, including social and environmental issues that impact on health and well-being and provide a context for how we live our lives.

'Beyond the individual': why context matters

As a future health-care professional, it will be very important that you 'connect' with each of your patients at an individual level to provide the best possible person-centred care (McCormack & McCance, 2010). However, it is equally important to realise that individuals do not exist in a bubble. They are part of friendships, families, communities, cultures and societies, all of which exert their own influences and affect the way in which people live their lives.

Read more about this topic in Chapter 4.

The physical environment is also an important factor to consider, as explained by Clarke and Nieuwenhuijsen (2009, p. 14):

Population health outcomes are shaped by complex interactions between individuals and the environments in which they live, work and play. Environments encompass streets and buildings (physical environment), attitudes, supports and relationships with others (social environment), as well as social and political systems and policies.

One framework that encompasses both social and environmental influences on health and illness is the International Classification of Functioning, Disability and Health (known as the ICF), which was developed by the World Health Organization (see Figure 1.1).

FIGURE 1.1 The WHO framework

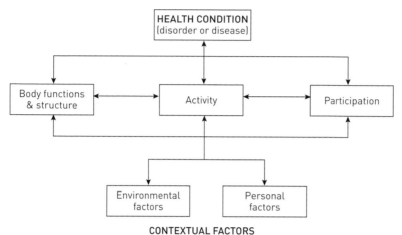

Source: World Health Organization, 2013.

The ICF is based on the understanding that social functioning and health, *activities* (such as dressing oneself and driving a car) and *participation* (such as attending public events, voting or socialising with friends) are affected by complex interactions between:

- *environmental factors* (including both *physical* environmental factors such as climate and building design, and *social* environmental factors such as laws and institutions)
- *body functions/structures* (i.e. physiological and psychological functions, organs and anatomy)
- *personal factors* (such as gender, age, education, race, fitness and coping styles).

This simple framework is helpful for thinking holistically about our patients/clients, and also highlights the importance of policies, laws and the wider environment. Let's now consider applying the ICF to ageing.

The ICF alerts us to the fact that the extent to which an individual experiences 'disability' is influenced by a variety of factors, including the individual's personality and usual coping mechanisms, social support, physical environment, organisational policies and practices, and government regulations. In other words, the 'fact' of having a particular physical limitation does not determine the *impact* of the limitation on a person's life. This is definitely the case in ageing. To highlight this point, let's consider the situation of two of our case-study people.

Fran and Chakrii are both 'older people' living in Australia who sustained a hip fracture following a fall, Fran while rock climbing and Chakrii in his home. Both were hospitalised and underwent surgery. Both received multidisciplinary care and early rehabilitation and have now been discharged from hospital. Now let's consider various aspects of their individual situations. As you read, think about how various elements could function as either barriers or facilitators to Fran and Chakrii's ability to 'live well' during their initial recovery from the injury, as well as in the longer term.

1.4 Getting to know the person: Chakrii's story

Chakrii lives in a multi-storey apartment block with his wife, who works part-time and is used to helping Chakrii with activities of daily living as he is becoming increasingly incapacitated by Parkinson's disease. If Chakrii needs help with something when his wife is at work, he can call their adult daughter, who lives a five-minute drive away. Their apartment block has an elevator, ramps and handrails. The surrounding area has an extensive network of well-formed footpaths with kerb crossings suitable for wheelchairs enabling access to road crossings. Chakrii is hoping to regain enough fitness to return to his daily short walk to the local café using his walking stick. He likes to enjoy a coffee in the outdoor area if the weather is fine. The accident has not impacted the family finances as they have a comfortable retirement income.

1.5 Getting to know the person: Fran's story

Fran and her small dog live in a caravan on a large property in rural Victoria. Fran does garden clean-up work on a casual basis to supplement her finances. She has a number of regular customers she was afraid of losing during her absence.

Once she was back home, Fran focused on regaining her fitness. She needed to be careful though because the ground is rough and uneven on her rural property. She has been advised to only walk on sealed surfaces. She is even worried about walking her dog. Since she cannot work, her budget is now very tight. Fran wonders whether she will ever regain the level of fitness that would allow her to join her usual rock-climbing group and get back to marathon running. She is feeling down about her future as she looks ahead to possible declining health and finances, but is thankful for a good network of friends.

FOCUS QUESTIONS

These two case studies show how two people with the same surgical intervention can have completely different psychosocial and environmental contexts that impact their recovery and life journey.

Think about both Chakrii and Fran:

- What are the strengths in their situations, and what barriers do you see for them?
- What are the different supports they might need after their hip surgery and any services you might be able to refer them to?

The wider context: Australia's ageing population

Let's now transition from thinking about the situation of specific individuals to the wider context of older people in this country. As you are probably aware, Australia's population is ageing. This is a global phenomenon among developed countries that is attributed to a sustained increase in life expectancy throughout the twentieth century and the first decades of the twenty-first century as well as sustained lower fertility during the past decades.

These demographic changes have arisen from large-scale changes in health and society, some of which are:

- the success of public health measures
- improved standards of living
- social changes that have enabled fertility control
- education and employment opportunities for women.

These are remarkable achievements of modern societies that are rightly celebrated. However, the demographic outcome has resulted in proportionally fewer children (under 15 years of age) in the population and a larger proportion of adults aged 65 years and over.

Population growth in Australia has also been driven by targeted immigration, which has increased the working-age population and numbers of children, though not to the extent of disrupting this ageing trajectory. ABS data show that the proportion of Australia's population aged 65 and over increased from 12.3 per cent to 15.9 per cent between 1999 and 2019. This tells us that this group is projected to increase more rapidly during the coming decade, as further cohorts of the **baby boomer generation** (people born between 1946 and 1964 and during a period of elevated birth-rates that have since dropped) reach their 65th birthdays (ABS, 2020).

baby boomer generation
People born between 1945 and the mid 1960s.

Within this ageing population, the proportion of people aged over 85 is growing more rapidly than the overall population. Over the decades 1999 to 2019, the number of people aged 85 years and over increased by 117 per cent, compared to a total population growth of 34.8 per cent over the same period (ABS, 2020). The number of people aged 85 and over in Australia is projected to increase from 493 000 in 2017 to between 1.5 million and 2.2 million in 2066. As a proportion of the population, those aged 85 years and over is projected to increase from 2.0 per cent in 2017 to between 3.6 per cent and 4.4 per cent in 2066, as reported by the Royal Commission into Aged Care Quality and Safety (RCACQS) (Commonwealth of Australia, 2021a).

The 'dependency ratio' is often used by economists as a guide to the sustainability of an ageing population. It uses the number of people of non-working age (using the traditional working-age range of 15 to 64) per 100 people to estimate the proportion of the population unlikely to be in paid employment in relation to the whole population. The ABS projects an increase in the dependency rate from 52 in 2017 to 58 by 2042 (ABS, 2018).

What these data tell us is that in the next decades, the ageing of the Australian population will continue to grow and the ageing of the older adult cohort of 85 and over is also predicted to increase. This indicates a significant increase in the need and demand for health services and aged care, while the projected increase in the dependency ratio suggests that the proportion of the population in paid employment funding services for the entire population will decrease.

This is the nub of the 'ageing population crisis' discourse that has dominated media and, to some extent, government representations of the implications of our ageing population. However, the situation is much more complex and nuanced than this crisis claim would suggest. It is important to examine the assumptions underpinning this discourse. We also need to consider evidence about factors such as the health status, social structures, level of contributions to community that are not captured in the paid workforce (e.g. in roles such as volunteer, carer, mentor, leadership of community organisations, etc.) and potential opportunities that are provided by the ageing population in relation to growth of the health workforce in order to come to a more balanced understanding of what the ageing population could mean for Australia. A deeper analysis will be addressed in further chapters of this book. What the ageing population means for trainee health professionals is that there is ample and growing scope for interesting, challenging and rewarding work roles.

PLACE AND HOUSING

Where and how we live are important factors in either supporting or creating barriers to health and well-being at any age. As we saw in the case studies of Chakrii and Fran, for older adults the home and community environment is of even greater significance. Supportive and well-designed environments can assist an older person to maintain independence despite losses of function or the onset of a chronic condition. The suitability of house design – for example, without steps, with access for mobility devices, with fitted handrails in bathrooms and/or with new smart technology purpose designed to assist with operating doors, heating, lighting and appliances – can support an older adult in their own home for longer than would otherwise be possible. This is very important because not only does research show that most Australians wish to remain in their own homes as they grow older – for reasons of identity, comfort, familiarity, neighbourhood links and as a place of family memories – but this is also economically favourable for the individual and for the public cost of care services in the home as opposed to residential care.

The wider physical and social environments in which we live are also important in enabling health and well-being as we age. The World Health Organization (WHO), in aiming to respond effectively to global population ageing, has developed a framework for Age Friendly Cities and Communities that provides information and resources to help local governments and their communities to better meet the needs of their older residents and enable them to maintain active participation in those pursuits and activities that are meaningful to them (see Box 1.1). In Australia there are currently fourteen age-friendly cities/communities listed on the WHO network. Examples of the activities and practical changes those communities have undertaken are inspiring and provide guidance on what can be done to support older citizens at the community level. As a health professional working with older adults, you too can play an important role in your community by getting involved in age-friendly co-design with older people, local governments and other organisations to support health and well-being. As a bonus, age-friendly communities are people friendly: parents, children and people with disability also benefit from these environments.

Box 1.1 The WHO Age Friendly Cities and Communities framework

Age-friendly environments support the individual capacities of older people and compensate for any functional limitations they may develop in order to enable individuals and older population cohorts to fully participate in their communities as they grow older.

'In practical terms, age-friendly environments are free from physical and social barriers and supported by policies, systems, services, products and technologies that:

* promote health and build and maintain physical and mental capacity across the life course; and
* enable people, even when experiencing capacity loss, to continue to do the things they value.

Age-friendly practices help build older people's abilities to:

* meet their basic needs;
* learn, grow and make decisions;
* be mobile;
* build and maintain relationships; and
* contribute [to their families, networks and communities].

In doing so, age-friendly practices:

* recognise the wide range of capacities and resources among older people;
* anticipate and respond flexibly to ageing-related needs and preferences;
* respect older people's decisions and lifestyle choices;
* reduce inequities;
* protect those who are most vulnerable; and
* promote older people's inclusion in and contribut[ion] to all areas of community life.' (WHO, n.d., 'Age-Friendly in Practice')

Values of the program include:

* respect for diversity
* equity
* participation
* rights.

Principles of the program (based on age-friendly practices) are:

* co-design
* collaboration
* participatory processes
* life-course approach.

Eight domains have been identified as key areas for communities to address in order to better adapt their structures, services and processes of consultation to the needs of older citizens. These are:

1 outdoor spaces and buildings
2 transportation

CLARISSA HUGHES, CHRISTINE STIRLING AND ROBIN HARVEY

3   housing
4   social participation
5   respect and social inclusion
6   civic participation and employment
7   communication and information
8   community and health care. (WHO, n.d., 'Global Network for Age-Friendly Cities and Communities')

HOUSING OPTIONS

In general, older Australians have the same housing options as all Australians. Owning one's own home has long been seen as the 'great Australian dream' and the majority of older Australians do own their own home with access to familiar environments, neighbours and gardens. However, there are societal changes impacting this vision of retirement, with older Australians increasingly deciding to move as they age for changes in lifestyle such as downsizing for less maintenance, a sea change or a tree change. This flexibility provides greater lifestyle options because people live longer and healthier lives, but it does mean that increasing numbers of older Australians don't live near family or long-time neighbours and friends. As well, while currently only around one-fifth of older Australians rely on less secure housing such as rentals or caravans, this portion of the housing market is projected to increase over the next few decades (AIHW, 2018)

One housing option available for older people but not other age groups is Australia's system of residential aged care facilities (RACF), which provides subsidised accommodation with access to care and support services. Housing options become important for the older person if they experience declining function, need additional assistance or housing adaptations, or if their retirement income becomes very limited. The following section takes a closer look at housing options other than owner-occupied housing.

Insecure housing

'Ageing in place' has been an Australian policy focus for several decades as the benefits of being able to stay in a familiar environment and live in the community are recognised. This works well for the majority of older Australians who own or are buying their own home, but not so well for the increasing number of Australians living in low-cost or insecure housing. For those older Australians living in private rental and/or marginal housing situations, such as caravan parks and boarding houses, there is a risk of homelessness, particularly if they develop morbidities such as dementia, Parkinson's disease or a chronic illness needing home modifications. The older person may have problems maintaining the house and garden, or confusion may lead to missed lease arrangements or rental payments. Housing such as caravan parks and boarding houses can also make personal care difficult to manage and may prevent access to home-based support. In 2020, Emma Power highlighted the problems of high rents and utility bills for Australian renters on fixed incomes such as the pension and how this can lead to housing instability as well as the impact of having to move house. Some housing service providers are increasing their focus on collaboration and case management for older people with conditions such as dementia to help prevent or reverse homelessness (Power, 2020).

Residential aged care

Residential aged care facilities are places where older people needing significant levels of assistance go to live. They become the residence of the older person, but they are also institutions. The Australian Royal Commission into Aged Care Quality and Safety (Commonwealth of Australia, 2021b) has been outspoken in highlighting some of the problems for this care sector. Residential aged care takes a large portion of the aged care budget, yet more than two-thirds of aged care service users are living in the community.

Residential Aged Care (RAC), and the state of residential aged care in Australia, is a topic of discussion among older as well as younger people. As with the examples of diversity of experiences, there is considerable variability regarding how people think about, and experience, the move into the RAC setting. For some people, their geographical location, financial resources and social supports mean they are able to exercise choice regarding their living arrangements in older age. RAC may be just one of several options for them to consider. Some people look forward to moving to RAC because they will no longer have the pressure to maintain gardens or do their own housework – or because there will always be someone nearby for a chat. Some like the idea of having easy access to activities or being 'less of a burden' on their family members. For other people, the thought of moving into RAC fills them with dread. They may have heard stories of older people being neglected or not having their needs adequately catered for. They may grieve the loss of independence or the familiarity of living in the family home.

Some of the ways people think about RAC is influenced by wider societal factors. Around the world, cultures differ significantly in terms of the place of older people in the community, and what is considered 'appropriate' care for people later in life. You will learn more about cultural differences in later chapters of this book.

Think back over recent media coverage of the RAC 'industry' both in terms of privately- and government-run facilities. What springs to mind? What sorts of impacts do you think the Aged Care Royal Commission has had on:

- people currently living in RAC or considering moving into RAC in the future?
- people with family members living in RAC or whose family members may be moving into RAC in the future?
- people currently working in RAC or considering working in RAC in the future?

You might like to jot down some thoughts about what the Royal Commission has revealed and what you know of the recommendations.

FOCUS QUESTIONS

Conclusion

Read more about the recommendations of the Royal Commission in Chapter 2.

In this chapter we have provided an overview of some key aspects of ageing in Australia, many of which will be explored in subsequent chapters in the book. Our focus has been on revealing the diversity of experiences of ageing within the Australian population; the social, community and environmental contexts of ageing and some age-associated changes; and the ways in which individuals and their communities may adapt to these. Our aim has been to provide you with an introduction to the opportunities and rewards of growing older as well as to the challenges of this life stage for older Australians. Some challenges and opportunities of an ageing population have also been introduced, including awareness of ageism and the need to challenge it, and the opportunities to develop communities that are age friendly (and consequently more people friendly for all ages). This is an exciting time to be preparing to enter the health workforce, given the growing opportunities to work with older adults to increase their ability to age adaptively, and with health and well-being, for as long as possible.

REVISION QUESTIONS

1   What is ageism and how might it affect older Australians?
2   How do ageing theories help to guide our practice in working with older people?
3   What are some of the major life changes people are likely to experience as they age?
4   What are some key factors that might impact a person's experience of ageing?

Learn more
Access additional resources – such as weblinks, further readings and podcasts – to broaden your understanding of this chapter. See the Guided Tour for access details.

REFERENCES

Allende, I. (2014). 'How to live passionately – no matter your age'. TEDx Talk. https://youtu.be/5ifMRNag2XU

Australian Bureau of Statistics (ABS) (2018) Workforce participation measures. www.aph.gov.au/About_Parliament/Parliamentary_Departments/Parliamentary_Library/pubs/rp/BudgetReview201819/Workforce

Australian Bureau of Statistics (ABS) (2019). Informal carers. www.aihw.gov.au/reports/australias-welfare/informal-carers

Australian Bureau of Statistics (ABS) (2020). Voluntary work and unpaid work support. General social survey: Summary results. www.abs.gov.au/statistics/people/people-and-communities/general-social-survey-summary-results-australia/latest-release

Australian Institute of Health and Welfare (2018). Older Australia at a glance. People at risk of homelessness. www.aihw.gov.au/reports/older-people/older-australia-at-a-glance/contents/diverse-groups-of-older-australians/people-at-risk-of-homelessness

Bertoldo, M. J., Listijono, D. R., Ho, W. H. J., Riepsamen, A. H., Goss, D. M., Richani, D., ... & Wu, L. E. (2020). NAD+ repletion rescues female fertility during reproductive aging. *Cell Reports*, *30*(6), 1670–81.

Butler, R. (1969). Ageism: Another form of bigotry. *The Gerontologist*, *9*(4), 243–6.

Carstensen, L. L. (2006). The influence of a sense of time on human development. *Science*, *312*, 1913–15.

Charles, S. T. & Carstensen, L. L. (2010). Social and emotional aging. *Annual Review of Psychology*, *61*, 383–409.

Clarke, P. & Nieuwenhuijsen, E. (2009). Environments for healthy ageing: A critical review. *Maturitas*, *64*(1), 14–19.

Commonwealth of Australia. (2021a). Royal Commission into aged care quality and safety. Final report: Executive summary, p. 61. https://agedcare.royalcommission.gov.au/publications/final-report-executive-summary

Commonwealth of Australia. (2021b). Royal Commission into aged care quality and safety. Final report: Care, dignity and respect. Vol. 1, Summary and recommendations. https://agedcare.royalcommission.gov.au/sites/default/files/2021-03/final-report-volume-1_0.pdf

E-Shien, C., Kannoth, S., Levy, S., Shi-Yi, W., Lee, J. E. & Levy, B. R. (2020). Global reach of ageism on older persons' health: A systematic review. *PLoS One, 15*(1). doi:http://dx.doi.org.ezproxy.csu.edu.au/10.1371/journal.pone.0220857

Fung, H. (2013). Aging in culture. *The Gerontologist*, *53*(3), 369–77.

Hooyman, N. & Kiyak, H. (2018). *Social Gerontology: A multi-disciplinary perspective* (10th edn). Pearson.

Jung, C. G. (1933). *Modern Man in Search of a Soul*. Harcourt, Brace & World.

Kane, A. E. & Sinclair, D. A. (2019). Epigenetic changes during aging and their reprogramming potential. *Critical Reviews in Biochemistry and Molecular Biology*, *54*(1), 61–83.

Kane, A. E. & Sinclair, D. A. (2019). Frailty biomarkers in humans and rodents: Current approaches and future advances. *Mechanisms of Ageing and Development*, *180*, 117–28.

Martin, P., Kelly, N., Kahana, B., Kahana, E., Willcox, B.J., Willcox, D. C. & Poon, L.W. (2015). Defining successful aging: A tangible or elusive concept? *Gerontologist, 55*(1), 14–25.

McCormack, B. & McCance, T. (2010). *Person-Centred Nursing: Theory and practice*. Wiley.

Perry, T. E., Ruggiano, N., Shtompel, N. & Hassevoort, L. (2015). Applying Erikson's wisdom to self-management practices of older adults: Findings from two field studies. *Research on Aging, 37*(3), 253–74.

Power, E. R. (2020). Mobility-based disadvantage in older age: Insecure housing and the risks of moving house. *Ageing & Society*, pp. 1–23.

Pressman S. & Cohen S. (2007). The use of social words in autobiographies and longevity. *Psychosomatic Medicine. 69*, 262–9.

Robertson, M. (2020). If you've seen one older adult, you've seen ONE older adult. The complexity & variability is profound and should be respected. 14 February. [Mariah Robertson MD MPH @MLRobertsonMD].

Subramaniam, P. & Woods, B. (2012). The impact of individual reminiscence therapy for people with dementia: Systematic review. *Expert Review of Neurotherapeutics, 12*(5), 545–55.

Tavares, J. & Cohen, M. (2019). A view of older adults' demographic, health and economic profiles by retirement choice status. *Innovation in Aging,* Vol. 3 (Supplement 1).

Taylor, P. & Earl, C. (2016). The social construction of retirement and evolving policy discourse of working longer. *Journal of Social Policy, 45*(2), 251–68.

Taylor, P. & Smith, W. (2017). What's Age Got to Do with It? Towards a new advocacy on ageing and work. Percapita. https://percapita.org.au/wp-content/uploads/2018/05/AgeingReport_Final-1.pdf

Westerhof, G. (2015). Life review and life-story work. In S. Krauss (ed.). *The Encyclopedia of Adulthood and Aging.* Wiley.

World Health Organization (WHO) (2013). How to use the ICF: A practical manual for using the International Classification of Functioning, Disability and Health (ICF). Exposure draft for comment.

World Health Organization (WHO) (n.d.). Age-Friendly in Practice. Age-friendly world. https://extranet.who.int/agefriendlyworld/age-friendly-practices/

World Health Organization (WHO) (n.d.). Global Network for Age-Friendly Cities and Communities. Age-friendly world. https://extranet.who.int/agefriendlyworld/age-friendly-cities-framework

Yeung, J. W. K., Zhang, Z. & Kim, T. Y. (2018). Volunteering and health benefits in general adults: Cumulative effects and forms. *BMC Public Health 18*, 8. https://doi.org/10.1186/s12889-017-4561-8

2

Policies Influencing Aged Care in Australia: Past, Present and Future

J. MICHAEL WYNNE, LYNDA SALTARELLI AND DENISE WINKLER

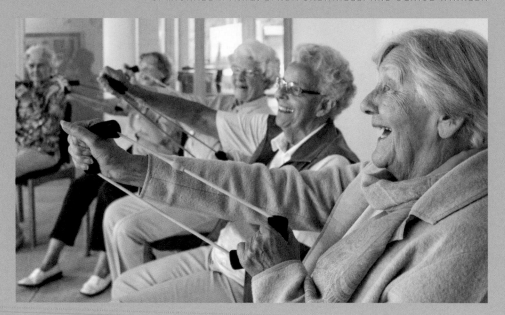

LEARNING OBJECTIVES

After reading this chapter, you will:

» understand the evolution of policy related to the provision of aged care in Australia

» recognise that the Royal Commission has exposed the failure of policies and be able to critically analyse the outcomes of recommendations

» recognise that all political parties have played a role in the evolution of the current aged care system

» understand that aged care policy can be subjected to policies that impact caring and caring relationships

» acknowledge that as responsible individuals in society, we have a role to advocate for the quality of life and safety of older people, wherever they choose to live.

Introduction

Stories of older people suffering from malnutrition and dehydration in aged care facilities because there wasn't enough staff, and viral videos of staff members screaming at, hitting and abusing older people showed us the grim realities of being an older person in need of care. By 2017, Australians were begging their political leaders to investigate these stories and videos. In early September, *Four Corners* announced a two part series exposing the mistreatment of older people would air on 17 and 24 September. Prime Minister Scott Morrison quickly announced a Royal Commission into aged care. The Governor General formally established the Royal Commission on 8 October 2018. When the first choice announced, Justice McGrath was unable or unwilling to serve, Justice Richard Tracey and long-term bureaucrat Lynelle Briggs were appointed. Even during the Royal Commission investigations, mistreatment continued, with reports of older people dying alone because their families weren't allowed to see them due to quarantine restrictions and suffering neglect because staff were afraid they might pass on COVID-19.

So began two long years of testimonies, expert evidence, surveys of people receiving care, hearings and workshops about the neglect, mistreatment and abuse of older people. The two royal commissioners appointed were Honourable Richard Tracey AM RFD QC and Ms Lynelle Briggs AO. In establishing the Royal Commission, the governor-general required them to provide an interim report by 31 October 2019. Commissioner Tracey died of cancer in October 2019 and was replaced by retired judge Tony Pagone.

During the inquiry into aged care quality and safety, the commissioners also commissioned research into aged care. They commissioned the National Ageing Research Institute (NARI) to investigate integrated care and accommodation (NARI, 2020). The University of Wollongong provided data on how much residential aged care services should cost (Commonwealth of Australia, 2020a). This data and the powerful stories from older people resulted in a five-volume final report (Commonwealth of Australia, 2021). You can access the entire document online. In this chapter, we will summarise and highlight the recommendations applicable to health-care professionals.

The chapter is split into three sections: the first section details applicable recommendations of the final report; the second section is dedicated to the history of aged care policy in Australia; and the final section prompts you to consider the type of aged care you want for yourself or your loved ones and all older people who live in Australia. It is vital that you, as a health-care professional, understand the past so that you may learn from it as you develop a career in this sector. If we don't learn from our history, we face the danger that it will repeat itself – and this is never more clearly demonstrated than in aged care. As you read through the timeline, you'll find the same issues apply today as those encountered by colonialists, despite many millions of dollars having been spent on inquiries.

The Royal Commission into Aged Care Quality and Safety (RCACQS)

Commissioners Lynelle Briggs and Richard Tracey commenced their investigations in January 2019 and heard evidence from older people, families, carers and staff across the country. Many failures were exposed by the Royal Commission, the media and the Aged Care Quality and Safety Commission (ACQSC). The problems in staffing, care, management and regulation were exposed. The Royal Commission handed down its findings in an interim report titled 'Neglect' in October 2019 (Commonwealth of Australia, 2019). It had detected widespread neglect and abuse – an appalling situation. The report promised radical reform. Sadly, Commissioner Tracey died after compiling an initial report to inform the ongoing work of the Royal Commission. The reform was left to Commissioner Briggs and the new commissioner, Tony Pagone.

The final report, titled 'Care, Dignity and Respect' (Commonwealth of Australia, 2021) was released at the end of February 2021. In redesigning the system, the Royal Commission engaged principally with the aged care industry, government departments and officials, economists and community groups that had been involved with government in designing the system under scrutiny during the inquiry.

FINDINGS AND RECOMMENDATIONS

The final report consists of 26 chapters outlining 148 recommendations, each with two or more subsections. Interestingly, the two commissioners disagreed strongly. Commissioner Pagone sought to rebuild the aged care system by making it more independent from government and by creating regional managers to manage and oversee the care. Commissioner Briggs wanted to renovate the existing system. They differed in how their agreed objectives should be accomplished. They wrote separate chapters with separate recommendations.

There are five key recommendations from the Royal Commission that we will look at in detail. Our purpose is to provide theme threads for you to look out for while you read through the timeline of aged care. By following these theme threads, you may see a pattern of reoccurring answers to the fundamental questions of who should provide care; what quality care looks like; where the best place is to provide it; and how it will be funded and by whom. The context and motivation for political decisions and policies created to answer these fundamental questions can be understood by following these theme threads. The five key Royal Commission recommendations that we will detail in this chapter are:

1 Informal carers and volunteers (Final Report, Chapter 5, pp. 237–9)

2 Aged care accommodation (Final Report, Chapter 6, pp. 239–40)

3 Aged care for Aboriginal and Torres Strait Islander People (Final Report, Chapter 7, pp. 240–4). ('Aboriginal and Torres Strait Islander People' is the official term used in the recommendation in the final report and it is used here to assist you in accessing further information in the official document. However, in this chapter and the remainder of this book the term 'First Nations peoples' will be used.)

4 Aged care in regional, rural and remote areas (Final Report, Chapter 8, pp. 245–6)

5 The aged care workforce (Final Report, Chapter 12, pp. 258–64).

Informal carers and volunteers

The Royal Commission's recommendation in Chapter 5 of the final report answers the fundamental question of who should care for people who are less able to contribute to our communities, culture and economy. The time, energy and finances that families, friends and volunteers provide to care for older people is recognised by this recommendation for informal carers. It states that support for them should be improved by the Australian Government. Three actions should be taken:

1 *Recommendation 42:* Support for informal carers should include that the two current online platforms (My Aged Care and the Carer Gateway) should be linked as a single

system that provides information; requests and receives training and support services; and secures respite care. This online platform should enable direct referral between the carer, care finders and assessment services. This recommendation should also establish and fund a community-based carers network.

2 *Recommendation 43:* This directive is to investigate the impact that changing the *Fair Work Act 2009* to entitle additional unpaid carer's leave might have on care, businesses and the economy.

3 *Recommendation 44:* By increasing funding, the Australian Government should promote volunteers and volunteering to support older people to live a meaningful life either in their own home or in a residential care home. Funding to the Volunteer Grants under the Families and Communities Program would assist communities and organisations to recruit volunteers, and to provide training and ongoing support for volunteers. The training should include pathways for complaints to be managed and clear ways to report suspected abuse or neglect. The increased funds for volunteering would require aged care providers and services that have volunteer programs to designate a staff member for the role of volunteer coordinator.

This recommendation to the Australian Government to provide funding to support informal carers and volunteers is evidence that there is validation and incentive for older people to age in place and not be forced to move into residential care. The next recommendation addresses the building and designing of residential aged care facilities for older people.

Aged care accommodation

In the next recommendation, outlined in Chapter 6 of the final report, the commissioners begin to answer the fundamental question of where older people should live. In the 'Timeline of aged care policy in Australia' section of this chapter, you will see how the government began taking more and more responsibility for the care of people who could no longer care for themselves by housing them in state hospitals. This recommendation specifically details a plan for the architectural and functional design of the spaces where older people should live.

1 *Recommendation 45:* The design of appropriate residential aged care accommodations should be guided by the Australian Government. Appropriately designed accommodation would follow the 'small household' model. This model encourages small-scale congregate living that is accessible and dementia friendly. A national aged care design containing principles and guidelines should be developed and published.

2 *Recommendation 46:* The number of capital grants for providing more 'small household' models of accommodation should be increased. Aged care providers with a majority of residents in certain categories should be given priority. The prioritised categories are:
   a people with low income, concessioners or supported and assisted residents
   b people with special needs
   c people who live in an area where there are limited residential care services
   d people living in rural and remote areas.

The aged care accommodation recommendation details the plan to create more physical spaces where older people can live that provide safety. Homes that minimise falls risks, that can easily contain the spread of viruses/pathogens and that can be navigated with mobility aides would be considered safe. Homes that contain familiar furnishings and are close

See Chapter 5 for a comprehensive look at the challenges and benefits for informal carers.

The invaluable role of volunteers, and strategies to manage and support them, are detailed in Chapter 8.

Dementia-friendly housing is discussed in Chapter 13.

to familiar carers provide emotional and psychological safety. Homes located in people's chosen community provide consistency, access to friends and family and connection to Country. Allowing older people to live where they choose should be funded and supported by the Australian Government.

Aged care for Aboriginal and Torres Strait Islander People

What quality care should look like now and into the future begins to be addressed by the recommendations in Chapter 7 of the Royal Commission's final report (Final Report, Chapter 7, pp. 240–4). For First Nations peoples, who age faster than non–First Nations peoples, this recommendation acknowledges and addresses the changing and diverse needs of those communities' elders. The commissioners outlined a comprehensive plan for the care of older First Nations peoples that includes ongoing funding, appointing a First Nations person as aged care commissioner to the **System Governor**, building flexibility into program streams, prioritising First Nations health and aged care organisations, and providing **trauma-informed care** and culturally safe care through training and education. A summary of the seven recommendations for improving the lives and care of First Nations peoples in Australia is outlined next.

1 *Recommendation 47:* A 'Pathway' should be created for First Nations peoples within the new aged care system. No matter where they live, First Nations peoples should have aged care services that are:

   a   culturally safe and respectful

   b   high quality

   c   trauma informed

   d   needs based

   e   flexible.

2 *Recommendation 48:* This states that the System Governor and the Australian Government should require all aged care system employees and care finders to be trained regularly about trauma-informed service delivery and cultural safety. It also requires that care finders within First Nations communities be local First Nations peoples who are culturally trained and familiar with services that are trusted by the local population. Aged care assessments should be done by First Nations peoples or health professionals trained in cultural safety and trauma-informed care. Establishing culturally appropriate advanced care directive materials, processes and training that reflect the diversity and cultural practices should be done in collaboration with state and territory governments.

3 *Recommendation 49:* Within the System Governor, a First Nations aged care commissioner should be appointed to develop, promote and nurture culturally safe, flexible and bespoke aged care services across Australia. This commissioner should be a First Nations person.

4 *Recommendation 50:* The System Governor and Australian Government should prioritise First Nations organisations as care providers by ensuring that First Nations organisations are not disadvantaged in the approval and regulation process, and that new organisations moving into aged care services are given special consideration. Encouraging and supporting these First Nations organisations will require the system to be flexible in its approving and regulating process. Flexibility should include additional time to meet requirements and demonstrate capabilities by alternative

System Governor
Refers to the overall management function of the controlling Independent Australian Aged Care Commission in Pagone's model and the Department of Health in Brigg's. An Aged Care Advisory Council appointed by the minister would advise on policy matters concerning the performance of the aged care system and on matters of importance from the perspectives of older people who need and use aged care services, the workforce, providers, educators and professionals involved in the provision of aged care.

trauma-informed care
Care that is aware of trauma symptoms and accepts the role it plays in a person's life.

means, as well as building capacity with exemptions in rare cases. There is also a statement about building capacity within these First Nations organisations with financial assistance.

5   *Recommendation 51:* The Australian Government should develop a national plan for the First Nations workforce. This would include fine-tuning of employment and training for First Nations aged care programs, creating targets across the full spectrum of aged care roles for First Nations peoples. Funding is to be provided to implement the national plan and meet the training and employment targets. In urban, rural, regional and remote areas of Australia, training facilities, instructors and courses should be made available to meet these targets.

6   *Recommendation 52:* Blocking out funds for three to seven years in an assessment-based funding cycle should set up the First Nations Pathway to provide high-quality, culturally safe aged care services.

7   *Recommendation 53:* The funds specifically designated for the First Nations Pathway should be dispersed in flexible program streams. Flexible grant funds should provide for home and community care, residential care and respite care. Aged care providers could apply for funds for expenditures, capital development and provider development. Residential aged care providers could apply for funds to facilitate First Nations residents to stay connected to Country. This would cover the costs of three situations:

> For the story behind these recommendations and the First Nations peoples who made them, see Chapter 3.

1   for the resident, and anyone they need to assist them, to travel to and from Country

2   for a family member to travel to visit an older person in a residential care facility in a distant location

3   for infrastructure installation and maintenance of technology (video conferencing) to facilitate communication between the residential facility and communities in Country.

The last recommendation in Chapter 7 of the final report begins to address the practicality of travelling the vast distances across Australia. It also acknowledges the findings that aged care services are lacking in rural, regional and remote areas of Australia.

Aged care in regional, rural and remote areas

In Chapter 8 of the final report, the fundamental question of where aged care should be available and what quality care looks like is explained (Final Report, Chapter 8, pp. 245–6). Many older Australians choose to stay in rural or remote areas after their children leave to pursue opportunities in urban areas. Others desire a change from the pace of life in the city and choose to retire in less populated areas. Leaving choice aside, economic realities are forcing older people to reside where the cost of living is affordable. With ever more older people living outside urban areas, where most of the health services are located, the demand for health services in rural, regional and remote areas is increasing. The findings and recommendations of the Royal Commission recognise the lack of aged care services in non-urban areas and aim to investigate the extent of the needs of older people, and then propose a solution that should meet most of these needs. The two recommendations for aged care in regional, rural and remote areas are:

1   *Recommendation 54:* The System Governor and Australian Government should ensure the equable provision of aged care in regional, rural and remote areas of Australia. First, an investigation should be launched to identify areas with an inadequate supply of services and plans should be developed for an active response. Then, aged care services should be

supplemented to meet the needs of the community and fulfil the entitlements of older people living in the identified areas.

Multi-Purpose Services Program
Provides integrated health and aged care services to regional and remote communities in areas that can't support a hospital and a separate aged care home.

2   *Recommendation 55:* Working with state and territory governments, the Australian Government should boost the **Multi-Purpose Services Program**. This should be done by the Systems Governor, along with the community, to create new multi-purpose services in two areas: where an aged care provider already exists and both the demographics and market make it feasible; and where health services for acute patients do not exist but a combined aged care and acute care service would meet the needs of the community. This recommendation also aims to ensure that people receiving multi-purpose services are meeting the same needs assessments and eligibility requirements as all other people already getting aged care services. This would require these people to pay for the cost of their care and accommodation by meeting the same financial means test as all the other people in aged care. Multi-purpose service providers should also be allowed to access all aged care funding programs on the same basis as other aged care providers. A funding model should be devised to guarantee that older people will get the care they need over a financial year based on the changes to and acuity of their needs for services. Multi-purpose services that need to be rebuilt or refurbished to ensure the infrastructure meets aged care design standards (as outlined in Chapter 6 of the final report) and supports residents with dementia should be able to apply for cost-shared capital grants.

See Chapter 6 for the facts and stories of older people ageing outside of the capital cities in Australia.

Once the demand for aged care services in regional, rural and remote areas is determined, and the implementation of recommendations 54 and 55 is enacted, a trained, skilled workforce will be required. To this end, there will be many job opportunities for health-care professionals according to the findings and recommendations of the Royal Commission.

The aged care workforce

Of all 148 recommendations in the final report, Chapter 12 will have the biggest impact on you as a health-care professional (Final Report, Chapter 12, pp. 258–64). The 2020 Aged Care Workforce Census reports there were 277 671 people working in residential aged care and 80 340 people providing home care (Department of Health, 2021). There are thirteen separate recommendations stating that the Australian Government should make changes to and improve the aged care workforce by:

1   gathering data in order to plan for the demand for trained aged care workers
2   working with industry to improve competencies, qualifications and accreditation requirements
3   establishing a national registration scheme for personal care workers
4   including minimum qualifications
5   reviewing courses for aged care certificates
6   ensuring all aged care workers receive training in palliative care and dementia
7   offering ongoing professional development to upgrade the workforce
8   reviewing the accreditation standards and curricula for undergraduate health profession students

9   providing funding for teaching aged care

10 increasing the wages of aged care workers

11 providing a guarantee that aged care workers are getting equal pay to workers doing comparable work

12 requiring residential aged care service providers to engage staff for a minimum period of time (200 minutes per day; for 40 minutes of this time there must be an RN present) to guarantee quality and safety standards

13 enforcing labour standards as a condition of ongoing approval for delivering aged care services.

By detailing these key recommendations from the final report of the Royal Commission, the fundamental questions of who should provide care, what quality care looks like, where the best place is to provide it, and how it will be funded, and by whom, have been addressed. The changes that these recommendations, if implemented, should bring to the lives of older people in Australia are hugely impactful.

Before we look too far into the future, let's first look at how we got here by following the theme threads of aged care policy through time. The following section includes information on the dramatic impact Florence Nightingale had on improving the skills of women caring for the ill, frail and aged. There are also other references to periods of time when the training and skills of nurses and other health professionals was less valued.

Timeline of aged care policy in Australia

The story of aged care in Australia has a poor beginning, a messy middle and a dramatic climax. The end of this story is yet to be written. Will it be a happy ending? A satisfying ending? Or a sad, bittersweet ending? The best part of the story of aged care is that you will have a part in writing the ending. Whatever health profession you choose to work in, you will be working with people who are ageing. Your family members, loved ones and neighbours may be in aged care at some point in their life. You yourself will age and may spend some time in aged care. In small and potentially large ways you will be involved in writing the next chapter of aged care.

As you read through each of the time periods of Australia's aged care history, ponder what it would have been like to be a carer and an older person. Put yourself in each of these roles and look for the theme threads to ask and answer some reflective questions:

- Who was taking care of older people in each period of time?

- What did aged care look like in each period of time?

- Where was care of older people taking place?

- Who paid for it?

FOCUS QUESTIONS

1788–1900: THE COLONIAL PERIOD

From the beginning of the aged care story in Australia, people who could no longer contribute to establishing a colony were abandoned and placed away from everyone else. The early colonial period, after colonisation in 1788, was characterised by military rule. The British military did not see itself as having a major role in care. Few people became old, and care for the old and destitute was provided by families or a benevolent community in poor houses funded by colonial government grants. In 1821, the governor funded a benevolent society asylum for the destitute. Care for the sick, dying and aged was mostly provided by convict women in these asylums.

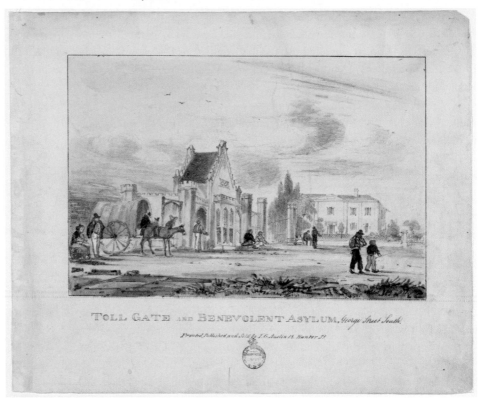

A benevolent society

In the 1850s, the New South Wales (NSW) Government took over management of the Benevolent Asylum and established the state hospital system. These state hospitals cared for most of the impoverished aged into the twentieth century. Families assumed a role in caring for their own older people. The wealthy employed servants to help care for their ageing family members.

Later, when transportation of convicts ceased and the gold rush attracted immigrants, social consciousness grew. There were several inquiries into the care of the poor and the states assumed greater responsibility for their care. During the Crimean War in Europe (1853–1856), English social reformer Florence Nightingale initiated the formal training of nurses. By the late 1870s, these trained nurses were staffing state asylums for the aged. They brought skills, humanity and ethical traditions to care.

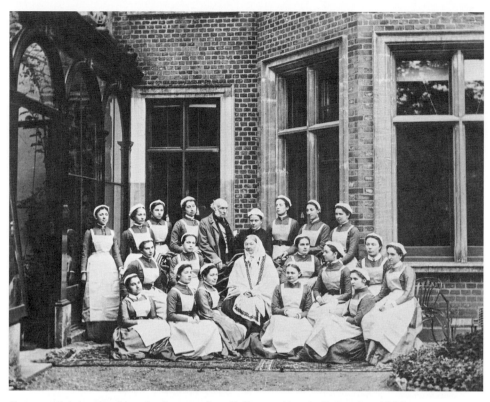

Florence Nightingale with trained nurses from St Thomas Hospital in London, 1886

Concern about the plight of the destitute spread through the community. Church and charitable institutions started providing more services. There was growing concern for the destitute elderly. The inappropriateness of institutional care for the poor in asylums was recognised. This resulted in multiple inquiries and agitation for pensions. These changing attitudes towards the role of the state were reflected in the new Australian Commonwealth Constitution.

1901–1914: THE POST-FEDERATION PERIOD

In 1901, the states responded by creating pensions for the indigent elderly and it became the responsibility of the Commonwealth in 1908. Life was short during this period, with the average life span being 55 years. Pensions were initially only for the 'deserving poor': those who were over 65 years of age (60 for females), who had lived in Australia for 25 years and who were of 'good character'. It is no surprise that only 34 per cent of those over 65 qualified. Further support for older people was provided when the district nursing services were established in 1910 (Baldwin, 2014, pp. 19–24; Coleman, 1975, pp. 30–2; Fine, 1999, pp. 11–16).

1914–1945: THE WORLD IN CRISIS

There were enormous upheavals in the first half of the twentieth century with World War I and the 1918 flu pandemic. Ten years later, **marketplace** excesses resulted in the Great Depression and a period of profound social upheaval, accompanied by a loss of confidence in the structures

marketplace
A place where goods and services are supplied and purchased.

for-profit
An organisation that operates in the private sector with the aim of making a profit for its owners.

regulated
Business activity controlled by means of rules or regulations.

of society. Undemocratic ideologies such as communism and fascism became very appealing. The growth of these ideas led to World War II (1939 to 1945). During this period, older people continued to be cared for by families, district nurses, hospitals, an increasing number of charitable bodies and the occasional **for-profit** owner who secured a livelihood by serving the wealthy. Aged care was not **regulated** during this period.

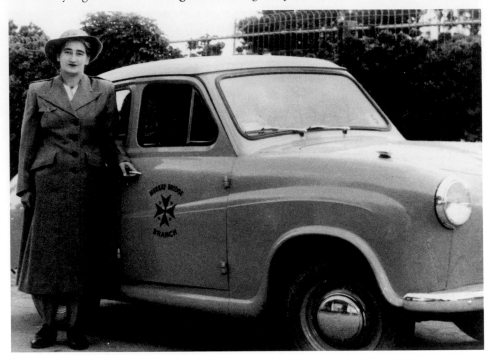

A Murray Bridge (SA) district nurse, 1953

1946: THE POST–WORLD WAR II PERIOD

The global war effort, hardship and loss of life drew people together and helped to rebuild civil society. This led to a period of social responsibility and economic stability in Western countries. A new economic approach developed by John Maynard Keynes, a British economist, was developed in response to the excesses that resulted in the Great Depression of the 1930s. The Keynesian approach – a radical new economic model that regulated the economic **market** – followed the Great Depression, and wealth was more evenly distributed. Society responded to the extensive suffering by becoming more socially conscious.

market
An arena where commercial dealings are conducted.

1945–1949: THE LABOR (CHIFLEY) GOVERNMENT

Post-war socialism saw government in the United Kingdom take greater control of welfare (the welfare state), providing services for the needy. The United States went in a more market-focused direction, while Australia tried to steer a middle course between market forces and altruistic approaches.

In Australia, the post-war Labor Government adopted a strong social reform policy that followed the policies in the United Kingdom. It funded housing and pensions, but its efforts to nationalise health and the banks were unpopular. It did not address aged care.

1949–1972: THE LIBERAL/COUNTRY PARTY COALITION GOVERNMENT

Following World War II, Australia voted the newly created Liberal Party into leadership. Its first prime minister, Robert Menzies, formed a coalition with the Country Party that radically shifted the focus of Australian politics and had two decades to develop social reform policies.

In Menzies' own words it was a move from placing 'the emphasis on state action' to 'the emphasis on the encouragement of prosperity in industry and business'. The Menzies Government continued to fund social services. It established a pensioner medical service in 1951 (Fine, 1999, pp. 12–14).

The Keynesian approach was growing globally. It challenged both big central government and Australia's protectionist policies. By the late 1960s the Liberal Party was divided as the Keynesian thinking of its leaders was challenged. Prime Minister William McMahon presided over a divided and fractious party, which meant that very little meaningful policy could be put in place.

Through the changes in leadership within the Coalition, the focus was economics rather than care. As evidenced, during this period there were no ministers for aged care, but a pro-market aged care policy was gradually adopted.

Thinking changed in the early 1960s. Government felt that for-profit nursing homes would be cheaper. Regular nursing home funding for care was provided to encourage this. The market-driven approach and the amount of government funding had progressively increased over the years (Le Guen, 1993, pp. 2–3).

Private investors saw nursing homes as 'low risk, high profit financial ventures' (Giles, 1985, p. 13) and the sector expanded rapidly. Ninety-five per cent of growth over the first six years was non-government nursing homes and most of these were built by for-profit groups looking to make money (Fine, 1999, p. 14). Many older people admitted to these homes did not need nursing care and private nursing homes were unwilling to accept residents needing costly, intense nursing care. Governments responded by providing extra funding for specialised nursing care.

To contain spiralling costs, governments tried to control admissions to aged care and funded less costly hostels to house older people who needed help but not skilled nursing (Le Guen, 1993, p. 4; McLeay, 1982, pp. 12–23). More funding was provided for home care and for meals delivered by volunteers. 'Senior citizens' centres' staffed with welfare officers were established to address fragmentation by integrating social and nursing care in the community.

During this period, the system was **unregulated** and exploitation of the system to increase profits became a problem. It was suggested that 25 per cent of nursing home residents did not need to be there. By 1972, for-profits owned almost twice as many nursing home beds as **non-profits** (Le Guen, 1993, p. 4). Care in nursing homes was still more profitable. Despite multiple attempts to control this, growth was only temporarily contained and it continued into the early 1980s when major reforms came into existence (Fine, 1999, p. 14).

unregulated
Not controlled or supervised by government regulations or laws.

non-profits
Organisations with a social mission and not seeking a profit for any individual.

1972–1975: THE LABOR (WHITLAM) GOVERNMENT

Gough Whitlam inspired Australia and swept to victory, bringing rapid social change. The flood of social reforms, including those to medicine and education, have improved the lives of many. They proved so popular that coalition governments have been forced to accept them and work within them ever since. However, the Whitlam Government's political and economic ineptitude was such that the Liberal Party persuaded the Governor-General to dismiss it after only three years.

In 1974, the Whitlam Government introduced a 'participating (fees control) scheme' to control for-profit facilities. Non-profits were encouraged by a 'deficit financing scheme', which was based on the actual money they spent, giving them a considerable advantage over the for-profits.

Policies that favoured non-profit facilities resulted in major confrontations with the for-profit nursing homes, which formed an association to act on their behalf. At the government's suggestion, the non-profit providers formed their own association to work with government.

Non-profits had increased their share of new beds to 54 per cent by 1983 but were providing care to the middle class rather than the poor as government had intended. The problem of **overservicing** of nursing homes was not solved by these new policies. An attempt was made to contain staffing costs by basing them on resident dependency, but the levels were hopelessly inadequate, and three states refused to comply.

1975–1983: THE LIBERAL (FRASER) GOVERNMENT

Malcolm Fraser adopted the established Keynesian economic model and supported industry with funding and tax breaks. He dismantled the Medibank health-care reforms but did not abolish all the social reforms of the Whitlam era. He increased fiscal restraint and dissolved the National Social Welfare Commission created by the Whitlam Government in 1972.

Conflicts occurred again when treasurer John Howard abandoned **protectionism** and supported free trade and a **neoliberal** approach to markets. He commissioned a committee of senior businessmen to examine the economy (Campbell, 1981) but its findings were not supported by Prime Minister Fraser. Many in the party supported Howard, opening up divisions within the Liberal Party.

There was little real change made to aged care by the Fraser Government and Australia still had one of the highest rates of residential care in the world (Le Guen, 1993, p. 1). Many older people were admitted to nursing homes when they did not need to be there and those who did need to be there were not getting the care they needed.

1983–1991: THE LABOR (HAWKE) GOVERNMENT

Bob Hawke worked closely with Treasurer Paul Keating to do what Fraser would not. He adopted some of the new global **free-market** policies, joining the **open market** and abandoning protectionism. At the same time, he initiated an extensive social program that targeted the poor and the vulnerable so that there was less inequality. He reinstated Whitlam's health reforms, calling them Medicare. He focused on developing consensus in the fractured industrial relations, reaching an '**accord**' with the unions.

Inquiries leading to reform

There were four major inquiries into aged care during the 1970s and 1980s. Inquiries and reviews commissioned by the Whitlam and Fraser Governments had identified what the major problems in aged care were. Hawke set out to address them and initiated several inquiries himself (Le Guen, 1993, pp. 11–29). The Giles report (Giles, 1985) was the first report on private nursing homes. This exposed extensive failures in care and is reminiscent of the October 2019 interim report of the Royal Commission into Aged Care Quality and

overservicing
Market weaknesses are exploited to make profits by providing more services than are needed as and to those who don't need them.

protectionism
Refers to government policies that restrict commercial activity with the aim of improving safety and/or quality.

neoliberal
Refers to market-oriented policies with minimal regulation and reduced government interference and influence.

free market
A situation where supply and demand are free from any form of regulation by government or any other authority.

open market
Refers to economic situations where there is free trade.

accord
An official agreement between two or more parties.

Safety titled 'Neglect'. Multiple subsequent inquiries, including those by Ronalds, were part of a 10-year reform plan. These inquiries and reviews are relevant to the Royal Commission into Aged Care Quality and Safety. The inquiries are:

1 The Social Welfare Commission 'Care of the Aged' inquiry (Coleman, 1975)

2 The House of Representatives Standing Committee on Expenditure 'In a Home or at Home' inquiry (McLeay, 1982)

3 A Senate select committee chaired by Senator Giles, 'Private Nursing Homes in Australia: Their conduct, administration and ownership' inquiry (Giles, 1985)

4 The 'Residents' Rights in Nursing Homes and Hostels' inquiry (Ronalds, 1989).

All four inquiry reports accepted the thrust of the argument that because of the complexity and wide variation between the requirements of individuals, ethnic groups and cultural groups, regions and even states, 'planning and delivery of programs should be conducted at the regional level' (McLeay, 1982, p. xiii), concluding that considerable flexibility was required. Next, we will examine each report.

The Coleman report (1975)

Coleman wanted the focus to be on local and regional involvement. She wanted integration to include public participation at the local level with integration through regions and states using joint coordinating committees – finally leading to a central coordinating body. The system was to be integrated with regional hospitals. Specialist assessment teams were recommended for rehabilitation, nursing homes and hostels.

There was a strong focus on care in the community, but it was difficult to get support for this as it was less profitable. The system was uncoordinated and therefore not effective. These inquiries saw the role of central government as the creation of services that integrated and supported the regional and local authorities in managing aged care services while the Commonwealth and states simultaneously battled to avoid responsibility for aged care (Coleman, 1975, p. 32).

The McLeay report (1982)

McLeay supported the Fraser Government in trying to persuade states to take responsibility for the care of their citizens, arguing that the Commonwealth was too far away and incapable of doing so. However, the states resisted. While Coleman was critical of for-profits and supported the non-profits, the McLeay report and other reports accepted that non-profits were advantaged by the funding introduced in 1974 and so able to provide better care.

The Giles report (1985)

The Giles report investigated private nursing homes. It exposed neglect, abuse, understaffing, maladministration and regulatory failure. Her report recommended the establishment of 'Community Standards Committees in each region, with the task of monitoring the quality of care in nursing home(s) within the region' (p. xxiv). They would be the local arm of the complaints system and would have 'the effect of opening nursing homes to public view' (p. 133). They would report back to central government bodies, which would support them and act. The report also recommended resident councils within nursing homes.

Giles focused on transparency, condemned the staffing levels advised at that time, urged strategies to assess what was needed and supported 'uniform minimum staffing levels' (p. 118) and quality indicators. In 1985, Giles recognised the importance of having enough staff in aged care and in 2021 the Royal Commission into Quality and Safety in Aged Care identified the same issue.

The Ronalds report (1989)

The Ronalds inquiry represented a government commitment 'to social justice: enhancing people's rights, ensuring that the benefits of a growing economy are distributed equitably, and improving equality of opportunity – in short, giving all Australians a fair go' (p. v). As a lawyer, Ronalds was charged with developing a bill of rights. She also recommended a trained community visitors' scheme that would get to know residents and watch over them, providing knowledge and support. These visitors would have access to documents and case records and would pass information up the system, including to advocates. Industry strongly opposed the visitor and advocacy proposals, describing the empowered visitor's scheme as a 'community busy bodies scheme' (Braithwaite et al., 2007, p. 186). What ultimately eventuated fell well short of what Ronalds wanted.

Ronalds also wanted an independent local advocacy service, as well as an 'advocacy, advice and network agency' in each state and territory. This service would provide information to all those who needed it and would address all identified issues, support test court cases, address policy issues and advise governments – a very different advocacy service from the one we have today. Despite strong opposition from church groups and the Liberal Party, the Human Rights Bill that Ronalds recommended was passed in 1991 (Le Guen, 1993).

FOCUS QUESTIONS

- List the commonalities between these four reports and the recommendations from the Royal Commission's Final Report.
- What evidence can you find in the recommendations that supports or disputes the statement, 'These inquiries saw the role of central government to be the creation of services'?
- How might aged care look today if findings from these four historical inquiries had been implemented and funded? Choose a single issue in aged care that was brought to light in the Royal Commission into Aged Care Quality and Safety and trace it to one of these inquiries.

Major reforms commence

In 1986, a 10-year reform program with eight stages commenced (Le Guen, 1993, p. 11–29). Many of the recommendations made in the reports were strongly resisted by industry and only some were implemented. Industry unsuccessfully challenged the planned reforms in the courts in 1986 (*The Sydney Morning Herald*, 1987). The reform program addressed administrative problems identified by previous reports, such as:

1   The bulk of the funding for aged care was still going to nursing homes. Steps were taken to restrict the number of nursing home beds and 'Geriatric Assessment Teams (GATs)' were created to limit unnecessary admissions. They were later renamed 'Aged Care Assessment Teams (ACATs)'.

2   The 'Home and Community Care (HACC)' program (Queensland Government, 2017) was set up. It put the focus on home-based care. Changes encouraged care in hostels rather than nursing homes. In 1990, for-profits were encouraged to invest in hostels and they were allocated 20 per cent of new hostel bed approvals. The rapid growth in nursing home beds stopped (Fine, 1999, p. 14).

3   Special attention was paid to specific groups including the disabled young, culturally diverse, First Nations peoples and remote communities. It was acknowledged that people with dementia had special needs and sometimes required separate facilities.

4   A 'Joint Commonwealth–State Working Party on Nursing Home Standards' was created. It was to 'formulate national standards of care for nursing home residents and to develop a funding system for uniform nursing home staffing standards throughout Australia' (Le Guen, 1993, pp. 16–20). One major reform was the introduction of oversight of the care provided within aged care. While funding came from the Commonwealth, care standards were assessed by states, which was problematic in many ways including that the standards were not consistent across the states, each having different requirements for care provision. After a review and extensive negotiations, 31 unified agreed outcome standards were gazetted in 1987 with a subsequent and separate set introduced for hostels in 1991.

    a   A vigorous inspection program used trained state inspectors who assessed the standards and drilled down into failures to identify the causes. Findings were reported publicly from 1990.

5   Another reform was made to the funding of aged care. A Resident Classification Instrument assessed the degree of service needs into five levels for funding purposes, with level 5 requiring personal but not nursing care. It abolished the inequitable deficit funding system and replaced it with the SAM and CAM funding systems:

    a   The 'Standard Aggregated Module (SAM)' was calculated using an occupied bed indexed formula to cover 'infrastructure costs such as transport, laundry, food and also return on investment'. SAM commenced on 1 July 1987.

    b   The 'Care Aggregated Module (CAM)' was based on the Resident Classification Instrument. Care, and particularly nursing care, was specifically protected from commercial profit pressures. Profits could not be taken from this money and any unspent funds had to be returned to the Commonwealth. CAM started on 1 July 1988.

    c   There was additional ongoing funding for:
        •   more respite beds in nursing homes and hostels
        •   day therapy centres to provide treatment and rehabilitation to the community
        •   dementia
        •   training staff.

6   The government-reimbursed industry for long service leave, superannuation and workers compensation. In 1990, government started an annual audit of expenditure for each nursing home to ensure funds had been properly spent and that any overpayments were repaid.

7   Another reform was centralisation of funding so that it became a one-size-fits-all model. It lacked flexibility so it was not problem free. There were problems with the documentation required and a review by a consultant supported government (Le Guen, 1993, p. 17). It identified problems with documentation and urged industry to fix the problem.

8   The states provided regulatory oversight, but it was centrally integrated. A review of regulation (Braithwaite et al., 1993) found it to be superior to that in the United States, United Kingdom, Canada and Japan because of its shift to a greater focus on outcomes. It concluded that much more needed to be done.

    a   Jenkins and Braithwaite (1993) examined failures identified by the new regulatory system. They found that, as in other sectors and in aged care in the United States, failures were a result of pressure from the top to 'get this done, but don't tell me how you do it' (p. 222). This was more common in for-profits. They also found that some church groups performed very poorly in respecting residents' rights, often due to an 'ideology of paternalistic caring'.

1991–1996: THE LABOR (KEATING) GOVERNMENT

The relationship between Hawke and his more economically aggressive treasurer broke down and, after a successful challenge, Paul Keating became prime minister in 1991. He pursued his 'neoliberal' reform policies of free markets, globalisation, deregulation and privatisation, while paying some attention to social issues.

He immediately set about restructuring society along neoliberal lines, passing legislation and setting up bodies such as the National Competition Council to implement and manage National Competition Policy. Both major parties were supportive, but minor parties condemned it (Australian Competition Law, 2014). Consultation with the public was poor and the policies were unpopular. Articles in the medical press warned of the negative consequences for healthcare.

Keating commissioned economist Professor Bob Gregory to examine aged care to assess the potential for labour market efficiencies using the new neoliberal management processes. This would have meant abolishing the CAM funding system that protected staffing and care from profit taking. Gregory (1993, p. 79) found that if this happened neither the current system nor any possible alternatives would be able to prevent the diversion of funding from care. Keating took his advice but Prime Minister John Howard did not.

Aged care reform falters

In 1988, the owner and operator of a large, for-profit aged care business, Doug Moran, formed a new anti-regulation organisation, the National Association of Nursing Homes and Private Hospitals, and it rapidly increased its influence. Moran's focus was on protecting the rights of for-profit organisations and building the profit potential of the sector, which was more aligned with Keating's position. As the pressure from industry increased, the momentum of the Hawke 10-year reform plan, and the closer and more frequently on-site regulation, waned (Braithwaite et al., 2007, pp. 188–9). The system became more centralised and supportive of the market, but there was a steady decline in the number of trained nurses.

1996–2007: THE COALITION (HOWARD) GOVERNMENT

Keating's policies were so unpopular that the Howard Government was elected in 1996 without fully explaining its policies. Neoliberal policies and a privatisation agenda were vigorously pursued. Policies included free markets, privatisation, small government, minimal regulation, competition and efficiency. These economic and political priorities soon replaced altruistic ethics as the driving force in care.

Starting in 1997, major changes were made in aged care and a new model of reform was adopted. These 'reforms' were continued over the next 20 years. Those responsible for the changes were well educated and trained and skilled in law, economics, management and psychology. They were leaders in government, in the public service, in the marketplace and in the community.

A policy of small government saw the public service radically reduced. Career bureaucrats were replaced by politically appointed industry representatives. The public sector's capacity to advise government independently or to regulate effectively was markedly reduced. Instead, research and policy development were contracted to private sector consultants that operated within neoliberal and managerial paradigms.

A revolving door of industry advisers were appointed to government bodies and a network of industry-dominated bodies liaised with governments. Politicians and government officials moved into senior positions in industry (Wood & Griffiths, 2019). Conflicts of interest were ignored. Alternative views and democratic processes that protected the public interest were undermined. The behaviour of ministers changed, and Howard was forced to replace or not reappoint several who behaved inappropriately, including those in aged care.

With the priority shift of the Howard Government, health and aged care were the two most vulnerable sectors. Doctors were aware of the privatisation of aged care in the United States and warned of the consequences (Arnold, 1996; Leeder, 1996; Wynne, 1996). Healthcare and aged care followed divergent paths and there are important lessons to be learnt.

Healthcare

In healthcare, marketisation started in the 1990s. Large mega corporations, which had successfully neutralised doctors' capacity to resist in the United States, were welcomed into Australia. Doctors and some citizens were aware of the changes caused by the mega corporations in the United States. With the help of US citizens, data was collected and lodged with state **probity regulators**. They acted responsibly, finding that these companies' conduct showed that they could not be trusted. None of them stayed in Australia.

> **probity regulators**
> Authorities who undertake an assessment of an applicant's trustworthiness before licensing them to operate in vulnerable sectors.

When, in 1998, Michael Wooldridge (Minister for Health & Ageing, 1996–2001) introduced changes that copied the United States and undermined doctors' market power, the doctors united and won the battle. Relationships with the minister broke down entirely. In 2002, when Australia's largest private hospital company adopted practices that threatened care, doctors took their patients elsewhere and put it out of business.

There are lessons here: health-care professionals and communities had united and prevented the marketisation of healthcare. If the same pressure were applied within the aged care sector and a community-led aged care system insisted on it, then a similar outcome could be achieved.

Aged care

Within aged care, the Australian Government and industry were influenced by Andrew Turner, a successful US businessman who brought his health-care company (Sun Healthcare) to Australia in 1997. Sun Healthcare had been exploiting a funding loophole in the United States allowing it to provide lucrative **step-down care** in its nursing homes rather than skilled care for its older residents. Turner claimed that you did not need skilled staff in aged care and that money was being wasted. Governments should mind their own business and leave it to the market, which would soon fix the problem. The government was obsessed with the costs of care, and this is exactly what it did: it supported any attempts to reduce staffing.

> **step-down care**
> Hospitals receiving payment to provide rehabilitation care transferred patients to nursing homes where the payment system allowed more therapy and much larger profits.

Since the mid 1980s, studies in the United States and Australia had shown that for-profit corporations staffed more poorly and provided inferior care. Despite this, to justify the abolition of probity regulations that vetted the trustworthiness of new owners, the government described owners as passive investors who had no impact. After this became untenable, it was claimed that providers, not owners, provide the care and must meet Australia's rigorous accreditation standards – concluding that ownership does not matter. In 1997, Labor Senator Brenda Gibbs (a vocal opposition critic of the Howard Government) warned that accreditation would not work referring to Gregory's warning in 1993.

Aged care marketised

The *Aged Care Act 1997* was developed in close cooperation with the for-profit groups that had supported government. Doug Moran, who had led the for-profit revolt against Labor's reforms, 'boasted that he had played a leading role in designing nursing home policy' (*The Sydney Morning Herald*, 2011). This close alliance between industry and government has persisted. Some of the key features of the Aged Care Act were free-market practices, industry-friendly accreditation and profit impacts on staffing.

Competition policy and free-market practices were imposed on aged care. Non-profits had no choice but to bring in market managers and compete in the same way, changing their culture to survive in the new context. Residents were expected to pay more themselves if they had the money to do so. The distinction between nursing homes and hostels was abolished and a policy of 'ageing in place' was adopted. Care was divided into **low care** and **high care**.

low care
Care for older people who can manage their daily chores with minimal assistance from a nurse or carer.

high care
Care for older people who require almost complete assistance with most daily living activities including meals, laundry, room cleaning and personal care.

The introduction of bonds was another sign of the marketisation of aged care. The Federal Government planned to fund aged care by requiring residents to pay bonds, which were interest-free loans refunded when the resident left or died. Residents usually had to sell their homes to do so. When the legislation was introduced in 1997 there was an angry backlash from the public that threatened the Coalition Government's re-election in 1998. The government backed down and bonds were only imposed on low-care residents.

Effective regulations were replaced with an industry-friendly accreditation agency to assist providers. In 2011, the accreditation agency (Aged Care Standards & Accreditation Agency, 2011) repeatedly stressed that it was not a regulator and that the two processes were incompatible. It quoted Minister Judi Moylan, who in 1998 had made it clear that accreditation was not a 'policing style system', but served to assist 'facilities to improve service'. For this reason, the agency resisted pressure to become part of a single aged care regulatory body; consequently this didn't happen until 2018.

The funding streams for aged care were in keeping with free-market principles; Gregory's 1993 warnings were ignored and the CAM funding, which protected staffing and care, was abolished. Accountability for how public money was spent was no longer required and existing requirements and accountability for staffing were removed. Providers were free to take profits wherever they could. Government encouraged the for-profit sector to invest with the promise of profits and favoured them in the allocation of bed licences.

Cost cutting to increase profits focused on staffing. Staffing comprises 70 per cent of the costs of nursing home care, so it is a focal point for those who want to maximise profits. In 1997, Senator Gibbs warned of the consequences of for-profit organisations determined staffing levels and skill mix (Gibbs, 1997). Government allocated most of the money for care and decided how much to pay so that income was fixed. The market was unwilling to invest unless it could compete by controlling its largest cost: staffing.

Senate inquiries, which identified major problems in nursing and care in 2002 and 2005, were ignored. At the same time, companies that had invested large sums in aged care after 1997 found that they could not make the profits they expected because the unions were still able to resist pressures to reduce staff even further. The big banks and private equity were unwilling to invest because of this. Government passed the unpopular WorkChoices legislation, which reduced union power in 2005. The banks and private equity invested heavily in aged care during 2006–2007.

In 1997, the government 'liberated' the market for investors by quietly abolishing probity requirements for new owners. These had evaluated their trustworthiness (probity) by examining their past behaviour before granting a licence to own or operate in vulnerable sectors. Any multinational with a bad track record was now able to invest in aged care and then appoint managers who would do what the corporation wanted. Even when it was supplied with information, the Federal Department of Health was unable to assess the trustworthiness of multinationals buying Australian aged care companies.

There were multiple reports of failed care in the press and a major scandal at the Riverside Nursing Home in Victoria under Bronwyn Bishop (Minister for Aged Care, 1998–2001). The number of reports increased steadily. This culminated in the rape scandal, which exposed the rape of four 90 year olds at one facility, triggering more reports of rape and sexual abuse in others. Those devoting so much effort to market reform could not accept that it was failing. They claimed that failures and abuse were rare exceptions, but it is clear that care was steadily deteriorating.

2007–2010: THE LABOR (RUDD) GOVERNMENT

After engaging with industry stakeholders, the Aged Care Amendment (2008 Measures no. 2) Bill did not address the problems in ownership the minister had claimed it would. The party, which had been so critical of aged care marketisation in opposition, did nothing about the deteriorating situation. The ideological divide in the Labor Party resurfaced during this period. It came to the surface in 2009, when – after the 2008 recession – Prime Minister Rudd wrote a scathing article (Rudd, 2009) attacking neoliberalism and claiming its time was over. He threatened to increase taxes on the profitable mining companies. Then he came under pressure and was deposed by his own party in June 2010. A few weeks earlier, in April, the party had referred aged care to the Productivity Commission asking it to address the business models needed in the sector.

2010–2013: LABOR (GILLARD) GOVERNMENT

The new leadership walked away from Rudd's ideas. It focused on social issues and initiated the National Disability Insurance Scheme (NDIS), which was implemented using market principles. The Productivity Commission's 'Caring for Older Australians' report in 2011 supported more centralised control and management (Productivity Commission, 2011). Its recommendations were market focused and what the industry wanted.

Living Longer Living Better (LLLB) reforms

The 2011 Productivity Commission report was the basis for the Living Longer Living Better (LLLB) reforms. Mark Butler (Minister for Aged Care, 2010–2013) was responsible for policy and developed these 'reforms' in close consultation with the **National Aged Care Alliance (NACA)** and the **Council on the Ageing (COTA)**. It recommended that bonds be reintroduced into high care. The Labor Government, which had been so critical of bonds in 1997, now brought them back, calling them 'Refundable Accommodation Deposits' (RADs). The distinction between low care and high care was abolished. The new reforms increased the market pressures in the system and there were soon many more failures reported in the press.

National Aged Care Alliance (NACA)
An alliance of a number of providers and other groups involved in aged care formed in 2000 and designed to lobby and work with government. It supported a focus on individual choice and control within government-free market policies.

Council on the Ageing (COTA)
A group claiming to represent seniors having a central role in policy development in NACA.

2013–2015: THE LIBERAL COALITION (ABBOTT) GOVERNMENT

The Abbott Government adopted an aggressive neoliberal approach. Regulation was targeted under a policy of 'red tape reduction', which aimed to save $1 billion a year. Privatisation, market competition, market consolidation and closer cooperation between the market and government were the objectives. Trade agreements were negotiated with China, and these specifically included aged care.

The 2011 Productivity Commission's recommendations were implemented more aggressively. The objective was a consumer-driven system that provided 'consumers' with choice and control. It believed that a competitive market was required. The Abbot Government created partnerships with industry to drive their competitive market.

Aged care was not considered to be health care and was moved from the Department of Health to the Department of Social Services. A new advisory body, the Aged Care Sector Committee, comprising industry and supportive seniors groups was established. One of the first tasks of this committee was to reduce red tape in aged care and it cooperated with NACA to do this. The number of visits by regulators to nursing homes decreased, as did scrutiny and oversight. The second task of the Aged Care Sector Committee working with NACA was to develop a new Aged Care Roadmap (Wynne, 2016) based on free-market principles. Home care was made more competitive by encouraging for-profit groups to invest. This was marketed to the public as providing more choice and control. Funding packages were allocated to the customer, who could decide how the money they were allocated was spent. This was called **Consumer Directed Care (CDC)**.

Consumer Directed Care (CDC)
An approach to service delivery where the individual receiving the service determines the types of services, from whom, when and how these services will be delivered, giving individuals choice and flexibility.

However, the market was considered to be fragmented and immature. A policy of competitive commercial consolidation was adopted. This policy ignored long-established international data showing that for-profit status, company size and facility size were all associated with poorer staffing and more failures in care, while research published in 2014 (Baldwin et al., 2014) showed that Australian for-profit facilities were sanctioned for poor care more than twice as often as non-profits. The evidence was ignored. The industry received record funding from the RADs now being paid. In addition, there was more government funding and more payments by residents. This large profit stream enabled companies to borrow money for acquisitions and growth.

Companies competed aggressively to make more money to increase market share by acquiring smaller groups and non-profits. Hundreds of nursing homes changed hands (Belardi, 2014). Those that became large enough and more profitable listed on the share market, where they were able to raise more money for expansion. The more profitable they became, the more money they could raise. Any weaknesses in the funding system were exploited to improve profitability. The number of trained staff continued to decline as money was diverted from care to the business of competing.

As home care became more popular, the age of nursing-home residents increased and they were frailer, needing more care. The proportion of skilled staff needed to provide this care continued to decrease. Complaints and adverse publicity increased steadily. At the same time, visits to investigate complaints and monitor standards decreased. The success rate in achieving perfect accreditation outcomes had steadily increased from 64 per cent in 2000 to 97.8 per cent in 2015. The demand for home care increased and while recipients of Consumer Directed Care felt more empowered, administration fees increased and there were other problems.

2015–2018: THE LIBERAL COALITION (TURNBULL) GOVERNMENT

Abbott's policies were unpopular and opinion polls plummeted. He was replaced by Malcolm Turnbull in September 2015. Turnbull moved away from the hard-line conservatives, who were dropped from his ministry. This created tensions in the party. He tried to reduce government expenditure – and aged care was not immune.

Aged care once again became the responsibility of the Department of Health, and funding that had been created for some special problem areas was abolished because it was being extensively misused. Sussan Ley (Minister for Health and Aged Care, 2015–2017) was vocal about this. The funding bonanza was over. Big companies attempted to manipulate extra charges to squeeze more from their residents, but the regulators blocked this. The prices for nursing homes fell and companies had less income to pay off their loans, so the quality of care continued to deteriorate.

Consequences of profit over people

The unhappiness about aged care was steadily increasing. Between 1997 and 2016, there had been well over 20 consultations, reviews and inquiries into aged care or aged care–related matters, including some that were part of the Abbott reforms. Very few issues were addressed, and market policies were not challenged. As the aged care system collapsed, the inquiries multiplied in number. Federal Government went through the motions of reforms, but not those that were needed.

In December 2016, an independent state investigation revealed appalling care, neglect and abuse at the Oakden government-owned facility in South Australia. The facility had been fully accredited during the 10 years that the abuse and neglect had been happening. Available data suggested that regulators had been more concerned about protecting the system than the residents they was supposed to serve.

In June 2017, a Senate Workforce Inquiry report identified major problems in staffing. An industry-led task force chaired by a prominent businessman made recommendations and set up processes to improve staffing. These depended on a voluntary code and there was little overall improvement.

The reforms that followed these inquiries rearranged the failed regulatory system without addressing the causes of the problems. The multiple failed government bodies were amalgamated into a single body: the Aged Care Quality and Safety Commission (ACQSC) in 2018. The 44 accreditation standards were reduced to eight broad standards and a new charter of rights was developed.

2018– : LIBERAL COALITION (MORRISON) GOVERNMENT

Tension with the Abbott faction had been growing and in August 2018 they challenged Turnbull. Scott Morrison emerged as the new Prime Minister, subsequently winning the May 2019 election.

Publicity and unhappiness about aged care increased and there were calls for a Royal Commission. Then, in October 2018, the ABC program *Four Corners* televised a two-part exposé of the many failures in aged care. Many more failures and problems were exposed by the ABC program and, with the situation out of control, Morrison called a Royal Commission.

As the scandals in residential care grew, the demand for home care increased. Yet funding and capacity lagged a long way behind demand. Soon there were more than 100 000 citizens on the waiting list for home care. CDC, an appealing concept, was not working as well as expected. Too much of the money was being taken in management fees. Many older people were not using the money they had been given so that those needing support either experienced inadequate service provision or went without.

The COVID-19 pandemic interrupted hearings and the final report of the Royal Commission was delayed until February 2021. The pandemic exposed the inadequacy of staffing and the plight of underpaid, poorly trained carers who worked part time at multiple facilities, spreading the infection. They did not have the training in infection control that was needed. The ineptitude of the Federal Government and aged care regulators was exposed for all to see. Too many older people died alone in aged care facilities without the support of their families. The Royal Commission investigated and its report was scathing (Commonwealth of Australia, 2020b).

Government response to the report

In May 2021, the government released its response to the Royal Commission into Aged Care Quality and Safety's final report (Commonwealth of Australia, 2021). It accepted the recommendations that ensured the government remained in control. The 2021 budget did provide considerable additional funding for providers, but without real accountability. The system remained primarily a market-led system rather than a community-led and organised one.

This next chapter in the story of aged care continues to be written. The Australian Government has responded to the findings and recommendations of the Royal Commission with policies, programs and funding. The evidence that any of these will positively impact the lives of older people, their carers or the aged care workforce will take time to surface.

The main force impacting the implementation of any of the government's responses is the COVID-19 pandemic. This health crisis has caused political and economic crises. The government's actions in the health crisis are evidence of its values. Three examples are included here for your consideration and contemplation.

- Mirroring the arrival of the First Fleet laden with influenza, measles and whooping cough into the population of First Nations peoples without antibodies to these diseases, the Australian Government did not vaccinate the First Nations peoples against COVID-19 first.

- Aimed at righting the abuse and neglect that was brought to light during the Royal Commission's investigation into safety and quality, the policy of new standards for aged care facilities requires more documentation. The Serious Incident Scheme now requires that police investigate and report all incidents of aggression. The logical reaction is for administrators of aged care facilities to calculate the risks and benefits to the older person, the cost of additional time and paperwork to report the incident based on the severity, and consequences of the aggressive behaviour. The outcome of this policy is that residential aged care facilities are simply not accepting residents that might incur risk. Residents who have disabilities, are a falls risk or are inclined to aggression are not able to find accommodation in aged care facilities

- Older people living in residential aged care facilities were some of the first publicised deaths from COVID-19. The government promised that the aged care workforce would be the first to receive the vaccine in order to keep older people from dying. That did not happen.

These three examples offer evidence of the government's response to the practical aspects of aged care safety and quality. The changes in policy to improve the aged care system require more regulation and paperwork. They also show how industry is adapting to changing policy rather than the people in its care. We continue to wonder if the underlying issues are being addressed and if history will continue to be repeated.

- Of the five key recommendations, out of 148, in the Final Report, how many were accepted, approved and funded? Are there inferences that can be made by identifying where the funds to support older people are going? What message is the Australian Government sending about its attitude towards older people?

- What aspects of the government's response provides hope to you as a health professional? In the time that has passed since the Royal Commission, what changes in aged care policy and/or history have you seen?

- How can we, as responsible individuals in society, look critically at the recommendations and government response? What actions can we take to make our viewpoints and values known to the different political parties?

Offering another paradigm in relation to providing quality and safe aged care

The following section presents another way of thinking about how to reform aged care. It is offered for your consideration as you begin and further your professional practice in healthcare. We are providing you with the opportunity to read further and consider how you would like future aged care to look.

Academics studying social and socio-ecological systems have examined the way balanced forces in complex social systems can cause the forces to respond to changes. At the same time, the systems operate within boundaries so that they function well (Walker & Salt, 2006). These systems can operate over a wide range of social systems (governmental, commercial, societal, healthcare) so they are flexible and responsive. There is also sufficient redundancy to allow the system to adapt and be resilient to unpredictable challenges such as the COVID-19 pandemic. Figure 2.1a illustrates how these different forces might act in a functional aged care system (red ball) as the forces respond to changes.

FIGURE 2.1A A balanced aged care system

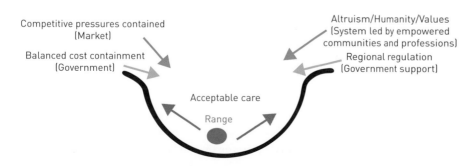

FIGURE 2.1B An unbalanced aged care system

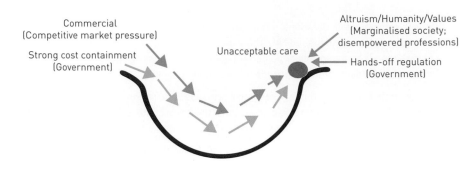

Unbalanced system
(Inflexible, unresponsive, not adaptable, not resilient)

Commercial
(Competitive market pressure)

Strong cost containment
(Government)

Unacceptable care

Altruism/Humanity/Values
(Marginalised society;
disempowered professions)

Hands-off regulation
(Government)

Source: Walker & Salt (2006).

When, as in Figure 2.1b, these forces are unbalanced – as has happened in aged care – the system is pushed into a different situation where it cannot function effectively. It is unable to change or respond effectively. When forces become unbalanced, complex systems behave differently and no longer function properly. This situation is usually difficult to reverse. The system is unable to adapt to change, lacks resilience and fails badly when confronted by unexpected developments (e.g. COVID-19).

When unbalanced social systems fail, there can be multiple attempts to fix them. One way to analyse failed social systems was created by Walker and Salt (2006), who analysed the recurrent cycles through which failing, unbalanced, complex systems often progress as attempts are made to address their failure. Figure 2.2 graphically represents the phases involved in the cycles of recurrent failure as they rebuild after failure (fore loop) and then fail again (back loop).

FIGURE 2.2 Cycles of recurrent failure

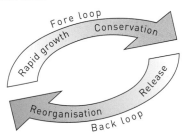

Fore loop
Rapid growth   Conservation
Release
Reorganisation
Back loop

Source: Walker & Salt (2006).

In many situations, the rapid growth phase involves increased centralised management and the development of more efficient processes. In the conservation phase, these rigid structures are continually refined until there is no redundancy (e.g. staff). During these phases, the system fails to adapt to changes (e.g. increased frailty) or to unexpected challenges (e.g. the COVID-19 pandemic). They are resistant to evidence and challenges to their effectiveness or legitimacy.

In the release phase, the system comes apart as its failures are exposed (e.g. Oakden, *Four Corners*, Royal Commission Interim Report). This is followed by a phase of reorganisation (e.g. Royal Commission) before the cycle starts again and keeps repeating itself with overall long-term deterioration.

The phase of reorganisation provides the best opportunity for advocates to make fundamental changes that will break the cycle. These are likely to be strongly resisted by powerful vested interests in the system (e.g. industry and government).

Restoring a balanced system has been achieved once centralised management is regionalised and these regionalised systems work closely with social networks of local businesses (e.g. providers), local staff, local professionals and local communities that know what is happening. Alternative points of view from civil society that restrained those of vested interests became legitimate and were debated, which restored balance. If this did not happen, the cycle repeated itself.

These new balanced systems were less efficient because of more redundancy (e.g. staff). They became more adaptable to changed circumstances and more resilient to challenges, and so more durable. Central management's task became to integrate and support this.

APPLYING A BALANCED SYSTEM TO AGED CARE

In aged care we can see a first cycle going from growth to failure between 1960 and 1985. We can see the Hawke reforms as a period of reorganisation for aged care, in which these decentralisation changes with community involvement were advocated but ultimately defeated by the vested interests of the powerful industry and a new ideology. Instead, greater centralisation, more processes and greater efficiency was the solution, creating an even bigger problem to address later.

The Royal Commission's reforms have not rebuilt empowered communities and their altruistic values. They have not effectively balanced the forces in the system. The same vested interests responsible for the previous system have played a role in designing the new system. The membership of the Aged Care Sector Committee advising government is unchanged.

Despite all the useful recommendations, we are entering the fore loop of the cycle of failure again. The reputation of this industry and government, both responsible for failure, is still seriously compromised, but window of opportunity is still open.

- Can the aged care system be rebalanced? What would create resiliency in the system?
- How can we in the caring professions and the community work together to build on the Royal Commission's recommendations in ways that rebalance the system?

FOCUS QUESTIONS

ADVOCATES FOR CHANGE

The reorganisation through regionalism is another way to create balance in the system. Many groups have been advocating for 'deliberative democracy' and greater citizen involvement in our democracy (Curato & Parry, 2017; Feenstra, 2018; Moore, 2019). Professor Hal Kendig, an eminent gerontologist, advocated for a regional approach to aged care over the last 20 years of his life (Kendig, 2010). Others have pressed for regions, local areas and diverse cultures to play a greater role in their own affairs (Hawkes, 2001; Local Government Review Panel, 2014; Sansom, 2019; Sansom & Robinson, 2019). Here are some examples of groups advocating for a regionalised approach to balance the aged care system:

- Advocacy group Aged Care Crisis (2021) has been pressing for a decentralised system where management and oversight are done locally. In a restructured system that was 'community-led' rather than 'industry-led', community would work closely with local government management. They would participate in planning regional or local services, in contracting for the building of facilities and in selecting those who would be their agents in providing care. They would license or contract the providers of services they need.

  Community would help in deciding who can be trusted to provide the service locally. In a restructured system, community and local management would be able to replace any provider who betrayed their trust by not meeting their expectations with another and do so without disrupting staffing or residents. They would also work closely with local managers and staff and be able to influence decisions made by their agents. This can be described as both community- and place-based governance. It would be governance backed by the power to act. The intention is to create the situation illustrated in Figure 2.1a.

- A representative from the Municipal Association of Victoria gave evidence to the Royal Commission on behalf of the Australian Local Government Association (Hargreaves, 2019a, 2019b). She pressed for regionalism and explained the central role that local governments had always played in managing the care of vulnerable members of their communities. She shared how frustrating it had become working with the centrally managed aged care system. A report prepared for the Royal Commission by academics from Flinders University pressed for increased involvement of local or regional authorities (Dyer et al., 2020).

- In November 2020, the Grattan Institute issued the report 'Reforming Aged Care: A practical plan for a rights-based system' (Duckett et al., 2020). It proposes a centrally integrated but regionally managed and overseen system. Its staff would work across local services and watch what was happening. It aims to protect care and staffing from profit taking. It advises the creation of local as well as central representative community bodies to participate in aged care locally and advise both regional and central management.

If adopted, this regionalised system should enable and encourage regional managers and social networks to develop and have input into residents' assessments (with payments based on them), along with oversight, complaints handling, data collection and research. Complex system analysis suggests that it has the potential to restore balance and then become flexible, resilient, able to adapt to local circumstances and respond to change, and weather unexpected crises.

Conclusion

Learn more
Access additional resources – such as weblinks, further readings and podcasts – to broaden your understanding of this chapter. See the Guided Tour for access details.

This chapter detailed key recommendations from the Royal Commission's Final Report and encapsulated a long and complex history of aged care provision in Australia. The chapter has no ending as the story of aged care is ever evolving and changing. What you need to continually ponder is the extent to which government policy supports the humanity, autonomy, dignity and individuality of any person living in Australia who needs to engage with health and care systems.

The information provided is aimed to empower you to be engaged in debate about policy, recognise that despite numerous government enquiries we continue to face the same challenges, and think about how we can achieve the type of aged care system you would like to have for your loved ones and for yourself.

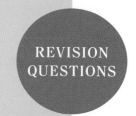

REVISION
QUESTIONS

1 Compare the needs of older people and their options in the time period prior to World War I to the needs and options of older people today. How has policy related to the provision of aged care in Australia evolved? What were the influences on policy?

2 In the column headings of a table, write the different political parties that have an interest in an aged care system. What are the different approaches, different priorities and different levels of authority that these parties had in the decade between 2011 and 2021?

3 List three indicators that aged care is a complex part of society that has responsibility for our most vulnerable citizens. What are three policies that are not suited to caring and caring relationships?

4 Personally reflect on the ways this chapter has made you look critically at the aged care system and understand what is happening to care. How will you react to political parties and policies that impact your career as a health-care professional?

5 Critically analyse the outcomes of the recommendations of the Royal Commission into Aged Care Quality and Safety. How has the Royal Commission exposed the failure of current policies?

REFERENCES

Aged Care Crisis (2021). Make aged care accountable. https://agedcarecrisis.com/resources/make-aged-care-accountable

Aged Care Standards & Accreditation Agency (2011). Response to the Productivity Commission: Caring for Older Australians. Inquiry Draft Report. http://bit.ly/2La4Ydv

Arnold, P. C. (1996). Price competition, professional cooperation and standards. *Medical Journal of Australia, 165*(5), 272–3. https://doi.rg/10.5694/j.1326-5377.1996.tb124965.x

Australian Competition Law (2014). *Competition Policy Reform Act 1995 (Commonwealth)*. www.australiancompetitionlaw.org/legislation/1995cpra.html

Baldwin, R. (2014). *The future of residential aged care in Australia: A mixed methods analysis of the relationship between policy, structure and the provision of care*. Doctoral dissertation Vols 1 & 2.

University of Technology. Open Publications of UTS Scholars. https://opus.lib.uts.edu.au/handle/10453/34391

Baldwin, R., Chenoweth, L., dela Rama, M. & Liu, Z. (2014). Quality failures in residential aged care in Australia: The relationship between structural factors and regulation imposed sanctions. *Australasian Journal on Ageing, 34*(4), E7–E12. https://doi.org/10.1111/ajag.12165

Belardi, L. (2014). Investor appetite builds in aged care. *Australian Ageing Agenda*. 3 October. http://bit.ly/32fGRPN

Braithwaite, J., Makkai, T. & Braithwaite, V. (2007). *Regulating Aged Care: Ritualism and the new pyramid*. Edward Elgar. https://doi.org/10.4337/9781847206855

Braithwaite, J., Makkai, T., Braithwaite, V. & Gibson, D. (1993). Raising the Standard: Resident Centred Nursing Home Regulation in Australia. Department of Health, Housing and Community Services.

Australian Government Publishing Service. www.anu.edu.au/fellows/jbraithwaite/_documents/Reports/Raising_standards_resident_home.pdf

Campbell, J. K. (1981). Australian Financial System – Final Report of the Committee of Inquiry. Australian Government Publishing Service. https://treasury.gov.au/publication/p1981-afs

Coleman, M. (1975). Care of the Aged: Social Welfare Commission Report. Government Printer. https://nla.gov.au/nla.obj-1362224402

Commonwealth of Australia (2019). Royal Commission into Aged Care Quality and Safety. Interim report: Neglect. Vol. 1. https://agedcare.royalcommission.gov.au/sites/default/files/2020-02/interim-report-volume-1.pdf

Commonwealth of Australia (2020a). Royal Commission into Aged Care Quality and Safety. Research Paper 10 – Technical mapping between ACFI and AN-ACC.

August. https://agedcare.
royalcommission.gov.au/
sites/default/files/2020-08/
research_paper_10_-_
technical_mapping_between_
acfi_and_an-acc.pdf

Commonwealth of Australia
(2020b). Royal Commission
into Aged Care Quality
and Safety. Aged Care and
COVID-19: A Special
Report. https://agedcare.
royalcommission.gov.au/
publications/aged-care-and-
covid-19-special-report

Commonwealth of Australia
(2021). Royal Commission
into Aged Care Quality and
Safety. Final report: Care,
dignity and respect. https://
agedcare.royalcommission.
gov.au/publications/final-
report

Curato, N. & Parry, L. J. (2017).
Deliberative democracy must
rise to the threat of populist
rhetoric. *The Conversation.* 7
June. https://theconversation.
com/deliberative-democracy-
must-rise-to-the-threat-of-
populist-rhetoric-76576

Department of Health (2021).
2020 Aged Care Workforce
Census. Australian
Government Department
of Health.

Duckett, S., Srobarr, A. &
Swerissen, H. (2020).
Reforming Aged Care: A
practical plan for a rights-
based system. Grattan
Institute Report no. 2020-17.
https://grattan.edu.au/wp-
content/uploads/2020/11/
Reforming-Aged-Care-
Grattan-Report.pdf

Dyer, S. M., Valeri, M., Arora, N.,
Ross, T., Winsall, M., Tilden,
D. & Crotty, M. (2020).
Review of International
Systems for Long-Term Care
of Older People. Research
Paper 2. Report prepared for
the Royal Commission into
Aged Care Quality and Safety.
Flinders University. https://
agedcare.royalcommission.
gov.au/sites/default/
files/2020-01/research-paper-
2-review-international-
systems-long-term-care.pdf

Feenstra, R. A. (2018). Kidnapped
democracy: How can citizens
escape? *The Conversation. 26*
April. http://bit.ly/2Lc7GPC

Fine, M. (1999). The
Responsibility for Child and
Aged Care Shaping Policies
for the Future. Social Policy
Research Centre Discussion
Paper no. 105.

Gibbs, B. (1997). *Aged Care Bill
1997.* Senate Hansard, 24
June, p. 5042. http://bit.
ly/2rfThau

Giles, P. (1985). Private Nursing
Homes in Australia: Their
Conduct, Administration
and Ownership. Senate
Select Committee on Private
Hospitals and Nursing
Homes. Parliamentary Paper
no. 159/1985. Australian
Government Publishing
Service. https://nla.gov.
au/nla.obj-2085072989/
view?partId=nla.obj-
2088428334#page/n0/
mode/1up

Gregory, R. G. (1993).
*Review of the Structure of
Nursing Home Funding
Arrangements, Stage 1.* Aged
and community care service
development and evaluation
reports; no. 11. Australian
Government Publishing
Service.

Hargreaves, C. L. (2019a).
Statement to the Royal
Commission into Aged
Care Quality and Safety.
Flinders University. https://
agedcare.royalcommission.
gov.au/system/files/2020-06/
WIT.0071.0001.0001.pdf

Hargreaves, C. L. (2019b).
Transcript of Proceedings
in the Matter of the Royal
Commission into Aged
Care Quality and Safety.
Flinders University, pp.
787–803. https://agedcare.
royalcommission.gov.au/
sites/default/files/2019-12/
transcript-19-march-2019.pdf

Hawkes, J. (2001). The Fourth
Pillar of Sustainability:
Culture's essential role in
public planning. Cultural
Development Network
(Vic). https://apo.org.au/
sites/default/files/resource-
files/2001-06/apo-nid253826.
pdf

Jenkins, A. & Braithwaite, J.
(1993). Profits, pressure and
corporate lawbreaking. *Crime,
Law and Social Change, 20*,
221–32. www.anu.edu.

au/fellows/jbraithwaite/_
documents/Articles/Profits_
Pressure_1993.pdf

Kendig, H. (2010). Submission
to the Productivity
Commission's Inquiry:
Caring for Older Australians.
www.pc.gov.au/inquiries/
completed/aged-care/
submissions/sub431.pdf

Leeder, S. (1996). Mad-cow
thinking – how far has
it spread? *Australian
Medicine*, p. 6.

Le Guen, R. (1993). Residential
Care for the Aged: An
overview of Government
policy from 1962 to 1993.
Background paper no. 32.
Parliamentary Research
Service. www.aph.gov.
au/binaries/library/pubs/
bp/1993/93bp32.pdf

Local Government Review Panel
(2014). Community-level
Governance: What provision
should be made in local
government legislation?
McKinlay Douglas. www.
lgnz.co.nz/assets/In-
background/bf38e040f4/
Community-Governance-
Report-.pdf

McLeay, L. (1982). In a Home or
at Home: Accommodation
and home care for the aged.
Report from the House of
Representatives Standing
Committee on Expenditure.
Commonwealth Department
of Community Services,
Australian Government
Publishing Service. www.
aph.gov.au/parliamentary_
business/committees/house_
of_representatives_committ
ees?url=reports/1982/1982_
pp283report.htm

Moore, N. (2019). Co-design and
Deliberative Engagement:
What works? Report no. 3.
Democracy 2025. https://
apo.org.au/sites/default/files/
resource-files/2019-05/apo-
nid239236.pdf

National Ageing Research Institute
(2020). Research Paper 7:
Models of Integrated Care,
Health and Housing. https://
agedcare.royalcommission.
gov.au/publications/research-
paper-7-models-integrated-
care-health-and-housing

Productivity Commission (2011). Caring for Older Australians. Report no. 53. Final Inquiry Report. www.pc.gov.au/inquiries/completed/aged-care/report/aged-care-volume1.pdf

Queensland Government (2017). What is the Home and Community Care (HACC) Program? http://conditions.health.qld.gov.au/HealthCondition/condition/12/69/656/what-is-the-home-and-community-care-hacc-prog

Ronalds, C. (1989). Residents' Rights in Nursing Homes and Hostels: Final report. Office for the Aged. Australian Government Publishing Service.

Rudd, K. (2009). The global financial crisis. *The Monthly*. February. http://bit.ly/32cWveV

Sansom, G. (2019). Is Australian local government ready for localism? *Policy Quarterly, 15*(2), 25–32. https://doi.org/10.26686/pq.v15i2.5366

Sansom, G. & Robinson, T. (2019). Place-Based Governance and Local Democracy: Will Australian Local Government Deliver? LogoNet, Australia. https://logonetdotorgdotau.files.wordpress.com/2019/06/the-logonet-dialogue-2017-19-report-final-designed.pdf

The Sydney Morning Herald (1987). 'Tight law on aged homes upheld', 11 March.

The Sydney Morning Herald (2011). 'Philanthropist who shaped elderly care', 3 December.

Walker, B. & Salt, D. (2006). *Resilience Thinking: Sustaining ecosystems and people in a changing world*. Island.

Wood, D. & Griffiths, K. (2019). Submission to the Senate's 'Revolving Door' Inquiry. Grattan Institute. https://grattan.edu.au/wp-content/uploads/2019/08/Grattan-submission-to-revolving-door-inquiry.pdf

Wynne, J. M. (1996). The impact of financial pressures on clinical care: Lessons from corporate medicine. In P. K. Donnelly & L. Wadhwa (eds). *Access to Surgery: A national symposium on the planning and management of health care programs under Medicare*. University of Queensland Press, 23–24 May, pp. 98–127. www.corpmedinfo.com/corpmed.html

Wynne, J. M. (2016). Aged care roadmap. Inside Aged Care. www.insideagedcare.com/introduction/aged-care-roadmap

3

Healthy Ageing and Aged Care of First Nations Australians

JAYNE LAWRENCE

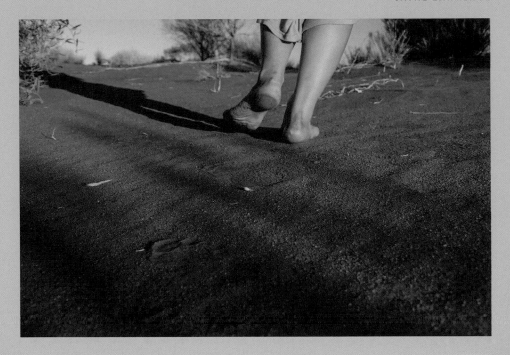

LEARNING OBJECTIVES

After reading this chapter, you will:

» reflect on providing culturally safe care to older First Nations peoples

» identify the role of nurses and other health professionals in First Nations aged care

» explore techniques to build culturally safe communication

» understand the perspectives of First Nations peoples about concepts of healthy ageing and aged care.

Introduction

First Nations Australians are the world's longest existing race, having survived for more than 60 000 years. Older First Nations people in Australia are living longer and have a high burden of chronic diseases. As a result, all health-care providers must be aware of the attitudes, skills and knowledge required to care for this population. Older people, like people of any age, are entitled to high-quality, person-centred care. This chapter examines the health and well-being of older First Nations Australians, as well as the factors to consider when caring for them, so they can experience culturally safe and high-quality aged care. We present reasons why some First Nations Australians are perceived to be non-compliant or disengaged in the health system by various health professionals when in fact they are making conscious choices in relation to their ongoing care that can be culturally defined and seen as a cultural determinant of health. We aim to provide you with information and insight so that you are aware of how to be culturally sensitive with communication and interpretation of responses from First Nations peoples.

Traditionally, aged care services have offered a 'one-size-fits-all' solution. As our communities become more culturally diverse, services must be responsive to the many beliefs, values and traditions of individuals seeking assistance. At the time of writing, there are 51 303 First Nations Australians aged 60 and over, with that number predicted to rise to 89 495 by 2026 (AIHW, 2018). As stated in the Aboriginal and Torres Strait Islander Health Plan 2013–2023, older First Nations peoples should be entitled to choose the setting in which they feel most at ease as they age, especially if they are troubled by illness or incapacity. For those who wish to age on Country and require access to suitable services, options for the growing number of older First Nations peoples will be required (Australian Government, 2013, p. 38).

As with many other health issues, the solution lies in our ability to provide high-quality, culturally sensitive, long-term aged care for our community, in our community, so that aged care services may be delivered on Country (Maguire & Wenitong, 2012). Providing you with information about a **strengths-based approach** as a basis for delivering aged care services is another of our aims.

strengths-based approach
A social work theory that focuses on an individual's self-determination and strength.

Culturally sensitive communication to provide culturally safe, high-quality aged care must begin with person-centred care. We begin this chapter with insight into the persons who are First Nations Australian Elders and their significant role. We then discuss cultural factors influencing the health of First Nations peoples as well as the challenges of providing services for them. Some insightful information about residential aged care and end-of-life care is included at the end of the chapter.

The importance of the First Nations Australian Elders

First Nations Australian Elders play a vital role in sustaining strong **cultural practices** and traditions within their communities with important roles and responsibilities such as passing on knowledge, languages and customs, participating in decision-making ceremonies, and 'looking after Country'. As such, First Nations Elders play an important role in the health of their communities, including maintaining cultural connections to Country, caring for

cultural practice
The traditional and customary practices of a particular ethnic or other cultural group.

JAYNE LAWRENCE

extended family members, including grandchildren, and offering leadership and support within communities (LoGiudice, 2016). Elders and older First Nations peoples are regarded as 'cultural knowledge holders' in modern Australia, and they act as the 'social glue' in their communities. Nonetheless, there is a deficit of understanding of what it means to 'age well' in a First Nations culture. The World Health Organization recognises that ageing well for all people involves 'optimising opportunities for good health, so that older people can take an active part in society and enjoy an independent and high quality of life' (WHO, 2015). Yet identifying what good health and quality of life means, taking into account culture and how culture is enacted and lived, is dependent on the individual. There is a lack of understanding among health-care providers and planners about how to fulfil the specific needs of individual First Nations peoples. This is the motivation for the chapter – to support you to learn more about the most culturally safe ways to support Elders, families and community.

There is a growing body of knowledge about the ageing of First Nations peoples to inform our practice as health professionals and we acknowledge the importance of the input of Elders who have contributed to this chapter to enhance your learning. Their thoughts and wisdom, as well as insights from First Nations health-care professionals, are presented throughout this chapter. We hope you find these insights beneficial on your journey as a health-care professional.

Box 3.1

Robert's thoughts/wisdom

Robert is culturally connected to the Wiradjuri, Morowarri and Kunja Nations through his mother's line and grew up in Brewarrina, a small rural town in North Western New South Wales. Robert has twenty-seven years of work experience in a range of community service roles, including education (school and tertiary), Aboriginal health and community development.

Pre-Invasion – before the systemic changes were introduced by the British – we valued those who were called Elders. Male and female Elders were an integral part of society with roles that were expected and fulfilled. This contributed towards longevity in regard to their physical, mental and emotional well-being. Elders felt like they were important and not a surplus within society. These roles were a preventative approach to many of the health issues elders experience today: obesity, heart disease, dementia, depression, anxiety and feeling unloved.

Children listened to the Elders for wisdom and guidance in a land that could be harsh and cruel. Their lessons, learnt from their Elders and experiences, provided sustenance, conservation for the land and rules to ensure society continued.

FOCUS
QUESTIONS

- What significant consequences might there be when people are ignorant of the status of the traditional place of Elders in the community?
- What are some social, spiritual and psychological impacts on the person when Elders feel they are unimportant and a surplus within society?

Cultural safety

Healthy living, as well as healthy ageing, involves cultural safety. The National Aboriginal and Torres Strait Islander Health Plan 2013–2023 (NATSIHP) draws attention to 'the centrality of culture in the health of Aboriginal and Torres Strait Islander peoples and the rights of individuals to a safe, healthy and empowered life' (Australian Government, 2013, p. 4). A safe, healthy and empowered life is what we all want. As health professionals, we can diligently practise ongoing critical reflection to keep healthcare free of racism.

'Cultural safety is determined by Aboriginal and Torres Strait Islander individuals, families and communities. Culturally safe practice is the ongoing critical reflection of health practitioner's knowledge, skills, attitudes, practising behaviours and power differentials in delivering safe, accessible and responsive healthcare free of racism' (AHPRA, 2020, p. 9). In an unpublished thesis, Irihapeti Merenia Ramsden (2002) outlined a three-step strategy for establishing cultural safety and suggested that such work should be ongoing. She said that health professionals should start with **cultural awareness** and work their way up to **cultural sensitivity** before learning how to practise **cultural safety** (Best & Fredericks, 2021).

cultural awareness
The emotional, social, economic and political context in which people exist.

cultural sensitivity
Alerts practitioners to the validity of difference and starts a self-exploration process of their own experience and realities of life and the effect this could have on others.

cultural safety
An outcome that enables safe service to be determined by those who receive the service. Cultural safety is determined by First Nations individuals, families and communities.

FOCUS
QUESTIONS

- What context do you live in right now? Reflect on what is happening in your social, emotional, economic and political contexts. How culturally aware are you? What action can you take to become more culturally aware?
- How are people different? What differences are you keenly aware of? Is there validity in these differences? What impact does this have on others?
- Have you begun the process of self-exploration? Are you culturally sensitive?
- How do we as health professionals build critical reflection into our busy lives? Brainstorm several ways you can make time and space for this to sustain yourself throughout your career.

Providing culturally safe care is the expectation of the Australian Government. The Council of Australian Governments (COAG) emphasised that health-care services must be available, accessible and culturally safe to implement suitable and effective measures to reduce unnecessary deaths (Best & Fredericks, 2021). COAG also acknowledged that Aboriginal and Torres Strait Islander community-controlled health services (ACCHS) can achieve greater results than mainstream care by reducing unintentional racism, removing access barriers and improving health outcomes.

Strategies to improve access to healthcare for First Nations peoples include:

- employing more First Nations peoples within the health-care settings, which may provide better engagement and promote willingness of attendance at that health-care service
- creating a health-care service that belongs to and is a part of the community. Outreach services, which deliver care in the community, have also been demonstrated to boost rates of client participation in remote regions (Davy et al., 2016)
- providing culturally safe care. Care is not always a priority due to conflicting obligations and the stress of being diagnosed with a chronic disease. When faced with an acute health problem, however, First Nations peoples have prioritised care provided in a health-care facility that was able to provide culturally safe care
- encouraging health professionals to create strong and trusting connections with their clients and care about more than just their physical needs has been proven to encourage First Nations peoples to seek treatment (Davy et al., 2016).

Cultural factors influencing health

holistic concept
A concept that health requires a view of the individual as an integrated system – including physical, cognitive, spiritual and emotional – rather than one or more separate parts.

For First Nations peoples, health has always been a **holistic concept**. It refers to an individual's and a community's physical, social, emotional, spiritual and cultural well-being. The community's health depends on the health of the individual as well as the other way round. Health is founded in relationship to Country, culture, family and community for many First Nations peoples (LoGiudice, 2016).

From this holistic view, we can better understand the reason older First Nations peoples do not always put their own needs above the needs of the community. Kinship, family commitments and responsibilities are often prioritised over personal health needs. These circumstances commonly lead to individuals discharging themselves against medical advice, resulting in adverse health consequences.

First Nations peoples may view health differently and have a world view that is largely different from the biomedical model of health that forms the basis of Australia's health-care system. Understanding of this difference is fundamental to providing culturally safe healthcare for First Nations peoples (Taylor & Guerin, 2010). What may at first be perceived as barriers or obstacles to interacting with a health-care professional, is often due to cultural and historical issues, as we learn from Robyn's experience.

Box 3.2

Robyn's experience

Robyn's cultural connection is to the Kamilaroi Nation on her mother's side. She has been on the Cancer Council committee for five years and a board member of Dubbo Health Service and Lourdes Hospital. She shares with you what she has heard from older First Nations peoples.

I have spoken to a number of Elders about their ageing process. Some said it is a part of the life cycle. Some don't like it as they say it comes with many aches and pains and more visits to the 'white' doctor. When they visit the doctor, they don't listen to them as they are always at the computer. Most of the Elders I spoke with said they would like to go back to Country but can't as they have no money. They also commented that they would be buried in the town where they have lived for many years.

They don't like going to hospital as they say that their culture and age is not respected, and they would rather have Aboriginal nurses looking after them. For me, my own experience in the local hospital was not a pleasant one and I was left in a ward without a drink of water for over 24 hours. My friend made a complaint about my treatment and I received an apology. One thing, as a health professional, you must remember is that the current generation of older Aboriginal people may have never learnt to read as they were raised on Aboriginal missions and reserves.

- Older First Nations peoples want to return to Country. What were the implications of the lockdowns caused by the COVID-19 pandemic on this strong desire to return to Country?

- What can we learn about communicating with First Nations older people from what Robyn has been told?

- How do these experiences promote or detract from First Nations peoples' willingness to engage with the health system?

FOCUS QUESTIONS

First Nations age distribution

In the following section, we outline demographics related to the profile of the First Nations older people. Although the First Nations population is relatively young, the older population is expected to grow rapidly due to population growth in general as well as a shift in the age composition of the population, including that due to increasing life expectancy. The ageing population expansion in Australia may be unevenly distributed, with significant implications for health demand in regional and remote locations as well as high-growth urban areas (Temple et al., 2020).

When compared to non-Indigenous Australians, First Nations Australians are the most socially and economically disadvantaged and have the worst health (AIHW, 2021). Early onset of chronic disease and an anticipated earlier need for care, including in-home care and the prospect of residential care, as well as a reduced life expectancy, are essential to consider.

There are two major and noticeable disparities in the age structure of First Nations and non–First Nations Australians, as seen in Figure 3.1. The First Nations Australian population has a relatively young age structure compared to non–First Nations Australians. In 2020, a projected 33 per cent of First Nations Australians were aged under 15 (compared with 18 per cent of non–First Nations Australians), and only 5.2 per cent of First Nations Australians were aged 65 and over (compared with 16 per cent of non–First Nations Australians) (ABS, 2018, 2019). First Nations peoples in various locations within Australia have varying life situations, as well as linguistic and cultural requirements. When compared to the non-Indigenous population of 75 years and older, First Nations peoples over 50 are deemed 'aged'. In the near future, improvements in First Nations peoples' life expectancy is expected to result in a boom of First Nations seniors.

FIGURE 3.1 Australian population distribution projection by Indigenous status and age group, 2020

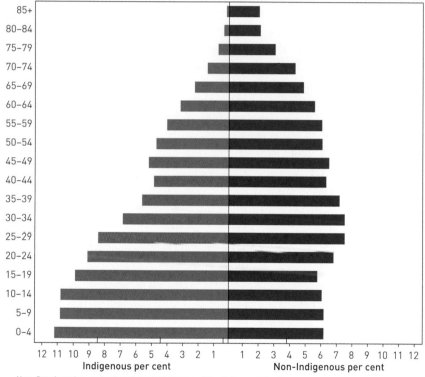

Note: Data based on projections from 2016 Census of Population and Housing.
Sources: ABS 2019a, ABS 2018a. http://www.aihw.gov.au/

Compared with non–First Nations Australians, First Nations Australians are:

- 2.9 times as likely to have long-term ear or hearing problems among children
- 2.7 times as likely to smoke
- 2.7 times as likely to experience high or very high psychological distress
- 2.1 times as likely to die before their fifth birthday
- 1.9 times as likely to be born with low birth weight
- 1.7 times as likely to have a disability or a restrictive long-term health condition (AIHW, 2021).

FIRST NATIONS PEOPLES AND SERVICE ENGAGEMENT

First Nations Australians are twice as likely as non–First Nations Australians to be in residential care when they are 65–75 years old (AIHW, 2021). In 2018, there were 1700 First Nations people living in permanent aged care institutions (AIHW, 2021) and approximately 49 per cent of First Nations peoples over the age of 75 resided in assisted living facilities.

According to the findings of the Royal Commission into Aged Care Quality and Safety in Australia, First Nations Australians are also more likely to utilise community-based supported services, with three times the likelihood of using home support and seven times the likelihood of using home care (AIHW, 2021). This clearly illustrates that community-based services are being significantly relied upon to care for Australia's elderly First Nations population. Community members have pushed for, organised and established specific aged care services for Elders and older persons in various places. Non-governmental organisations (NGOs) may be formed specifically for this purpose, or they may be sponsored by existing First Nations or community organisations (Commonwealth of Australia, 2021).

> There is more information about the Royal Commission into Aged Care Quality and Safety in Australia in Chapter 2.

Initiatives and services such as the Multi-Purpose Service (MPS) and the National Aboriginal and Torres Strait Islander Flexible Aged Care Program (NATSIFACP), as well as other home and community care (HACC) programs, provide care to Elders across Australia. Packages of care for older people are supplied to people's homes. Centre-based respite care, residential hostels (with some personal care), and nursing homes that specialise in supporting First Nations peoples are also available. These services are offered as culturally safe services with culturally safe practices, and they are in high demand. As a result, especially as the Indigenous community's life expectancy improves and there is a growing older population, there is a rising struggle to care for Elders and the aged (Commonwealth of Australia, 2021).

Box 3.3

Jordan's experience

Jordan is a First Nations aged care support worker who provides high-quality supports to both Aboriginal and non-Aboriginal elders. He states:

The Elders look forward to my visits as they do not often receive visitors for days, sometimes weeks. They are friendly and often provide refreshments such as a cup of tea or lunch. I feel this is a way for them to show hospitality, a result of their upbringings and where they come from – a different generation where people looked out for each other. The Aboriginal Elders like to share their knowledge once they know I am Aboriginal. They like to yarn about who they know in your family and cultural linkages.

- What could be the factors inhibiting First Nations peoples visiting relatives and friends in a health care or aged care facility?
- Consider how institutions could be more welcoming of First Nations peoples to visit.
- What can we learn from Jordan's experience about how to build rapport with First Nations peoples?

FOCUS QUESTIONS

Even though various government publications and sources mention that the First Nations population is ageing, a full investigation of the underlying determinants of health such as housing, income and employment, and implications of these on ageing in the First Nations population, remains lacking (Temple et al., 2020). For a variety of reasons (e.g. increased demand for primary and allied health services, formal aged care and **informal care** provision), these underlying determinants and implications of ageing in the First Nations population must be recognised and understood (Temple et al., 2020).

informal care
Unpaid care provided by family, friends, neighbours and other community supports without support from a government agency or service provider.

Influences and challenges on service provision for First Nations peoples

The Australian Institute of Health and Welfare (AIHW, 2021) estimates that 49 per cent of First Nations peoples aged over 75 years of age live in residential aged care and many are reliant on community services. With increasing numbers of First Nations peoples requiring culturally safe assessment, support and care, it is the responsibility of those of us working in or learning about ageing to ensure the services provided and the approach we take to working with First Nations peoples is delivered in a way that is appropriate to their way of living and respecting culture. The following sections of the chapter provide guidance about how to deliver culturally safe services and care.

From the standpoint of service provision, the following factors can influence the quality and degree of healthcare:

- gaps in the health-care system's performance (including access) in meeting health-care needs
- a lack of cultural competence (which research demonstrates is linked to risks and poor-quality health outcomes)
- a breakdown in communication (which research demonstrates may lead to adverse events and poor quality of care).

The following are some of the challenges that First Nations families may face:

- living in rural and remote locations, which have the worst socioeconomic disadvantage and the highest disease burden due to a lack of access to prevention and health management services
- residing in major cities/urban communities in the most disadvantaged areas
- poor socioeconomic level, as well as socio-political and environmental issues
- an increased risk of developing health problems
- distrust and fear of mainstream health services, which can be intimidating and alienating, especially if no consideration is made to include cultural elements in the health-care environment
- a perception of a power imbalance due to historical factors and disadvantage
- vulnerability, isolation, shame and powerlessness – feelings that many people have
- misunderstandings, stereotypes and contempt based on culture (racism)
- insufficient time for service providers to provide effective healthcare
- financial stressors

- issues with accommodation and transportation
- protocols and practices that are culturally and gender specific.

Box 3.4

Jan's experience

Jan is a First Nations woman who worked in aged care as a registered nurse and as an administrator.

I worked in an aged care facility, feeling very passionate about whether those in our care were or were not being cared for in an appropriate manner. My employment spanned over a 21-year period, where I worked in a management/admin role in a small facility. It had been pretty much a hands-on approach at this facility in earlier years and most staff were multi-skilled, in so much that most of the staff helped each other with the many tasks that were to be undertaken. In this regard, we got to know most of the residents on a personal level and regarded that many of them were more like family. Many did not have family in town, so we (the staff) became their family.

As a passionate advocate for people in aged care, I think that person-centred care should be at the forefront. Having cared for both my parents in their later years, I like to think I have an appreciation for the life of an older person as a whole unit. Many older people are cared for in their homes, in the community, where they have much more autonomy, choice and the right to contribute to decisions about their lives.

- What are the key points that Jan makes about residential aged care that resonate with you as a health professional?
- Can you imagine working at the facility Jan describes? What might be the best and worst thing about working there?
- How would you feel about having fewer choices, less autonomy and minimal rights to contribute to the decisions about your own life?

FOCUS QUESTIONS

Focusing on the person

The following section of the chapter will develop your understanding of what being focused on the person means for First Nations peoples and the means of enacting this in a culturally safe way. Using a person-centred approach (i.e. looking at the whole person) will allow First Nations people to be directly involved and empowered in their care while also considering their cultural and individual needs, preferences, beliefs and values, as well as their comfort and surroundings. Person-centred care can be defined as care that is 'respectful of and responsive to individual client preferences, needs and values and ensuring that client values guide all clinical decisions' (Institute of Medicine (US), 2001, p. 6). Adopting this practice will improve the person's experience and health outcomes while also benefiting clinical and organisational health services (Queensland Health, 2014). Person-centred care begins with building rapport with the person and using effective communication strategies to work together on their chosen health outcomes.

We discuss some of these communication strategies here.

> ## Implications for practice
>
> As a health-care professional, it is crucial to pay attention to the first few minutes of your contact with patients and their families. Individual barriers, such as anxieties or preconceptions that the patient and their family may have, may be overcome through efforts to develop the appropriate rapport (Queensland Health, 2015).
>
> Strategies to build rapport with First Nations older people can include:
> - making them feel welcome by greeting them with warmth and friendliness
> - using non-threatening body language and tone of voice
> - asking them where they come from. Linking people is important in establishing rapport (you may know of a place that you have in common)
> - sharing some background information with them about yourself
> - giving a simple explanation of the processes or procedures
> - showing empathy and asking how they are feeling
> - providing clarity or information if they raise concerns.

LANGUAGE

Many First Nations people speak English as a second or third language rather than their first. Furthermore, just because an older person and their support worker communicate in English does not mean that the individual understands the language in its entirety. Due to the need to communicate in a language other than English, accessing and using the aged care system may be problematic for First Nations Australians (Queensland Health, 2015).

First Nations peoples often use stories or discussion about a topic to demonstrate a point in conversational/narrative approaches. For some people, direct contact can be intimidating, and it may discourage them from participating in any further conversations.

'SHAME'

'shame'
An uncomfortable feeling of humiliation or distress caused by being aware of wrong or reckless behaviour.

men's and women's business
The separate responsibilities of men and women to families, communities, culture and Country that traditional Australian Indigenous cultures had numerous laws governing and which are sacred and remain secret.

Older First Nations Australians may experience **'shame'** while discussing personal or private concerns; they may not grasp the medical issue being discussed and the 'shame' prevents them from articulating their confusion; they may believe there has been a breach of confidence. This is especially important in smaller communities. Avoid discussions in open or public settings and take a discreet approach. Maintain confidence and take into account both **men's and women's business**.

THE MEANING OF EXTENDED PERIODS OF SILENCE

Many First Nations people employ silence, and it is common in conversations. Each person, location and community may have different interpretations of silence. Silence may show respect; silence may be needed to contemplate what has been said; silence may allow for translation of information into their own language; and silence may indicate discomfort in an unfamiliar environment.

During medical assessment, First Nations peoples may:

- smile and nod to signal that they are paying attention
- show respect for the authority and status of the staff members by acting like a good patient (power imbalance and historical authority figures)
- agree or say yes or be nodding throughout the consultation to indicate that they want the discussion to end or that they comprehend what has been discussed
- be hesitant to publicly argue with authoritative figures.

This does not always imply that the information presented has been received; therefore, it is important to utilise your interviewing techniques in order to establish a successful nurse–patient relationship. This could include asking the patient to repeat the information you just delivered to ensure that what you're expressing is comprehended. Listen actively and utilise verbal and non-verbal cues to encourage your patient to elaborate on the information being provided. Using empathy, validation and reassurance in your clinical assessment demonstrates that you understand and care about what your patient may be experiencing.

INABILITY TO MAKE EYE CONTACT

In Western culture, avoiding someone's eyes is often seen as dishonest, disrespectful or uninterested, but this is not the case among First Nations peoples. Eye contact avoidance among First Nations peoples is linked to a variety of characteristics, including gender, 'shame', disrespect, aggressiveness, mistrust and previous traumatic experiences. Follow their lead and adjust your level of eye contact as needed.

Implications for practice

Ways to build rapport with First Nations older people include:

- introducing yourself in a polite and warm manner
- giving yourself time to develop a rapport
- allowing time for silence while listening and being present
- using non-threatening body language and voice tone
- maintaining a non-judgmental mindset and approach
- speaking in plain English and being thorough in your explanations
- staying away from jargon and technical terms
- inquiring about people's backgrounds, sharing personal stories or looking for other topics of mutual interest
- asking non-direct probing questions that are open-ended
- making forms or written information as simple as possible
- using visual aids to help with understanding explanations
- always double-checking that they understand what you're saying
- summarising and repeating what your patient has stated in order to aid in clarity and demonstrate that you've been paying attention

---

- stressing the importance of confidentiality, while also being clear about its limitations
- seeking assistance from local First Nations staff if necessary.

Assistance with communication and cultural support may be provided by other First Nations staff (e.g. a First Nations health worker), and staff from your local First Nations community may be able to assist you with cultural knowledge and information interpretation.

TIME

Time is valued highly in Western culture in order to achieve deadlines and schedules. However, in First Nations cultures, time is perceived differently, with a higher priority put on family responsibilities and community relationships.

When interacting with older First Nations people, assigning flexible consultation times is a good idea (this is seen widely in the ACCHS space, and we must ask ourselves why this can't be replicated in the Western health-care systems). Also, take your time explaining everything to the person and don't rush them – this is so important to ensure they understand what is required.

NON-VERBAL COMMUNICATION

First Nations people are skilled at reading body language and non-verbal communication. Always be aware of your non-verbal communication through the use of hand signals, facial expressions and body language.

Your body language, for example, may express annoyance, which will be recognised. Personal space is also important: be aware of the gap between you and the person you're standing near. Standing too near to someone you don't know or who is of the opposite gender can make someone feel frightened. Always ask for permission before touching someone and explain why you need to.

TITLES

The terms 'Aunty' or 'Uncle' are used in First Nations cultures to convey respect for someone older than you. This individual does not have to be blood related or an Elder. Only address someone with these titles if they have granted you permission and/or if you have a good relationship with them.

DECISION MAKING

Decisions are frequently made with input from other family members due to family kinship patterns and relationships. Find out if the person's decision necessitates family consultation. Allow enough time for the information to sink in. If you're asked to leave a room or a meeting so that the family may discuss anything alone, do so politely.

Good health care outcomes for Aboriginal and Torres Strait Islander peoples require health professionals to be both clinically and culturally capable. (Australian Government, 2013, p. 4)

Strengths-based approach

It's critical to distinguish between practices that arose because of the trauma of colonisation and those that were founded on traditional cultural beliefs. Governance by fear and threat, or for personal gain, is not a cultural norm, and in most cases, governance was a collaborative effort aimed at achieving a balanced, harmonious and respected community life. Individuals and communities must be empowered to speak up about concerns or participate in discussions without fear of retaliation and for true consensus to be reached (Behrendt et al., 2017).

One of the vestiges of the colonial legacy is **powerlessness**. To redress this, pathways to promote and develop self-determination are required. Being able to make decisions and be responsible for oneself, family and community; having choice; and being able to participate effectively in society is important for development and well-being. It is crucial for children to perceive their parents and Elders in positions of responsibility and respect in society, as decision makers and leaders. Parents and Elders must, in turn, have a sense of self-efficacy, control and self-determination (Behrendt et al., 2017).

powerlessness
A lack of influence, ability or power.

The following are some ideas for implementing a strengths-based approach to providing culturally safe care:

- Focus on the pre-Invasion health status of First Nations peoples – 60 000 years versus 236 years. The state of health today in Australia is not the natural state for First Nations peoples.

- Instead of focusing on 'what's wrong', focus on the strengths and resilience of First Nations peoples; present historical and contemporary instances of strengths and healing.

- Identify and investigate the wide range of resources and capabilities present in First Nations Australian communities.

- Understand the relationship between First Nations peoples' self-determination and improved health and socioeconomic outcomes.

- Educate health-professional students on the notion of a strengths-based approach, as well as on how to use critical reflection to assess their own reactions to employing a strengths-based approach in practice.

- Find evidence of effective strengths-based approaches for enhanced health and social outcomes.

- In the context of First Nations Australians' healthcare, learn how to focus on strengths.

The strategies that systems could employ to support health-care providers include ensuring that providers have the time to connect with patients, their families and the community; providing cultural safety training and ongoing professional development to ensure that health-care professionals not only understand but take responsibility for their own cultural impositions to ensure they can provide culturally appropriate care to the community they serve; designing employment contracts that facilitate the flexibility necessary for providers to deliver the type of care that communities need; and creating employment contracts that allow caregivers the flexibility they need to provide the type of care that communities require. Health-care services could be better supported if the resources needed to engage with communities were available (Davy et al., 2016). Employing and providing educational and career opportunities for First Nations staff would assist with ensuring that patients feel welcomed and comfortable in engaging with services.

AN EXAMPLE OF COMMUNITY ENGAGEMENT AND EMPOWERMENT: DUBBO COMMUNITY FORUM

The following is an example of First Nations older people being actively involved in the future of aged care service provision directly to the Royal Commission. The outcomes were of benefit to the entire community.

In May 2019, an aged care community forum was held in Dubbo, hosted by the Three Rivers University Department of Rural Health (UDRH), School of Nursing, Midwifery, and Indigenous Health, Charles Sturt University, and sponsored by the Dubbo Regional Council. Representatives from a variety of community groups and organisations, as well as individuals with an interest in ageing and the older community, attended the forum and participated enthusiastically. The Dubbo community's submission to the Aged Care Royal Commission details how the community forum was organised, as well as the conversation, information and experiences that were gained from this forum. The community forum attracted about 51 attendees from the local community. Three Rivers UDRH assessed the event to gauge community participation, and replies revealed that residents thought they had 'ample chance to offer their views on aged care' and that 'the forum was an effective means to contribute local experiences to the Royal Commission'.

Access to aged care services in regional, rural and remote regions was a particular source of concern for us. In these locations, older people make up a larger proportion of the population than in major cities. Furthermore, those living in regional, rural and remote areas have many disadvantages, which can exacerbate the need for assistance as they get older. The forum highlighted the unique challenges, problems and consequences due to location, accessibility and affordability for the community living in a rural setting. The information provided by the Dubbo community indicates some of the positive features of ageing in a rural town, such as community spirit, support, connectivity and a willingness to participate in various kinds of technology – such as telehealth, Zoom meetings and other technologies – to overcome some of these challenges. Several obstacles, poor experiences and difficulties of inequitable access to care were also mentioned. The forum attracted First Nations participants who willingly shared their unique experiences with ageing and/or provided care to someone who is ageing. According to the data, the availability of aged care in rural and remote locations is much lower than in large cities and has been declining in recent years (Commonwealth of Australia, 2021).

This community forum resulted in the commissioners visiting Dubbo and organising a hearing in Mudgee to hear the voices of First Nations peoples. The forum informed the relevant recommendations in the Royal Commission's final report.

You can find further discussion about the challenges of ageing in rural Australia in Chapter 6.

Box 3.5

Jan's story

Jan, a proud First Nations woman who was one of the participants of the Dubbo community aged care forum, shares her experience.

As a participant of the Dubbo community aged care forum in 2019, it was encouraging to be given the opportunity to have an opinion about the care of our loved ones in aged care. At the forum, we were given stimulus questions, with most of the group I was in being registered nurses. The focus of their answers seemed to be about the nursing aspect of care, concentrating around the funding instrument of the time. My opinion didn't always correlate with theirs as I was trying to focus on the person being cared for as a whole.

The Dubbo community aged care forum was a positive step for the Dubbo and surrounding community. Personally, it gave me the peace of mind that the people we have working in the industry mostly have the best interest of their residents at heart in a medical sense; however, the staffing levels do not allow for the 'whole' person to be cared for in a meaningful way.

- Although the organisers of the forum were providing an opportunity for community members to share their stories, what lessons can be learnt about hearing the voices of First Nations peoples?

FOCUS QUESTION

 Elders and other senior community members should be engaged as key stakeholders to champion culturally appropriate choices and approaches to health and wellbeing. *Participant, Brisbane Community Consultation* (Australian Government, 2013, p. 38)

Residential aged care

Residential aged care in Australia is designed to offer high-quality care effectively and efficiently to all older or vulnerable people who are evaluated as needing assistance despite major regulatory requirements, staffing issues and rising client demands (Commonwealth of Australia, 2021). Traditionally, First Nations peoples have been cared for in their own communities; nevertheless, an increasing number of people in residential aged care facilities are now from these communities. Future planning is essential to support capacity and improve quality of life. Quality care entails more than just meeting a person's physical and psychological requirements. It must also provide culturally appropriate care that is compatible with a person's belief systems, history, culture and experiences.

While government agencies and communities alike are emphasising this, the unique skill set of the workforce and the resources required to facilitate this shift are grossly undervalued. This shift exacerbates gaps in the sector's ability to provide the finest and most practical support for this population. Funding initiatives to assist the needs of First Nations peoples in residential aged care facilities across Australia are urgently needed. To understand the demands of this population in such a specialised context, research activities must be sufficiently financed, and research into the development of cross-cultural relationships must be supported to better understand care strategies (Commonwealth of Australia, 2021).

In 2020, Larke and colleagues conducted a study to assess older First Nations Australians' preferences for health and aged care. First Nations peoples want to be looked after in their community, live near their families and die on their Country. First Nations peoples require aged care services at a younger age than non–First Nations Australians, and with more complicated requirements, such as dementia rates that are three to five times higher than the general population. In contrast to this, however, First Nations Australians make up fewer than 1 per cent of the available places in residential aged care institutions (Larke et al., 2021). The low rate contrasts with a significant need, raising questions about older First Nations Australians' access to aged care services.

People's primary preference for ACCHS provision arises when they engage with ACCHSs that supply services adapted to the needs of the ageing population (Larke et al., 2020). This is demonstrated by the huge growth in the use of First Nations aged care and disability support services, with 64 per cent of respondents claiming to use ACCO-provided services solely.

When considering the reported steady increase in the median age of the First Nations Australian population, as well as the number and proportion of older people, and also the younger age at which First Nations peoples may require aged care services, the apparent high demand for First Nations aged care and disability services is important. Larke and colleagues' (2021) findings support recommendations for the expansion of First Nations-specific aged care facilities.

ASSESSMENT OF AN OLDER FIRST NATIONS PERSON

With the likelihood of an increase of First Nations peoples into health-care services and aged care facilities, the need for accurate and appropriate assessment increases. With the emphasis on cultural safety, assessment of the older First Nations person becomes a soft skill to practise. In a health-care context, there are ways to improve the assessment of older people:

- Make time to speak with the older person and pay attention to them. Clinicians are frequently interrupted, making it difficult for them to interact in a safe manner. Side stories are sometimes seen as a waste of time, but they can actually aid your assessment by highlighting the older person's beliefs and desires for care.

- Being courteous and attentive, anticipating client needs and taking time to listen are all ways to demonstrate empathy. Instead of staring at a computer screen or notes, make eye contact with someone (if culturally appropriate).

- Use straightforward language that is neither colloquial nor patronising. Avoid endearing terms such as 'dear' or oversimplifying language, as this might make the older person feel disrespected and give the sense that the clinician assumes they are cognitively impaired.

- Remember that First Nations peoples are more likely to have hearing and visual impairments due to chronic diseases. Identify hearing and vision problems and, if possible, employ hearing and vision aids. Instead of conversing with the individual from the end of the bed, get closer to them. If they wear glasses, check that they are on and that they are clean. Make sure you have enough light and a quiet environment.

- Obtain information about the person's history from a variety of sources. It may be culturally appropriate to discuss the care with other family members and not just the client. You may also gain information from other long-term carers, GPs, medical experts, and friends and neighbours. Some will provide health information, while others may go into greater detail around their social and emotional well-being.

The following have been identified as guidelines for care for First Nations Australians within residential aged care facilities (Sivertsen et al., 2019; Brooke, 2011).

Care and communication

- Encourage community members to participate in care planning and activities.
- Understand that generalised care plans do not allow for an individualised or culturally appropriate approach.
- Informed consent must be documented and obtained in a culturally acceptable manner.
- Respect body language and eye contact (or lack thereof).
- Recognise the possibility of sensory impairment, with 30 per cent of First Nations peoples having vision problems and 12 per cent having hearing problems.
- Recognise and incorporate culturally appropriate foods, as well as preparation activities that are relevant to the residents' beliefs and traditions, into facility menus.

Activities

- Establish links with the residents' community in order to engage in culturally appropriate activities as part of the facility's regular programming.
- Encourage discussions with local Elders and residents to have a deeper understanding of their lifestyles and culture.
- Recognise and participate in First Nations Australian celebratory national dates such as 'Sorry' Day, Reconciliation Week, NAIDOC Week and so on.

Environment

- If feasible, provide access to good and private outside locations.
- As a symbol of respect, display the First Nations flag and artworks – this creates a more culturally appropriate and welcoming environment.
- To support spiritual ideas about the dying trajectory, First Nations peoples prefer a bed that allows a view of the outdoors to maintain cultural and spiritual beliefs (Brooke, 2011).

The current provision of culturally safe services is insufficient, according to the 2019 interim report of the Royal Commission into Aged Care Services (Commonwealth of Australia, 2019). These facilities are also often placed far from where people have lived for most of their lives, as well as their family and other community members. When people are cut off from their familial and cultural supports, this can cause additional stress and have an impact on their social and emotional well-being. Those that do exist are mostly created by First Nations communities in reaction to a shortage of mainstream services.

First Nations Elders, most importantly, want the following essential principles of care:
- easy access to information about their options so that they may make well-informed decisions

- active participation in all parts of their care planning and to feel empowered to do so
- access to culturally safe aged care services, regardless of location
- an aged care system that understands the impact of harmful colonisation policies and the trauma caused by the forced separation of children from their families
- aged care services that are not affiliated with organisations that supported the forced separation of children from their families, which could retraumatise survivors of colonisation practices
- an aged care system that makes it easy for them to use a trusted First Nations organisation/person to assist each of them – and represent them if they so decide – to navigate/work their way through MyAgedCare
- an aged care system where the providers and their employees recognise the significance of their role as informal caregivers in their communities, and ensure they are given assistance in attending cultural events and activities (Australian Government, 2019).

End-of-life care

Health-care professionals must have the expertise to fulfil the requirements of First Nations Elders, and aged care facilities must be culturally sensitive. This includes palliative care services to guarantee that First Nations individuals receive culturally appropriate end-of-life care. Families who are responsible for caring for older First Nations peoples with health issues or disability need support as well. Some people will choose to return home despite the difficulty and lack of treatment and care options. This is judged to be a higher priority than receiving treatment in a city or regional centre (Palliative Care Australia, 2009). This may be difficult to comprehend and confrontational for you as a health-care professional trying to provide care and treatment during this time (Best & Fredericks, 2021). It's important not to assume that everyone thinks the same way about palliative care and treatment, and to recognise that every First Nations person will handle this period of time differently. During this period, respect is essential in all interactions.

> You can find more information related to culturally safe palliative care in Chapter 19.

Conclusion

In this chapter we encouraged you to understand the holistic perspectives of First Nations peoples, which include the health of the community and the environment. Both the statistics and the lived experiences shared provide unique details of healthy ageing and aged care for First Nations peoples. Critically reflecting on this information over the course of your professional career will allow you to provide culturally safe care to older First Nations peoples. In your role as a nurse or other health-care professional in First Nations aged care, you must have strategies for assessment and communication to create culturally safe experiences. We hope you will benefit from the techniques to build culturally safe communication such as building a rapport, non-verbal communication and respecting silence.

Learn more
Access additional resources – such as weblinks, further readings and podcasts – to broaden your understanding of this chapter. See the Guided Tour for access details.

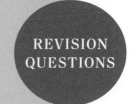

1   Identify aged care services in your area that are exclusively for First Nations peoples. Do these services cater to persons with diverse cultural, gendered and sexual identities?

2   What is the focus of the services and how do you refer clients/patients to them?

3   What factors should you consider while interacting with First Nations men and women, based on what you've learnt in this chapter?

4   Some First Nations men and women prefer to use services that are offered to all older people over First Nations-specific services. What may their motivations be for this choice?

REVISION QUESTIONS

REFERENCES

Australian Bureau of Statistics (ABS) (2018). Estimates of Aboriginal and Torres Strait Islander Australians. www. abs.gov.au/statistics/people/ aboriginal-and-torres-strait-islander-peoples/estimates-aboriginal-and-torres-strait-islander-australians/latest-release

Australian Bureau of Statistics (ABS) (2019). National Aboriginal and Torres Strait Islander Health Survey, 2018–19. www.abs.gov.au/ ausstats/abs@.nsf/mf/4715.0

Australian Government (2013). National Aboriginal and Torres Strait Islander Health Plan 2013–2023. Commonwealth of Australia. https://www. health.gov.au/sites/default/ files/documents/2021/02/ national-aboriginal-and-torres-strait-islander-health-plan-2013-2023.pdf

Australian Government (2019). Actions to Support Older Aboriginal and Torres Strait Islander People: A Guide for Consumers. Commonwealth of health. www.health. gov.au/sites/default/files/ actions-to-support-older-aboriginal-and-torres-strait-islander-people-a-guide-for-consumers_0.docx

Australian Health Practitioner Regulation Agency (AHPRA) (2020). Annual Report 2019/20. www.ahpra.gov.au/ Publications/Annual-reports/ Annual-Report-2020.aspx

Australian Institute of Health and Welfare (AIHW) (2018). Older Australia at a Glance. Summary. www.aihw.gov.au/ reports/older-people/older-australia-at-a-glance/contents/ summary

Australian Institute of Health and Welfare (AIHW) (2021). Profile of Indigenous Australians. www.aihw.gov. au/reports/australias-welfare/ profile-of-indigenous-australians

Behrendt, L., Jorgensen, M. & Vivian, A. (2017). Self-Determination: Background Concepts. Scoping paper 1 prepared for the Victorian Department of Health and Human Services. www2.health.vic.gov. au/about/publications/ researchandreports/self-determination-background-concepts

Best, O. & Fredericks, B. (eds) (2021). *Yatdjuligin: Aboriginal and Torres Strait Islander Nursing & Midwifery Care.* Cambridge University Press.

Brooke, N. J. (2011). Needs of Aboriginal and Torres Strait Islander clients residing in Australian residential aged-care facilities. *Australian Journal of Rural Health, 19*(4), 166–70. https://doi. org/10.1111/j.1440-1584.2011.01207.x

Commonwealth of Australia (2019). Royal Commission into Aged Care Quality and Safety. Interim report: Neglect. Vol. 1. https://agedcare. royalcommission.gov.au/ sites/default/files/2020-02/ interim-report-volume-1.pdf

Commonwealth of Australia (2021). Royal Commission into Aged Care Quality and Safety. Final report: Care, dignity and respect. Vol. 1, Summary and recommendations. https:// agedcare.royalcommission. gov.au/sites/default/ files/2021-03/final-report-volume-1_0.pdf

Davy, C., Cass, A., Brady, J., DeVries, J., Fewquandie, B., Ingram, S., ... & Brown, A. (2016). Facilitating engagement through strong relationships between primary healthcare and Aboriginal and Torres Strait Islander peoples. *Australian and New Zealand Journal of Public Health, 40*(6), 535–41.

Institute of Medicine (US) (2001). Committee on Quality of Health Care in America. Crossing the Quality Chasm. A New Health System for the 21st Century. National Academy Press.

Larke, B. M., Broe, G. A., Daylight, G., Draper, B., Cumming, R. G., Allan, W., ... & Radford, K. (2021). Patterns and preferences for accessing health and aged care services in older Aboriginal and Torres Strait Islander Australians. *Australasian Journal on Ageing, 40*(2), 145–53.

LoGiudice, D. (2016). The health of older Aboriginal and Torres Strait Islander peoples. *Australasian Journal on Ageing*, *35*(2), 82–5.

Maguire, G. & Wenitong, M. (2012). Indigenous Ageing: Walking Backwards into the Future. http://theconversation.com/indigenous-ageing-walking-backwards-into-the-future-7355

Palliative Care Australia (2009). Improving Access to Quality Care at the End of Life for Aboriginal and Torres Strait Islander Australians. Position Statement. https://palliativecare.org.au/wp-content/uploads/2015/08/PCA-Palliative-care-and-Indigenous-Australians-position-statement-updated-16-8-11.pdf

Queensland Health (2014). Aboriginal and Torres Strait Islander Patient Care Guidelines. www.health.qld.gov.au/__data/assets/pdf_file/0022/157333/patient_care_guidelines.pdf

Queensland Health (2015). Aboriginal and Torres Strait Islander Cultural Capability. Communicating Effectively with Aboriginal and Torres Strait Islander People. www.health.qld.gov.au/__data/assets/pdf_file/0021/151923/communicating.pdf

Ramsden, I. M. (2002). Cultural Safety and Nursing Education in Aotearoa and Te Waipounamu. Unpublished PhD thesis, Victoria University of Wellington.

Sivertsen, N., Harrington, A. & Hamiduzzaman, M. (2019). Exploring Aboriginal aged care residents' cultural and spiritual needs in South Australia. *BMC Health Services Research*, *19*(1), 1–13.

Taylor, K. & Guerin, P. (2010). Health Care and Indigenous Australians: Cultural Safety in Practice. Palgrave Macmillan.

Temple, J. B., Wilson, T., Taylor, A., Kelaher, M. & Eades, S. (2020). Ageing of the Aboriginal and Torres Strait Islander population: Numerical, structural, timing and spatial aspects. *Australian and New Zealand Journal of Public Health*, *44*(4), 271–8.

World Health Organization (WHO) (2015). World Report on Ageing and Health. https://apps.who.int/iris/handle/10665/186463

4

The Personal Perspective of Ageing in a Complex World

DENISE WINKLER

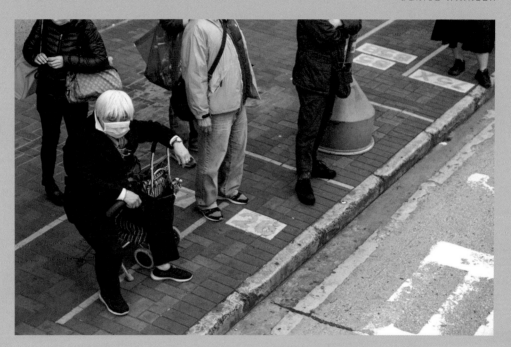

LEARNING OBJECTIVES

After reading this chapter, you will:

» conclude that the perspective an older person has about their ageing experience is ultimately the only one that matters

» value the unique perspective individuals have of their life events

» treat all people with respect and dignity no matter their age or stage of life

» compare development theories that explain people ageing differently and their unique experience

» use theories and research findings, balanced with the older person's unique viewpoint, to frame our daily professional practice.

OXFORD UNIVERSITY PRESS

DENISE WINKLER

Introduction

The world was a complex place before the bushfires, the protests against racism, the pandemic and the global economic consequences of closing down schools and businesses to stop the spread of COVID-19. These world events have caused us to notice our perspective of the world and ourselves. Simultaneously, both perspectives are being influenced by these world events. Each person's perspective on their personal, national and global events is unique and depends on many factors. Some of these are the society, culture and historical era from which the person experiences the events. Each person's self-esteem and mental well-being are important too, as these factors influence the way they perceive world events. Personal perspectives include information from the physical senses, experienced **life events** and the person's reaction and memory of them. Even though we have all experienced a world in which bushfires and pandemics have changed our lives, our personal perspectives are unique.

Throughout this chapter, the unique personal perspective of Darlene will help you to understand some of the theories of ageing and human development. As her life events are told through her story, the hope is for you to conclude that her perspective of her ageing experience is important. As you get to know how Darlene felt and reacted to the COVID-19 lockdowns and bushfires, perhaps your own perspective of global events will be influenced.

life event
A major change in a person's status or circumstances that affects interpersonal relationships, leisure and recreation activities, or work duties.

4.1 Getting to know the person: Darlene's story

During January 2020, Darlene was anticipating her eightieth birthday. Her four children were planning a big party at the local RSL club; the Chinese food there was her favourite meal. Three of her children, her grandchildren and great grandchildren would be travelling interstate and staying at the bed and breakfast on the street of the country village where she now lived.

She was really looking forward to having her family around her to celebrate a happy occasion. The last time they had all been together was for her husband's funeral two years earlier. Her life had been turned upside down after that and she was now living with her youngest son, his wife and their teenage son. After a year of appointments with new doctors, going to watch her grandson's footy and cricket games, adjusting to her daughter-in-law running the household and learning to live without her husband of 60 years, she was finally feeling settled.

Then the bad news began pouring in: bushfires were closing down the highways. Darlene's family was blocked from travelling to her party. She watched the news constantly in hopes that firefighters might get the fires under control. The stories about the property damage, loss of wildlife and heroism kept her glued to the television day and night. In the end, her children decided they would postpone the big party until Mother's Day. She was very disappointed.

Two days after her birthday, her daughter-in-law noticed that Darlene was wheezing when she brought the clothes in from the line. After a barrage of questions, taking her temperature and a call to the GP, Darlene was helped into the car and taken to the small local hospital. A thorough exam and a chest x-ray showed she had smoke-induced asthma and not pneumonia. The doctor gave her a breathing treatment and an inhaler to take home. Everyone told her that the smoke from the fires caused her breathing trouble. On the drive home she did notice the grey smoky skies.

A few facts have been shared in Darlene's story. She has recently turned 80, and is widowed. She lives with her son, his wife and their teenage son. Taking the clothes off the line is a household duty she still performs. Yet, not enough information has been provided for an evidenced-based opinion about whether or not Darlene is ageing successfully. A definition of 'successful ageing' (or 'healthy ageing') is outlined in the following section.

Defining successful ageing

Research over the decades has been searching for an understanding and definition of what constitutes healthy or **successful ageing** (Rowe & Kahn, 1987; Baltes & Baltes, 1990; Strawbridge et al., 2002; Vaillant, 2002; Tate et al., 2003; Lupien & Wan, 2004; Blazer, 2006; Urtamo et al., 2019). The centre of this search has expanded beyond physiological changes to include psychosocial, cultural and spiritual domains of development in older people (Schulz & Heckhausen, 1996; Crowther et al., 2002; Wagnild, 2003; Depp et al., 2007). An understanding of ageing is not limited to the passing of calendar days or only to the physiological changes taking place during those days. Minkler and Fadem (2002, p. 229) define successful ageing as 'low probability of disease and disease-related disability: high cognitive and physical functioning and active engagement with life'.

Some of the successful ageing research involved talking to older adults to gain the lay perception of healthy or successful ageing (Bowling & Dieppe, 2005; Montross et al., 2006). A study significant to the perception of successful ageing reported by Montross et al. (2006) found that 92 per cent of older adults rated themselves as ageing successfully even though they had a chronic illness or a disability. In fact, only 5 per cent of these older people met the criteria for successful ageing, which are absence of disease, freedom from disability and active engagement with life (Montross et al., 2006). Another study, by Reichstadt and colleagues (2010, pp. 569–70), used qualitative interviews to understand the lay perception of successful ageing. One of the participants explains successful ageing with these words:

 [Successful ageing is] accepting what you are at this time. Not dwelling on what you could have been or forgot to do or couldn't do or things you want to do that you are no longer capable of … Just being content. That's not the right word either because contentment I think can lead to stagnation. But to be satisfied with where you are.

The key findings from the Reichstadt et al. (2010) study indicated that older adults emphasise a balance between self-acceptance, self-contentedness, self-growth and engagement with life. To quote the researchers, '[t]his perspective supports the concept of wisdom as a major contributor to successful aging' (Reichstadt et al., 2010, p. 567).

successful ageing
Ageing where the person perceives themselves as healthy, disability (if any exists) is not impeding their enjoyment of life and they are functioning at a level that enables them to be actively engaged in activities they enjoy or find fulfilling.

Learn more
Watch Video 4.1:
George Elliot, the race
car driver, talks about
his ageing experience.

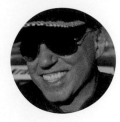

Wisdom as a key factor in successful ageing recognises the older person as the driver of their ageing experience.

The complex world we live in has changed in many, many ways since 2019. There has been abuse perpetuated on older people and the dysfunction of the aged care system has been brought to light in the Royal Commission into Aged Care and Safety, as well as the incidents that have caused us globally to recognise and address the systemic lack of inclusive discourse. Perhaps this complexity prompted the members of the Australian Association of Gerontology (AAG) to begin a discussion of the term 'successful ageing'. In a February 2021 discussion paper (Voigt, 2021), the term 'adaptive ageing' was proposed in a continued attempt to find an inclusive term describing the process of ageing that is respectful and all-encompassing of the diverse experiences of older people. Acknowledging that the construct of ageing is shifting, the criticisms of the term 'successful ageing' are that it is too focused on remaining healthy, active, fit and young; and that it lacks the emphasis or recognition of the needs of older people and the changes of circumstances they experience (Stephens, 2017). If the AAG can explore a term to bridge the gap between the theoretical definition of ageing and the operational definition, then health professionals will better understand their role. Defining ageing will benefit our growing understanding of this complex world. The context of the complex world we live in and the ways and reasons it affects human development are explored next.

Theories of ageing

Gerontology is the study of the physical, mental and social changes of people as they mature from middle adulthood to later life (Institute of Gerontology, n.d.). Professionals from many fields focus on the multiple and various aspects of ageing and development (Martin et al., 2014). Generally considered one large field of study, gerontology is actually many smaller fields (such as nursing, social work and genetics) working together in a united focus on older people. Currently this field is intensely studying the increasing global population as it matures and develops (Skinner et al., 2014). The next section provides three theories of ageing that will help to build your understanding of older people and to inform your communication and care as a health professional.

Learn more
Watch Video 4.1:
In his seventies,
George Elliot is a
living example of the
activity theory.

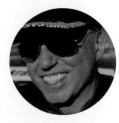

ACTIVITY THEORY

Activity theory dictates that, in order to age well or successfully, the individual must be active (Maddox, 1963). It is often summarised by the saying, 'the more you do, the better you will age'. The basis of activity theory is that people who remain engaged in activities tend to be happier, healthier and more aware of the world around them than those who don't (WHO, 2002). Many articles in the mass media support this theory with lists of things to do to keep people looking and feeling younger. The increasing participation into 'master' level sporting competitions as well as dance and martial arts by people in their middle years is evidence that this theory continues to be popular.

Providing evidence that this theory is employed by facilities and programs aimed at older people is the role of the activity director, an employee whose function is to keep clients engaged in activities to help them be happy, healthy and in touch with the world around them. Sometimes a facility's schedule may consist of only busy work rather than interesting and fulfilling activities. The intensity level of activities must be considered with respect to older people.

Activity and
continuity theories
in relation to older
people are referred
to in Chapter 9.

CONTINUITY THEORY

The basic premise of continuity theory is that older people continue to make choices, behave and socialise in much the same way they did throughout their lives (Atchley, 1989). If a person was happy and healthy as a child, adolescent and young adult, they will probably be a happy and healthy older person. Robert Atchley (1989, p. 185) summarises it this way: 'If you age successfully, it is because you made good choices and habits earlier'. Queen Elizabeth II is a well-known example of a person who has aged well, adapting to each **stage of life** by remaining true to herself.

stage of life
A period of human existence that has unique characteristics: infancy, early childhood, childhood, adolescence, adulthood, middle adulthood and advanced years.

DISASSOCIATION THEORY

Considered the first book to expound a theory of ageing, Cumming and Henry's *Growing Old* was published in 1961. Their theory is the direct opposite of activity and continuity theories. Cumming and Henry described ageing as 'an inevitable, mutual withdrawal or disengagement, resulting in decreased interaction between the ageing person and others in the social system he belongs to' (Cumming & Henry, 1961, p. 14). It is based on the perspective that as people age, they shrink away from social interaction as society forgets about them. Disassociation theory proposed that withdrawing from social interaction would eventually happen to everyone on the planet and, once started, could not be reversed (Silverstein et al., 2008). As more social, scientific and gene research has revealed different information, this theory has been shown to be problematic.

Table 4.1 outlines these three psychosocial theories. In the left-hand column, the theory is identified. The next column briefly describes the theory. The third column outlines some of the issues that result when the theory is firmly held as being true. The right-hand column acknowledges the researchers who proposed the theory.

Psychosocial theory is a tool that can assist health professionals to understand the reasons older people are the way they are. Taking time to explore the life of the older person you are

TABLE 4.1 Comparing psychosocial theories of ageing

THEORY	DESCRIPTION	ISSUES WITH THE THEORY	REFERENCES
Activity theory	People age in a healthier way if they are actively connected to groups and continue to contribute to society.	By advancing this theory, older people can be made to feel guilty if they do not engage in some form of activity. Well-meaning carers and health professionals can push older people into inappropriate groups or programs that are not suited to them.	Maddox (1963) World Health Organization (2002)
Continuity theory	Ageing is a continuity of life, so people age as they have lived. Attitudes, beliefs, values and personality remain the same throughout life and into older age.	This theory does not allow for the changes that occur throughout life and into old age. New opportunities may present themselves so that individuals can pursue an interest they previously did not have the time or capacity for.	Atchley (1989)
Disassociation theory	As people age, they tend to withdraw from society and become more introspective.	Older people might not be assessed for depression, loneliness, delirium and dementia if withdrawal is believed to be the norm.	Cumming & Henry (1961)

Source: Bernoth & Winkler, 2017 (1st edn), p. 77. Written & created by D. Winkler.

working with will provide some clues to their behaviour, personality and decision making. Seeing them as someone who has experienced many things, felt every emotion possible and accomplished significant achievements will show you their value. It is important to remember that before becoming the person you see in front of you, they lived through a multitude of life events: value the many years of life experience, stories and wisdom that they have accumulated.

These theories provide a framework for understanding ageing and each contributes to our knowledge of the ageing experience. However, ageing is about the individual person so it is problematic to rigidly hold to any particular theory. What is significant is appreciating every person as an individual and understanding the importance of skilled, individual assessment of each older person and their circumstances. Older people change as they age so there is a need for health professionals to engage in ongoing assessment as circumstances change.

4.2 Getting to know the person: Darlene's story

In the following months, the news from China about a new virus began to be talked about. Darlene, didn't really pay too much attention to the illness in a land so far away, but did wonder if this new virus was as bad as polio. Memories of her childhood and those sad, frightening months that her mother had been away from the farm with her older brother in the infectious disease ward came back, but she shook them off. Darlene just hoped the RSL wouldn't stop serving her favourite Chinese food.

Then, the day came when a friend who lived in the aged care centre called. The hot gossip was that two of her friends had come back from a cruise and were sick with COVID-19. The same day, her daughter-in-law came home to say that her workplace was making all the employees work from home, on their computers. Then her grandson came home saying that he would be doing his school work from home too – only for a few weeks. Darlene felt that was the day her freedom ended.

The weeks of too many people in the kitchen, imposed silence because her daughter-in-law or grandson were meeting 'online' and constant cleaning turned into months. Easter came and went. The phone calls with her daughters drained her hope of a party on Mother's Day weekend. One evening, she overheard a conversation between her son and his wife in which they discussed the possibility that Darlene may have had the virus rather than asthma. She began to worry that the virus was worse than polio and the world was no longer a safe place to live in.

In June, it finally rained for the first time since the destructive bushfires and Darlene felt momentary relief and joy. The news still focused on the virus and the daily count of new cases. She had given up hope of seeing her children and grandchildren anytime soon. When the Chinese restaurant at the RSL closed, she sank into a deep depression. She spent more time in her room reading and doing wordsearch puzzles. One evening, when she ventured out to make a cuppa, she overheard her son say that he thought it wasn't healthy for her to spend so much time in her room and that she needed to be more active. Her daughter-in-law responded that she thought Darlene had never been very active and liked her books and puzzles better. Darlene wished they would talk *to* her rather than *about* her.

Perceptions and experiences are ways of teaching us about ageing and helping us move into a person-centred focus. We are learning *about* older people and *from* older people while at the same time learning about our practice and ourselves as health professionals. If we can be open to the stories of older people, they can enhance our own lives and our professional practice.

- Is there validity in Darlene's perspective of her current situation? Which of her life experiences support your answer?

- Is Darlene ageing successfully?

- To what extent do activity, continuity and disassociation theories explain Darlene's experience of ageing?

- What are the implications for clinical practice if health professionals hold to the disassociation theory?

FOCUS QUESTIONS

Theories of human development

Throughout an individual's lifespan, age-related changes happen in a series; this is called development. Each individual passes through these stages in a unique way. Human development involves all aspects of a person's being. The aspects, called domains, of human development include the physical, cognitive, linguistic, spiritual, psychological and social. The parameters of these domains have merged, giving way to sub-domains such as psychosocial, social emotional and psycholinguistic.

In this chapter we will focus on two theories of human development in the domain of psychosocial development. Psychosocial development involves the cognitive, emotional and personality changes of people affected by their social relationships and the world around them. The two theories we highlight have been named after the men who developed them through observation, study, research and deep thinking. Erik Erikson's theory of psychosocial development and Urie Bronfenbrenner's ecological systems theory explain some of the reasons people think, behave and react the way they do during the ageing process.

ERIKSON'S THEORY OF PSYCHOSOCIAL DEVELOPMENT

In the early 1960s, Erikson developed a theory that people's personalities continued to develop throughout their lifetimes. Before this theory, the common belief was that children developed personalities during childhood and once people matured into adults their personalities did not change – except in cases of a brain injury or psychosis. From his work with Anna Freud, the daughter of the famous psychologist Sigmund Freud, he was offered a teaching position at Harvard Medical School. Erikson is considered a neo-Freudian psychologist. His theory proposes that humans go through eight stages of identity crisis (see Table 4.2). Indeed, Erikson coined the phrase 'identity crisis' that is commonly used today. His stages were different from Sigmund Freud's because they went beyond early adulthood and factored in the person's social experiences (Charles Scribner's Sons, 2008).

TABLE 4.2 The eight stages of Erikson's theory of personality development

INFANCY: 0–18 MONTHS	EARLY CHILDHOOD: 18 MONTHS–3 YEARS	PLAY AGE: 3–5 YEARS	SCHOOL AGE: 5–13 YEARS	ADOLESCENCE: 13–21 YEARS	YOUNG ADULTHOOD: 21–39 YEARS	MIDDLE ADULTHOOD: 40–65 YEARS	OLD AGE: 65 YEARS AND OLDER
							Ego integrity vs despair
						Generativity vs stagnation	
					Intimacy vs isolation		
				Identity vs confusion			
			Industry vs inferiority				
		Initiative vs guilt					
	Autonomy vs shame						
Trust vs mistrust							
Hope	Will	Purpose	Competence	Fidelity	Love	Care	Wisdom
			LIFE VALUE GOALS				

Source: Bernoth & Winkler, 2017 (1st edn), p. 81 (adapted from Agronin, 2013).

ERIKSON'S SEVENTH AND EIGHTH STAGES

Erikson's theory provides insight into healthy ageing. During middle adulthood (40–65 years) people are busy generating a legacy (Hearn et al., 2012). Families, careers and creating a positive change that benefits other people preoccupy this stage of life. In this seventh stage, the crisis is **generativity** versus **stagnation**, or self-absorption, which means people either create or nurture things that will outlast them, or become selfish (Erikson, 1959). When adults feel they are successful in life, they feel useful and full of accomplishment (Villar, 2012). However, when older adults feel they have failed to influence the world, they feel depressed and useless. The transition from stage seven may, but does not necessarily, dictate the outcome of **despair** in stage eight. The reason each stage has two options is that as humans develop, they can make choices by relating to other people in an ever-changing world. It is the element of **free will**, an individual's ability to choose freely, that provides options.

The eighth stage – ego **integrity** versus despair – is the one that most people over the age of 65 experience (Erikson, 1959). Older people are in the process of examining their lives in the context of their relationships and current society (Hearn et al., 2012). When older people look back at their lives and feel a sense of fulfilment, their outcome is wisdom and knowing deep within themselves that they are valuable individuals. However, when older people look back at their lives and feel a sense of regret or longing for another chance, their outcome is bitterness and despair.

generativity
Focusing on perpetuating and moulding the next generation.

stagnation
Lack of progression.

despair
To be without hope.

free will
The ability to act as you choose without being confined by fate.

integrity
Being true to yourself, honest and undivided.

4.3 Getting to know the person: Darlene's story

The long days of isolation, when everyone at her house spent the day in separate rooms on computers, gave Darlene time to examine her life in the context of her relationships and current society. Every part of their lives was based around the computer: work, communicating with family – even visits with their GP! And if she wanted to talk to and see her other children and grandchildren it was only possible via a phone or computer. She felt dumb because she could barely use the devices. And then, if everyone was trying to do something at once, there was yelling when the internet went down. Her son kept harping on the lack of connectivity. Darlene tried to ease the tension in the house by doing the only things she knew how to do: laundry and baking.

During quiet times, Darlene reflected on the past and wished she had taken an interest in computers when they first came out. She remembered there were workshops offered by the local farming system to teach farmers how to use technology. Her husband had gone to most of them and he was pretty good with the computer before his dementia set in. Darlene, however, had been too busy keeping everyday life rolling along: raising teenagers and paying for boarding school, then uni, then weddings and finally the payoff when the grandbabies arrived. Compared to the long, empty days she had now, the past seemed to have flown by in a flash. Sometimes she would think about the years during which

DENISE WINKLER

she had taken care of her husband while his personality slowly faded away with dementia. She didn't like to dwell on all the sadness or the guilt around being relieved he was gone. Admittedly, she still loved him and missed their life, even if he hadn't been himself. She wondered if he would have come down with the virus and died alone in an aged care facility. Most days, Darlene was relieved that she didn't have to worry about that, at least. She didn't have to worry about being alone either.

One good thing about the periods of isolation imposed by the government was the dinners that brought the family together once a day. Seeing how exhausted everyone was after being in front of a computer all day, Darlene dusted off her cook books and made dinner for everyone. She liked the challenge of using ingredients from the pantry and the herb garden. Her son, daughter-in-law and grandson really appreciated her cooking. They took turns doing the washing up and stayed to chat or play cards. Darlene felt lucky that she was living with her family during this awful time in history.

FOCUS QUESTIONS

Use Erikson's last two stages of psychosocial development to understand Darlene's perspective.

- How did Darlene transition from stage seven, where she was obviously in stagnation, into stage eight?

- What could she choose to do in the next stage of her life that would lead her into ego integrity?

- Considering the last stage of Erikson's theory, what can be learnt about interacting with older people? Do you think there are implications for interacting with a person who has a cognitive impairment such as dementia?

Learn more
Watch Video 4.2: George talks about his life experience as he navigated Erikson's eight stages.

Bronfenbrenner's theory is described further in Chapter 6.

Erikson's eight stages of psychosocial development help us understand the reason each individual develops differently. Any two people from anywhere on the planet at any given age or stage will be similar because the stages happen in the same order (Erikson, 1959). However, the way each individual passes through the stages as they interact with people in the world is unique. Individuals have value as they contribute their uniqueness to the world.

BRONFENBRENNER'S ECOLOGICAL THEORY

Urie Bronfenbrenner was a renowned developmental psychologist who taught for over 50 years at Cornell University. He developed the 'human ecology theory', which is based on many years of study examining both naturally occurring and deliberately designed experiments in the real world. In the 1979 publication *The Ecology of Human Development*, along with John C. Condry Jr., Bronfenbrenner delivered a theory that human development unfolds in a nested set of systems that involve cultural, social, economic, political and chronological influences. This theory expanded the aspects of personality beyond the psychological ones.

Bronfenbrenner's model of concentric circles symbolising four nested systems (the microsystem, mesosystem, exosystem and macrosystem) best illustrates his theory. Figure 4.1 shows these systems, along with the chronosystem of time as the individual ages, shown at the bottom of the diagram.

FIGURE 4.1 Bronfenbrenner's theoretical model

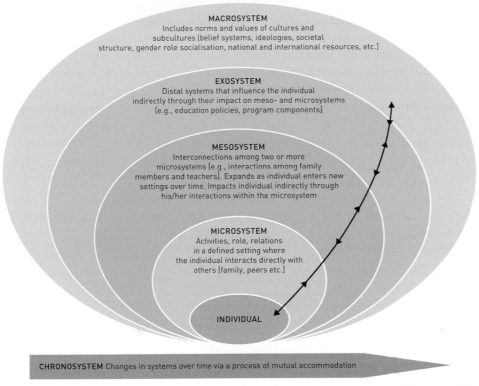

Source: Bernoth & Winkler, 2017 (1st edn), p. 83 (adapted from McEathron & Beuhring, 2011, based on Bronfenbrenner, 1989, 2006).

THE HUMAN ECOLOGY THEORY WITH THE OLDER PERSON AT THE CENTRE

Bronfenbrenner theorised that a person is influenced by other people and events in their microsystem, mesosystem, exosystem and macrosystem over time. Bronfenbrenner's fifth system, which encompasses the concept of time, is called the chronosystem. All of these influences affect an individual's development, and the individual has the choice and power to affect all of the systems (Bronfenbrenner, 1993). In Figure 4.1, the arrows have heads pointing into and away from the individual, indicating the factor of free will. No matter the age or stage of an individual, their impact on the world around them is as powerful as the impact the world has upon them. An explanation of the systems with an older person at the centre of an ecological model is shown in Table 4.3.

World events during 2020 and beyond most definitely influenced the microsystems, mesosystems, exosystems and macrosystems of Darlene and her family. Prior to the global pandemic, few people considered macrosystem influences on their daily lives and livelihoods. At the same time, the lockdowns were evidence that each individual had influence on the macrosystem. Bronfenbrenner's human ecological model offers a way to make sense of the chaos that we all experienced during the global pandemic.

TABLE 4.3 The older person in the centre of the human ecological model

SYSTEMS WITHIN THE MODEL	INFLUENCES WITHIN EACH SYSTEM	EXAMPLES OF INFLUENCES	
Individual	Gender	Genetics	
	Health	Comorbidity	
	Age	Physiological changes	
Microsystem	Living arrangements	Home with spouse or partner	
		Home but spouse or partner is in aged care	
	Family	Married or de facto relationship	
		Widowed	
		Children	Involved or uninvolved in person's life
			Live nearby
			Live interstate
			Live overseas
		No living children	
		Grandchildren	
		Siblings	
		Extended family	
	Health services	Public	
		Private	
		Metropolitan	
		Rural	
	Religious group	Involved in a community of faith	
		Uninvolved in an organised religion	
	Social group	Rotary	
		RSL	
		Sports clubs (golf, tennis, bowls, etc.)	
		Culture	
Mesosystem	Aged-care facility	Interconnection of living arrangements and health services	
	Church-supported aged care	Interconnection of religious group and living arrangements	
	Retirement village	Interconnection of social or sports groups with living arrangements	
	Relative's home	Interconnection of family and health	
Exosystem	Community	Funding for locations and services	
		Access to healthcare, chemists, allied health services	
	Government policies	Registered nurses in aged-care facilities	
		Funding of pensions	
	Social welfare services	Qualification standards	
		Funding schemes	
		Waitlist length	
	Laws	Elder abuse laws	
	Mass media	Feeds the value of youth	
		Terrorist attacks around the world	
	Social media	Requires connectivity, devices and skill set	
		Global influence	
		Algorithms determine items on personal feed	

TABLE 4.3 Continued

SYSTEMS WITHIN THE MODEL	INFLUENCES WITHIN EACH SYSTEM	EXAMPLES OF INFLUENCES
Macrosystem	Governments	International and national border restrictions
		Quarantine protocols and requirements
		Vaccine production, approval, dispersal
		Royal Commission into Aged Care Quality and Safety: recommendations
	Religion	Judaism, Christianity, Buddhism, Islamism, atheism, spiritualism
	Values	Traditional values versus secular/rational values
		Survival values versus self-expression values
	Beliefs	Gender roles, liberty, democracy, racism, ageism
Chronosystem	History	Intergenerational trauma
		World War II generation
		Baby boomers
		Wide use of technology and the internet

Source: Bernoth & Winkler, 2017 (1st edn), pp. 84–5 (adapted). Created by D. Winkler.

4.4 Getting to know the person: Darlene's story

In spring, Darlene had an odd experience getting up from the dinner table. She could hear her grandson talking to his mother at the kitchen sink, but she couldn't see him. It was like the lens on her eyes wouldn't open all the way. She felt tipsy, but had had no wine with dinner. Reporting that she felt unwell brought on a big discussion about whether or not they should go to the ED and whether anyone would be permitted to go in with her due to the coronavirus. After an hour, Darlene had worried herself into her first panic attack. Her son took her to the nearest base hospital.

After three people tried to get blood from her veins and start an IV, she was left alone to worry about all the things that could be seriously wrong. Just as she was convincing herself she'd had a stroke, a doctor came to look at her eyes and ordered a CT scan of her brain. A few hours later, they told her she was having a migraine headache and to see her GP in the next few days.

This incident started a string of twenty-two telehealth visits. Darlene also started taking medication regularly: antidepressant, anti-anxiety, high blood pressure meds. She had asked for a sleeping pill, but no one, except her, thought it was a good idea. The new medications made her feel flat and one of them increased her urgency to use the toilet. As the weather warmed up, she was relieved to wear housedresses again, which were easier to raise when she was in a hurry to get to the toilet. The urgency increased and her daughter-in-law asked if she thought she might have an infection. Phone calls were made and a sample cup and urine test were dropped off. She was grateful to her daughter-in-law for running to the surgery and the chemist, and for organising the delivery of pads along with groceries. Mostly she was appreciative to her daughter-in-law for not embarrassing her about the incontinence.

Her son had to help her with the devices for her telehealth visits. He was also verbal about his discomfort with hearing about his mum's bladder problems. He stated he would rather drive into town to pick up the medications. Sometimes, he offered for her to ride along and have a coffee at Maccas. One time on the car ride into town, her son talked about how lucky she was to not have to pay full price for her medications. He explained how it made paying taxes a little less painful knowing she benefitted from them. It surprised her when he said he was very glad that she was living with them during the pandemic. He even confessed that he didn't tell her often enough that he loved her cooking.

FOCUS QUESTIONS

- Put Darlene in the centre of the human ecological model. What are some of the influences in her systems that are affecting her? How is she affecting her systems?
- Never forget that the interaction you have with an older person is one of those experiences. As a health professional, you are a part of their microsystem. How will you contribute to their development?

Humans evolve throughout their lives, and the changes in their personality can be understood by recognising how the world influences them. An individual's choices about these changes and the final outcome of their life can be explained through psychosocial theories. Erikson's and Bronfenbrenner's theories offer insight for human development across the lifespan – however, they lack the specifics for a favourable outcome. Narrowing the focus to the social and psychological aspects of successful ageing prompted the field of gerontology.

FOCUS QUESTIONS

- How would you use one of these theories to devise a plan of care to ensure that an older person ages the way they want to? Create a plan of care for now and into the future.
- What are the consequences for an older person if health professionals hold too firmly to a particular theory?

Learn more
Access additional resources – such as weblinks, further readings and podcasts – to broaden your understanding of this chapter. See the Guided Tour for access details.

Conclusion

Successful ageing has been defined by social science researchers as arriving at a high number of calendar years with a low chance of contracting a disease, or a disability related to a disease, and the ability to function physically and cognitively in order to engage actively in life (Minkler & Fadem, 2002, p. 229). Other researchers (Reichstadt et al., 2010) have delved into what successful ageing means and the older people in that study consider wisdom to be the most important factor. The reasons older people age successfully are determined by them, but can be understood by using several psychosocial theories, particularly the activity and continuity theories. Activity theory can explain older people who are engaged in social and/or physical activities and contributing to society. Continuity theory can explain older people who have not changed their attitudes, beliefs, behaviour or personality throughout their life. Erikson's and

Bronfenbrenner's psychosocial theories explain human development over the lifespan, including the advanced years. Erik Erikson developed a theory that included eight stages. The seventh stage, 'generativity versus stagnation', begins around middle age (40–65 years) and deals with the identity crisis of building a legacy or self-absorption. The eighth stage, 'integrity versus despair', begins after age 65 and deals with the older person looking back at life and feeling positive about their achievements or feeling despair over all the regrets. Bronfenbrenner developed a theory of five interrelated systems with the individual in the centre. The systems that influence the individual and that are affected by the individual are the microsystem, mesosystem, exosystem and macrosystem; there is also a fifth system called the chronosystem. All of these systems offer explanations for a person's development over their lifespan. These psychosocial theories offer understandings about how and why older people contribute to society.

1   Research older people who inspire you to compare and contrast their life events with the psychosocial theories presented. What do these people teach us about ageing successfully?

2   Identify all the systems and where you as the health professional fit into Bronfenbrenner's systems.

REVISION QUESTIONS

REFERENCES

Agronin, M. E. (2013). From Cicero to Cohen: Developmental theories of aging, from antiquity to the present. *The Gerontologist*, *54*(1), 30–9. https://doi:10.1093/geront/gnt032

Atchley, R. C. (1989). A continuity theory of normal aging. *The Gerontologist*, *29*(2), 183–90. https://doi:10.1093/geront/29.2.183

Baltes, P. B. & Baltes, M. M. (eds) (1990). *Successful Aging: Perspectives from the behavioral sciences*. Cambridge University Press. https://doi:10.1017/CBO9780511665684

Bernoth, M. & Winkler, D. (eds) (2017). Healthy Ageing and Aged Care. Oxford University Press.

Blazer, D. G. (2006). Successful aging. *American Journal of Geriatric Psychiatry*, *14*(1), 2–5. https://doi:10.1097/01.JGP.0000195222.93655.d1

Bowling, A. & Dieppe, P. (2005). What is successful ageing and who should define it? *BMJ*, *331*(7531), 1548–51. https://doi:10.1136/bmj.331.7531.1548

Bronfenbrenner, U. (1979). *The Ecology Of Human Development: Experiments by nature and design*. Cambridge University Press.

Bronfenbrenner, U. (1993). Ecological models of human development. In M. Gauvain & M. Cole, (eds), *Readings on the Development of Children* (2nd edn). Freeman, pp. 37–43.

Charles Scribner's Sons (2008). Erikson, Erik Homburger. *The Complete Dictionary of Scientific Biography*. www.encyclopedia.com/topic/Erik_Erikson.aspx#1

Crowther, M. R., Parker, M. W., Achenbaum, W. A., Larimore, W. L. & Koenig, H. G. (2002). Rowe and Kahn's model of successful aging revisited: Positive spirituality – the forgotten factor. *The Gerontologist*, *42*(5), 613–20. https://doi:10.1093/geront/42.5.613

Cumming, E. & Henry, W. E. (1961). *Growing Old: The process of disengagement*. Basic Books.

Depp, C. A., Glatt, S. J. & Jeste, D. V. (2007). Recent advances in research on successful or healthy aging. *Current Psychiatry Reports*, *9*(1), 7–13. https://doi:10.1007/s11920-007-0003-0

Erikson, E. (1959). *Identity and the Life Cycle*. International Universities Press.

Hearn, S., Saulnier, G., Strayer, J., Gienham, M., Koopman, R. & Marcia, J. E. (2012). Between integrity and despair: Toward construct validation of Erikson's eighth stage. *Journal of Adult Development*, *19*(1), 1–20. https://doi:10.1007/s10804-011-9126-y

Institute of Gerontology (n.d.). What is Gerontology? College of Public Health, University of Georgia. www.publichealth.uga.edu/geron/what-is

Lupien, S. J. & Wan, N. (2004). Successful ageing: From cell to self. *Philosophical Transactions of the Royal Society B: Biological Sciences*, *359*(1449), 1413–26. https://doi:10.1098/rstb.2004.1516

Maddox, G. (1963). Activity and Morale: A longitudinal study of selected elderly subjects. *Social Forces*, *42*(2), 195–204. https://doi:10.2307/2575692

Martin, P., Kelly, N., Kahana, B., Kahana, E., Willcox, B. J., Willcox, D. C. & Poon, L. W. (2014). Defining successful aging: A tangible or elusive concept? *The Gerontologist*, *55*(1), 14–25. https://doi:10.1093/geront/gnu044

McEathron, M. & Beuhring, T. (2011). Postsecondary education for students with intellectual and developmental disabilities: A critical review of the state of knowledge and a taxonomy to guide future research. *Policy Research Brief*, *21*(1).

Minkler, M. & Fadem. P. (2002). Successful aging: A disability perspective. *Journal of Disability Policy Studies*, *12*(4), 229–35. https://doi:10.1177/104420730201200402

Montross, L. P., Depp, C., Daly, J., Reichstadt, J., Golshan, S., Moore, D., ... Jeste, D. V. (2006). Correlates of self-rated successful aging among community dwelling older adults. *American Journal of Geriatric Psychiatry*, *14*(1), 43–51. https,//doi:10.1097/01 JGP.0000192489.43179.31

Reichstadt, J., Sengupta, G., Depp, C. A., Palinkas, L. A. & Jeste, D. V. (2010). Older adults' perspectives on successful aging: Qualitative interviews. *American Journal of Geriatric Psychiatry*, *18*(7), 567–75. https://doi.10.1097/

JGP.0b013e3181e040bb

Rowe, J. W. & Kahn, R. L. (1987). Human aging: Usual and successful. *Science*, *237*(4811), 143–9. https://doi:10.1126/science.3299702

Schulz, R. & Heckhausen, J. (1996). A life span model of successful aging. *American Psychologist*, *51*(7), 702–14. https://doi:10.1037/0003-066X.51.7.702

Silverstein, M., Bengtson, V. L., Putnam, M., Putney, N. M. & Gans, D. (eds) (2008). *Handbook of Theories of Aging*. Springer Publishing.

Skinner, M. W., Cloutier, D. & Andrews, G. J. (2014). Geographies of ageing: Progress and possibilities after two decades of change. *Progress in Human Geography*, *39*(6), 776–99. https://doi:10.1177/0309132514558444

Stephens, C. (2017). From success to capability for healthy ageing: Shifting the lens to include all older people. *Critical Public Health*, *27*(4), 490–8.

Strawbridge, W. J., Wallhagen, M. I. & Cohen, R. D. (2002). Successful aging and well-being: Self-rated compared with Rowe and Kahn. *The Gerontologist*, *42*(6), 727–73. https://doi:10.1093/geront/42.6.727

Tate, R. B., Lah, L. & Cuddy, T. E. (2003). Definition of successful aging by elderly Canadian males: The Manitoba follow-up study.

The Gerontologist, *43*(5), 735–44. https://doi:10.1093/geront/ 43.5.735

Urtamo, A., Jyväkorpi, S. K. & Strandberg, T. E. (2019). Definitions of successful ageing: A brief review of a multidimensional concept. *Acta bio-medica: Atenei Parmensis*, *90*(2), 359–63. https://doi.org/10.23750/abm.v90i2.8376

Vaillant, G. (2002). *Aging Well*. Little, Brown and Company.

Villar, F. (2012). Successful ageing and development: The contribution of generativity in older age. *Ageing and Society*, *32*(7), 1087.

Voigt, T. (2021). AAG Discussion Paper: 'Adaptive Ageing' versus 'Successful or Positive Ageing'. Draft for member consultation.

Wagnild, G. (2003). Resilience and successful aging: Comparison among low and high income older adults. *Journal of Gerontological Nursing*, *29*(12), 42–9. https://doi:10.3928/0098-9134-20031201-09

World Health Organization (WHO) (2002). Active Ageing: A Policy Framework. A contribution of the World Health Organization to the Second United Nations World Assembly on Ageing, Madrid, Spain, April. https://extranet.who.int/agefriendlyworld/wp-content/uploads/2014/06/WHO-Active-Ageing-Framework.pdf

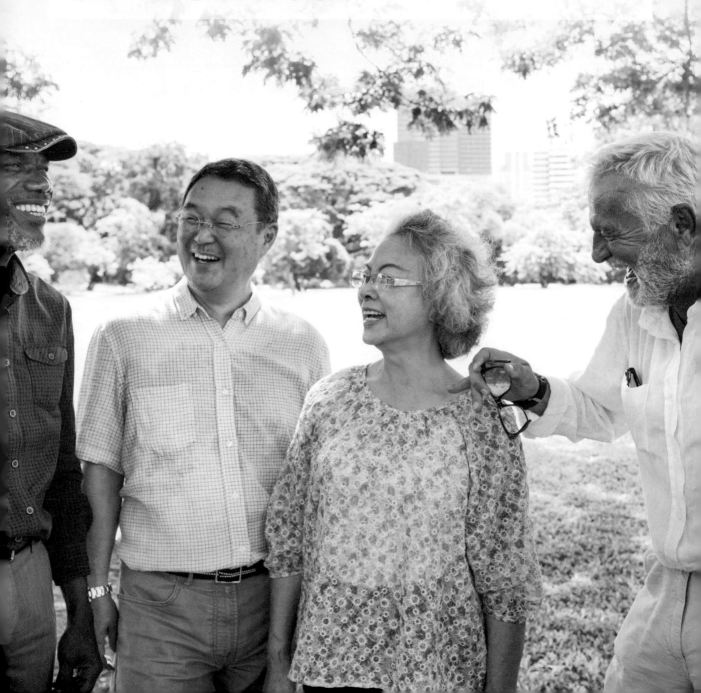

PART 2
THE SOCIAL ASPECTS OF AGEING

5 Family Relationships and Informal Care

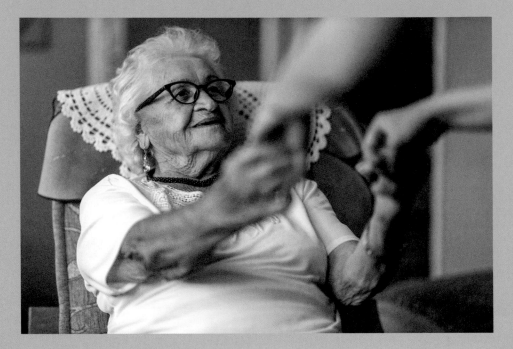

LEARNING OBJECTIVES

After reading this chapter, you will:

» have considered the impact of changing family dynamics on older adults and informal caregivers, including how cultural and social diversity can influence expectations of familial care

» have explored how the complex and diverse nature of family relationships can impact the individual experience of ageing

» have considered how social determinants contribute to opportunities and barriers to healthy ageing

» have identified the significant risks to the health and well-being of families and caregivers of older adults, including spousal caregiving and co-dependence in older couples

» have explored why assessment and practice with older adults should occur within a family and social context.

Introduction

This chapter explores the integral role that family and informal caregiving plays in supporting and enabling healthy ageing in Australia. Everyone has their own unique family background and experiences, which provide the lens through which they view the world. These experiences and expectations can also have a significant impact on the availability and provision of support to older adults. As well as encouraging you to learn about the ways that family relationships can impact ageing and informal care, this chapter also asks you to reflect on your own personal views and experiences openly and critically, as these can have important implications for your practice with older adults, their families and caregivers. This chapter draws on many of the other chapters in this book, as we explore the impact of demographic shifts, social policy, ageing in a rural area, cultural diversities and other diversities on families and **informal care**. Developing an understanding of family context will provide a good foundation for future practice with older adults and their caregivers.

> **informal care**
> Unpaid care provided by family, friends, neighbours and other community supports without support from a government agency or service provider.

The role of informal care

Care and caregiving are essential social phenomena, often regarded as a central function of families across countries and cultures. Despite this, care work has historically been quite invisible, with the provision of care for children and older family members typically an unpaid domestic responsibility of women (Fine & Davidson, 2018). While this disproportionate gendering of care is still evident in current times, population ageing has prompted discussions of caregiving to move from the private to the public domain (Fine & Davidson, 2018). Planning for the care needs of growing numbers of older adults in Australia has required a significant shift in thinking for families, communities, health and social service providers, policymakers and governments. Understanding this changing social and policy context will help health professionals to successfully navigate practice with older health-care consumers and their caregivers.

As people age, the likelihood of needing some form of care or support increases markedly, with most of the care provided by family, friends and other informal supports in both developed and developing countries (WHO, 2015). In Australia, it is estimated that there are more than 2.8 million informal caregivers providing care for family and friends (Deloitte Access Economics, 2020). These unpaid caregivers provide more than 80 per cent of all aged care, enabling older adults to remain in their homes and connected to their community longer.

Australia's health and aged care systems are heavily dependent on the availability of informal caregivers, a reliance that can place a significant burden of care on families and friends. It is estimated that if the informal care currently provided by unpaid family and friends was replaced by **formal care** arrangements, the cost would be in excess of $77 billion per annum (Deloitte Access Economics, 2020). This estimate does not reflect the anticipated increase in numbers of older adults and their subsequent needs in coming years, which highlights the essential role of families and informal caregivers in successfully meeting the care needs of an ageing population.

> **formal care**
> Services and supports provided by paid healthcare, aged care and other professionals.

This reliance on informal care is overtly acknowledged within contemporary social policy, with the health and aged care systems built on the premise of **familial** caregiving. While familial models of care have long been established in many countries and cultures,

> **familial**
> Relating to or involving a family.

this concept is not as simplistic in practice as it sounds. Families provide a complex and increasingly diverse context for ageing, caregiving and practitioners. Understanding and working effectively with families as partners in care is an essential aspect of practice for all health and aged care professionals.

Who provides informal care?

Informal care is provided to older adults by their spouses, family, friends, neighbours and other community supports. As shown in Table 5.1, most primary caregivers in Australia are either the partners, children or parents of individuals requiring care.

TABLE 5.1 Profile of informal caregivers in Australia

| | RELATIONSHIP OF CARER TO MAIN RECIPIENT OF CARE | | | | |
	PARTNER OF RECIPIENT	CHILD OF RECIPIENT	PARENT OF RECIPIENT	OTHER RELATIONSHIP TO RECIPIENT	TOTAL
Male primary carers (estimate '000)					
15–24 years	0.0	4.4	0.0	0.0	7.0
25–44 years	11.8	17.6	6.4	3.8	39.0
45–64 years	46.2	36.6	15.8	11.4	108.2
65 years and over	73.4	6.1	5.2	6.4	89.4
Total	129.6	62.7	27.1	22.1	241.9
Female primary carers (estimate '000)					
15–24 years	1.3	2.4	1.2	8.0	13.7
25–44 years	20.7	31.5	99.8	16.9	165.6
45–64 years	64.2	110.8	88.3	34.4	208.2
65 years and over	99.0	15.6	18.1	7.7	139.3
Total	185.7	161.4	205.6	65.2	618.8
All primary carers (estimate '000)					
15–24 years	1.3	7.8	1.9	8.1	18.6
25–44 years	32.0	48.6	104.0	20.5	205.6
45–64 years	111.4	146.6	102.2	45.7	406.0
65 years and over	172.8	20.3	21.8	12.1	228.3
Total	**315.2**	**226.0**	**233.5**	**89.6**	**861.6**

Source: ABS, 2018, Table 34.1.

One consequence of an ageing population is the significantly increased demand for informal caregivers in the future, yet demographic predictions suggest that, at this time of increased need, there will also be fewer informal caregivers available (Deloitte Access Economics, 2020). While the reduced availability of caregivers is in part due to the shift in population demographics, there are also several significant sociological changes happening that will influence the availability of informal caregivers in the future. These changes include:

- changing and more diverse family structures, which are less like the traditional or nuclear families that care assumptions are often based on

- increased rates of divorce, meaning that more older adults will experience later life without a partner who might provide care

- more individuals and couples deciding not to marry or have children, or to have fewer children, which is resulting in fewer adult children being available to provide care in later life

- increased geographic mobility, which is seeing lots of migration away from family, so older adults are not necessarily living near family in later life

- increased workforce participation by women, meaning they are no longer available to provide unpaid care.

These sociological developments, as well as changes in intergenerational attitudes and perceptions of providing care, are contributing to a reduced propensity to care, which will further compound issues of future caregiver availability (Deloitte Access Economics, 2020). These changes in both availability and willingness to care will impact professionals who work within policy and organisational frameworks that rely heavily on the family to provide support and care for older adults, an assumption that may not be viable in the future.

SPOUSAL CAREGIVING

As demonstrated in Table 5.1, the largest subgroup of informal care providers are older adults themselves, who are most often providing care to a partner. It is also within this subgroup that men make their largest contribution to informal care.

Co-residence and existing interpersonal relationships often result in a spouse being the most logical provider of care, though it is important to consider the unique nature of this relationship and the potential impacts that can arise in a **spousal** care **dyad**. Co-residence in later life can enable couples to remain together longer in the home by providing mutual support; however, this close relationship also presents a range of unique challenges.

Later-life spousal care often means that caregivers are providing care at a time when their own frailty may be increasing and their health needs are becoming more complex. Spouses are thought to be particularly susceptible to depression as a consequence of providing the most extensive range of care to their partner (Butler et al., 2005) and the sense of obligation and family responsibility to take on a caring role (ABS, 2018). It has also been demonstrated that providing care within your own household is around four times more intensive than providing care to someone living outside of your home, with looking after a spouse the most intensive type of care relationship for both men and women, close only to mothers caring for a sick or disabled child (Hirst, 2005). Studies have also shown that spousal caregivers are more likely than those in other relationship types to have unmet support needs, which places them at increased risk of poor health outcomes and psychological distress (Temple & Dow, 2018).

Beyond the psychological and physical risks of caregiving, the spousal caregiver is in a life partnership with the care recipient, consequently also experiencing the financial and social implications of the frailty or disability. These contextual factors place spousal caregivers at a much greater risk of negative psychological and physical impacts than other carers and non-carers.

spousal
Relating to marital or de facto relationships.

dyad
A social group that consists of two members – for example, husband and wife – or a caregiver and a care recipient.

Learn more
Watch Video 13.1: Listen to Ronita talk about the challenges of becoming a carer for her husband David.

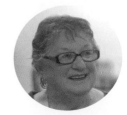

The story of Robert and Olive explores some of the challenges that can arise in this situation.

5.1 Getting to know the couple: Robert and Olive's story

Robert (82) and Olive (79) have been married for 59 years. They continue to live together in the family home where they raised their three children, though the children have long since left the local area to pursue employment and raise their own families. Their eldest daughter, Cheryl, lives an hour's drive away and visits regularly to check in with her parents and provide support as required.

Twelve months ago, Olive slipped in the garden while watering her flowers. She sustained significant injury to her left side, fracturing a hip and wrist. While her recovery initially progressed well, she has experienced several setbacks and has not fully regained strength in her left side. She continues to experience severe pain and difficulty with mobility, which affects her ability to stand for extended periods and shower independently.

Upon discharge from hospital, Olive returned home with a plan for Robert to provide the help she required with personal care and household tasks. While this worked well for several months, Robert recently had a fall while trying to help Olive in the shower, resulting in cuts and bruises to his face and arm. Cheryl contacted the local health-care service and requested additional support for her parents, expressing concerns at their ability to remain safely together in the family home. She told the service that on her recent visit home she observed that the house has become increasingly unkempt, and Olive's personal hygiene is declining. She also reports that Robert has lost a significant amount of weight and appears withdrawn.

The local district nurse has arranged to visit Robert and Olive at home to assess the situation. After conducting a preliminary assessment, the nurse offers to investigate options for further help to the couple. Robert immediately refuses help and insists they are coping well together. He tells the nurse that Olive is his wife and that they are committed to caring for one another without outside support. The nurse asks Olive for her thoughts and she readily agrees with Robert.

While walking the nurse to the car, Robert admits that he is struggling to cope with the caregiver role and says he would never tell Olive as she would be heartbroken. He adds that his recent injury has left him fearful of providing physical assistance to Olive as he is worried that one of them will be seriously injured should another accident occur. When the nurse reiterates her offer of support, Robert states that he is fine, and they will be OK. He proudly tells the nurse that he and Olive have plans to celebrate their upcoming sixtieth wedding anniversary and have promised one another that they will do whatever they can to stay together at home to avoid being separated in residential care.

OBLIGATIONS AND EXPECTATIONS TO PROVIDE CARE

Assumptions and expectations about the provision of informal care are clear in both social policy and in wider social norms, hence the need to consider how this is managed in practice. Supportive relationships are complex; they intertwine tension, affection, hostility, respect and empathy (Rummery & Fine, 2012; Cash et al., 2019). By the time an older person requires care and support, a lifetime of family history, relationship interactions and reciprocity has already occurred.

It is important that health professionals do not assume that informal caregiving happens because of love. There are many complex reasons that caregiving occurs, including obligation and lack of alternatives, as demonstrated in Figure 5.1. This survey found that 70 per cent of primary caregivers identified a sense of family responsibility as the reason for taking on a caregiving role, with reasons also weighted heavily towards emotional obligation, feeling that they could provide better care, that no one else was available or that there was no other choice (ABS, 2018). These findings demonstrate the importance of asking respectful questions and exploring the dynamics of each individual situation rather than making assumptions about relationships.

FIGURE 5.1 Complex reasons for caregiving

PRIMARY CARERS, REASONS FOR TAKING ON CARING ROLE, BY RELATIONSHIP TO MAIN RECIPIENT OF CARE (A)(B), 2018

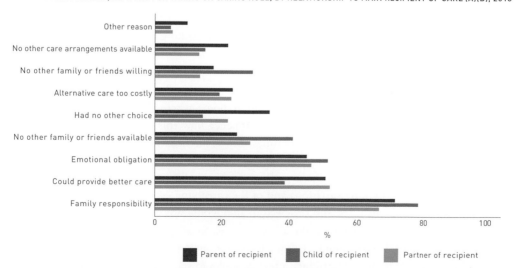

a. Proportions have been calculated using totals that exclude 'not stated' responses

b. Respondents may have provided more than one reason for taking on caring role

Consumer Directed Care
An approach to service delivery where the individual receiving the service determines the types of services, from whom, when and how these services will be delivered, giving individuals choice and flexibility.

Health professionals play an important role in enabling choice for older adults and their caregivers by helping them to access complex service systems and to overcome issues of health literacy. The complexity of changing policy and practice systems also requires professionals to have a critical understanding of the impact policy directions such as **Consumer Directed Care (CDC)** initiatives can have on families and caregivers (Cash et al., 2016). The complexity of familial obligations and social norms can mean that caregivers are often reluctant to discuss an unwillingness to provide informal care or admit to difficulty in coping with this role (Burridge et al., 2007; Cash et al., 2016, 2019), which is an important consideration for health professionals working with older adults and their families.

Implications for practice

It is common in practice for assessments to be conducted either directly with the care recipient or with both recipient and caregiver present. It is suggested that opportunities are also provided for the caregiver to speak openly about their care role while not in the presence of the family member receiving care, in order for them to have a safe space to discuss any concerns or reluctance around this role (Cash et al., 2016). Inclusion of caregivers within assessment and planning processes was also highlighted in the Royal Commission into Aged Care Quality and Safety report as being key to building a new and more holistic approach to aged care (Commonwealth of Australia, 2021a, p. 38). A final key point is to consider the changing and evolving nature of care needs and caregiving. As a health professional you must ensure that regular discussions take place with caregivers to ensure that as care tasks increase over time, the ongoing provision of informal care is still acceptable.

The impact of individual and family diversity on care

When thinking about ageing, the diverse nature of both older adults and their families is often overlooked. It is essential to develop a sound working understanding of the impact family relationships can have on the individual experience of ageing, on caregiving and for health-care practice.

Older Australians often rely on caregiving from family, spouses and other informal supports so that they can continue living at home where they are connected to their community. There are many factors that influence how this informal care is distributed, experienced and perceived within families, hence the need for work with older adults to be framed within their family and social context. These factors can contribute positive and protective factors for older adults, as well as creating challenges and risks. The changing and evolving nature of family situations and of the caregiving experience also mean that these dynamics must be revisited and reviewed in an ongoing way.

This chapter does not have the scope to consider all possible family, cultural, sexual, geographic, social and economic factors that can influence informal caregiving. This section is instead going to briefly introduce a few examples to start you thinking about the impact of diversity on families and caregivers in later life.

GENDER

Unpaid care work has historically been gendered as 'women's work', with past generations of women less likely to be in the workforce and seen as responsible for the unpaid care needs of children and older family members. Although women now increasingly participate in the workforce, the gendered nature of care continues to see disproportionate numbers of women in both informal and formal care roles (WHO, 2015).

As the revolution of women's roles in society continues to shift, health professionals navigating work with informal caregivers need to be aware of gender biases and remain open to all potential care support, not only that dictated by traditional social norms. Longevity is contributing to increasing numbers of male caregivers providing care to partners, and researchers are beginning to consider the dissimilar needs and experiences of men in caregiving roles (Shu et al., 2017). Awareness of evolving attitudes and expectations is important to ensure that health professionals do not inadvertently reinforce gendered expectations of care.

FAMILY SOCIO-ECONOMIC STATUS

The socio-economic status (SES) of individuals and families can play an important role in the experience of ageing and on the provision of care. Research has demonstrated that intergenerational exchanges are significantly affected by SES, with families in higher SES groups more able to finance external support if required and subsequently expecting little or no care from their children (Timonen et al., 2013). This sentiment is often expressed by a desire for independence and a wish not to burden adult children with expectations of care (Productivity Commission, 2011). Interestingly, children in this higher SES bracket correspondingly demonstrate less **filial** obligation to provide care (Timonen et al., 2013).

filial
Referring to a child's relationship with or feelings towards their parents.

On the other hand, families in lower SES groups often focus on distributing resources towards children in the hope that this will benefit the next generation. Lower SES groups demonstrate much stronger and often unquestioned obligations around **intergenerational care**, for reasons of reciprocity and the financial inability for this care to be outsourced (Timonen et al., 2013). Women from lower SES backgrounds are often required to give up opportunities to pursue work or education in order to provide care to ageing relatives, creating further inequalities within an already disadvantaged group. This is important to consider when working with older adults and their families, as the financial ability to outsource care will significantly affect the requirements and obligations experienced by family caregivers. Challenges emerging from the privatisation of care can result in even greater inequities for already disadvantaged social groups who cannot afford to engage in 'user pays' systems.

intergenerational care
The exchange of care and support across generations.

Implications for practice

The implications of SES for informal care obligations are significant, particularly considering the enormous health gaps already created by social determinants across an individual's life course (Marmot, 2015). Many older adults and their family members are unfamiliar with available services and supports, so it is important for you as a health professional to be aware of government programs and initiatives that

> clients with lower SES can be referred to for additional support. This might include government-provided supports such as carer payments and utility concessions or the practical assistance provided by programs such as the National Continence Program for Australia (Department of Health, n.d.).

CULTURAL AND FAMILY BACKGROUND

An awareness of cultural diversity and the effect of this on informal care expectations is also useful for health professionals. One of the fastest growing sections of the Australian population is migrants, with almost 30 per cent of Australians born overseas (ABS, 2020). This creates considerable cultural diversity within the ageing population, with the values and influences of cultural origins continuing into later life.

Cultural traditions and expectations can play a significant role in how families conceptualise and enact care for older family members. Within Western societies there are pervasive issues of ageism, with older adults often devalued and perceived as a burden (Hughes & Heycox, 2010). Within Australia, policy and practice has increasingly focused on individualised approaches to ageing, encouraging preventative and healthy ageing approaches, and promoting financial independence and preparedness for older age and for ageing at home. This focus contrasts with the overt reliance on traditional models of familial care and the long-held normative and societal expectations of spousal and filial care responsibilities (Cash et al., 2013).

individualised values
Values that emphasise independence and personal fulfilment.

The role of informal caregiving can also be perceived very differently at the family level, with some families demonstrating more **individualised values** and placing less emphasis on intergenerational care. These families tend to have more focus on independence between family members, fewer expectations of intergenerational care, greater reliance on formal supports if required and may have lower levels of contact.

Many cultures, however, have strongly held values that place great emphasis on the provision of intergenerational exchanges and care for older family members as a means of maintaining family solidarity. These cultural expectations can significantly alter family views on providing care and on familial expectations and willingness to do so. These patterns are not always evident and can be influenced by the degree to which families experience their relationships as being either rewarding and meaningful or strained and difficult. Individuals can also belong to more than one cultural group, so it is key that health professionals actively discuss how each individual and their family conceptualise ageing and caregiving rather than make assumptions about this.

THE IMPACT OF GEOGRAPHY ON CARE

While Australia is geographically one of the largest countries, it has one of the lowest population densities in the world, with considerable distances between metropolitan cities. Around one-third of the total population resides outside of major urban centres, with older adults less likely to live in major cities than other age groups (AIHW, 2018, 2020).

As mentioned earlier in this chapter, demographic predictions suggest that while an ageing population means the demand for informal caregivers will inevitably increase, there will be fewer informal caregivers available (Productivity Commission, 2011). The shortage of informal caregivers is likely to be more evident in rural areas, as younger generations are more inclined to relocate to cities for education and employment opportunities (McDonald, 2017). This may mean that traditional providers of informal care will not reside in the same rural location as ageing family members, reducing the potential pool of support. This will be compounded by fewer people of working age to provide care to older adults and a shortage of residential care facilities (Commonwealth of Australia, 2021b).

Chapter 6 will further your understanding about ageing in rural areas.

It is important, however, to consider that rurality is complex. While there may be fewer health services, rural areas can be richer in social capital, with potentially greater support for older adults and their carers within the community. The challenges of geographic distance require practitioners to be creative in developing solutions to local needs and problems.

This discussion touches only briefly on some examples of diversity and difference in families and older adults to illustrate that older Australians cannot be conceptualised as a homogenous group. Diversity can contribute to different expectations of ageing and caregiving for families, caregivers and older adults requiring care. The nature of diverse family and social networks also requires health professionals to recognise non-traditional supports and relationships that may be available for older adults, such as same-sex partners, neighbours and colleagues.

Implications for practice

These are some useful reflections for you as a health professional to consider in relation to the impact of family diversity on care:

- Health professionals should hold a stance of curiosity and awareness about diversity in all assessment and practice contexts to encourage asking questions without making assumptions about how an individual or family might understand and approach ageing and caregiving.
- All health professionals should continue reflecting on their own cultural and family experiences to understand how these can influence assumptions and expectations of care in practice.
- The richness of an individual's family and social background enables health professionals to respectfully identify potential risks while enhancing and utilising existing strengths.

While some aspects of diversity might appear to be overt, it is key not to make assumptions about the experiences and preferences of families and individuals. Consider the case of Luisa and Rosa, who are part of a family experiencing the intergenerational exchanges that are often evident between family members.

5.2 Getting to know the family: Luisa and Rosa's story

Luisa (42) is married to John (46). They have three children: David (16), Emilia (13) and Violet (11). Luisa works full time as a receptionist at a local accounting firm. She enjoys her job, but often finds it difficult to manage full-time work with the needs of the kids, who attend various school and sporting activities. Luisa also provides an increasing amount of support to her mother Rosa (72), who lives 20 minutes' drive away in another suburb. Rosa was left a widow when her husband Francesco died suddenly 10 years ago, and she has not re-partnered. Luisa has an older brother who lives in another state and visits infrequently.

Rosa has always been active and enjoyed good health, though it has become increasingly evident recently that her physical condition is no longer as good as it once was. Rosa has developed mild arthritis in her knees and wrists, which has worsened significantly in recent months. Changes to her mobility are making it very difficult for her to get out and enjoy her walks in the local neighbourhood and to get to the shops. She is also having difficulty managing cooking tasks that involve bending to the oven or lifting heavy pots or pans on the stove top. As her pain and reflexes worsened, Rosa was forced to surrender her driving licence after a couple of near misses, which has significantly restricted her independence. Luisa now drives Rosa to the shops weekly and spends a day each week helping with meal preparation so that Rosa can reheat meals in the microwave, reducing the risk of an injury in the kitchen. Luisa also accompanies Rosa to medical appointments and on a weekly visit to the cemetery to refresh flowers at Francesco's grave.

Luisa feels very ambivalent about providing care to her mother as it impacts heavily on both her work and time with her husband and children. While she and Rosa have always been close, Luisa describes feeling like she 'has to' provide support to her mother as there is no one else available to do so. Luisa also feels guilty that Rosa often provided care to her grandchildren when they were younger so that Luisa was able to return to work or to have a break. Luisa and John have discussed moving Rosa into their family home to reduce the amount of travel to support her, though they are unsure if this would place too much strain on their own family, particularly with David completing his final years of high school. Rosa has clearly stated that she does not want to leave her own home as she would be a burden to Luisa and her family. As Rosa continues to age, Luisa is becoming increasingly anxious about Rosa being alone and is keen to discuss possible options that might help alleviate this situation.

- Think about intergenerational care and reciprocity within families. Do you have a personal view on whether families are obligated to provide care?
- What impact do you think feelings of reciprocity and obligation have on family members' decisions to provide care?
- Consider the impacts of care on the 'sandwich generation' of adults, who have care responsibilities for both ageing parents and their own children. How might this be affected by other sociological changes?

FOCUS QUESTIONS

The challenges of informal care

Research has repeatedly highlighted the significant risks and challenges to physical, psychological, social and financial well-being that informal caregivers experience. These are important considerations for health professionals, who are often involved in the journey of family members commencing and continuing in informal care roles. It is also important to acknowledge the strongly held expectations and obligations that are often evident around familial care, and which can make it very difficult for family members to relinquish care, even when experiencing the significant personal costs that result from this role. It is necessary for health practitioners to regularly review informal care situations to ensure that supports reflect the changing nature of care and family relationships.

Some key impacts to be aware of are:

- the responsibility of providing care often falling onto families with little preparation or professional support
- caregivers repeatedly demonstrating that they experience greater levels of risk to their physical, social, mental and financial health and well-being (Temple & Dow, 2018)
- a growing body of evidence that demonstrates that the chronic stress associated with caregiving increases the vulnerability to and progression of illness, triggers physiological reactions, increases risky health behaviours and decreases engagement in preventative health activities, subsequently compromising the physical health of caregivers (Bauer & Sousa-Poza, 2015; Brimblecombe et al., 2018; Butler et al., 2005; Hartke et al., 2006)
- research demonstrating a significantly higher incidence of psychological disorders, levels of stress and poorer general well-being in carers compared to non-carers, with a strong correlation between deterioration in mental health and the transition to a significant caring role (Temple & Dow, 2018; Mohanty & Niyonsenga, 2019; Butterworth et al., 2009)
- informal caregivers often being financially disadvantaged by the costs of caregiving, which can include things like increased utility expenses, medication or medical care, transport and other incurred costs. These expenses can be borne by either the care recipient or the caregiver, though in the instance of spousal care it is inevitable that this will have an impact on both parties, regardless of who the costs are being accrued for
- that caregivers of working age are also often required to forgo paid work in order to provide the required unpaid care needs of family members; this has impacts on caregiver income and cumulative disadvantages regarding employment opportunities (Bittman et al., 2007; Schofield et al., 2014).

ABUSE AND NEGLECT OF OLDER ADULTS

A significant spotlight was cast on the abuse and neglect of older adults during the most recent Royal Commission into Aged Care Quality and Safety, which identified that 'substandard care and abuse pervades the Australian aged care system' (Commonwealth of Australia, 2021a, p. 78). The inquiry revealed the shocking extent of physical and sexual abuse perpetrated on older adults within residential aged care settings. These findings and associated recommendations will hopefully present an important turning point for addressing issues within the residential and formal care systems.

Alongside addressing harm by paid care staff, it is crucial that responses to the mistreatment of older adults also tackle abuse and neglect of older adults within the family environment (Joosten et al., 2017). While there has not been a population-wide study in Australia to determine the prevalence of abuse towards older adults, estimates suggest abuse prevalence is between 2 and 14 per cent, with rates of neglect likely to be much higher (AIHW, 2019). Abuse outside of care facilities occurs largely within families, with risk factors including caregiver stress and burden and the intersection of care with existing family conflict and family violence (Joosten et al., 2017).

Elder abuse is defined by the WHO as being 'a single, or repeated act, or lack of appropriate action, occurring within any relationship where there is an expectation of trust which causes harm or distress to an older person' (WHO, 2018). Some of the more recognised forms of abuse to older adults related to caregiving relationships are:

- inadequate caregiving or care-receiving
- theft or fraud conducted by family members
- family violence and interpersonal relationship problems that extend into older age for both caregivers and care receivers
- conflict or aggression that is associated with dementia.

As with all situations of this complexity, it is important for health professionals to engage with older adults in a way that supports their right to make decisions about how to proceed. This might include empowering and supporting an individual and their family to understand and navigate domestic violence protection procedures, criminal sanctions, and other safety and future planning options.

The story of Anna and Barry highlights some of the complexities that can contribute to the context of decision making for older couples and the professionals working with them.

> Read more about strategies for identifying the abuse of older people in Chapter 7.

5.3 Getting to know the couple: Anna and Barry's story

Anna (69) and Barry (74) have been married for 48 years. They have three adult children, two of whom live overseas and a third whom they rarely see. Anna and Barry have had a difficult marriage, which included the loss of a child at a young age in a tragic accident. They continue to live together on the family property, which Barry farmed for most of their married life. They no longer run any stock on the property, and it is becoming increasingly difficult for them to manage the upkeep as they grow older.

Anna describes Barry as a difficult man, detailing how he controlled the family with an iron fist. While he was not physically violent towards her, his level of control over the family finances and emotional abuse of Anna has clearly taken its toll. When Barry began to experience confusion and early signs of cognitive decline four years ago, Anna sought help from the family GP. It became increasingly evident that all was not well with Barry, and he was eventually diagnosed with a form of dementia.

Barry has deteriorated progressively in the past few years to the point that Anna is becoming increasingly anxious about his safety on the farm. Barry has wandered off several times and become disoriented while in the paddocks and Anna feels unable to leave him unattended for even short periods of time. He is sleeping less and will often move about the home during the night. This is affecting Anna significantly; she is tired, anxious and becoming increasingly resentful of her caregiving of Barry.

With all their finances tied up in the farm, they do not have the financial means to move closer to town. They have been unable to sell the property and this has proven problematic in attempting to create the financial freedom to pursue other care options for Barry. Barry has become increasingly difficult for Anna to manage at home and on two occasions he has struck out in frustration. She is becoming increasingly fearful of him. Anna openly states that she no longer loves Barry and that whatever was there in the early days of their relationship has long since gone. Despite this, she feels strong feelings of guilt at wanting to place him into residential care and shame at not being able to fulfil her marriage vows and set an example to their children. While Anna would be pleased to relinquish her care role, she feels it is all too hard to do and sees the death of herself or Barry as the only possible way out of her predicament.

FOCUS QUESTIONS

- What are your initial responses to this situation?
- What are some of the barriers (both physical and emotional) that prevent Anna from relinquishing care?
- How might the health professionals involved in this situation be able to help?
- What impacts might living in a rural area contribute to this situation (both positive and negative)?
- What are some of the unique challenges to caregivers of people with dementia?
- What is the relationship between burden of care and vulnerability to abuse?

Working with informal caregivers in practice

See a summary of the inquiries and reviews into aged care in Chapter 2.

Although informal caregivers are an essential component of Australia's health and aged care systems, they are not always well integrated into care planning and assessment processes. The most recent Royal Commission into Aged Care Quality and Safety pointed out that supports for caregivers continue to be inadequate and often not available until the situation has hit crisis point (Commonwealth of Australia, 2021a, p. 103). This is an issue that has been acknowledged in numerous reviews and inquiries into aged care in recent years, though little meaningful change has been achieved at policy or practice levels to resolve it.

It is often difficult for families to engage with and navigate health and aged care systems, so the role of health professionals can be central to ensuring access to appropriate services and supports for older adults and their families. While formal services are very important in the provision of care to older adults, they essentially supplement informal care and provide a safety net for when this is no longer available or sufficient. It is therefore crucial that formal and informal supports work together for the benefit of the person receiving care.

Bronfenbrenner's ecological systems theory is discussed comprehensively in Chapter 4. See in particular Figure 4.1.

A useful way to conceptualise the many layers of the care system is with Bronfenbrenner's ecological systems theory, which encourages health professionals to understand people in their social environment.

Thinking about individuals as part of their broader context can help health professionals identify potential supports and risks for both the older person and their caregiver/s. It also encourages consideration of the role social systems play in contributing to individual and community well-being. Systems approaches recognise that environmental elements cannot be separated from one another, so impacts on one part of the system may subsequently put pressure on another part. This is important to keep in mind as situations evolve for an individual and their family navigating changing care needs.

An example of these impacts through different parts of the care system is evident in policy shifts towards greater independence and choice for older Australians. This shift provides benefits at the level of government expenditure and places greater emphasis on individual autonomy. A consequence of this, however, is a shift in the burden of caring to individuals and families. This demonstrates how a shift at a macro level of the aged care system can affect multiple levels, creating autonomy for older adults while potentially conflicting with the needs and best interests of their caregivers.

The systems approach also views problems as arising from a poor fit between a person and their environment. This provides practitioners with opportunities to explore how existing systems may need to be altered or how identifying potential new supports can adapt a system to better suit an individual's care and support needs.

Conclusion

This chapter has discussed informal care as being central to the experience of ageing for older Australians. Familial care has long been the primary source of care for older adults, with the unpaid work of family caregivers underpinning the success of community-based care. There can be many rewards and benefits inherent in the provision of family-based care, though it is important to acknowledge the extensive research that demonstrates significant risks to the health and well-being of informal caregivers.

Throughout this chapter, you have been encouraged to consider the impact of social, political and family contexts on the availability and provision of support to older adults. The evolving and changing nature of these contextual factors requires health and aged care professionals to maintain an active awareness of their effects on client groups, on family caregivers and on professional practice.

It is also important to continue to reflect on and critically challenge your own personal views and responses to these contextual changes. The journey of a health professional is one of continuing personal and professional development, with critical reflection being key to safe and effective practice with older adults and their caregivers.

The complexity and diversity of individual and family situations is an important consideration for health and aged care practitioners, as are the changing social demographics that will influence the availability of informal caregivers in the future. Considering older adults within their social and family environments enables health professionals to meaningfully consider these contexts of care.

Learn more
Access additional resources – such as weblinks, further readings and podcasts – to broaden your understanding of this chapter. See the Guided Tour for access details.

1   Consider the impact that changing family dynamics has on older adults and informal caregivers. How do cultural and social diversity influence expectations of familial care?

2   How does the complex and diverse nature of family relationships impact an individual's experience of ageing?

3   List both the opportunities and barriers to healthy ageing caused by social determinants of health.

4   Identify the significant risks to the health and well-being of families and caregivers of older adults, including spousal caregiving and co-dependence in older couples.

5   Explain why assessment and practice with older adults should take place within a family and social context.

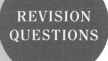

REVISION QUESTIONS

REFERENCES

Australian Bureau of Statistics (ABS) (2018). Disability, Ageing and Carers, Australia: Summary of findings. Table: Primary carers, reasons for taking on caring role by relationship to main recipient of care 2018. www.abs.gov.au/statistics/health/disability/disability-ageing-and-carers-australia-summary-findings/latest-release#carers

Australian Bureau of Statistics (ABS) (2020). Australian Migration Statistics, April. www.abs.gov.au/statistics/people/population/migration-australia/2018-19

Australian Institute of Health and Welfare (AIHW) (2018). Older Australia at a Glance.

Cat. no. AGE 87. AIHW. www.aihw.gov.au/reports/older-people/older-australia-at-a-glance

Australian Institute of Health and Welfare (AIHW) (2019). Australia's welfare 2019: Data insights. Australia's welfare series no. 14. Cat. no. AUS 226. AIHW.

Australian Institute of Health and Welfare (AIHW) (2020). Australia's Health 2020: In brief. Australia's health series no. 17. Cat. no. AUS 232. AIHW.

Bauer, J. M. & Sousa-Poza, A. (2015). Impacts of informal caregiving on caregiver employment, health, and family. *Journal of Population Ageing, 8*(3), 113–45. https://

doi:10.1007/s12062-015-9116-0

Bittman, M., Hill, T. & Thomson, C. (2007). The impact of caring on informal carers' employment, income and earnings: A longitudinal approach. *Australian Journal of Social Issues, 42*(2), 255–72.

Brimblecombe, N., Fernández, J., Knapp, M., Rehill, A. & Wittenberg, R. (2018). Review of the international evidence on support for unpaid carers, *Journal of Long-term Care, 1*(1), 25–40.

Burridge, L., Winch, S. & Clavarino, A. (2007). Reluctance to care: A systematic review and development of a conceptual framework. *Cancer Nursing, 30*(2), 9–19. https://doi:10.1097/01. NCC.0000265298.17394.e0

Butler, S. S., Turner, W., Kaye, L. W., Ruffin, L. & Downey, R. (2005). Depression and caregiver burden among rural elder caregivers. *Journal of Gerontological Social Work, 46*(1), 47–63.

Butterworth, P., Pymont, C., Rodgers, B., Windsor, T. D. & Anstey, K. J. (2009). Factors that explain the poorer mental health of caregivers: Results from a community survey of older Australians. *Australian and New Zealand Journal of Psychiatry, 44*(7), 616–24. https://doi:10.3109/00048671 003620202

Cash, B., Hodgkin, S. & Warburton, J. (2013). Till death us do part? A critical analysis of obligation and choice for spousal caregivers. *Journal of Gerontological Social Work, 56*(8), 657–74. https://doi:10.1080/01634372.201 3.823472

Cash, B., Hodgkin, S. & Warburton, J. (2016). Practitioners' perspectives on choice for older spousal caregivers in rural areas. *Australian Social Work, 69*(3), 283–96.

Cash, B., Warburton, J. & Hodgkin, S. (2019). Expectations of care within marriage for older couples. *Australasian Journal on Ageing, 38*(1), E19-E24.

Commonwealth of Australia (2021a). Royal Commission into Aged Care Quality and Safety. Final report: Care, dignity and respect. Vol. 1, Summary and recommendations. https:// agedcare.royalcommission. gov.au/sites/default/ files/2021-03/final-report-volume-1_0.pdf.

Commonwealth of Australia (2021b). 2021 Intergenerational Report: Australia over the next 40 years.

Deloitte Access Economics (2020). The Value of Informal Care in 2020. Deloitte Access Economics, Report for Carers Australia. www2.deloitte.

com/au/en/pages/economics/ articles/value-of-informal-care-2020.html

Department of Health (n.d.). National Continence Program. www.health.gov.au/initiatives-and-programs/national-continence-program-ncp

Fine, M. & Davidson, B. (2018). The marketization of care: Global challenges and national responses in Australia. *Current Sociological Monograph. 66*(4), 503–16.

Hartke, R. J., King, R. B., Heinemann, A. W. & Semik, P. (2006). Accidents in older caregivers of persons surviving stroke and their relation to caregiver stress. *Rehabilitation Psychology, 51*(2), 150–6. https://doi:10.1037/0090-5550.51.2.150

Hirst, M. (2005). Carer distress: A prospective, population-based study. *Social Science & Medicine, 61*(3), 697–708. https://doi:10.1016/j. socscimed.2005.01.001

Hughes, M. & Heycox, K. (2010). *Older People, Ageing and Social Work: Knowledge for Practice*. Allen & Unwin.

Joosten, M., Vrantsidis, F. & Dow, B. (2017). Understanding elder abuse: A scoping study. University of Melbourne and the National Ageing Research Institute. https:// socialequity.unimelb.edu. au/__data/assets/pdf_ file/0011/2777924/Elder-Abuse-A-Scoping-Study.pdf

Marmot, M. (2015). *The Health Gap: The challenge of an unequal world.* Bloomsbury.

McDonald, P. (2017). Population ageing: A demographic perspective. In K. O'Loughlin, C. Browning & H. Kendig (eds). *Ageing in Australia: Challenges and Opportunities.* Springer.

Mohanty, I. & Niyonsenga, T. (2019). A longitudinal analysis of mental and general health status of informal carers in Australia. *BMC Public Health. 19*, 1436.

Productivity Commission (2011). Caring for Older Australians: Overview. Report no. 53. Final Inquiry Report.

Productivity Commission. www.pc.gov.au/inquiries/ completed/aged-care/report/ aged-care-overview-booklet. pdf

Rummery, K. & Fine, M. (2012). Care: A critical review of theory, policy and practice. *Social Policy & Administration, 46*(3), 321–43. https:// doi:10.1111/j.1467-9515.2012.00845.x

Schofield, D., Cunich, M., Shrestha, R., Passey, M., Kelly, S., Tanton, R. & Veerman, L. (2014). The impact of chronic conditions of care recipients on the labour force participation of informal carers in Australia: Which conditions are associated with higher rates of non-participation in the labour force? *BMC Public Health, 14*(1). https://doi. org/10.1186/1471-2458-14-561

Shu, C. C., Cumming, R. G., Kendig, H. L., Blyth, F. M., Waite, L. M., Le Couteur, D. G., Handelsman, D. J. & Naganathan, V. (2017). Health status, health behaviours and anxiety symptoms of older male caregivers: Findings from the Concord Health and Ageing in Men Project. *Australasian Journal on Ageing, 36*, 151–7. https://doi.org/10.1111/ ajag.12376

Temple, J. & Dow, B. (2018). The unmet support needs of carers of older Australians: Prevalence and mental health. *International Psychogeriatrics. 30*(12), 1849–60.

Timonen, V., Conlon, C., Scharf, T. & Carney, G. (2013). Family, state, class and solidarity: Re-conceptualising intergenerational solidarity through the grounded theory approach. *European Journal of Ageing, 10*(3), 171–9. https:// doi:10.1007/s10433-013-0272-x

World Health Organization (WHO) (2015). Supporting Informal Caregivers of People Living with Dementia. WHO.

World Health Organization (WHO) (2018). Elder Abuse. Ageing and life-course. WHO.

6

Ageing in Rural Areas: Embracing Diversity

KAREN BELL AND SABINE WARDLE

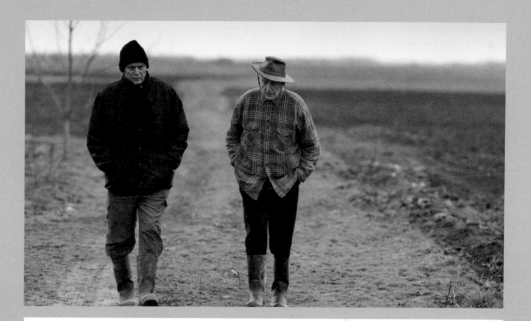

LEARNING OBJECTIVES

After reading this chapter, you will:

» describe ageing as normal yet contextual, individual and multidimensional by nature

» conclude that social justice and human rights are central to the experience of healthy ageing

» define what the terms 'rural', 'regional' and 'remote' mean in the Australian context and examine the heterogenous nature of rurality, regionality and remoteness

» contrast some positives and challenges of rurality including the nature of informal and formal care as well as service delivery models

» compare and contrast the biopsychosocial and biomedical models around ageing

» examine how health professionals require interprofessional communication and multidisciplinary approaches to:

    – healthy ageing

    – transition to residential care

    – culturally safe care

    – supporting those in caring roles

    – the management of trauma and crisis.

Introduction

This chapter uses two personal case studies to explore different aspects of ageing in rural areas. One story focuses on Harpreet Kaur (Preet), an immigrant Punjabi Indian woman for whom others are increasingly concerned; and the other on Aurora, a capable woman in her seventies who suddenly finds herself in challenging circumstances.

Learn more
Watch Video 6.1:
Preet talks about the
challenges of living in
rural Australia.

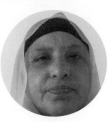

6.1 Getting to know the person: Harpreet Kaur's story

Harpreet Kaur, aged 78, is sitting on a low-back armchair in her son Sunny's home in a rural Australian town. As she looks out the window admiring the peace and tranquillity of the eucalypts swaying in the breeze, she feels the loss of her husband, Surjit, who died almost 40 years ago. A mixture of emotions and memories arise upon reflection that she was left to raise their two children alone in India.

Back then it was necessary for her to work, so she worked as an office manager in the Indian public service. Thinking about her co-workers and clients all speaking Punjabi warmed her heart and she smiled, just a little. They had called her 'Preet'. There was no one here to speak her local, regional language with, nor any need to read or write it either. Those were difficult years, but also ones filled with purpose and activity. Then, as per the Indian Government retirement policies, she had to accept compulsory retirement at the age of 58. Her smile faded. For the past 20 years she had not been as happy; she had felt restless and useless. It gave her some satisfaction to know that her hard work and savings had made it possible for her to pay for her children's education. She was very proud of her son, Sunny, who is an engineer and her daughter, Seerat, a medical doctor.

Looking around the lounge room, Preet thought about the house in India that she bought with her husband. This Australian house was so very different, fancy, new. In India, she had lived happily with Sunny and his wife Sonia. There she had loved cooking nice vegetarian meals for her family. It was wonderful having Seerat live only one hour away with her husband. They could visit every weekend. The memories of visitors brought back precious moments with extended family and friends who also lived nearby. Her heart swelled with the feelings of connectedness. But she shook her head with sadness because she had always assumed she would remain in her much-loved home for the last phase of her life. The sadness grew as she missed her Sikh community in India. Her heart sank at the thought that all her superannuation payments had been used to pay off the remaining debts on her much-loved house in India, and also for Seerat's wedding.

All of that was lost in 2009, when Sunny, Sonia and their newly born son, Ansh, migrated to Australia to pursue better career opportunities. She had tried to remain in her home in India, but being alone was very difficult and lonely. After a couple of years of waiting, she had been able to join her son's family in Australia. As she struggles to get out of the chair to make herself a cup of *chaa* (tea), she murmurs, 'I am so grateful to be able to see my son and his family, but I wonder how long before I could see Seerat?'

6.2 Getting to know the person: Aurora's story

As Aurora sips her first cup of tea for the day, sitting on her shady veranda admiring her verdant garden, she thinks about her partner, Chris. Chris died almost two years ago. They had moved to Smalltown (population about 9000) from the city when they were in their thirties. Aurora's family had not supported the relationship between her and Chris and had cut off all contact once they had moved out of the city. Chris was all the 'family' Aurora felt she had. She and Chris had worked so hard to build their mud-brick house, plant their orchard and develop their vegetable patch. They had both enjoyed scouring local tips, demolition sites, second-hand shops and recycling yards to source building materials. Chris had taken up leadlighting, so most of the windows in the house are original designs crafted by Chris. Their hard work over the years meant that they had been largely self-sufficient for much of their fresh food. What they could not grow they would usually try to barter from other eco-friendly producers in the area. The garden is a lot of work for Aurora now she is alone, but some of her friends and neighbours help out from time to time in exchange for fruit, vegetables and eggs.

This particular morning, Aurora is recovering from her seventy-fourth birthday party; it wasn't a huge party in terms of the number of guests, but the 35 or so people who did attend were quite exuberant and really wanted to celebrate Aurora's life. She has been scrolling through photos on her phone, taken the night before, and these photos make her smile. There had been many speeches about her artistic endeavours, her community work and her dedication to the local pioneer women's museum. Aurora and Chris had been instrumental in establishing and then maintaining the museum; they had used their links with women's groups in the city to gather artefacts and stories of women's lives.

Aurora really misses Chris; she visits the cemetery most weekends to ensure there are always flowers from the garden on the grave. The local council does a good job maintaining the cemetery grounds; it's a peaceful place with picturesque views of the surrounding hills and valleys.

Learn more
Watch Video 1.1: To assist your thinking about rural issues, listen to Ray's comments.

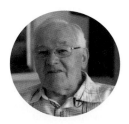

KAREN BELL AND SABINE WARDLE

Although we have only just been introduced to Preet and Aurora, their respective situations raise quite a few issues about the broader context of ageing. Before we learn even more about Preet's and Aurora's circumstances, and before practice issues are discussed, it is important to consider some basic demographics about ageing and diversity in contemporary Australia.

The context and diversity of ageing

cultural diversity
Having a mix of people from different cultural backgrounds (Diversity Council of Australia (DCA)).

culturally appropriate care
More than just awareness of cultural differences, this focuses on the capacity of the health system to improve health and well-being by integrating culture into the delivery of health-care services.

culturally safe residential aged care
A concept that aims to ensure service users of a different cultural background from the caregiver/ practitioner can feel safe in their experience of care; where there is no assault, challenge or denial of identity of who they are and what they need.

You will find more detail about the experience of ageing for First Nations peoples in Chapter 3 and more information about cultural traditions and family backgrounds in Chapter 5.

The Australian Bureau of Statistics (ABS) defines 'older person' as someone aged 65 years and over (ABS, 2018a). More than a century ago, the proportion of older people in the population was 4 per cent; now, older people make up 15.9 per cent of the total population, which equates to one in every six people. The growth in the proportion of older people has been steadily increasing over the years, with a 35 per cent increase in the number of older people in the years between 2009 and 2018 (ABS, 2018a).

While First Nations peoples make up 2.8 per cent of Australia's total population, they comprise just 1.5 per cent of older people, reflecting the lower life expectancy of this population group (ABS, 2018b). Australians born overseas make up 24 per cent of the general population and 36 per cent of the population aged 65 years and over. The majority of older people born overseas are from non–English speaking countries, with two in 10 still predominantly speaking a language other than English (AIHW, 2018). This **cultural diversity** reflects Australia's migration patterns since the late 1940s (ABS, 2018b).

In terms of aged care services, 25.7 per cent of all recipients of home care services in 2018–19 were from culturally diverse backgrounds. In general, older people from culturally and linguistically diverse (CALD) backgrounds have a relatively lower socio-economic status and may face language barriers in accessing the care services they need (FECCA, 2015, p. 87). One of the challenges of ensuring the provision of **culturally appropriate care** is the changing make-up of the migration population. People from CALD communities may also find it difficult to be seen, heard and understood (Commonwealth of Australia, 2019, p. 114).

Language and cultural barriers are common, and misunderstandings between staff and residents further complicate the transition into **culturally safe residential aged care** (FECCA, 2015, p. 10). Indeed, the Australian Government's Royal Commission into Aged Care Quality and Safety heard evidence to indicate that while aged care providers are able to access cost-free translation and interpretation services for people from culturally and linguistically diverse backgrounds, this does not extend to First Nations languages (Commonwealth of Australia, 2019, p. 175).

Ageing and disease should not be equated and, while ageing does increase our vulnerability to a range of biopsychosocial issues, significant disability is not inevitable (Sinclair & LaPlante, 2019). Of all people aged 65 years and over, 49.6 per cent experience disability. The majority of older people (95.3%) live in households, while 4.6 per cent live in care accommodation. Of those living in households, two-thirds report having a level of disability significant enough to require some assistance with activities of daily living (ABS, 2018a).

Perspectives on ageing

The following section outlines two different models of assessing older people. The aim is to provide you with an understanding of the various paradigms that underpin the models and why there may be disparity in different approaches used by health professionals from a variety of disciplines.

MEDICAL MODEL

Sometimes referred to as the biomedical model, or biomedicine, the medical model still dominates medical practice. It focuses on biological determinants of disease such as pathogens and dysfunctions of bodily organs. It is narrowly focused on individual deficits and emphasises diagnosis, treatment and cure (Havelka et al., 2009; Munford & Bennie, 2013). Unwell people are defined as 'patients' and a 'good patient' is a passive, compliant individual. The model comes from a positivist paradigm and relies on observed clinical data as a basis for individual diagnosis and treatment (Beddoe, 2013). The model certainly has an important place in healthcare, but it also has some significant limitations. The medical model emphasises biological aspects of health, but not psychological and broader social factors influencing the health of individuals, groups, communities and wider populations.

Within the medical model, health professionals are organised hierarchically, with specialist medical doctors at the top, followed by general medical practitioners, then nurses and then a range of allied health professionals (occupational therapists, speech therapists, social workers, psychologists, physiotherapists). While professional collaboration may be valued, control of the treatment team and of 'patients' is still the medical doctor's terrain (Beddoe, 2013).

Not only does the medical model influence how people's situations are viewed, but it also has impacts at broader levels such as funding and service provision. For instance, health and welfare services were traditionally delivered for the most part through large institutions. Institutional care is very expensive compared to community and alternative forms of care. As broader perspectives on health and welfare have gained influence, approaches to service delivery have likewise broadened to include a larger proportion of services providing care in the community rather than in institutional settings such as hospitals and residential aged care facilities (Beddoe, 2013). There will always be a need for some level of institutional care in health and welfare, but ideally, there should be a mix and a range of services available to meet a variety of health and social needs. Indeed, the World Health Organization (WHO, 2013) advocates a continued shift from the 'disease and deficit' model of healthcare to a biopsychosocial model, with policy priorities in health and welfare, sustainability, wellness, prevention and primary healthcare (Burnham, 2014).

THE BIOPSYCHOSOCIAL MODEL

The biopsychosocial model recognises the social determinants of health and well-being and constructs 'health' as 'interplay between environment, physical, behavioural, psychological, and social factors' (Beddoe, 2013, p. 25). Biological factors include physical factors such as disease, disorders, genetics, nutrition, medication, musculoskeletal issues and physiological factors. Psychological factors include emotions, cognition, anxiety, stress and memory. Social factors include family relationships, group membership, community involvement and connections, income, education, housing, employment, life experiences, loss and grief, gender,

KAREN BELL AND SABINE WARDLE

and culture. These interdependent and interrelated factors are also situated within the broader context of the natural environment. Factors such as pollution, sustainability, climate change, clean air, fresh water, fertile soil and natural disasters also have an impact in various ways on the biological, psychological and social aspects of human experience (Heinsch, 2012).

For example, the biopsychosocial model can be applied to the case of a person with short-term memory loss. The person may be assessed and diagnosed as having dementia, with some of the biological factors contributing to dementia being understood (genetic factors and cardiovascular factors, for example). The disease of dementia then has impacts on the individual at the psychological level (e.g. frustration, personality, memory loss and changes in cognitive ability). There will also be social impacts of the disease on the person's partner, family, friends, employment and community engagement. In terms of the natural environment, at an individual level, a person with advanced dementia might find being in nature or being able to look out at nature soothing. At a broader level, all people benefit from a clean, safe, natural environment. Figure 6.1 is a graphic representation using the biopsychosocial model of a person with dementia.

See Chapter 4 for information on Bronfenbrenner's ecological systems theory.

FIGURE 6.1 A biopsychosocial model of a person with dementia

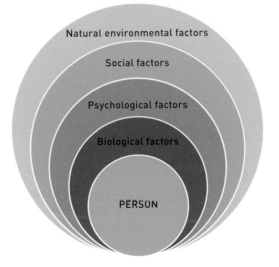

Ageing as a continuum

As highlighted by the different experiences of ageing outlined in the case studies so far, ageing is a dynamic, lifelong process shaped by biopsychosocial, environmental, locational, political and cultural processes (Hughes & Heycox, 2010). Hughes and Heycox (2010) advocate a 'life course' approach to ageing, whereby experiences of ageing are seen in the context of a person's whole life and their past experiences; ageing is not viewed as a disconnected or diseased/abnormal state, but instead is part of normal human experience. Some say that 'old age' covers the biological age from 40 years of age and that most health and welfare services focus on the later phases of old age – 'old-old' age – 85 years and over (Naughtin & Schofield, 2013, p. 207).

Hughes and Heycox (2010, pp. 31–5) also discuss phases of ageing including:
- the 'sandwich generation' (40–60 years)
- the 'young-old' (over 60 to 74 years)

- the 'old-old' (over 74 to 85 years)
- the 'old-old-old' (over 85 years).

During the mid-life years (the forties and fifties), many people find themselves 'sandwiched' between caring for their own (and/or others') children as well as taking on caring roles in relation to ageing parents. Around 13 per cent of all parents living in a family with children under 15 provide unpaid care to a person because of a disability, long-term illness or issues related to old age (ABS, 2009) These multilayered caring roles, combined with the demands of other unpaid and paid work, can create stress for the 'sandwich generation'.

The proportion of 'old-old-old' people in Australia's population has tripled in the past 100 years and 63 per cent of those aged 85 years and over are women. In 2017, 497 000 (13%, or 0.5 million) older people were aged 85 and over. By 2047, it is projected that one in five older people will be aged 85 and over (20%, or 1.5 million) (AIHW, 2018). In the 'old old' population, 18.5 per cent of the 80 and over population living in Australia were born in non–English speaking countries (FECCA, 2015, p. 6).

This lifespan or life-course approach fits well with the biopsychosocial model of care in that it positions ageing as a normal part of human life affected by social, political, environmental, cultural and economic factors. 'Older people' as a population category are also very diverse in terms of life experiences, health status, lifestyle and cultural background (Naughtin & Schofield, 2013). In some cultures, older people are regarded with increased respect and have greater community expectations placed on them as providers of guidance and wisdom to younger community members (Martin, 2014).

Let's return to the case studies to explore some of these issues in more detail. As you read the next instalments in Preet's and Aurora's lives, try to use a life-course approach and think about the biopsychosocial aspects of each situation, as well as the environmental, locational and political elements of each situation. The framework illustrated in Figure 6.2 might assist you to view each scenario holistically; it is based on Healy's (2014) framework for social work practice. It draws on early social work theory (Richmond, 1917) about the 'person-in-environment' perspective as well as the 'first wave' of general systems theory (Von Bertalanffy, 1968), and 'second wave' ecosystems perspectives (e.g. Meyer, 1976 and Bronfenbrenner, 1979, as cited in Healy, 2014). Figure 6.2 is a framework for understanding the personal stories as they become more complex.

FIGURE 6.2 Framework for understanding the continuing personal stories

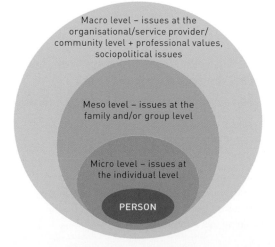

KAREN BELL AND SABINE WARDLE

6.3 Getting to know the person: Preet's story

When Preet came to Australia to live with Sunny, his wife Sonia and their young son Ansh in rural New South Wales, she knew that her son believed the move was a sensible decision. She knew he was always worried about her living on her own in India.

Although she would have preferred not to spend the last phase of her life in a 'foreign' land, she also knew she could not accept ongoing assistance from her married daughter. Her deep-rooted cultural traditions made the move to Australia more of a need than a desire.

In spite of this understanding, she often felt very sad and homesick for India; she missed her daughter, Seerat, as well as close family and friends. Mostly, she missed conversations in Punjabi: the flow, the ease, the words that meant how she felt. Although she could speak a bit of English, she is not confident about speaking in English. She would like to be able to talk with others, but it takes a lot of effort. Just understanding what people are saying is hard work. If people make the effort to speak slowly and clearly, she can understand a few words. Mostly, she makes effective use of body language and other forms of non-verbal communication to get her message across.

When Preet first moved in with Sunny and Sonia, she was very independent and did not need any help with activities of daily living. As she loved cooking and had always cooked for her family, Sunny expected that his mother would do a lot of cooking for his family in Australia. But this has not transpired, primarily because she always relied on local *rickshaws* (three-wheeled passenger carts) to commute to food markets and shops in India and never felt the need to hold a driver's licence. Now, she does not often venture far from the house, except for short walks in the local neighbourhood.

Recently, she heard about the Sikh prayer meetings held once a month at the local community centre by a handful of local people from the Sikh faith. She has enjoyed attending the prayer meetings with her family, who also try to provide her with opportunities to chat with people within the Sikh community. Most days, however, are very quiet for Preet; other than playing with her grandson, she generally stays in her bedroom.

See Chapter 5 for more information about cultural traditions and family backgrounds.

FOCUS QUESTIONS

- Brainstorm the micro-, meso- and macro-level issues in Preet's situation. Were you able to identify at least three issues at each of these levels?

- Did you find one or other level of analysis more challenging? If so, why do you think that might be?

- What are some of the strengths, positives and potential resources, as far as you can tell at this stage in this situation?

- Based on the information in the chapter and Video 6.1, do you have any particular concerns about Preet? If you were involved with Preet on a professional level, what sort of additional information would you need to assess the situation more thoroughly? How might you go about gaining this information?

- If this individual and family happened to be First Nations peoples, how might this influence the situation?

6.4 Getting to know the person: Aurora's story

Aurora still earns a steady income from the art and craft gallery she established and continues to run in the main street of Smalltown. She runs the gallery as a cooperative and this collective approach to the business helps to support a range of local artists. She sells most of her own handmade silver jewellery, paintings and sculptures through the gallery, but also has a growing online business. She's also part of the newly formed local branch of 'Seniors Creating Change' and is about to start filming a clip for YouTube.

As Aurora finishes her cup of tea, she decides she'd better feed the chickens, as they're used to being fed much earlier in the morning. As she fills the chickens' feeding tray with vegetable scraps left over from the party, some of the new chickens she recently received escape the enclosure. Aurora's old dog Blanche is usually uninterested in the chickens, but the fuss the escapees are creating has attracted her attention and she starts to chase them around the backyard. Aurora is worried that Blanche might harm the chickens. She yells at Blanche to stop, but the dog is very excited by the commotion, ignores Aurora and continues to run after the chickens. Aurora runs after Blanche, knowing that if she can reach her, she will soon settle her down and get the chickens back to their yard. As Aurora pursues the dog, she slips over, hitting her head.

- Brainstorm the micro-, meso- and macro-level issues in Aurora's situation. Were you able to identify at least a few issues at each of these levels?

- Did you find one or other level of analysis more challenging? If so, why do you think that might be?

- What are some of the strengths, positives and potential resources, as far as you can tell at this stage in this situation?

- If you assume Aurora is a First Nations Australian, how might this influence the situation? What are some of the loss/grief and change issues in this scenario?

- How might a crisis such as a traumatic injury impact Aurora's life?

FOCUS QUESTIONS

Rural context

Since the 1950s, aged care service delivery has changed from a system based largely on the medical model whereby care services were predominantly delivered via large residential institutions to a system where the bulk of care is delivered at a community and home-based level.

KAREN BELL AND SABINE WARDLE

Indeed, a 'relatively small proportion of older adults seek services from community agencies' and most human services practitioners (such as nurses, doctors and social workers) often only interact with the minority of older people who need significant external support for complex care needs such as chronic disease, disability, dementia, practical issues or loss (Chenoweth & McAuliffe, 2021, pp. 178–9). Services to older people are delivered by government, commercial and not-for-profit entities (Naughtin & Schofield, 2013).

Community expectations about aged care in contemporary Australia also reflect the growing visibility, cultural diversity and political power of older people and human-rights-based arguments for policy reform. In short, people expect to have a reasonable choice of and access to decent services; they prefer community care and participate in aged care as active citizens rather than as dependants (Giles et al., 2010).

Other factors influence the provision of aged care in Australia. Along with shifts in community expectations, there is a necessity to contain costs in the sector. Traditional approaches to aged care involving institutional, residential and hospital care are also very costly. Community-based, primary-health-care approaches emphasise health education, prevention and chronic disease management, and reduce the need for and reliance on high-cost acute care (Giles et al., 2010).

In regional and rural areas, there are generally not enough aged-care services. This is particularly the case in smaller rural towns (Bernoth et al., 2012). This often means that people from farms and small rural towns are forced to travel long distances to access the aged care services they need. For some people, this could mean a journey of five hours or more to reach the required service (Bernoth et al., 2012). The need to travel long distances is another disadvantage for older people seeking healthcare in regional and remote locations (Gardiner et al., 2019). Bernoth, Dietsch and Davies (2012) explored the distress this causes to older people, their partners, families and their communities as people are disconnected from their home and familiar networks.

In addition, the final report of the Royal Commission into Aged Care Quality and Safety (Commonwealth of Australia, 2021, p. 71) notes that people in regional and remote locations often have to wait longer for the services they need, especially residential aged care. There is also emerging evidence that in the current aged care system people in non-metropolitan areas seeking home care packages are also waiting longer to receive support (Commonwealth of Australia, 2021, p. 71).

These locational disadvantages are significant enough, but when you consider that most rural areas also experience higher fuel prices, poorer roads and lack of public transport options, the degree of cumulative disadvantage is exacerbated (Baldwin et al., 2013; Commonwealth of Australia, 2019, p. 184). These locational disadvantages are typically experienced to an even greater degree by people living in remote locations.

RURAL PRACTICE ISSUES

Australia has a highly urbanised population, with 71 per cent of all Australians living in major urban areas. In terms of older Australians, people aged 65 years and over are less likely to live in urban areas, with 24 per cent in smaller cities and towns, and 8.5 per cent in rural areas (ABS, 2018a). This concentration of the population in major urban areas often means that service delivery models are developed to suit this majority. Sometimes the dominant models of service delivery do not effectively translate to smaller towns, rural areas and remote settings. As a result, these areas continue to experience a relative

You can find more information about policy in Chapter 2 and more detail about the experience of ageing for First Nations peoples in Chapter 3.

disadvantage compared to the metropolitan areas (Massey & Parr, 2012, p. 15). This population distribution also affects the availability of skilled health-care providers in non-metropolitan areas, with rural and regional service providers often finding it difficult to attract skilled workers, including qualified interpreters (Commonwealth of Australia, 2019, p. 186). In small towns with a growing number of migrant populations, health providers can find it challenging to overcome language and cultural differences (Wardle & Mungai, 2018). Structural forces such as funding and resourcing are the contributing factors for the compromised psychosocial care in rural locations (Johns et al., 2019).

6.5 Getting to know the person: Preet's story

Preet has recently received terrible news. She has been diagnosed with breast cancer. Many people explained her condition to her, but all she knew was that she was going to die. The inevitability and despair are a weight she is struggling to carry. She tries very hard not to let anyone see her tears and sadness. But she knows Sunny worries about her care and wants to spend more time with her. He often takes days off work to drive her to medical appointments. When the appointments are in the city, he has to take additional time off work. Preet also cringes at the expense of accommodation while they are in the city.

Sonia tries to help with the local medical appointments when she's not taking care of Ansh. A Punjabi interpreter is needed at every medical appointment, and often Sunny or Sonia help Preet convey her message by interpreting for her. This embarrasses and frustrates her because she has always been an independent woman and managed to deal with the major challenges of her life on her own. She doesn't like relying on other people.

Lately, she hates that she needs help with a range of everyday activities such as going to the toilet, showering and getting dressed. It feels like another layer of humiliation.

One evening, she overhears a conversation between Sonia and Sunny. They are worried that Preet can no longer safely manage her daily routine in their rental house. They also worry about the options for long-term care as the local town has only low-care, independent-living aged care facilities. If Preet is not suitable for this type of care, she would have to relocate to the regional city, some two hours away. She returns to her room and cries herself to sleep.

This conversation causes her to be reluctant to attend check-ups with the local general practitioner (GP) and the specialist in the nearest regional city for her cancer treatment. When Sunny visits the local GP with her for her regular health check, the doctor has a lot to say, and his voice is sad and urgent. She's not sure she wants to hear all of what he has to say. Her son doesn't interpret the rest of the doctor's words.

The GP indicates concern about Preet and asks whether the palliative care team should assess the situation. Sunny seems confused about 'palliative care'. But at the same time, he appreciates the doctor's concern for Preet's well-being. Sunny wonders how he will explain palliative care to his mother and how he will persuade her to see someone from the palliative care team.

See Chapter 19 for more information about palliative care.

FOCUS QUESTIONS

- What are some of the political and community-level issues at this stage?
- How is Preet's rural location a potential disadvantage to her in the circumstances?

6.6 Getting to know the person: Aurora's story

Aurora is awakened by Blanche licking her face and nudging her. She isn't sure how long she's been on the ground, but her head and neck really hurt. After taking a few more moments to regain her senses, she tries to get up – it's not going to do her any good to be out in the hot sun for much longer. As she tries to move her arms to support herself, she feels a stabbing pain in her right wrist and fears it is broken. She manages to manoeuvre onto her side but, as she rolls over, she experiences a sharp pain in her hip as well.

She calls out for help a few times in the hope that someone might hear, but she knows her neighbours' houses are too far away for them to hear her yelling. She had always enjoyed living on the big house block, but in this moment she's not so sure.

After quite some time, Aurora uses her 'good' arm to drag herself back to the veranda. Fortunately, her mobile phone is within reach and she calls her close friend, Sam, to come and help. Sam arrives about 10 minutes later and is shocked by how much pain Aurora is in. Sam also notices a swelling and a nasty bruise emerging on Aurora's forehead and calls the ambulance. Aurora is taken to Smalltown Multipurpose Health Centre. She's very worried: does she have some broken bones? Does she have osteoporosis just like her mother did? What if she's out of action for a long time: who will look after Blanche and the garden? The gallery? Who will upload the YouTube clip?

Once she arrives at the health facility and her injuries are assessed, she is asked in a loud voice, 'Do you still live at home, dear? Can we give your husband a call to let him know what's happened?'

heteronormativity
Consciously or subconsciously using heterosexuality as standard human behaviour, thereby leaving non-heterosexual peoples out of the frame of reference.

FOCUS QUESTIONS

- What are the stereotypes and attitudes being held by the health professionals?
- What assumptions are being made about Aurora's circumstances? For example, think about the **heteronormative** assumption underpinning the question about contacting Aurora's next of kin. In your reflection on Aurora's situation, had you assumed Aurora's partner Chris was a man?
- What would be the impact of these attitudes and stereotypes on Aurora?
- How might you avoid making assumptions about people's circumstances?

GEOGRAPHIC LOCATION

For older Australians, their geographic location is a major factor influencing the range of services on offer and access to services (Giles et al., 2010). Since the mid 1980s, the agricultural sector of Australia's economy has declined and this, in turn, has affected the range of health and welfare services in regional and rural areas (Alston, 2010). Services in such locations can be limited in scope, difficult to access, costly or simply unavailable (Commonwealth of Australia, 2019, p. 184).

Older people living in rural areas often experience cumulative disadvantage because of chronological age as well as geographic location. Despite the fact 'the further people live away from major cities, the less healthy they are likely to be', regional and rural areas typically have fewer health and welfare agencies and even fewer specialist agencies and primary care professionals (AIHW, 2018; Chenoweth & McAuliffe, 2021). This affects service users as well as service providers – not only does it restrict options for clients, but it also impacts the nature of service provision. Health and welfare practitioners in regional and rural areas often have to perform a wider range of professional duties to fill these service system gaps and meet client needs. This potentially means a more creative, tailored approach to professional practice, thereby benefitting clients as well as practitioners. There are practice opportunities for 'fly-in-fly-out' models of practice, telecommuting, video and online client consultation (Alston, 2010). There are, however, potential drawbacks to these opportunities, including difficulties in recruiting and retaining students, slow staff recruitment processes, turnover of staff, skills gaps, professional isolation, challenges to confidentiality, lack of anonymity and a lack of referral options, especially as the level of isolation and remoteness from major population centres increases (Chenoweth & McAuliffe, 2021).

Typically, in regional and rural areas, aged care services tend to be smaller in size compared to services in major urban centres. In major cities, 1.4 per cent of aged care facilities have 20 'beds', or fewer, while in regional and rural areas 47 per cent of aged care facilities accommodate 20 or fewer people (Baldwin et al., 2013). This has implications for service users and service providers: for service providers, smaller facilities can affect financial viability and sustainability, as funding is often based on economies of scale achievable only by larger service providers. It can also be more difficult to recruit and retain qualified, experienced staff (Bernoth et al., 2012).

Along with formal care provided by health and welfare services, informal sources of care have always been important elements of the aged care sector. Informal (unpaid) care is often provided by an older person's partner, family and/or friends. Despite the importance of informal care and support, the value of informal care and the idea of individual choice in informal caregiving has often been 'invisible' to policymakers (Cash et al., 2013; Pickard, 2010). Some key social changes have also affected people's capacity to provide significant levels of unpaid care to people in need. As mentioned in Chapter 5, these factors include an increase in the number of sole parent and sole person households, decreased fertility rate, increased numbers of women in paid work and increased geographic mobility. The current aged care system relies on informal carers self-identifying as 'carers' and knowing where to go for support. This makes it difficult for carers to access respite care and other support for themselves. Carers have also expressed concern about the complexity they encounter in the aged care service system; the inadequacy of financial support; limited access to support services (especially respite care); lack of flexibility in the paid workforce and lack of recognition of care responsibilities (especially for rural carers); and a need for greater access to technology and assistive devices (Commonwealth of Australia, 2021, pp. 66–7; Giles et al., 2010).

MULTIDISCIPLINARY APPROACHES TO PRACTICE

human rights
Individual and collective rights to food and shelter; rights that are inherent to being human, universal and indivisible.

multidimensional
Containing a number of different levels, including micro (individual), meso (family, group) and macro levels (community, policy, research).

multidisciplinary team
A team that includes professionals from a range of disciplines consisting of a group of experts whose goal is comprehensive patient-centred care.

A **human rights** approach to the health and welfare of older people underpins contemporary biopsychosocial approaches to human services practice. Service provision for older people is strengths based and emphasises social connectedness, client self-determination, inclusion, prevention, early intervention and community care. Most services aim to build on people's existing capabilities and resources to maximise client wellness and improve quality of life. To achieve these aims, a **multidimensional** approach is needed to holistically assess a person's situation and to implement an appropriate support plan (Giles et al., 2010). Ideally, an older person in need of health and welfare services would have a **multidisciplinary team** available to assess their needs, as well as a reasonable range of accessible services within their local community. This is a challenge in many metropolitan areas and particularly challenging in non-metropolitan areas.

Multidisciplinary teams in health-care settings are generally made up of nursing, medical and allied health professionals (Portsmouth et al., 2008). For multidisciplinary teams to work well, different professions must be able to work together respectfully and collegially *with* clients to best serve clients' needs (Martin, 2014). Indeed, the client and/or their family should be active team members in their own right. Hierarchical, competitive models of practice are not effective or efficient and are less likely to result in positive, multidimensional outcomes for clients and team members alike.

Implications for practice

As a member of a multidisciplinary team in a health-care setting, it is important for you to be aware that effective teamwork is achieved when team members appreciate their interdependence – a range of professional skill sets is needed to comprehensively assess and respond to clients' needs. Dominance or unwarranted over-reliance on one professional skill set is unlikely to produce satisfactory outcomes. Success within teams is achieved through mutual trust, collaboration, respect and open communication. Successful outcomes for clients, families and carers are more likely if the team's activity is comprehensive, coordinated, organised and integrated (Portsmouth et al., 2008).

> Indicators of effective communication in teams include shared power, autonomy, reciprocal and multidirectional communication between team members. Indicators of ineffective teamwork include hierarchical patterns of communication, dominance by one or two professional perspectives, authoritarian decision-making and exclusion of the client's perspective. Even in problematic teams, when clients' needs are explicitly discussed as central to the team's purpose, communication problems may quickly recede as common ground and an overall shared goal becomes the focus, rather than inter-professional competition.
>
> *Source:* Portsmouth, Coyle & Trede, 2008.

Portsmouth, Coyle and Trede (2008, p. 235) outline indicators of team functioning such as:

- *attendance:* who is at the meeting, and who is not?
- *exchange:* are there patterns in who speaks most? Who asks questions? Who answers questions? Are some professionals privileged at the expense of others?
- *perspective:* are some aspects of health discussed more than others? Are some aspects of health ignored, silenced or minimised?

Returning to Aurora's situation, what did you imagine or assume about Aurora's partner, Chris? Did you assume Aurora's partner was male – a heteronormative assumption? Are there other assumptions you made that would influence working with Aurora in her healing process? As a health-care professional on a multidisciplinary team, what unique skill set might you contribute to comprehensively assess and respond to her needs?

6.7 Getting to know the person: Aurora's story

Due to her injuries, Aurora is told she will need to spend quite a long time in hospital before she can be assessed by the discharge planner. If she recovers well enough, she might need some home nursing and support for a while. Aurora is worried she might be not be able to manage at home – there are quite a few stairs inside the house and she does have a large garden to care for. She couldn't bear to live anywhere else but at the place she and Chris built for themselves. Since Chris' death, the home is the only physical reminder of Chris – every time the sun shines through the leadlight, she feels Chris' presence. She worries about being forced into a nursing home – she's not ready for that yet! She gets a bit upset from time to time, but doesn't want to 'burden' her friends or the nursing staff with her concerns.

The nursing staff and ward attendants are usually very attentive and Aurora has a steady stream of visitors throughout her hospital stay. She worries a lot about Blanche and hopes the neighbours keep a good eye on the old dog while Aurora is not there. She would love to see Blanche – it would be a real tonic.

- Using a biopsychosocial approach, how might some of Aurora's needs be addressed? Specifically: her 'bio' needs are being addressed, but how might some of the psychosocial aspects of her well-being be improved?
- How might a multidisciplinary team approach this situation? Using Figure 6.3 and Aurora's story to guide you, brainstorm some of the issues a multidisciplinary team might consider in assessing Aurora's situation.

FOCUS QUESTIONS

FIGURE 6.3 Provision of care for Aurora using a multidisciplinary approach

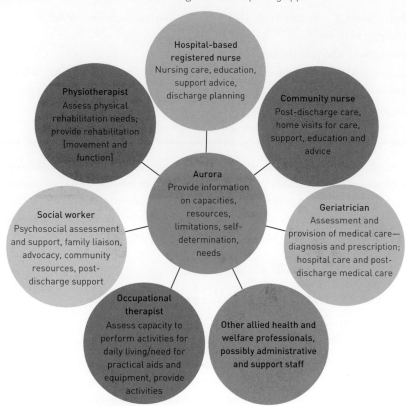

ETHICAL ISSUES IN PRACTICE

Using human rights, a biopsychosocial approach in aged care brings the principle of client self-determination into sharp focus. Professional practice for client self-determination involves respecting older people's autonomy and providing honest and accurate information about all aspects of care as well as alternatives, risks and options for care. Client self-determination can be challenging to operationalise for people experiencing an impaired capacity to act for themselves. In such cases, human services professionals should aim to maximise client self-determination, reduce barriers to disadvantage, reduce dependence and recognise the influence of a range of factors including age, disability, culture, past trauma and location (AASW, 2010).

The notion of 'risk' is another ethical consideration for practice: what is acceptable in terms of risk? For example, looking at Preet's case study, at what stage might the risks of Preet remaining in her son's house begin to outweigh the benefits of staying at home (such as her autonomy and her self-determination)? Is there a growing intolerance of risk? Is there such a thing as the dignity of risk?

ATTITUDES, ASSUMPTIONS AND POSITIONALITY IN PRACTICE

Along with a human rights approach to service provision and biopsychosocial models of practice, another important aspect of contemporary practice in aged care is reflective practice. How does who you are as a person influence how you think and act as a human service professional? How do your personal values and beliefs influence your practice on a day-to-day basis? How do your personal characteristics, experiences, beliefs and values 'fit' (or not) your professional code of ethics and/or your employer's code of conduct and also the client's situation (positionality)? Reflective practice in the context of ageing occurs when a professional consciously examines their own attitudes to ageing and ageism along with their own experiences of ageing (Hughes, 2013).

In Western societies, ageism and negative stereotypes about older people are all too common. The language we use, images in the media and a general preference for youthfulness over age all contribute to this negativity.

- Thinking about the two case studies, are there aspects of Preet's situation that reinforce some stereotypes about ageing?
- What do you think about Preet's regional location?

FOCUS QUESTIONS

6.8 Getting to know the person: Preet's story

Sonia had a gentle conversation with Preet to see if she'd ever considered moving out of their home so that she'd have more company and people could take more care of her. Preet responded quite decisively saying that it just 'wouldn't be right' to leave her family to be with strangers in a strange place.

Increasingly, Preet appears to be agitated and she complains a lot about being uncomfortable and unable to get a good night's sleep: 'I am worried someone will come to take me away in the night!'

Sunny and Sonia have more and more discussions about the situation and they try to think of alternatives to residential care for Preet – they really don't want to be responsible for moving her into an aged care or a palliative care facility if it's not absolutely necessary. They both have a fair idea of what's available in the local area, and know that the two community nurses are very, very busy. They wonder about home and community support services. They think that if Preet had someone to visit every once in a while, she would be safe and happy enough in their home for a while longer. They're keen to look after Preet at home for as long as they possibly can – they had made this promise to her family.

Sunny scours the internet, looking for private home care options – they're not well off, so they probably couldn't afford to pay someone. Nonetheless, in desperation Sunny telephones a couple of city-based private services. While they're sympathetic to the situation, they do not provide any rural outreach, nor do they know of any outreach rural service providers.

FOCUS QUESTIONS

- Using the reflective practice framework represented in Figure 6.4, identify your own values and beliefs about the Kaur family's situation. What might you do in the circumstances?
- Consider the ethical aspects of the situation: are there any ethical issues relating to professional practice with Preet and her family?
- Then, consider models of professional practice, perspectives on ageing and policy issues. How might this critical reflection affect your practice?

FIGURE 6.4 A reflective practice framework

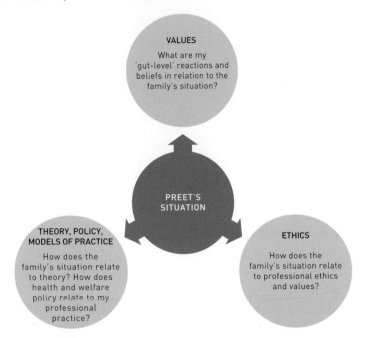

6.9 Getting to know the person: Aurora's story

After finding Aurora sobbing quietly to herself one day, one of the nurses asks her if she'd like to speak with a social worker in more depth about her situation. The nurse finds it frustrating that there's never enough time to sit with people and to comfort them, as there are always so many other people to care for on the ward. Aurora isn't keen to 'see a counsellor' at first, but eventually agrees that it can't do any real harm. She finds the social worker easy to talk to and she's able to discuss her current circumstances and plans to return home, along with how she's dealt with Chris' death.

Each day Aurora feels her strength returning and she increasingly feels she's closer to being discharged from hospital. Aurora can't wait to express her artistic urges once again – she's missed her creative pursuits terribly and, in some ways, this has been the most frustrating part of the whole experience.

The multidisciplinary team (the nursing staff, the social worker, the physiotherapist, the occupational therapist and the doctor) has discussed Aurora's case during team meetings and a discharge plan is emerging. Once the physiotherapist and occupational therapist are satisfied with Aurora's recovery, she can return to her home. The community nurse and social worker will provide some follow-up visits in the first few weeks after discharge.

Aurora is happy about the discharge plan and is confident that there's finally some light at the end of the tunnel.

See Chapter 11 for more information on discharge planning.

- How do you feel about the outcome in Aurora's situation?
- What ongoing issues might there be for Aurora?
- In what ways do you think the multidisciplinary team approach has been positive in this scenario?
- What else could have been done for Aurora to enhance her hospital stay, recovery and general well-being?

FOCUS QUESTIONS

Implications for practice

1   Encourage interprofessional communication and multidimensional approaches to practice with older people.
2   Encourage reflection on your own ageing, positionality, assumptions and stereotypes.
3   Encourage reflection on how biomedical **discourse** and biopsychosocial approaches differ and affect professional practice.
4   Encourage a strengths approach to practice and a thorough, holistic assessment of older people and their situations.
5   Appreciate the issues in rural service delivery.
6   Use tailored, dynamic and positive approaches to your practice rather than a generic approach.

discourse
Foundational ways of understanding the world and how these influence what we see, what we value and how we act.

Conclusion

In Australia, inland rural, regional and remote populations are dispersed over a large area, resulting in challenges to service delivery in health and welfare. Significant issues affecting aged care service delivery include urban-based policy and funding models, recruitment and retention of a skilled workforce, and often a scarcity of translators and interpreters. In addition, the medical model – or biomedical discourse – is still highly influential in framing

Learn more
Access additional resources – such as weblinks, further readings and podcasts – to broaden your understanding of this chapter. See the Guided Tour for access details.

the delivery of health and aged care services. The conventional biomedical discourse has a relatively narrow focus on individual disease, and it typically lacks focus on the broader psychosocial and environmental context. In contrast, the biopsychosocial model has a greater capacity to embrace diversity and holistically assess a situation, taking into account a more comprehensive range of factors such as culture, gender, age, religion and spirituality affecting individuals, groups, communities and organisations. Given the multidimensional nature of ageing with added complexities in rural, regional and remote locations, a multidimensional approach to service delivery is desirable. High-functioning multidisciplinary teams can assist people as they age in the community and in their transition to formal care when needed. The centrality of social justice and human rights – the basic tenets of professional practice – should not vary according to the field of practice, the client group or the location in which human service professionals are engaged.

REVISION QUESTIONS

1 What are some of the potential benefits and drawbacks for older people living in non-metropolitan areas?

2 How does a multidimensional approach to working with older people in a rural setting impact practice?

3 Define, compare and contrast the biomedical model and the biopsychosocial model.

4 Identify the challenges to service provision for rural older people and suggest strategies to address these.

REFERENCES

Alston, M. (2010) *Innovative Human Services Practice: Australia's changing landscape.* Palgrave Macmillan.

Australian Association of Social Workers (AASW) (2010). Code of Ethics. AASW. www.aasw.asn.au/document/item/1201

Australian Bureau of Statistics (ABS) (2009). Volunteers: Everyday people, extraordinary contribution. www.abs.gov.au/ausstats/abs@.nsf/Latestproducts/4918.0Main%20Features5May%202009

Australian Bureau of Statistics (ABS) (2018a). Disability, Ageing, and Carers, Australia: Summary of findings, 2018: Older people. www.abs.gov.au/ausstats/abs@.nsf/Latestproducts/4430.0Main%20Features62018?opendocument&tabname=Summary&prodno=4430.0&issue=2018&num=&view=

Australian Bureau of Statistics (ABS) (2018b). Estimates of Aboriginal and Torres Strait Islander Australians. www.abs.gov.au/ausstats/abs@.nsf/mf/3238.0.55.001

Australian Institute of Health and Welfare (AIHW) (2018). Older Australia at a Glance. www.aihw.gov.au/reports/older-people/older-australia-at-a-glance/contents/diverse-groups-of-older-australians

Baldwin, R., Stephens, M., Sharp, D. & Kelly, J. (2013). *Issues Facing Aged Care Services in Rural and Remote Australia.* Aged and Community Services Australia.

Beddoe, L. (2013). Health Social Work: Professional identity and knowledge. *Qualitative Social Work,* *12*(1), 24–40. https://doi:10.1177/1473325011415455

Bernoth, M., Dietsch, E. & Davies, C. (2012). Forced into Exile: The traumatising impact of rural aged care service inaccessibility. *Rural and Remote Health,* *12*(online), 19–24. www.rrh.org.au/journal/article/1924

Burnham, J. C. (2014). Why sociologists abandoned the sick role concept. *History of the Human Sciences,* *27*(1) 70–87. https://doi:10.1177/0952695113507572

Cash, B., Hodgkin, S. & Warburton, J. (2013). Till death us do part? A critical analysis of obligation and choice for spousal caregivers. *Journal of Gerontological Social Work, 56*(8), 657–4. https://doi.org/10.1080/01634372.2013.823472

Chenoweth, L. & McAuliffe, D. (2021). *The Road to Social*

Work and Human Service Practice (6th edn). Cengage Learning.

Commonwealth of Australia (2019). Interim Report: Neglect. Vol. 1. Royal Commission into Aged Care Quality and Safety. https://agedcare.royalcommission.gov.au/sites/default/files/2020-02/interim-report-volume-1.pdf

Commonwealth of Australia (2021). Royal Commission into Aged Care Quality and Safety. Final report: Care, dignity and respect. Vol. 2, The current system. https://agedcare.royalcommission.gov.au/sites/default/files/2021-03/final-report-volume-1_0.pdf

Federation of Ethnic Communities Councils of Australia (FECCA) (2015). *Review of Australian Research on Older People from Culturally and Linguistically Diverse Backgrounds*. http://fecca.org.au/wp-content/uploads/2015/06/Review-of-Australian-Research-on-Older-People-from-Culturally-and-Linguistically-Diverse-Backgrounds-March-20151.pdf

Gardiner, F., Richardson, A., Bishop, L., Harwood, A., Gardiner, E., Gale, L. et al. (2019). Health care for older people in rural and remote Australia: Challenges for service provision. *Medical Journal Of Australia, 211*(8), 363–4. https://doi.org/10.5694/mja2.50277

Giles, R., Irwin, J., Lynch, D. & Waugh, F. (2010). *In the Field: From learning to practice*. Oxford University Press.

Havelka, M., Lucanin, J. D. & Lucanin, D. (2009).

Biopsychosocial model: The integrated approach to health and disease. *Collegium Antropologicum, 33*(1), 303–10.

Healy, K. (2014). *Social Work Theories in Context: Creating frameworks for practice*. Palgrave Macmillan.

Heinsch, M. (2012). Getting down to earth: Finding a place for nature in social work practice. *International Journal of Social Welfare, 21*(3), 309–18. https://doi:10.1111/j.1468-2397.2011.00860.x

Hughes, M. (2013). Sexuality and social work. In M. Connolly & L. Harms (eds). *Social Work Contexts and Practice*. Oxford University Press (pp. 99–110).

Hughes, M. & Heycox, K. (2010). *Older People, Ageing and Social Work: Knowledge for practice*. Allen & Unwin.

Johns, L., McAuliffe, D. & Dorsett, P. (2019). Psychosocial care provision for terminally ill clients in rural Australian communities: The role of social work. *Rural and Remote Health*. https://doi.org/10.22605/rrh5285

Martin, J. (2014). Building a culturally diverse and responsive aged-care health workforce. In L. H. Kee, J. Martin & R. Ow (eds). *Cross-cultural Social Work: Local and global*. Palgrave Macmillan, pp. 197–212.

Massey, S. & Parr, N. (2012). The socio-economic status of migrant populations in regional and rural Australia and its implications for future population policy. *Journal of Population Research, 29*(1), 1–21. https://doi.org/10.1007/s12546-011-9079-9

Munford, R. & Bennie, G. (2013). Social work and disability. In M. Connolly & L. Harms (eds). *Social Work Contexts and Practice*. Oxford University Press, pp. 194–205.

Naughtin, G. & Schofield, V. (2013). Working with older people. In M. Connolly & L. Harms (eds). *Social Work Contexts and Practice*. Oxford University Press, pp. 206–18.

Pickard, S. (2010). The 'Good carer': Moral practices in late modernity. *Sociology, 44*(3), 471–87. https://doi.org/10.1177/0038038510362482

Portsmouth, L., Coyle, J. & Trede, F. (2008). Working as a member of a health team. In J. Higgs, R. Ajjawi, L. McAllister, F, Trede & S. Loftus (eds). *Communicating in the Health Sciences* (2nd edn). Oxford University Press, pp. 230–8.

Richmond, M. (1917). *Social Diagnosis*. Russell Sage Foundation.

Sinclair, D. A. & LaPlante, M. D. (2019). *Lifespan: Why We Age – and Why We Don't Have To*. Atria Books.

Von Bertalanffy, L. (1968). *General System Theory: Foundations, development, applications*. George Braziller.

Wardle, S. & Mungai, N. (2018). Emerging ageing and age-related issues amongst migrant population in regional Australia. *Social Work: Innovations and Insights*.

World Health Organization (WHO) (2013). *Research for Universal Health Coverage: World Health Report 2013*. WHO. www.who.int/whr/2013/report/en/

7

Elder Abuse

BIANCA BRIJNATH, KATE O'HALLORAN AND BRIONY DOW

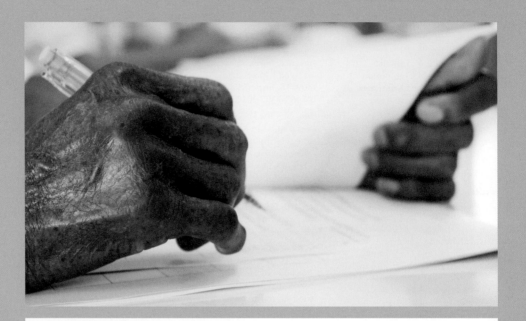

WARNING

This chapter includes content that some readers may find disturbing and/or traumatising. We encourage you to prepare yourself emotionally before reading.

LEARNING OBJECTIVES

After reading this chapter, you will:

» understand what elder abuse is, its prevalence and the different types of abuse

» recognise the drivers and risk factors of elder abuse

» identify and respond to elder abuse professionally

» know about effective interventions to prevent and/or resolve elder abuse.

Introduction

The World Health Organization (WHO, 2008) defines elder abuse as 'a single or repeated act or lack of appropriate action, occurring within any relationship where there is an expectation of trust which causes harm or distress to an older person … Elder abuse is a violation of human rights and a significant cause of injury, illness, lost productivity, isolation and despair'.

Another definition, commonly used in Australia and the UK specifies that elder abuse is 'Any act occurring within a relationship where there is an implication of trust, which results in harm to an older person' (Kaspiew et al., 2018, p. 2).

Common across both definitions is an understanding that elder abuse comprises:

- an older person being abused (a victim)
- acts or lack of action (as in neglect)
- a person who perpetrates the abuse
- relationship characteristics or pre-conditions, including a relationship of trust
- the impact on the older person, usually including harm or distress (Kaspiew et al., 2016).

However, questions remain about these sub-components of the definition. For example, should abuse be considered elder abuse because of the age of the victim? In Australia and other high-income countries, people are defined as older if they are aged 65 years and over. However, recognising the premature mortality experienced by Australia's First Nations peoples, those aged 50 years and over from Indigenous communities are considered older people (AIHW, 2018). Similarly, how should a relationship of trust be defined? Does carer stress play a role in elder abuse? Should behaviours that result in harm or distress of the older person that are unintentional constitute abuse?

Most importantly, older people themselves define elder abuse in much broader terms than these widely accepted definitions. They describe elder abuse as also inclusive of ageist attitudes from the wider community – for example, a lack of respect, especially from younger people; a lack of warmth; and being ignored (O'Brien et al., 2011):

 The older person becomes almost invisible in the corner or wherever, and even touching you know, the whole withdrawal of human kindness almost. (Amy, p. 37)

 I would extend it [the meaning of abuse] to … where you retire at 65 or so and you have got grey hair and suddenly one day you are capable of holding down an important job and the next day you are considered as having no valued opinion, you're not clever enough to understand what we are doing and we're here to help you and we have a whole organisation to help you rather than thinking that you still have a lot of life left in you. (Jack, p. 43)

Thus, while the WHO definition is the most generally accepted, in Australia there are a range of definitions and frameworks to describe the abuse of older people. In this chapter, we will present you with strategies for detecting and dealing with elder abuse situations that you may come across in your career when working with older people. We will also help you to identify the drivers and risk factors of elder abuse, as well as effective interventions to prevent and/or resolve elder abuse, to help create a world where older people feel respected, healthy and included.

7.1 Getting to know the person: Agnes' story

Emily, a home-care caseworker who works for the local council, arrives at the home with a 'For sale' sign out front. The owner of the home is her client, Agnes, an older person with early stage dementia of Italian background. Upon entering the home, Emily finds boxes piled in the lounge. Agnes barely acknowledges the caseworker, who let herself in as the door is unlocked. Distraught and tearful, Agnes says she is looking for a photograph of her late husband, but in all the chaos she can't find anything. Emily escorts Agnes into the kitchen, where there are papers and clutter covering the table. As they chat, Agnes shares that she has to move from the house her husband loved because her daughter Lucy says she can't afford it anymore.

Lucy arrives and is surprised to find someone in the house. When Lucy opens the cupboard door, Emily notices there is very little food in it. As Lucy insists that everything is fine, Agnes gets more upset and leaves the kitchen. On her way out, she bumps Lucy's handbag, which falls on the floor and a few items spill out: unpaid bills, and Keno and lottery tickets. While Lucy is picking up the Keno tickets and unpaid bills and putting them back in her bag, Emily asks about Agnes' proposed living situation once the house is sold and Lucy rudely responds by informing the caseworker that it is none of her business, but that her mother will be living with her. Emily sees Agnes wipe away tears as she goes to walk out the door. Agnes is still looking for things including a photo of her and John.

FOCUS QUESTIONS

Financial abuse is one form of elder abuse that may or may not be easy to recognise. Financial abuse involves the illegal or improper use of a person's finances.

- What are the signs of financial abuse in this case?
- What are the risk factors for Agnes?
- What are the risk factors for Lucy?
- What are the warning signs of abuse?
- What should be done to help Agnes and Lucy?

Types of abuse

Sadly, the case of Agnes and her daughter, Lucy, is all too common, as the available evidence suggests that people living with dementia are particularly vulnerable to abuse (Cooper et al., 2010; Dong et al., 2014; Hansberry et al., 2005; Spector & Nguyen, 2016). Elder abuse often happens at the hands of a trusted person and can be perpetrated by family members, a formal or informal caregiver or an acquaintance, and can occur in the home, community or institutional settings (Dong, 2017; Gorbien & Eisenstein, 2005; Kurrle & Naughtin, 2008).

Agnes and Lucy's case also demonstrates one of the most frequent types of elder abuse: financial abuse (Australian Longitudinal Study on Women's Health, 2014). As per the WHO (2008) definition, there are various forms of abuse, including financial, physical, psychological/emotional, sexual, social and neglect (Levine, 2003; Yon et al., 2019). These are described in more detail in Figure 7.1.

FIGURE 7.1 Types of abuse

PSYCHOLOGICAL/ EMOTIONAL	Any act that causes emotional pain, anguish or distress, or is demeaning to an individual. For example, verbal threats or forced isolation that prevent or restrict the older person's contact with friends, family or the community.
FINANCIAL	The illegal mismanagement or improper use of the older person's finances. It includes stealing money or possessions, controlling their finances without permission, threats or coercion to gain power of attorney, or pressuring them for early inheritances.
PHYSICAL	Describes any deliberate act that causes pain, injury to, or intimidation of, an older person. This includes all forms of physical assault, along with the use of restraint by physical or chemical methods.
NEGLECT	The failure of a carer to provide basic necessities such as food, shelter or medical care, or preventing someone else from providing them.
SEXUAL	Any sexual contact, language or display of pornography without the older person's consent, or through coercion. For example, making obscene phone calls in the person's presence, inappropriate handling when undertaking personal care activities, or making the person perform a sexual act they don't want.

Source: Compass: Guiding Action on Elder Abuse (2021a).

Prevalence of abuse

There is little evidence about prevalence of elder abuse in Australia, although a national population-level prevalence study was conducted in 2020. Extrapolating from international data, which estimates the global prevalence of abuse of older people in community settings at 15.7 per cent (Yon et al., 2017), we may assume an annual prevalence rate of between 2 per cent and 14 per cent of older Australians experiencing elder abuse, with the rate of neglect likely to be even higher (Kaspiew et al., 2016; Kurrle & Naughtin, 2008; Yon et al., 2017).

We have very little data on the abuse of older people in residential aged care. However, the most recent findings from the Royal Commission into Aged Care Quality and Safety (Commonwealth of Australia, 2021) have found that estimates for abuse in residential aged care are much higher than the prevalence of elder abuse in the community. These findings are discussed later.

International data synthesising 52 prevalence studies across 28 countries estimates the rates of psychological abuse and financial abuse to be 11.6 per cent and 6.8 per cent respectively, and lower for neglect, physical abuse and sexual abuse at 4.2 per cent, 2.6 per cent and 0.9 per cent respectively (Yon et al., 2017). This is also supported by an analysis of seven years of Senior Rights Victoria (SRV) helpline data from 2012 to 2019 by the National

Ageing Research Institute (NARI) into the nature of the problem in the state of Victoria (see Figure 7.2) (Joosten et al., 2020). However, these statistics should be interpreted with caution given the dataset is limited to those who sought help through this particular service (Joosten et al., 2020).

FIGURE 7.2 Types of abuse reported over time

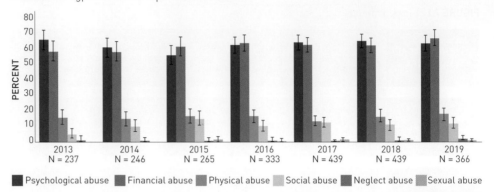

Source: Senior Rights Victoria (Joosten et al., 2020).

Family relationships and the pressure of caring for family members is discussed in Chapter 5.

Analysis of data from Senior Rights Victoria suggests that most elder abuse is committed by adult sons against their mothers. However, other forms of interfamilial and intergenerational abuse are also common, including abuse by daughters and abuse of fathers and/or grandparents. The SRV-NARI data also shows that an extremely high percentage (91%) of abuse experienced by older people is perpetrated by a family member, most commonly sons (39%) or daughters (28%). The same data shows that women are most often the victims of abuse (as 72% of callers seeking advice), and that men are most often the perpetrators of such abuse (at 54%) (Joosten et al., 2020).

Unfortunately, these figures are likely to be an underestimation as elder abuse is frequently underreported (Dow & Brijnath, 2019). This is often because older people fail to recognise the situation as abusive, are ashamed or embarrassed, or fear consequences for the perpetrator. This may especially be the case when the perpetrator is their child or another family member. Thus, while victims want the abuse to stop, many express ambivalence towards taking action about it because of the potential fallout for the family member who has harmed them, and out of concern for their relationship (Dow & Joosten, 2012).

In the context of population ageing, the problem of elder abuse is of increasing concern. By 2050, we can expect to see more than one-fifth of the Australian population aged 65 years and over, and approximately 5 per cent of the population will be aged 85 and over (Wilson et al., 2020). Therefore, we must act now to identify and effectively respond to elder abuse.

Elder abuse in diverse communities

Older people are not a homogenous group and therefore elder abuse may present differently in diverse groups – for example, older people from culturally and linguistically diverse (CALD) backgrounds, First Nations peoples, and older people who identify as lesbian, gay, bisexual, transgender, gender diverse, intersex, queer, asexual and questioning (LGBTIQ+) (see Table 7.1).

TABLE 7.1 Elder abuse in diverse communities

DIVERSE COMMUNITY	TYPES OF ABUSE ENCOUNTERED
People from culturally and linguistically diverse (CALD) backgrounds	People from CALD backgrounds may be at greater risk of financial abuse due to language and literacy barriers (Wainer et al., 2011) and risk factors for abuse such as social isolation (Brijnath et al., 2018; Zannettino et al., 2015). Older immigrants may experience financial and housing stresses, changes in social status and stress associated with trying to meet their traditional cultural expectations in a different cultural environment. These stresses can have an impact on abuse, especially if they lead to family members becoming frustrated or impatient with their older relative (Petosic et al., 2015).
People identifying as LGBTIQ+	The types of elder abuse experienced by older LGBTIQ+ people may include deliberate misuse of pronouns or mis-gendering of trans and gender-diverse people; refusal by services to recognise a person's sexuality including their partner(s); lack of understanding of non-biological or 'chosen' families; and discrimination against someone on the basis of their sexuality or gender identity (e.g. from religious aged care providers). Indeed, for many LGBTIQ+ people, such issues are so terrifying that they may avoid aged care by looking into alternatives such as renovating their homes, relocating to areas with specific trans-inclusive (or LGBTIQ+ – friendly) services and potential voluntary assisted dying (Waling et al., 2020).
First Nations peoples	In First Nations communities, financial abuse appears to be the most common form of elder abuse (Boldy et al., 2005; Kurrle & Naughtin, 2008). Colloquially, such abuse is commonly referred to as 'humbugging'. Humbugging is where an older person is hassled by members of their family or wider community to hand over their pension or other belongings. While open sharing of resources is a widely held value among First Nations communities, elder abuse occurs when the older person feels they do not have a choice about what or how much they share (Kimberley Birds, 2020).

We note the evidence is very limited in this space but highlight what is known in Table 7.1 in order to draw your attention to the differences across diverse communities. While it is important for you as practitioners and **intervention designers** to consider that emotional connections with family, community and culture are likely to be of great importance to an older person (Zannettino et al., 2015), it is also important to consider the different values held by various cultural groups and how these might influence the way elder abuse is perceived and responded to. For example, you may believe that elder abuse is an infringement of an individual's rights and seek to empower them to understand and claim those rights. However, in some communities greater value is placed on collective well-being and decisions may be made in the best interests of the family as a whole, rather than in the best interests of the older person as an individual (Wainer et al., 2011). In this case, a family-oriented approach such as family mediation (discussed below) might be more appropriate.

Similarly, where previous histories of trauma and **disenfranchisement** have left long-lasting scars on communities, including **lateral violence**, an **individual rights-based approach** may not work and instead collective efforts from communities, government and industry are required to create deep, safe and meaningful relationships (Gooda, 2011). For example, many older First Nations peoples may have reason to distrust interventions that come from outside their communities and are more likely to respond positively to recognised community representatives and custodians of culture in safeguarding them against abuse (Gooda, 2012). These preferences are derived from the historical trauma resulting from land and cultural dispossession and the Stolen Generations, which also increase the social and financial hardship faced by many First Nations peoples today.

intervention designers
The people responsible for designing interventions to prevent or respond to elder abuse.

disenfranchisement
The state of being deprived of a right or privilege, often the right to vote.

lateral violence
Displaced violence directed against one's peers rather than adversaries.

individual rights-based approach
An approach that privileges the human rights of the individual over the group or community.

 BIANCA BRIJNATH, KATE O'HALLORAN AND BRIONY DOW

As such, it is important to be sensitive to the needs of diverse older Australians and their communities, and further research is needed to better understand how diverse cultural norms and expectations can affect help-seeking behaviours and the reporting of elder abuse (Dow & Brijnath, 2019).

Impacts of abuse

Elder abuse can ravage the lives of older people, and is associated with decreased quality of life, morbidity and mortality (WHO, 2011). Elder abuse has been associated with increased mental health conditions, including depression, anxiety, fear, stress and feelings of unworthiness (Dong et al., 2013), drug and alcohol addiction, and suicide (Kaye et al., 2007). A 14-year follow-up study in the United States found elder abuse was associated with a 40 per cent increased mortality risk and confirmed elder abuse was associated with a more than two-fold increased all-cause mortality risk (Dong et al., 2009). A related study also found that the increased mortality risk associated with confirmed elder abuse applied not only to older people with high levels of depression and low levels of social connection and social engagement, but also to older people with moderate levels of depression and moderate levels of social connection and engagement (Dong et al., 2011).

In Australia, the financial costs of hospital admissions for maltreatment of older people were estimated to be between A\$9.9 million and A\$30.7 million for 2007–2008 (Jackson, 2009). These figures exclude costs incurred through the legal and social systems, such as adult social services agencies; in 2004 in the United States alone this amounted to approximately US\$500 million (Dyer et al., 2007; National Center on Elder Abuse, 2006). Indirect costs as a consequence of elder abuse include an inability to continue with activities of daily life, diminished quality of life, lost investment in social capital and loss of productivity of carers (Butchart, 2008). As a result of these devastating effects, the Australian Government committed \$18.3 million in 2018–2022 to support the delivery of frontline services to older people experiencing elder abuse (Attorney-General's Department, 2019b).

Drivers of abuse

As a health-care professional, it is important to be aware of the drivers of elder abuse because these are where primary prevention efforts are targeted. Primary prevention aims to stop elder abuse from occurring in the first place by changing the attitudes and social conditions that drive it.

Drivers of elder abuse are the 'social norms, practices and structures that influence individual attitudes and behaviours' (Respect Victoria, 2019). Ageism – that is, the stereotyping and/or discrimination against a person because of their age (Eastern Community Legal Centre, 2019; Lord et al., 2019; Senior Rights Victoria & Think Impact, 2019) – is considered one of the main drivers of elder abuse as it perpetuates ideas that older people are frail, cognitively slow, helpless or weak, and a burden on society or the economy (Officer et al., 2016). Such beliefs may significantly affect older people, who may be prevented from actively participating in everyday life in their communities (WHO, 2012).

Other drivers include gender inequality and other intersecting forms of discrimination such as racism, classism, homophobia and **ableism** (Dow & Brijnath, 2019; Dow & Joosten, 2012). More recently, capitalism – or a society where a person's worth is defined by their capacity to contribute financially – has also been considered as a potential driver of elder abuse (Eastern Community Legal Centre, 2019).

ableism
Discrimination in favour of able-bodied people.

Risk factors for elder abuse

Being able to identify the risk factors for elder abuse is also important for you as a health-care professional. Risk factors refer to the characteristics of individuals or groups that make them more likely to experience or perpetrate abuse (Our Watch & VicHealth, 2015). Unlike drivers, which refer to social norms (see above), risk factors directly impact either the perpetrator or the victim of abuse, or both, and increase the likelihood of abuse occurring within that relationship. There are some similarities between the risk factors for older people and perpetrators (see below).

RISK FACTORS FOR THE OLDER PERSON

Risk factors vary according to the type of abuse, but a review of the literature by Joosten and colleagues (2017) revealed the following as increasing a person's risk of elder abuse (Joosten et al., 2017, p. 21):

- cognitive impairment and dementia
- functional dependency and disability
- poor physical health or frailty
- psychiatric illness or psychological problems
- social isolation, or a lack of social networks and support
- co-residency with the perpetrator (except for financial abuse)
- loneliness
- traumatic life events, including past abuse
- low income and income dependency
- belonging to a minority or non-dominant culture
- substance abuse.

Very often, different types of elder abuse may occur concurrently. Similarly, risk factors can coalesce, differ or be amplified, depending on an older person's family situation, care relations, living arrangements, and socio-economic and cultural background. For example, living alone increases the risk of financial abuse, especially for older men (Jackson & Hafemeister, 2015). In relation to financial elder abuse, risk factors may include the perpetrator feeling entitled to the older person's assets and property; the older person feeling frightened of a family member (Bagshaw et al., 2013); not being aware of their legal rights (Bagshaw et al., 2013); and/or having limited social support (Beach et al., 2018).

RISK FACTORS FOR THE PERSON OF TRUST, OR THE PERSON PERPETRATING THE ABUSE OF THE OLDER PERSON

There is a scarcity of evidence about the experience of elder abuse from the perpetrator's perspective. Based on the available evidence, for perpetrators the risk factors can include (Joosten et al., 2017, p. 23):

- psychiatric illness or psychological problems
- substance abuse

- social isolation and a lack of social support
- childhood experience of family violence
- caregiver stress
- domineering personality traits
- financial problems
- dependency on the older person.

Understanding the relationship dynamics between the perpetrator and the older person is important for you as a health-care professional because it facilitates the development of a more person-centred response that meets the needs and wishes of older people. Elder abuse is perpetrated not only by adult children (though this is the most common form), but may also incorporate longstanding intimate partner violence, abuse by a carer, abuse by another older person (e.g. an older person with dementia) and abuse while in institutional care (Joosten et al., 2017). Table 7.2 outlines examples of how elder abuse may present in different relationships.

TABLE 7.2 Examples of how elder abuse may present in different relationships

	THE PERPETRATOR LIVES WITH THE OLDER PERSON	THE OLDER PERSON IS DEPENDENT ON THE PERPETRATOR FOR CARE	THE OLDER PERSON BEING CARED FOR HAS DEMENTIA
The perpetrator may:	» Have disability or behavioural issues » Have drug or alcohol dependence » Rely on the older person for child care	» Be a carer who is not coping with the demands of caring » Have no previous history of abusing an older person » Be un/intentionally abusive of an older person » Use restraints (both chemical and physical)	» Be trapped in a stressful caring situation » Feel frustrated and become abusive towards the person with dementia » Use restraints (both chemical and physical)
The older person may:	» Feel responsible for the perpetrator's or grandchildren's welfare	» Have a physical, cognitive and/or other impairment/ disability	» Have cognitive impairment or dementia » Act out of character because of their dementia and/or unmet needs (e.g. unrecognised pain)

7.2 Getting to know the person: Mulchand's story

Mulchand is 72 years old, of Indian background, and lives with dementia. The dementia has caused personality changes in Mulchand, who has gone from being a loving husband to a sometimes-violent man who can be both verbally and physically abusive towards his wife of 52 years, 70-year-old Reshma. He is also verbally abusive with hospital staff when he is admitted for a chest infection. June, a hospital social worker, expresses her concern for Reshma's safety. People with dementia can have changed behaviours. Physical abuse is very rare, but even in these circumstances, carers may want to keep caring. They may find it difficult to talk about the abuse and worry what will happen to their loved one living with dementia.

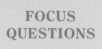

- How might relationship dynamics influence abuse in this case?
- What types of abuse may be occurring? What are the warning signs?
- What might the impacts of abuse be in this case?

FOCUS QUESTIONS

Identifying abuse: recognising the warning signs

Elder abuse often goes unreported. It is frequently missed by health professionals because of varying levels of understanding; limited training on the signs of abuse, especially financial abuse; inadequate access to routine screening and assessment tools; and insufficient institutional support to facilitate the reporting of suspected cases (Cooper et al., 2009; Dow et al., 2013; Penhale, 2010; Schmeidel et al., 2012; Tilse & Wilson, 2013).

Older adults also experience several barriers to revealing abuse. For example, they may not always understand what counts as abusive behaviour and may therefore be unable to recognise it (Taylor et al., 2014). Alongside this, they may fear retribution from the perpetrator (Roulet et al., 2017), feel guilty if the perpetrator is their child (Moon & Benton, 2000) or wish to protect the perpetrator from adverse outcomes that may result if the abuse were reported (Jackson & Hafemeister, 2015).

There are several screening tools available to aid you in identifying whether a client is at risk of or experiencing elder abuse. However, to date, no clear and concise screening tool is recommended to be used consistently (Neave et al., 2016). The Royal Australian College of General Practitioners recommends use of the Elder Abuse Suspicion Index (EASI) (Yaffe et al., 2008), which aims to assist doctors in identifying elder abuse to the point where a referral to a social support service would be appropriate. But the accompanying guidelines for reporting and documentation of cases of elder abuse only provide advice for elder abuse of a criminal nature; cases relating to professional malpractice; and cases requiring guardianship intervention. For cases in which an older person may be experiencing other forms of abuse – such as financial, psychological or social abuse, or neglect – no referral guidelines are provided to general practitioners (RACGP, 2019).

Regardless of the availability of an effective screening tool, elder abuse is everyone's business and there are several established warning signs you can look out for if elder abuse is suspected. These signs are listed in Table 7.3.

Please note that Table 7.3 includes highly confronting material.

TABLE 7.3 Signs of abuse

TYPE OF ABUSE	WARNING SIGNS
Financial	» An unexplained disappearance of belongings » An unexplained inability to pay bills » Significant bank withdrawals » Changes to wills » Access to bank accounts or statements is blocked » An accumulation of unpaid bills » An empty fridge » A disparity between living conditions and money » No money to pay for home essentials like food, clothing and utilities

(Continued)

BIANCA BRIJNATH, KATE O'HALLORAN AND BRIONY DOW

TABLE 7.3 Continued

TYPE OF ABUSE	WARNING SIGNS
Emotional/psychological	Any one of the following: » Resignation, shame, depression, tearfulness, confusion, agitation » Feelings of helplessness » Unexplained paranoia or excessive fear » A change in appetite or sleep patterns, such as insomnia » Unusual passivity or anger » Sadness or grief at the loss of interactions with others » Withdrawal or listlessness due to a lack of visitors » A change to levels of self-esteem » Worry or anxiety after a visit by a specific person/people » Social isolation
Physical	» Internal or external injuries, including sprains, dislocations and fractures, pressure sores, unexplained bruises or marks on different areas of the body; pain on touching » Broken or healing bones » Lacerations to the mouth, lips, gums, eyes or ears » Missing teeth and/or eye injuries » Evidence of hitting, punching, shaking or pulling (e.g. bruises, lacerations, choke marks, hair loss or welts) » Burns (e.g. from rope, cigarettes, matches, iron and/or hot water)
Sexual	» Unexplained STD or incontinence (bladder or bowel) » Injury and trauma (e.g. scratches, bruises etc. to face, neck, chest, abdomen, thighs or buttocks) » Trauma including bleeding around the genitals, chest, rectum or mouth » Torn or bloody underclothing or bedding » Human bite marks » Anxiety around the perpetrator and other psychological symptoms
Neglect	» Inadequate clothing » Complaints of being too cold or too hot » Poor personal hygiene and/or an unkempt appearance » Lack of medical or dental care » Injuries that have not been properly cared for » Absence of required aids » Exposure to unsafe, unhealthy and/or unsanitary conditions » Unexplained weight loss, dehydration, poor skin integrity, malnutrition

Source: Compass: Guiding Action on Elder Abuse 2021b.

Resolving elder abuse

Multidimensional responses such as counselling, case management, legal interventions, medical care and financial controls (Joosten et al., 2017) are needed to adequately resolve cases of elder abuse. For example, a social-worker–lawyer team in New York found 68 per cent of clients using their service had a reduced risk of abuse (Rizzo et al., 2015). Another US study compared a team comprising a nurse and a social worker versus a social worker alone (Ernst & Smith, 2012) and found that a multidisciplinary team reduced the risk of abuse.

Improving the education and training of health-care professionals is another effective way to prevent and stop elder abuse (Ayalon et al., 2016). Universal screening of all older people may be one option. It is very important for you to obtain information about this sensitive subject by building trust and rapport with the older person (Brijnath et al., 2018).

If initiated early, family mediation can also help resolve abuse because it can empower the older person to recognise the problem and seek help; identify the abuse and the perpetrator's behaviour; and explore options (Bagshaw et al., 2015). Older people often prefer family mediation over legal avenues because it is not perceived as being as confrontational and in fact appears to be geared towards a resolution of conflict (Braun, 2012; Hobbs & Alonzi, 2013).

Finally, using interventions such as psycho-education to support family carers may work (Hebert et al., 2003; Phillips, 2008). The STrAtegies for RelaTives (START) study used a one-to-one, in-person, eight-week psycho-education intervention for family carers of people living with dementia. Depression and anxiety were reduced following the intervention, but no statistically significant reductions were found regarding conflict (Cooper et al., 2016). Given that mental health issues are a risk factor in the experience and perpetration of elder abuse, this approach may be promising for reducing the likelihood or severity of abuse occurring within care relationships.

To assist you in gaining a better understanding of elder abuse and the responses required in your role as a health-care professional, there are numerous educational resources available in Australia, including online courses, videos, service pathways and screening tools. Look up the Australian Institute of Health and Welfare (AIHW), the National Ageing Research Institute (NARI) and Compass for more information.

The Attorney-General's Department (2019a) has published a detailed synopsis of legal, policy and service responses available for elder abuse in Australia called *Everybody's Business: Stocktake of Elder Abuse Awareness, Prevention and Response Activities in Australia*. Services targeted at individuals experiencing abuse include:

- helplines for confidential advice, information and referrals
- specialist elder abuse and general community legal centres
- collaborative practice models that bring together lawyers, health workers, social workers and advocates
- family mediation, counselling and other family inclusive services
- advocacy for the rights of older people
- other case management services.

Implications for practice

Thinking about the case study of Agnes and Lucy, what could be done to help them? Sometimes families find themselves in difficult circumstances, and it is hard to know what's OK and what's not OK. If you suspect financial abuse in your role as a health-care professional:

1 Talk to your supervisor. Be sure to take notes of any concerns you have, so that your information is accurate.

2 Have a conversation with the person you suspect is a victim of financial abuse:
- Remember that the person with dementia has rights and is often still capable of making their own decisions.
- This conversation should take place with the person on their own and in a place where they feel safe to talk. For example, the home may not be the

BIANCA BRIJNATH, KATE O'HALLORAN AND BRIONY DOW

safest place if they live with the person you suspect is financially abusive, or if that person is caring for them in their home.

- It is also wise for the person impacted to get independent financial and legal advice before making any decisions.

3   Refer the victim for financial counselling:

- This could be through Centrelink, My Aged Care or a community financial counsellor.
- Be sure the person has all of the information they need to make an informed decision. This includes laws and rules about gifting assets that may impact both parties' financial situations.
- It is important that both parties seek separate and independent legal advice.

4   Refer the victim for legal advice:

- The victim may also wish to discuss enduring power of attorney with a legal professional to make sure their financial and legal rights are protected in the future.
- There are services that provide free legal advice.
- Financial abuse often occurs alongside psychological abuse, with the older person denied the opportunity to make choices and decisions.
- This type of conflict can have an impact on the whole family.

5   Refer the victim for mediation and counselling:

- Be sure to ask the victim if they would like to talk to someone about their concerns and if they understand what their options are.
- Sometimes issues can be resolved within the family, especially if everyone knows their rights. In other situations, family relationships do break down.

Preventing elder abuse

The adage 'prevention is better than cure' applies in cases of elder abuse and, whenever possible, it is critical to stop abuse from occurring in the first place. This requires primary prevention efforts. Primary prevention is defined as work (including interventions) that addresses the 'underlying causes – or drivers – of violence. These include the social norms, practices, and structures that influence individual attitudes and behaviours' (Respect Victoria, 2019). By contrast, early intervention (secondary prevention) targets risk factors (which can be defined as putting someone at higher risk of perpetrating or experiencing violence), while response (or tertiary prevention) supports survivors of violence and aims to prevent the recurrence of such violence by holding perpetrators to account (Our Watch & VicHealth, 2015).

By addressing the drivers of abuse, you can contribute to creating a culture that encourages respectful relationships. This requires multiple strategies and a collective effort from older people, children, families and the public. By providing diverse communities with evidence-based tools, including role modelling respectful behaviour and strategies for how to safely call out disrespectful behaviour, the cultures that underpin family violence may be changed over time.

A systematic review of the elder abuse prevention literature has identified four primary or secondary prevention strategies that appear to have the potential for targeting the drivers or risk factors of elder abuse (Owusu-Addo et al., 2020). These are:

- intergenerational programs
- caregiver psycho-educational programs
- educational programs for professionals
- multisectoral/multidisciplinary team interventions.

These interventions target carer risk factors, ageism and social isolation, with one having an additional focus on the **marginalisation** of LGBTIQ+ older people. Two interventions focus on addressing organisational-level risk factors for the abuse of older people (i.e. reducing the incidence of abusive care environments). Three interventions focus on addressing risk factors specific to older people (Owusu-Addo et al., 2020).

marginalisation
The treatment of a person, group or concept as insignificant or peripheral.

Effective interventions to prevent the abuse of older people are contingent on partnerships across organisations, collaborative partnerships (alliance among professionals; and alliance between health-care professionals, older people and caregivers), co-design and person-centred approaches in optimising the impacts of programs. Interventions that are most likely to be successful incorporate social interactions (largely via group-based interventions), multi-component interventions, tailoring of interventions, motivational interviewing, booster sessions or calls, and a multi-professional team approach to program design and delivery. As a health-care professional working in policy and/or practice, you should be aware of these factors, which are crucial to successful implementation. You also need to pay attention to the development, implementation and evaluation of macro-level primary prevention interventions such as policies fostering positive attitudes to ageing, and addressing gender inequality and other forms of discrimination or marginalisation, which are identified drivers of the abuse of older people (Owusu-Addo et al., 2020).

Legislation and policy frameworks

See Chapter 2 for a timeline of laws and policies influencing the lives of older people and their care.

By law, in Australia elder abuse is not considered to have occurred where there is age discrimination, an estranged relationship with a relative, a crime committed by a stranger, or self-neglect or self-mistreatment. Rather, other laws and strategies determine responses to these activities.

Laws relevant to elder abuse vary by state and territory, with most undertaking or recently completing reviews of their existing legislation. The majority of these reviews canvass a range of issues such as matters to do with guardianship law, models of supported decision-making, substitute decision-making (including powers of attorney), and the roles and powers of key agencies (Attorney-General's Department, 2019b).

The Australian Law Reform Commission (ALRC) completed one of the most far-reaching reviews of elder abuse laws and legal frameworks. This review investigated Commonwealth laws and legal frameworks interacting with state and territory laws with regard to safeguarding older people from abuse (ALRC, 2017). The ALRC recommended that the Commonwealth and state and territory governments develop a national plan to reduce elder abuse, which integrated national service, policy and legal responses. The ALRC also recommended improving responses to elder abuse in aged care, better protection of older people from financial abuse and adult safeguarding processes. Accordingly, in March 2019, the Attorney-General's Department launched the *National Plan to Respond to the Abuse of Older Australians (Elder Abuse) 2019–2023* (Attorney-General's Department, 2019b). The plan describes the priorities over four years, including strengthening service responses, improving future planning and strengthening safeguards for vulnerable people. The plan represents a joint effort by the Commonwealth and state and territory governments.

Alongside the National Plan, there are several other recent reviews and inquiries of note. For example, the Carnell-Paterson *Review of National Aged Care Quality Regulatory Processes* (Carnell & Paterson, 2017) examined regulatory practices relating to monitoring the quality and standard of care in residential aged care facilities. On the basis of this report, the Royal Commission into Aged Care Quality and Safety, which was tasked with regulating the residential aged care sector, was established in 2019.

Similarly, in 2018, the Board of Taxation undertook a review of the tax treatment of granny-flat arrangements in an attempt to develop formal and legally enforceable family agreements as a measure to prevent elder abuse. Based on its recommendations (Board of Taxation, 2019), the Commonwealth government announced a targeted capital gains tax exemption for the creation, variation and termination of granny-flat arrangements where a formal, written agreement is put in place (Board of Taxation, 2019).

Other parliamentary inquiries have also taken place in recent years (see Attorney-General's Department, 2019a). These include the report of the Senate Community Affairs References Committee (2015) into violence, abuse and neglect against people with disability in institutional and residential settings; and the report of the House of Representatives' Standing Committee on Health, Aged Care and Sport (2018), *Report on the Inquiry into the Quality of Care in Residential Aged Care Facilities in Australia.*

THE TENSION BETWEEN ELDER ABUSE AND FAMILY VIOLENCE

Chapter 5 has information about the complexity of family relationships and informal caregiving.

Some state and local governments address elder abuse through broader policies on healthy ageing and ending family violence, while others have implemented specific elder abuse policies. Civil society organisations – such as researchers, community sector organisations, peak bodies and philanthropic organisations – are also developing policies and strategic frameworks to address elder abuse.

These efforts may un/intentionally create tension. For example, the relationship between elder abuse and family violence is contested – in particular, whether elder abuse is a subset of family violence and should therefore be included within family violence policy and service frameworks, and/or whether it should be seen as a specialist area requiring separate policy and service responses. For example, in the state of Victoria, elder abuse is recognised as a form of family violence that may occur between the older person and an adult child, intimate partners, family carers and/or other family members (Victorian Government's Elder Abuse Prevention and Response Initiative, 2020). This policy focus differs from the views of other state jurisdictions and international perspectives that recognise elder abuse as occurring within and outside institutional settings, as well as perpetrated by non-family members where there is an expectation of trust. In addition, because it is linked to family violence, the elder abuse response in Victoria is also influenced by a paradigm that is strongly focused on the gendered nature of violence (e.g. sexism, male partner violence against women and children, and gender divisions of household labour) (Our Watch & VicHealth, 2015; State of Victoria, 2016).

These latter focuses are very important but likely to have different manifestations when it comes to violence against older people. This is for three reasons: first, women are just as likely to be the perpetrators in elder abuse; second, perpetrators are more likely to be adult children than intimate partners, which means different family dynamics will shape the reporting and response; and third, perpetrators may not be a single individual but various family members (e.g. adult children and their partners).

At the same time, there are clear overlaps between elder abuse and family violence (Joosten et al., 2017). This includes the fact that elder abuse overlaps with intimate partner violence, of which women are the overwhelming majority of victims and men the perpetrators. Women are also overrepresented as the victims of elder abuse, and gender inequality is an established driver of such abuse. Gender stereotypes and norms must also be considered as factors in how intergenerational abuse plays out, particularly as perpetrated by sons against their mothers. In terms of intimate partner violence experienced by older women, it is not clear whether in practice these women are being treated as victims of elder abuse or intimate partner violence, and indeed they often fall between the 'gaps' of both service systems and responses. This is one critical issue to address going forward, particularly with regard to the unacceptable levels of sexual assault experienced by older women, especially those living in aged care (discussed in the following section) (Commonwealth of Australia, 2021).

Royal Commission findings and recommendations

Most recently, the Royal Commission into Aged Care Quality and Safety (Commonwealth of Australia, 2021) handed down 148 recommendations on how to improve the quality of aged care services; how best to deliver aged care services; and how to address the challenges and opportunities for delivering accessible, affordable and high-quality aged care services in Australia.

WHAT THE COMMISSION FOUND

Estimates of elder abuse in residential aged care are much higher than the known prevalence of elder abuse in the community:

- One in three people in residential aged care experiences 'sub-standard care', including physical assault, overuse of chemical restraint, unanswered calls for assistance and widespread sexual abuse.
- The prevalence for neglect was estimated at 30.8 per cent with concerns expressed for how older people are helped to shower, eat, toilet, get around, groom and/or use continence aids; concerns about how medication is managed, wounds are looked after, catheters are used and/or pain is managed; concerns about accessing a GP, dentist, mental health services and/or other allied health services; and/or care staff rarely being able to spend enough time attending to the person's individual needs.
- The prevalence for emotional/psychological abuse was estimated at 22.6 per cent, with concerns expressed around how older people felt forced to be dependent on staff, were treated like a child, were forced to wear continence pads, were being shouted at by staff, and/or were not having their specific care needs thought about or listened to.

Learn more
Watch Video 7.1:
Mardi discusses the
abuse and neglect of
her grandmother in
residential aged care.

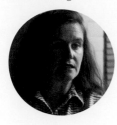

- The prevalence for physical abuse was estimated at 5.0 per cent, with concerns expressed around how older people were restrained, not allowed out of their bed/chair/room or outside, and/or being hurt or treated roughly by staff.

- More than 4 per cent of reportable incidents comprised unlawful sexual assault, including behaviours of rape, sexual assault and touching the resident's genital area without consent. Almost 58 per cent of these incidents were assessed by aged care staff as having 'no impact' on the victim. In real numbers, these percentages equate to 1700 assaults per year or 33 per week.

WHAT THE COMMISSION RECOMMENDED

Action is needed to give older people a real and loud voice. One way to achieve this is to ensure older people's voices are represented on a Council of Elders (Rec. 9), on the governing bodies of aged care providers and on any aged care advisory council established by government (Rec. 7 – Pagone Model), through regular independent reviews of user experiences (Rec. 94) and through the Aged Care Safety and Quality Authority (Rec. 10).

The commissioners also recommended stronger regulation around the use of restraints (Rec. 17) and an accessible complaints mechanism for reporting serious incidents (Rec. 100), along with an improved complaints management process (Complaints Commissioner) (Rec. 98). Individuals responsible for physical or sexual abuse of older people should face criminal charges and never be allowed to work in aged care again. The recommendation regarding a national registration scheme (Rec. 77) will help to address the latter and should be acted on as a government priority.

The majority of abuse and neglect is most likely a symptom of understaffing or staff with inadequate skills or expertise. This calls for a more systemic response. The proposed new Aged Care Act (Rec. 94) will see providers having a duty to provide high-quality and safe care. This, alongside the commissioners' recommendations for increases in award wages (Rec. 84), improved remuneration (Rec. 85), mandated minutes of care (Rec. 86), and staff education and training in dementia and palliative care (Rec. 114) will go some way to addressing these issues.

WHAT HAPPENS NEXT?

Chapter 2 includes
more information
about the history
of aged care policy
and the decisions
that led up to the
Royal Commission
into Aged Care
Quality and Safety.

The Commonwealth and state governments' responses to the recommendations from the Royal Commission are not comprehensive at the time of writing. However, there has been an initiative to address abuse in residential aged care facilities titled 'The Serious Incident Response Scheme'. The scheme is to clarify the obligations of management in response to a serious incident (ACQSC, 2021). The impacts of this initiative are yet to be determined. Whatever is implemented for community-dwelling older people has yet to be revealed and it is therefore too soon to predict what will happen. Overall, however, government must respond comprehensively to the commissioners' recommendations and go even further by enabling older people to have a voice in organisational governance and ongoing system reform. This will have both a symbolic and a practical impact in reducing ageism and improving aged care, and ultimately preventing elder abuse.

Conclusion

Elder abuse is a difficult subject, but it is of growing concern in Australian society due to our ageing population. This chapter has discussed definitions of elder abuse, its prevalence and the different types of abuse. We have also explored the drivers and risk factors of elder abuse, how to identify and respond to elder abuse, and effective interventions to prevent and/or resolve elder abuse. In the context of rapid legislative and policy change, the full effects of which will take time to realise, the key message remains that elder abuse is everyone's business – especially yours. It is a multidimensional problem that requires a multidisciplinary response. Health professionals have an obligation to prevent, intervene, respond to and mitigate abuse of older people and to create a world where older people are respected, healthy and included. You are empowered to create this world by reading and studying this chapter.

Learn more
Access additional resources – such as weblinks, further readings and podcasts – to broaden your understanding of this chapter. See the Guided Tour for access details.

1 What is elder abuse?

2 What are the different types of abuse?

3 How common is elder abuse in Australia?

4 What are the drivers and risk factors of elder abuse?

5 How could health professionals detect abuse?

6 What strategies could health professionals consider to resolve abuse?

7 What strategies could health professionals consider to prevent abuse from occurring?

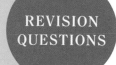

REVISION QUESTIONS

REFERENCES

Aged Care Quality and Safety Commission (ACQSC) (2021). Serious Incident Response Scheme. www.agedcarequality.gov.au/sirs

Attorney-General's Department (2019a). *Everybody's Business: Stocktake of Elder Abuse Awareness, Prevention and Response Activities in Australia.* Australian Government.

Attorney-General's Department (2019b). *National Plan to Respond to the Abuse of Older Australians (Elder Abuse) 2019–2023.* Australian Government.

Australian Institute of Health and Welfare (AIHW) (2018). Older Australia at a glance. Cat. no. AGE 87. www.aihw.gov.au/reports/older-people/older-australia-at-a-glance

Australian Law Reform Commission (2017). *Elder Abuse – A National Legal Response.*

Australian Longitudinal Study on Women's Health (2014). 1926–26 Cohort: Summary 1996–2013.

Ayalon, L., Lev, S., Green, O. & Nevo, U. (2016). A systematic review and meta-analysis of interventions designed to prevent or stop elder maltreatment. *Age Ageing, 45*(2), 216–27. https://doi.org/10.1093/ageing/afv193

Bagshaw, D., Adams, V., Zannettino, L. & Wendt, S. (2015). Elder mediation and the financial abuse of older people by a family member. *Conflict Resolution Quarterly, 32*(4), 443–80.

Bagshaw, D., Wendt, S., Zannettino, L. & Adams, V. (2013). Financial abuse of older people by family members: Views and experiences of older Australians and their family members. *Australian Social Work, 66*(1), 86–103. https://doi.org/10.1080/031240 7x.2012.708762

Beach, S. R., Schulz, R. & Sneed, R. (2018). Associations between social support, social networks, and financial exploitation in older adults. *Journal of Applied Gerontology, 37*(8), 990–1011.

Board of Taxation. (2019). *Review of Granny Flat Arrangements – Final Report.*

Boldy, D., Horner, B., Crouchley, K., Davey, M. & Boylen, S. (2005). Addressing elder

BIANCA BRIJNATH, KATE O'HALLORAN AND BRIONY DOW

abuse: Western Australian case study. *Australasian Journal on Ageing*, 24(1), 3–8.

Braun, J. (2012). Elder guardianship mediation: Threat or benefit to abuse victims? *International Perspectives on Victimology*.

Brijnath, B., Gahan, L., Gaffy, E. & Dow, B. (2018). 'Build rapport, otherwise no screening tools in the world are going to help': Frontline service providers' views on current elder abuse. *The Gerontologist*, 60(3), 472–82. https://doi.org/10.1093/geront/gny166

Butchart, A. (2008). New manual for estimating the economic costs of injuries due to interpersonal and self-directed violence. *Injury prevention*, 14(2), 143.

Carnell, K. & Paterson, R. (2017). *Review of National Aged Care Quality Regulatory Processes*. Department of Health.

Commonwealth of Australia (2021). Royal Commission into Aged Care Quality and Safety. Final report: Care, dignity and respect. Vol. 1, Summary and recommendations. https://agedcare.royalcommission.gov.au/sites/default/files/2021-03/final-report-volume-1_0.pdf

Compass: Guiding Action on Elder Abuse (2021a). Defining Elder Abuse. www.compass.info/defining-elder-abuse

Compass: Guiding Action on Elder Abuse (2021b). What to Look for: Signs and behaviours. www.compass.info/recognising-elder-abuse#link-5

Cooper, C., Barber, J., Griffin, M., Rapaport, P. & Livingston, G. (2016). Effectiveness of START psychological intervention in reducing abuse by dementia family carers: Randomized controlled trial. *International Psychogeriatrics*, 28(6), 881–7. https://doi.org/10.1017/s1041610215002033

Cooper, C., Selwood, A., Blanchard, M., Walker, Z., Blizard, R. & Livingston, G.

(2010). The determinants of family carers' abusive behaviour to people with dementia: Results of the CARD study. *Journal of Affective Disorders*, 121(1), 136–42. doi.org/https://doi.org/10.1016/j.jad.2009.05.001

Cooper, C., Selwood, A. & Livingston, G. (2009). Knowledge, detection, and reporting of abuse by health and social care professionals: A systematic review. *American Journal of Geriatric Psychiatry*, 17(10), 826–38.

Dong, X. (ed.) (2017). *Elder Abuse: Research, practice and policy*. Springer.

Dong, X., Chen, R., Chang, E.-S. & Simon, M. (2013). Elder abuse and psychological well-being: A systematic review and implications for research and policy – a mini review. *Gerontology*, 59(2), 132–42.

Dong, X., Chen, R. & Simon, M. A. (2014). Elder abuse and dementia: A review of the research and health policy. *Health Affairs* (Project Hope), 33(4), 642.

Dong, X., Simon, M., Mendes de Leon, C., Fulmer, T., Beck, T., Hebert, L., Dyer, C., Paveza, G. & Evans, D. (2009). Elder self-neglect and abuse and mortality risk in a community-dwelling population. *Jama*, 302(5), 517–26.

Dong, X. Q., Simon, M. A., Beck, T. T., Farran, C., McCann, J. J., Mendes de Leon, C. F., Laumann, E. & Evans, D. A. (2011). Elder abuse and mortality: The role of psychological and social wellbeing. *Gerontology*, 57(6), 549–58. https://doi.org/10.1159/000321881

Dow, B. & Brijnath, B. (2019). Elder abuse: Context, concepts and challenges. In Australian Institute of Health and Welfare (ed.), *Australia's Welfare in Brief 2019*, AIHW, pp. 143–61.

Dow, B., Hempton, C., Cortes-Simonet, E., Ellis, K. A., Koch, S. H., Logiudice, D., Mastwyk, M., Livingston, G., Cooper, C. & Ames, D.

(2013). Health professionals' and students' perceptions of elder abuse. *Australasian Journal on Ageing*, 32(1), 48–51. https://doi.org/10.1111/j.1741-6612.2012.00643.x

Dow, B. & Joosten, M. (2012). Understanding elder abuse: A social rights perspective. *International Psychogeriatrics*, 24(6), 853. https://doi.org/10.1017/S1041610211002584

Dyer, C. B., Pickens, S. & Burnett, J. (2007). Vulnerable elders: When it is no longer safe to live alone. *Jama*, 298(12), 1448–50.

Eastern Community Legal Centre (2019). *Older People: Equity, Respect & Ageing*: Phase 1 Findings.

Ernst, J. S. & Smith, C. A. (2012). Assessment in adult protective services: Do multidisciplinary teams make a difference? *Journal of Gerontological Social Work*, 55(1), 21–38.

Gooda, M. (2011). *The Social Justice Report 2011*.

Gooda, M. (2012). Speech given at the AAG Elder Abuse and Neglect Conference, Alice Springs, 5 September. Australian Human Rights Commission. www.humanrights.gov.au/news/speeches/aag-elder-abuse-and-neglect-conference

Gorbien, M. J. & Eisenstein, A. R. (2005). Elder abuse and neglect: An overview. *Clinics in Geriatric Medicine*, 21(2), 279–92.

Hansberry, M. R., Chen, E. & Gorbien, M. J. (2005). Dementia and elder abuse. *Clinics in Geriatric Medicine*, 21(2), 315–32. https://doi.org/10.1016/j.cger.2004.11.002

Hebert, R., Levesque, L., Vezina, J., Lavoie, J.-P., Ducharme, F., Gendron, C., Preville, M., Voyer, L. & Dubois, M.-F. (2003). Efficacy of a psychoeducative group program for caregivers of demented persons living at home: A randomized controlled trial [Abstract]. *The Journals of Gerontology*, Series B(1). https://academic.oup.

com/psychsocgerontology/article/58/1/S58/566226

Hobbs, A. & Alonzi, A. (2013). Mediation and family group conferences in adult safeguarding. *The Journal of Adult Protection*, *15*(2), 69–84.

Jackson, L. (2009). The Cost of Elder Abuse in Queensland: Who Pays and How Much. Report, Elder Abuse Prevention Unit.

Jackson, S. L. & Hafemeister, T. L. (2015). The impact of relationship dynamics on the detection and reporting of elder abuse occurring in domestic settings [Author abstract report]. *Journal of Elder Abuse & Neglect 2*, 121. https://doi.10.1080/08946566.2015.1008085

Joosten, M., Gartoulla, P., Feldman, P., Brijnath, B. & Dow, B. (2020). Seven Years of Elder Abuse Data in Victoria. https://seniorsrights.org.au/wp-content/uploads/2021/03/2020August26PolicySevenYearsEADataVictoriaSummary.pdf

Joosten, M., Vrantsidis, F. & Dow, B. (2017). Understanding Elder Abuse: A scoping study. https://socialequity.unimelb.edu.au/__data/assets/pdf_file/0011/2777924/Elder-Abuse-A-Scoping-Study.pdf

Kaspiew, R., Carson, R. & Rhoades, H. (2016). Elder Abuse: Understanding issues, frameworks and responses. Australian Institute of Family Studies.

Kaspiew, R., Carson, R. & Rhoades, H. (2018). Elder Abuse. Australian Institute of Family Studies. https://aifs.gov.au/publications/elder-abuse/export

Kaye, L. W., Kay, D. & Crittenden, J. A. (2007). Intervention with abused older males: Conceptual and clinical perspectives. *Journal of Elder Abuse and Neglect*, *19*(1–2), 153–72. https://doi.org/10.1300/J084v19n01_10

Kimberley Birds (2020). No More Humbug! Reducing Aboriginal Financial Elder Abuse in the Kimberley. Kimberley Community Legal Services Aboriginal Financial Elder Abuse Project. www.kcls.org.au/s/No-More-Humbug-final-report.pdf

Kurrle, S. & Naughtin, G. (2008). An overview of elder abuse and neglect in Australia. *Journal of Elder Abuse and Neglect*, *20*(2), 108–25. https://doi.org/10.1080/08946560801974521

Levine, J. M. (2003). Elder neglect and abuse. A primer for primary care physicians. *Geriatrics*, *58*(10), 37.

Lord, M., McMahon, K. & Nivelle, S. (2019). Preventing Elder Abuse: A literature review for the SMPCP Elder Abuse Prevention Network. Southern Melbourne Primary Care Partnership.

Moon, A. & Benton, D. (2000). Tolerance of elder abuse and attitudes toward third-party intervention among African American, Korean American, and White Elderly. *Journal of Multicultural Social Work*, *8*(3/4), 283–303. www.tandfonline.com/doi/abs/10.1300/J285v08n03_05

National Center on Elder Abuse (2006). The 2004 Survey of State Adult Protective Services: Abuse of Adults 60 Years of Age and Older.

Neave, M., Faulkner, P. & Nicholson, T. (2016). Royal Commission into Family Violence. www.rcfv.com.au/MediaLibraries/RCFamilyViolence/Reports/Final/RCFV-Vol-V.pdf

O'Brien, M., Begley, E., Anand, J. C., Killick, C. & Taylor, B. J. (2011). A Total Indifference to Our Dignity: Older people's understandings of elder abuse. Age Action Ireland.

Officer, A., Schneiders, M. L., Wu, D., Nash, P., Thiyagarajan, J. A. & Beard, J. R. (2016). Valuing older people: Time for a global campaign to combat ageism. *Bulletin of the World Health Organization*, *94*(10), 710.

Our Watch & VicHealth (2015). Change the Story: A Shared Framework for the Primary Prevention of Violence Against Women and Their Children in Australia. Our Watch.

Owusu-Addo, E., O'Halloran, K., Brijnath, B. & Dow, B. (2020). Primary Prevention Interventions for Elder Abuse: Results from a systematic review. Prepared for Respect Victoria on behalf of National Ageing Research Institute.

Penhale, B. (2010). Responding and intervening in elder abuse and neglect. *Ageing International*, *35*(3), 235–52.

Petosic, T., Guruge, S., Wilson-Mitchell, K., Tandon, R., Gunraj, A., Robertson, A., Roche, B., Di Zio, J., Ghosh, K. & Bauder, H. (2015). *Intergenerational Violence: The post-migration context in Canada*. Ryerson Centre for Immigration and Settlement.

Phillips, L. R. (2008). Abuse of aging caregivers: Test of a nursing intervention. *Advances in Nursing Science 2*, 164. https://doi.10.1097/01.ANS.0000319566.06879.e8

Respect Victoria (2019). Respect Victoria Strategic Plan 2019–2022. www.respectvictoria.vic.gov.au/sites/default/files/documents/201904/Full%20version_Strategic%20Plan.pdf

Rizzo, V. M., Burnes, D. & Chalfy, A. (2015). A systematic evaluation of a multidisciplinary social work–lawyer elder mistreatment intervention model. *Journal of Elder Abuse and Neglect*, *27*(1), 1–18.

Roulet Schwab, D. & Wangmo, T. (2017). Perceptions of elder abuse from community-dwelling older persons and professionals working in western Switzerland. *Journal of Interpersonal Violence*, 886260517732345. https://doi.org/10.1177/0886260517732345

Royal Australian College of General Practitioners (RACGP) (2019). *RACGP Aged Care Clinical Guide (Silver Book)* (5th edn). RACGP.

Schmeidel, A. N., Daly, J. M., Rosenbaum, M. E., Schmuch, G. A. & Jogerst,

G. J. (2012). Health care professionals' perspectives on barriers to elder abuse detection and reporting in primary care settings. *Journal of Elder Abuse and Neglect*, *24*(1), 17–36. https://doi.org/10.1080/08946566.2011.608044

Senate Community Affairs References Committee (2015). Violence, abuse and neglect against people with disability in institutional and residential settings, including the gender and age-related dimensions, and the particular situation of Aboriginal and Torres Strait Islander people with disability, and culturally and linguistically diverse people with disability. Parliament of Australia.

Senior Rights Victoria & Think Impact (2019). Older, Better, Together: The primary prevention of elder abuse by prevention networks.

Spector, K. & Nguyen, A. L. (2016). Expert perspectives on elder abuse among people with dementia. *The Gerontologist*, *56*(Supp. 3), 510. https://doi.org/10.1093/geront/gnw162.2058

Standing Committee on Health, Aged Care and Sport (2018). Report on the Inquiry into the Quality of Care in Residential Aged Care Facilities in Australia.

State of Victoria (2016). Royal Commission into Family Violence: Report and recommendations, Parliamentary Paper No. 132 (2014–16).

Taylor, B. J., Killick, C., O'Brien, M., Begley, E. & Carter-Anand, J. (2014). Older people's conceptualization of elder

abuse and neglect. *Journal of Elder Abuse and Neglect*, *26*(3), 223–43. https://doi.org/10.1080/08946566.2013.795881

Tilse, C. & Wilson, J. (2013). Recognising and responding to financial abuse in residential aged care. *The Journal of Adult Protection*, *15*(3), 141–52.

Victorian Government's Elder Abuse Prevention and Response Initiative (2020). Elder Abuse Prevention and Response. Victorian Government. www2.health.vic.gov.au/ageing-and-aged-care/wellbeing-and-participation/preventing-elder-abuse/elder-abuse-prevention-and-response

Wainer, J., Owada, K., Lowndes, G. & Darzins, P. (2011). Diversity and Financial Elder Abuse in Victoria: Protecting elders' assets study. Monash University.

Waling, A., Lyons, A., Alba, B., Minichiello, V., Barrett, C., Hughes, M., Fredriksen-Goldsen, K. & Edmonds, S. (2020). Trans women's perceptions of residential aged care in Australia. *The British Journal of Social Work*, *50*(5), 1304–23.

Wilson, T., McDonald, P., Temple, J., Brijnath, B. & Utomo, A. (2020). Past and projected growth of Australia's older migrant populations. *Genus*, *76*(1), 1–21.

World Health Organization (WHO) (2008). A Global Response to Elder Abuse and Neglect: Building Primary Health Care Capacity to Deal with the Problem Worldwide: Main Report. WHO.

World Health Organization (WHO) (2011). European

Report on Preventing Elder Maltreatment. WHO.

World Health Organization (WHO) (2012). World Health Day 2012: Ageing and health: Toolkit for event organizers. WHO. https://apps.who.int/iris/handle/10665/70840

Yaffe, M. J., Wolfson, C., Lithwick, M. & Weiss, D. (2008). Development and validation of a tool to improve physician identification of elder abuse: The Elder Abuse Suspicion Index (EASI)©. *Journal of Elder Abuse and Neglect*, *20*(3), 276–300.

Yon, Y., Mikton, C. R., Gassoumis, Z. D. & Wilber, K. H. (2017). Elder abuse prevalence in community settings: A systematic review and meta-analysis. *The Lancet Global Health*, *5*(2), e147–e156. https://doi.org/10.1016/S2214-109X(17)30006-2

Yon, Y., Ramiro-Gonzalez, M., Mikton, C. R., Huber, M. & Sethi, D. (2019). The prevalence of elder abuse in institutional settings: A systematic review and meta-analysis. *European Journal of Public Health*, *29*(1), 58–67. https://doi.org/10.1093/eurpub/cky093

Zannettino, L., Bagshaw, D., Wendt, S. & Adams, V. (2015). The role of emotional vulnerability and abuse in the financial exploitation of older people from culturally and linguistically diverse communities in Australia. *Journal of Elder Abuse and Neglect*, *27*(1), 74–89. https://doi.org/10.1080/08946566.2014.976895

8 Older People Volunteering

GAEL EVANS-BARR

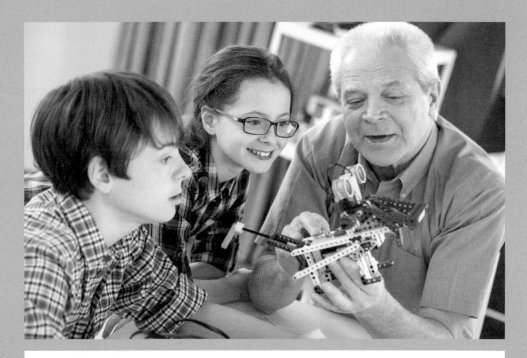

LEARNING OBJECTIVES

After reading this chapter, you will:

» justify various ways in which volunteers provide value to organisations, communities and families

» articulate reasons why volunteering is a key element to healthy ageing

» recognise ways volunteers may assist organisations to adapt in ever-changing environments and dynamic funding cycles

» appreciate the value of volunteering programs and how they support the viability of organisations and services

» choose to develop positive volunteer relationships of mutual benefit

» explain how registered nurses (and other health practitioners) play an important role in supporting older volunteers.

Introduction

Older people make invaluable contributions to society through their accumulated knowledge and life experiences. Older people benefit individuals, families, communities, organisations and charities who share in the older person's time, expertise, compassion, energy and talents. This chapter will focus on aged individuals who are involved in volunteering, with an emphasis on formal volunteering.

In this chapter, you will meet Morgan, a volunteer in a hospital. You'll learn, through Morgan's experiences, some of the common stages to volunteering and how volunteers can influence hospital programs, patient care and culture. In turn, you'll learn how volunteering has affected Morgan over many years. Throughout this chapter, you will read about situations that you will most likely encounter in your professional practice.

Volunteering

public good
A commodity or service that is provided without profit to all members of a society, either by government or by private individuals or organisations.

organisational viability
An organisation's ability to successfully adapt and manage business practices, finances and challenges over the long term.

Volunteers donate their time to achieve goals for the **public good**, often through an organisation's formal volunteer program. Volunteering contributes significantly to health and well-being, to family, community and **organisational viability**, and to the economy (Anderson et al., 2014; Volunteering Australia, 2016). It is a part of the social fabric in Australia, which boasts relatively high rates of volunteering, with over 31 per cent of the population reported to regularly volunteer (Volunteering Australia, 2016). Australia reports that aged individuals are most likely to volunteer, which is clearly an opportunity as ageing people will have dominant numbers in the population by 2050 (Volunteering Australia, 2016). Throughout this chapter, the features of volunteering will be illustrated through a series of vignettes based on a character named Morgan, constructed from my experiences with volunteers and volunteer management. This story is woven through the chapter to provoke thought and insight into the opportunity volunteers create, and how building a partnership of mutual benefit helps the volunteer, the organisation and health practitioners.

8.1 Getting to know the person: Morgan's story

Morgan retired five years ago from teaching at a local primary school at the age of 59. After retirement, Morgan's family noticed patterns of social isolation and encouraged connections in the community.

Morgan eventually looked in the local area to see what groups and activities were available, searching community noticeboards, social media pages, websites and local council information.

As a former primary school teacher, volunteering made sense; it aligned with Morgan's interest in contributing to community. With many volunteer roles available in the community, deciding what was best took some consideration. While reflecting on this, Morgan remembered a young student who had taken ill. At the time, Morgan was struck with the care the hospital staff provided, and how accommodating they were of the young child's peers, allowing mountains of their drawings to be stuck on the hospital walls and organising treatment and medication schedules in a way that the child could still engage in regular video calls with the school class.

Not knowing if anything would be available, Morgan tentatively enquired at this same hospital. Morgan was pleased to be greeted by friendly staff who described the volunteer positions available. They took Morgan's details and advised that the hospital's volunteer coordinator would call the following day.

The next day, the volunteer coordinator called to explain the process of application and provide information on some of the volunteer positions available. Morgan decided to assist at the admissions help desk. The position involved greeting patients, families and visitors at the hospital and assisting them to find their way to the relevant area. Being new to the hospital, Morgan felt that this was a nice introduction to volunteering.

- What are the features of Morgan's experience that are conducive to ensuring Morgan was enthusiastic about becoming a volunteer?
- What else could have been provided for Morgan to support the safe and effective commencement to his volunteer work?

FOCUS QUESTIONS

Why do we need volunteering?

It is indisputable that volunteering plays a significant part in the economic value of nations worldwide. Although calculating the true value is complex, in a well-known study Lisel O'Dwyer (Flinders University, 2014) reported that volunteering was worth more than $290 billion a year to Australia's economy. Her study also acknowledged the foreseeable trends and potential for growth, due to the ageing population in Australia. Such studies give credence to the importance of the **volunteering sector** and the value of understanding volunteer habits.

In keeping with the continuity theory of ageing discussed throughout this book, people's volunteering habits usually follow their personal interests so, not surprisingly, the most common sectors in which people volunteer are sport, recreation, community health, welfare, environment and religion (Volunteering Australia, 2016). The types of people who volunteer may vary, but their motives are generally shared. The majority of volunteers report that they want to make a difference and/or appreciate the feeling of personal worth their volunteering position provides (Volunteering Australia, 2016). It is this overwhelming sense of purpose, pride and social interaction that drives many of the health benefits associated with volunteering.

volunteering sector
Organisations that are not-for-profit and non-governmental.

To better understand continuity theory, see Chapter 4.

The benefits of volunteering

Research has told us over many decades now that volunteers derive various health benefits from volunteering, the most noticeable being reduced rates of stress, anxiety and reported mental health problems (Darja & Djurre, 2019; AIHW, 2018). Many health professionals and families attest to volunteering offering three factors that support these health benefits: increased physical activity, social interaction and regular meals (either directly or indirectly). These outcomes are especially beneficial for older, retired volunteers, as research shows that they may lose focus on these important areas of their health and well-being, especially during or after experiencing bereavement (Jang et al., 2018). Facilitating engagement in community and enabling older people to continue pursuing their interests fits with the activity theory of ageing that is elaborated on in other chapters of this book.

Interest and potential for volunteering is something to be considered when determining strategies to support an older person's physical, emotional and mental health (Lum & Lightfoot, 2005). The social involvement often created through volunteering can provide an informal support network, and promote healthy ageing by potentially reducing risks such as:

- social isolation
- inactivity
- an unhealthy diet (skipping meals and/or eating meals with limited nutritional content).

In many instances, volunteering encourages socialisation, mental stimulation, physical activity and healthy eating, influencing positive health (Stuart-Hamilton, 2012).

> Chapters 4 and 9 discuss the importance of activity theory.

8.2 Getting to know the person: Morgan's story

Morgan started volunteering one day a fortnight, and was surprised by the value of the volunteering role, so increased this to twice a fortnight. Patients and families were often very nervous when they arrived, and Morgan was astounded to see the difference volunteers could make through a friendly face and a few words of assurance.

Morgan also assisted the hospital staff by helping to relay hospital processes and protocols to patients and families. Visitors to the hospital were coming outside of visiting hours, and the staff found it difficult to keep them at bay. It was quite easy for Morgan to get people to adhere to visiting times, perhaps because people were pacified by the nature of the volunteer role. Visitors seemed less inclined to push the boundaries with someone who was volunteering their time and supporting a local service. Everyone was pleased, especially the nursing staff, who didn't have to worry about visitors arriving outside of visiting hours when Morgan was around, allowing them to concentrate on patient care.

Morgan enjoyed making a positive difference to people's lives, and the difference was noticeable with staff, patients and carers. Morgan's family was surprised to find out that Morgan had asked the volunteer coordinator if it was possible to take on an extra regular day of volunteering. They noticed that Morgan was forming friendships by often staying back to eat lunch or go out for dinner with the other volunteers.

Morgan's GP was also pleased with the changes in Morgan's health. Guiding people to and from different units had increased Morgan's physical activity and the difference was noticeable in some routine tests the GP performed during a check-up.

Creating a volunteer-friendly environment

In your professional work, there are always some stressful and busy days, but taking the time to give someone a friendly, affirming smile can offer them reassurance. Be positive and friendly with volunteers, especially new volunteers, who may be nervous and uncertain of their capabilities to fulfil the volunteer role. Small gestures contribute to the affirmative culture of a volunteer program and help the volunteer to feel positive about the organisation and their commitment to the role. A friendly, supportive organisational culture is vital to the success of any volunteer program.

Volunteers and employees hold very different roles and responsibilities in an organisation (Volunteering Australia, 2020). As their paths interweave, it is important for employees and volunteers to understand their respective roles and responsibilities (Commonwealth of Australia, 2021). Like employees, volunteers need education and orientation about policy and procedures, especially policies and procedures for which they are also accountable and responsible (e.g. occupational health and safety policy and procedures). It is important that employees are aware of volunteer rights and responsibilities so that they may provide support and advice when required. Such policies and procedures usually protect everyone within the organisation and provide a clear understanding of the organisation's expectations and processes.

A volunteer's perception of an organisation can be easily influenced, and employees should be mindful of their communication when speaking to volunteers. For example, negative comments may influence a volunteer's opinion of the organisation and their value in the role. In turn, this may impact their commitment to volunteering. It is also important for employees to speak positively about their workplace because volunteers often choose an organisation or volunteer role because of an emotional connection of some kind – whether this is due to a memory, family, culture, passion or sense of purpose – and negative comments may influence this emotional connection.

Volunteers will benefit from receiving as much information and communication as possible when they start a role, such as information on:

- the organisation, its purpose, business areas and relevant orientation information
- the operational responsibility of the volunteer role
- the scope or boundaries of their role
- the service standards of their role
- appropriate forms of tasks, communication and process
- how they may seek assistance or escalate concerns
- what they can expect overall from their volunteer coordinator/manager, such as reporting and communication.

There are differences in the roles of an employee and a volunteer. Employees and volunteers need to understand this demarcation to facilitate collaboration between the two and to ensure that there are no unrealistic expectations of either party. Volunteers generally appreciate clarity and guidance with the scope of their role. Table 8.1 encapsulates some of the differences often seen between the roles of volunteers and employed health professionals.

TABLE 8.1 Comparing the roles of health professionals and volunteers

EMPLOYED HEALTH PROFESSIONAL	VOLUNTEER
Recruited in a professional capacity	Acquired by defining a need, asking, word of mouth, volunteer interest, organisational promotion or succession planning
Extensive professional qualification and background checks	Limited background and, possibly, health, qualification and/or professional checks
Educated in their specific field	Widely varied education and training
Remunerated	Not remunerated, but willing to invest their own time in the organisation
May aspire to more senior positions	Motivated by altruism and personal interests
Have a specific lexicon	Often use layperson's language (especially when new to a role)
Higher level of responsibility and risk	Defers most responsibility and risk to employees
Prioritises their comment to the organisation as their employer	May have higher priorities and responsibilities elsewhere
Often committed to the organisation via an employee contract	May leave the organisation at any time
May be rewarded via pay rise, staff awards, industry awards and staff-related recognition programs	May be acknowledged and valued via volunteer recognition program or awards, state or local volunteer awards, and tailored low- or no-cost ways of valuing their contributions to the organisation
May wear a uniform	May wear civilian clothes, or be provided with clothing/items so people can identify their volunteer role

8.3 Getting to know the person: Morgan's story

Morgan was comfortable working at the admissions help desk. The halls were full of friendly faces that often chirped their greetings as they hurried to their next patient.

One day, a patient's family member was distraught and caused quite a ruckus in a hallway. Morgan brought the family member back to the help desk as it seemed that they hadn't followed the admission procedure. At one point, the family member was getting quite irate and was yelling at Morgan.

Morgan was quite taken aback, and an admissions clerk quickly stood in. The admissions clerk assertively informed the family member of the hospital's policy on verbal abuse and advised them that Morgan was not to be treated in such a manner. She was able to calm the family member and remind them of the care and excellent treatment provided in the hospital. The family member was mollified and apologetic, and Morgan was able to return to the desk.

Morgan went home that evening and discussed the event with family members. It was reassuring for the family that hospital policies covered volunteers, and that the admissions clerk was able to recognise that it wasn't Morgan's role as a volunteer to respond to irate family members.

Morgan reflected on what the admissions clerk had said in relation to the quality of care and treatment provided at the hospital. This affirmed the importance of the organisation and Morgan's role in contributing to it.

Supporting volunteers

Supporting volunteers is essential and quite easy. A common-sense, professional and courteous approach will ensure volunteers feel part of the organisation: happy, enthusiastic, comfortable, productive and safe (mentally and physically). Due to the nature of the service, health organisations often further support volunteers with specific policy and procedures, education and lines of communication, with all contributing to a safe and welcoming environment for all (Commonwealth of Australia, 2021; Volunteering Australia, 2020). These formal and informal efforts mount up to create a holistic support network, creating an environment that volunteers feel enthusiastic about working in. This means the organisation is more likely to retain valued volunteers in the long term (Oppenheimer & Warburton, 2014; Stuart et al., 2020).

Although many organisations have volunteer coordinators/managers employed to carry out the support process, every person in the organisation should contribute to the support and care of volunteers; after all, volunteers offer important services that would otherwise not be available and we all contribute to the culture of an organisation. Table 8.2 outlines a few suggestions on how to support volunteers. In addition to this, you should talk to the volunteers in your organisation to find out what resonates with them personally.

TABLE 8.2 Interacting with volunteers

	SPECIFICS OR ACTIONS	REFERENCES AND RESOURCES
Warm welcome	» Know when volunteers are present and acknowledge them. » Provide information that enables volunteer to feel welcome (e.g. name, position) and direct them to the correct area/task. » Be familiar with the volunteer programs and contacts in your organisation. » If a new volunteer identifies themselves, be friendly, acknowledge their time and take/point them to the area of best assistance.	» Volunteering Australia (2020) has numerous resources and professional development available for download. » Reach out to other nearby or like organisations that have volunteer programs. There may be a professional group that shares learnings. Or, if not, you might be able to set something up informally. » The Aged Care Royal Commission provides some strong insight into ways to support volunteers in Recommendation 44 (Commonwealth of Australia, 2021).
Orientation and induction	» Provide/contribute to the volunteer orientation/induction program. If possible, do this in a group as it creates instant camaraderie and support. » Provide clear guidelines and expectations for volunteer roles. » Make yourself familiar with the training provided. » Understand what the volunteer is capable of and their level of knowledge. » Take the time to understand why the volunteer wants to be involved and what drew them to your organisation. This will help you to identify additional skills, roles, processes and service improvements (for the individual and the organisation).	
Specific skills	» Provide opportunities for upskilling relevant to their volunteer role. » If possible, host training days with other volunteers to encourage a sense of belonging. » Consider volunteers who are unable to be present on the day.	» Workshops (e.g. public speaking, counselling, grief/bereavement, customer service, computer skills, fundraising) » Webinars, copies of literature

(Continued)

TABLE 8.2 Continued

	SPECIFICS OR ACTIONS	REFERENCES AND RESOURCES
Health and wellbeing	» Find out how volunteers are feeling on a regular basis, both informally and formally. » Offer support resources when needed and check back to see if they were used. » Volunteers in support/leadership roles are often contacted at all hours and this can be emotionally draining, especially when they are geographically dispersed roles. » Consider the potential for a volunteer to be affected during times of adversity. Provide them with some skills to assist with this and some resources for outreach (access to employee assistance programs may be helpful for all parties). Also consider other roles or opportunities for them to stay engaged if they need to take a break from their volunteer role. » If something happens that affects a volunteer's mental or physical well-being, report it, as you would for a staff member. » Remember that as medical professionals you may have a different level of emotional resilience from volunteers; volunteers may not be used to being exposed to situations that you are familiar with. » Ensure the volunteers are aware of work health and safety principles and maintain compliance.	» Know the organisation's available support resources/contacts. » If organisational support services aren't available, make sure you link the volunteer into their preferred support networks of external supports such as local, state or national mental health associations – for example, local GP or mental health services; Beyondblue Australia (2021).
Ways to interact with volunteers	» Be courteous and friendly, even when you are in a rush. A quick smile or simple acknowledgment is always appreciated and goes a long way. » Be genuine with volunteers, especially if you are asking for their feedback. » If you make a commitment, keep it, and if something changes let them know as soon as possible. » If the volunteers in your area operate autonomously or are geographically dispersed, try to organise different opportunities for them to gather with/without employees (even virtually). » Providing regular opportunities for updates on the program/organisation can be beneficial, but speak to your volunteers or review the readership data available to understand what the frequency should be. Sometimes we can overdo formal communications, creating unnecessary pressure and work for staff. » Including volunteers in staff social events is a good way of promoting cohesion and positive culture. » Hold joint meetings, when appropriate. » Highlighting staff and volunteer profiles in communications and on notice boards can be a nice way for everyone to get to know each other better.	
Communication tips	» Use your professional communication skills in the same way you would with a patient or their loved ones. » Be aware of the volunteer's preferred method of communication and use it. » Be aware of the timelines they require, and try to work within them when you can. » Keep volunteers informed, especially about program/process changes and, if you can, let them know why. » Provide friendly communications to the volunteer during periods of absence (e.g. newsletters, emails, handwritten notes). » Don't overlook social media as an effective communication and social cohesion tool, and don't assume that older volunteers won't engage with social media. » Ensure that you document the communications sent, and when, for future reference and good governance.	

TABLE 8.2 Continued

	SPECIFICS OR ACTIONS	REFERENCES AND RESOURCES
Emergency procedures	» Ensure that all volunteers know the correct procedures in case of emergency and have access to them. In the event that something does go wrong, knowledge of emergency procedures is vital. » If possible, include volunteers (or volunteer leaders) in emergency management exercises or preparation. They may be able to assist in times where surge capacity is required (hospital or emergency). » Ensure that volunteers understand their role or requirements in an emergency. » Don't overlook prior experience. Identify past experience or skills volunteers may have to be able to assist in other roles. Conversely, be aware if something makes them unsuitable for assisting in an emergency.	
Costs	» Be aware of the costs (especially hidden costs) associated with volunteering at your organisation. You'll find many volunteers don't want to be reimbursed, but no one likes to feel like they are being taken advantage of. Set up ways to track and reimburse volunteer out-of-pocket expenses, even if they aren't utilised. It's an important recognition, and helps you lessen the barriers to volunteering, making your programs more accessible. » Ensure that the volunteer is aware of what may or may not be reimbursed. For example, many hospitals offer free parking to their volunteers as parking is sometimes difficult and of significant cost. Or some organisations allow volunteers access to their patient/family shuttle service, so that volunteers who are unable to drive can still participate. » Provide information about company charges and payments appropriate to their role (e.g. volunteers providing official transport for patients may use a corporate credit card to purchase fuel for company vehicles, or to wash company vehicles). » Be cautious when providing benefits for volunteering. Organisations need to be mindful that offering certain privileges, money or gifts can alter the volunteering status and have implications for the organisation. It also takes away from the feeling of 'doing good' that volunteering is founded on. » Many organisational websites state the support they provide to volunteers, so check out what similar organisations are doing to find further best-practice examples. » Countries and states have different requirements, so make sure you review the workplace regulations and tax implications relating to volunteers before implementing benefit schemes and purchasing gifts.	Warburton, 2012 Stephens et al., 2015

8.4 Getting to know the person: Morgan's story

Morgan had been volunteering at the hospital for 10 years now and was looking forward to the upcoming volunteer morning tea, a celebration of the volunteers' contribution to the hospital. This year, Morgan would receive a 10-year service pin and special invitations for family to attend and be included in the celebration – a token gift, but something that Morgan was proud to receive. Morgan's family accepted their invitations to attend, and it was wonderful for them to see the valuable contribution Morgan was making by improving outcomes for staff, patients and visitors.

Morgan's reciprocal benefit from being involved was even greater now. The hospital had introduced a meal program that provided a free hospital cafeteria meal to all volunteers who volunteered for more than four hours during a day.

This couldn't have come at a better time as Morgan's life partner, Darcy, had died and he was grieving. When Darcy died, Morgan lost enthusiasm to cook regular meals at home. Eating alone only reinforced the absence of Darcy during what would ordinarily be their nice evening ritual. To receive a healthy meal on volunteering days was of great benefit and the distraction of the busy and social cafeteria was an added bonus. This was quite a relief to the family, who worried that Morgan was lacking basic dietary requirements. They had been trying to help by delivering regular meals, but increasingly noticed that the food remained untouched. Now, knowing that Morgan was eating at least one meal a day at the hospital gave them significant peace of mind. They had met some of the other volunteers at Darcy's funeral, so they knew that volunteering not only provided a meal, but also some support for Morgan during this time of great grief.

After the volunteer celebration, Morgan's family decided to speak to the hospital staff and let them know that they had some other concerns about Morgan's health and well-being, and how much they appreciated the new meal program. The empathy and time given to them made it overwhelmingly apparent that the hospital truly appreciated and cared about its volunteers. The staff assured the family that they kept an eye on volunteers, just as they did their staff and that Morgan was by no means socially isolated. In fact, it was quite the opposite. Volunteers, staff and even regular patients knew Morgan well and considered this volunteer part of the fabric of the services provided at the hospital. The family was thrilled to hear stories of Morgan being included in the hospital staff walking/fitness challenges, strategic planning days and social events. Having the family at this volunteer celebration gave them an insight into the fullness and richness of Morgan's life and the wonderful benefit volunteering is for everyone.

FOCUS QUESTIONS

- Reflecting on Morgan's last 10 years, how does engagement and communication benefit all stakeholders?
- Review Table 8.2. What other strategies can you identify that an organisation may provide to offer volunteer support?
- Involving volunteers in appropriate organisational staff and social activities is a way of boosting volunteers' sense of purpose, value and knowledge. Reflecting on your professional role, how do you believe this inclusion would benefit you?

Program diversification and supporting volunteers who lead delivery

As an organisation's volunteer program matures and grows, it is common for volunteers to be in a position of leading or mentoring other volunteers. Sometimes these lead situations also arise due to diversification – for example, perhaps funding changes mean that volunteers need to support a previously staffed program/function to ensure continuation of a service.

In such instances, sometimes a volunteer branch or committee forms. Often, these are a significant asset for the organisation. They can operate more autonomously, lead program/

process development from conception through to implementation and often run the day-to-day operation, assisting to reduce staff workload, improve sustainability and sometimes diversify geographic reach.

It is demonstrably important that such organisations retain strong lines of communication, support and training for these volunteer groups. It is also important to ensure that this happens holistically and on an individual member basis to assist in maintaining not only the volunteer relationship, but also continual improvement of the program/delivery. As mentioned, a volunteer coordinator may oversee this, but every employee in the organisation has a responsibility to ensure that they play a part in communications and improvements of mutual benefit.

Maintaining contact with the 'lead' volunteers also provides an opportunity to share information on important changes, activities and programs. Where possible, it is good to share with volunteers how their work has influenced this and/or even communicate to your colleagues how the volunteers have assisted. This is important, as volunteer leadership roles often take up extra time. Volunteer leaders are often considered a point of reference (especially when providing a geographically dispersed service) and therefore find themselves being contacted at home or during personal hours, so volunteer 'burnout' for these volunteers can be higher.

Organisations that demonstrate support, assist in removing barriers and offer professional/personal development to volunteers will, in turn, benefit from stronger volunteer commitment. Volunteers often feel valued in situations like this and longitudinal studies show this helps diminish the possibility of negative physical and mental health concerns that may arise in volunteer leadership (Stuart et al., 2020). Development will benefit the organisation as well, assisting with the provision of an improved volunteer program, volunteer retention and succession planning. Volunteers who are well trained and identified in succession planning may be able to offer additional support in times of need.

It is important to recognise that, much like employees, volunteers can easily become daunted by the workload, feel isolated in their activity area and feel pressured to take on too much in order to support their community, cause and organisation. This may be more prevalent in times of need or emergency management, where longer hours or greater responsibility has been incurred. Be aware of conversations with volunteers and, if it appears that a volunteer is struggling or feeling as though they need to overstep their role, report it to the volunteer coordinator or relevant personnel so they can assist.

However, many volunteers thrive with change, delivery pressures and autonomy. Experienced volunteers and/or volunteers with prior management experience may contribute to administrative tasks or be informal mentors to less experienced volunteers and health professionals. Such volunteers are obviously invested in the organisation and this should be celebrated. Setting these volunteers up for success and removing barriers to improve their effectiveness will mean that the majority should be able to work autonomously, allowing employees to complete core work.

This is especially important with volunteers working in regional areas, or those volunteering in communities remote from the organisation's centre (Oppenheimer & Warburton, 2014). Many health organisations have volunteer public health programs that fall into this category. The benefits of maintaining strong communication and support go beyond benefitting the volunteer. Strong communication with these volunteers will mean that they themselves will be able to convey the organisation's health messages to the community, and in turn keep you informed on how messages and programs are received at a grassroots level (Volunteering Australia, 2016). For instance, if an outbreak of a communicable disease has occurred, an organisation's geographically dispersed public health volunteer program may help to quickly inform the community of precautionary actions to limit infection rates.

Local volunteers are accessible and usually trusted in their community, so they are often more effective and efficient in such roles. In contrast, health professionals who aren't embedded in a community may have lower engagement levels due to their inability to build consistent rapport and personal connections.

8.5 Getting to know the person: Morgan's story

A member of the hospital staff asked about Morgan's career in education. After discussions, the staff member reported to the volunteer coordinator that Morgan was a school counsellor and staff mentor for many years. This was unknown to the volunteer coordinator and, coincidentally, during a formal review of the volunteer program later that month, it became evident there was a need for someone to mentor new volunteers.

The coordinator spoke to Morgan to get some more insight into the school counsellor role and Morgan's interest in this new role. It was evident that Morgan's skills offered more than just the ability to implement a mentor program for new volunteers. With Morgan's assistance, the volunteer manager formalised a Comfort Program: a volunteer-led service that would provide information and companionship to patients and their carers while they waited for appointments or treatment. This was a great benefit to the hospital as, in the upcoming financial year, they expected to lose some of the funding available for the in-situ patient and carer counselling service. The volunteers offer simple services such as a friendly welcome, tea or coffee, and information on the local area and support services.

The Comfort Program volunteers were given formal mental health training, specific training about the information nurses would like relayed and details on helpful information that would aid health-care professionals. This program also required further information and documentation to be signed in relation to patient/family privacy and confidentiality as this was of utmost importance, especially as some of the patients were familiar to the volunteers.

Morgan took on mentoring new volunteers easily, and the staff were always available as a sounding board to answer questions.

Being involved in the development of the Comfort Program challenged Morgan personally, but he found that learning new skills to provide the important patient/family support was interesting and rewarding. Morgan's role in this program was in the oncology ward, welcoming and sitting with patients (usually older people). Morgan also provided comfort to a small number of young children in this ward, especially when their parents were unable to be there during certain treatment or consultation periods. This was quite emotionally challenging at times, but due to Morgan's experience in education and counselling, past skills were reinvigorated and the benefits to the program and influence on positive health service outcomes were notable. Morgan had the ability not only to provide comfort to patients in need, but also to provide crucial patient information to nurses, who helped with diagnosis and treatment.

FOCUS
QUESTIONS

- Considering Morgan's story so far, what are the benefits to an organisation of identifying a volunteer's interests, skills and ambitions?
- What are the benefits to the volunteer?
- In your professional career, what can you do to identify volunteer opportunities?
- Reflecting on your knowledge of the health sector now, can you identify any opportunities?

Program evaluation and volunteer skills assessment

The relationship between employees and volunteers can be a fruitful one, filled with mutual learning and opportunities for all. Volunteers harbour a wealth of knowledge from their own career paths and life experiences. This is particularly so with ageing volunteers, who have valuable life experiences to share. The diversity in skills and qualifications provides organisations with rare access to improve facilities and increase networks (Commonwealth of Australia, 2021).

There are also opportunities to gain new perspectives and valuable insights about the organisation. To find out information about your volunteers, it is important to evaluate their volunteer experiences, aspirations and outcomes, both formally and informally. During this process, volunteers should be encouraged to provide details of their interests and experiences, as well as the program delivery and their perception of outcomes (positive or negative). In recent years, volunteer organisations have been improving their volunteer evaluation process (Nowland-Foreman, 2016). Many now ask for more details during the recruitment process, which will assist in the identification of appropriate volunteer roles from the outset, improving volunteer retention and future evaluation (individual and program).

In an ever-evolving environment, evaluation will help you identify changes in volunteer priorities, interests and skills, and importantly how they are coping. In turn, volunteers will be able to provide you with valuable information on the organisation, your role and the volunteer program.

8.6 Getting to know the person: Morgan's story

Morgan was thoroughly enjoying the new volunteer role, particularly the Comfort Program responsibilities. The volunteer coordinator arranged for Morgan to be involved in a formal evaluation of the program with other volunteers. Morgan had been involved in this process before so was comfortable and familiar with the process, but other volunteers who hadn't been involved were quite apprehensive.

Being familiar with the organisation, Morgan decided to speak to the volunteer coordinator about this. A simple solution was implemented: all volunteers were provided with an agenda and the questions before the evaluation, providing the information and reassurance they needed.

During the evaluation session, which was conducted in a safe and inclusive environment, the volunteers were able to discuss their ideas, constructive criticisms and positive feedback. At the end of the session, the key themes were mapped and reported back to the group by the volunteer manager. The hospital board and leadership team were provided with a de-identified report with the key themes raised. They appreciated the volunteers' time and honest evaluation, and let the group know this via a short email to the volunteer group.

One observation raised by Morgan was that the family and friends caring for patients didn't know much about the respite facilities available in the local area. They were reluctant to seek them out, thinking that others in the community would need them more, due to their sense of responsibility to their loved one, and some apprehension about the facilities themselves. A further point raised by the volunteers was that patients often got confused with the number of staff they see during the day. This was particularly the case in the Comfort Program, as the patients were either older or very young, and easily confused by the number of visitors. For those with family members caring for them, they themselves were worried; stress and sleep deprivation was often taking a toll and the rotation of staff through the ward/room was overbearing at times. Overall, the volunteers were thrilled with the impact of the program; they could see tangible benefits and enjoyed the interaction with staff and patients. They all hoped it would continue in the future.

A week after the evaluation, the feedback was provided to the hospital staff, and they thanked the volunteers for their observations. The two concerns raised about patient/family care were of real interest to staff and they wanted to investigate a way to improve this service. Each of the nursing units took different approaches to combat the issues identified, relative to their patients and the care they were providing. In the children's ward, the doctors and nurses better allocated staff rosters to patient stays/beds and tried to wear consistent, distinguishable accessories to help the parents and children identify them. They also made sure that they introduced themselves to the children and parents/caregivers before commencing treatment or tests, and reassured them that they knew the patient history and treatment plan.

The hospital provided staff and volunteers with an overview of the respite services and their facilities in the area. In response, the staff and volunteers talked more about the respite services in the local area, making sure that caregivers knew that this was a service available to them, and provided information on how the services could be accessed. Morgan was thrilled with the action taken by the hospital and staff, and the overall positive response to the feedback. After a matter of weeks, the volunteers made sure that the nursing staff received the praise patients and families gave throughout their stay, and everyone was very appreciative of the extra information and support.

Key points for interacting with volunteers

- Fear of the unknown is common and raises levels of anxiety in some individuals (Tanner, 2010). When asking for a change in processes, or asking for something out of the ordinary, make sure you explain why and how. It helps to provide context and allay fear, and is good communication practice.

- There are many free resources available to assist you with volunteer management and programs. Check out local, state or national volunteer websites to find these. Refer to Table 8.2.

- A sincere 'thank you' goes a long way. Rewards and gifts can take away from the volunteering act itself; a significant lesson to learn is the ability to allow someone to feel happy with their act of giving.

Volunteer absence

Ageing volunteers will inevitably need to interrupt or cease their volunteer involvement. This may be due to their own personal circumstances, such as health and family, or other events, such as an organisation's requirements or – as we have experienced in more recent years – a global pandemic resulting in various restrictions. Volunteers may experience a sense of loss during such periods; this aligns with role theory concepts that show a relationship between an individual's expectations and perceptions of themselves are often interrelated to their responsibilities and positions. Role theory states that a change in responsibility or role may affect health and well-being, especially if this change impacts the individual's sense of worth (Van Ingen & Wilson, 2017). For volunteers, this may be due to a variety of factors, such as their personal situations weighing on them, or social or physical isolation from the organisation and the people in it. Or it may be that not fulfilling their volunteer role is causing stress, emotional concern, social isolation, or a sense of failure or loss.

It is advisable that someone in the organisation keeps in touch with volunteers during these times. During COVID-19 we saw many volunteer programs cease operation for periods of time, and some organisations recognised the need to keep in touch with volunteers. Some did this exceptionally well, not only by sending regular communications, but also by using the current volunteers to set up their own support program to maintain social and organisational connection.

This chapter referred to the three positive by-products often associated with volunteering; however, during times of absence, health can decline, social isolation can occur, and cognitive and physical decline may accelerate (Guiney et al., 2021). Keeping in touch with volunteers and offering support where possible helps to further develop a longstanding relationship of mutual benefit and respect. The organisation is able to keep the volunteer informed about the organisation, and ready for a successful return to volunteering, if possible. You also increase the likelihood that the associated health benefits of volunteering are not negated and you, as an organisation, demonstrate that volunteering is not only a transactional process, but also a relationship to be valued and respected (Tanner, 2010).

Ways to keep in touch include:

- continuing to invite volunteers to volunteer gatherings
- if feasible, keeping them involved in the volunteer review/update process
- phoning, video calling or catching up face to face occasionally

- sending a message, or a 'shout out', via the organisation's social media channels
- asking the active volunteers to write a letter, card or email to the absent volunteers.

It may be worthwhile setting up a contact or support service during periods of longstanding volunteer absence or program disruption.

8.7 Getting to know the person: Morgan's story

Morgan had been volunteering for the hospital for 18 years, and although the impacts of ageing were becoming evident, Morgan was still an integral part of hospital life, maintaining the same volunteer hours and days.

Morgan had been unwell recently and the hospital staff had encouraged a visit to the GP. Morgan's family were grateful that the staff at the hospital had noted this deterioration as they were also encouraging a check-up. Eventually their persistence prevailed, and Morgan sought a medical review, with tests revealing cancer.

Morgan needed to reduce volunteer hours to allow for treatment, recovery and rehabilitation. Some treatment took place at the hospital, which offered a chance to catch up with staff and be on the receiving side of the Comfort Program. For Morgan, this eased a sense of loss in not being able to take part in volunteering.

Morgan's family would often stay during the treatments, but on the days when they weren't available there was comfort in knowing that Morgan was in familiar surrounds with people who cared.

The volunteer coordinator occasionally dropped in to visit Morgan. During one visit, Morgan announced that although volunteering was not possible at the moment, Morgan would like to contribute to the hospital financially. The next week, when Morgan's family came to offer support during treatment, they assisted in making a financial pledge – one that enabled the Comfort Program to diversify and continue into the foreseeable future.

FOCUS QUESTIONS

- What are the potential health impacts on aged volunteers who are unable to maintain their volunteering?
- What are the potential impacts to the organisation?
- What can be done to mitigate these impacts for both the volunteer and the organisation?

Appreciating and acknowledging volunteers

Respecting volunteers and appreciating the contribution they make to an organisation is really important for the ongoing viability of the volunteer program and so the volunteers understand their value. Most volunteers do so to make a difference; they, like all of us, need to understand their effort is valued. Communicating value to volunteers and individuals improves our self-worth and consequently our well-being (Alfes et al., 2015).

Just as we have performance reviews and feedback from our peers and managers, volunteers need to know how they are performing and, hopefully, that their contribution is helping the 'cause'.

Years of service is one way to acknowledge a volunteer's contributions; keeping accurate volunteer records is important to achieve this successfully. While a volunteer manager will often complete this, you can assist by providing added notes and achievements. This information can help to build comprehensive records to support volunteer awards and recognition programs, or national/state service awards.

A volunteer awards/recognition program can be a wonderful way to recognise the efforts of volunteers and publicly acknowledge the organisation's appreciation. It is important that a volunteer rewards scheme is transparent, and it is also important to personalise your recognition where possible. Many organisations structure their recognition program so that staff have a clear process to follow, showing them how to thank and when. As well as being useful, this structure helps to make sure people aren't missed and can be a cause of great celebration – like the 10-year service pin that Morgan received. However, it needs to be balanced. Research shows that authenticity over transactional reward is more valued and of greater benefit (Stirling et al., 2011).

The power of these acknowledgments can be significant, but make sure that each individual stands out from the crowd occasionally (Stirling et al., 2011). Simple ways to do this are:
- pop in for coffee on your way to a meeting
- ask them for their opinion on a relatable work matter
- ask how they are, or about their family
- ask them to review a new project proposal
- include them in a presentation at a staff conference
- send a card when their grandchild is born
- offer condolences and support if they are grieving
- remember anniversaries
- pick up the phone and have a chat
- write a handwritten 'thank you' letter – it's almost unexpected in this age of emails.

Or simply ask volunteers how they would like to be acknowledged and what makes them feel valued. Don't assume that ageing individuals won't use technology or forms of social media. This is a stereotype and you'll find that many more are accustomed to alternative forms of communication and interested in it (National Seniors Australia, 2019). Volunteering Australia has now included Virtual Volunteering as a defined type of volunteering, and many organisations are finding people with limited time or physical/mental capacity are choosing Virtual Volunteering as a way to be involved (Volunteering Australia, 2016). Virtual Volunteering may present an opportunity to keep older volunteers in your health service engaged for longer or diversify your programs to ease staffing pressures.

8.8 Getting to know the person: Morgan's story

Unfortunately, Morgan's health declined, and it was necessary to leave the volunteer program permanently. Staff and volunteers kept in contact and Morgan used online conference calls to participate in the hospital's events. At the annual Christmas morning tea, the team celebrated Morgan's nineteenth year of volunteer service. The hospital also announced that Morgan had won a regional volunteer award to be presented at the Australia Day awards the following month.

Morgan's family noticed a little more joy in Morgan after being told about the award; it was something to look forward to, a goal to achieve.

Morgan's health was deteriorating rapidly now, and the team decided to pick Morgan up in the bus for one last visit to the hospital. Many nurses took the time to chat and say 'thank you'. It meant the world to Morgan.

On the day of the Australia Day awards, the family drove Morgan to the local hall where the celebration was being held. To Morgan's surprise a number of current and former volunteers and staff where there to meet them. They cheered as Morgan was helped to receive a National Community Service medal. It was a day of great celebration and a show of the comradery and value in long-term volunteer, Morgan.

The next month, Morgan passed away. Many of the nurses, volunteers and managers attended the funeral. The volunteer coordinator spoke of Morgan's contribution to patient care and family support. They shared funny stories of how Morgan helped new nurses navigate their way through the seemingly endless corridors, and often ended up at the hospital café chatting with them instead.

After the funeral, the volunteer coordinator circulated a card for all of the staff to sign, and this was sent to Morgan's family. It was a small gesture filled with heartfelt words.

Three months later, the volunteer coordinator invited Morgan's family to attend their forthcoming 'Christmas in July' volunteer morning tea. The family said they would attend, but Morgan's two daughters wanted to meet with the director of nursing and the volunteer coordinator the week before.

The meeting took place two weeks later, and Morgan's two daughters announced that Morgan had left the hospital a significant bequest for the diversification and continuation of the Comfort Program. The two daughters thanked the hospital staff for the care they had provided over nearly 20 years. They spoke of the reassurance it gave them to know that Morgan was active, eating well, mentally stimulated, developing meaningful relationships and able to share stories of the past with peers, patients and families.

The following week, the hospital announced Morgan's legacy donation and eagerly revealed its plans to refurbish the lounges used for the Comfort Program and to extend the program into the palliative care unit. The donation also included a generous amount that was to be invested for the future. Morgan had set this up so that the hospital would be able to access funds in perpetuity and keep the program running and relevant.

After the announcement, the hospital presented the family with Morgan's 20-year service pin and, to their surprise, Morgan's eldest daughter announced her plan to join the volunteer program when she retired. The family felt like the volunteer program was an extension of their own family, as they too had made so many lasting connections through Morgan's involvement.

- Reflecting on the hospital's care and interaction with Morgan's family, what did they do to make it a supportive place for volunteers and their families?
  - How could these strategies be enhanced in the future?
  - What could you do in your capacity as a health-care professional?

FOCUS
QUESTIONS

Implications for practice

Strategies for valuing volunteers

- *Volunteer awards:* Many countries celebrate a national Volunteer Week. This is a good way for you to recognise the volunteers in your organisation. Investigate your local, state and national authorities as they often have avenues for nominating volunteers for prestigious awards, many of which support volunteering at the grass roots level.
- *Cyclical giving:* If cared for and supported, volunteers will share their experiences with others and often this results in further support for your organisation. This may be in the form of further volunteer acquisition and new volunteers recruited by current volunteers who are more likely to become regular volunteers in the future (Volunteering Australia, 2016).

  Respect and a bit of time will go a long way in helping you in your own career. But more importantly just doing the right thing helps make a volunteer's day a little bit brighter and more valued.

  As we have seen with Morgan, it may just give your community health-care facility the ability to offer levels of care previously unimaginable.
- *Time-poor trends:* Volunteers are now calling for more flexible volunteer hours and options. Many ageing Australians who volunteer also have other interests and responsibilities, such as caring for family or pursing their passions. Keep this in mind when you are discussing volunteer hours and planning volunteer programs.
- *Support for commencement costs:* Volunteers are required to undergo various police checks, depending on the area in which they choose to be involved, and some have mandatory vaccination responsibilities. These requirements incur costs that some volunteers can't afford. Consider having an incentive program that assists with some of these expenses.

Learn more
Watch Videos 8.1 and 8.2: Listen to John, Mary and the Wallsend Area Community Care volunteers' experiences and hear about what volunteering means to them.

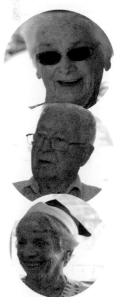

Learn more
Access additional resources – such as weblinks, further readings and podcasts – to broaden your understanding of this chapter. See the Guided Tour for access details.

Conclusion

Forging positive working relationships with volunteers can have significant benefits for everyone. Encouraging volunteers and building a longstanding working relationship will provide many benefits for your career and professional development. Developing a transparent volunteer program provides volunteers and staff with clear purpose, expectations, values and processes. Organisations that ensure they are aware of their volunteers' value are able to provide fulfilling opportunities that encourage volunteer retention and acquisition. Taking the time to communicate with the volunteers and, where appropriate, their support networks, provides avenues for further opportunities and program consistency. This in turn benefits you, the health professional, the patient or client, the volunteer and the community at large.

REVISION QUESTIONS

1   Interacting with volunteers as a registered nurse or other health-care professional may not have been part of the professional practice you anticipated. To better prepare yourself, look at Table 8.2 and identify at least two resources. Become familiar with these resources and create something for your professional portfolio as a reminder of these useful resources.

2   Morgan's story offers several lessons for the health-care professional and volunteer programs. State three points that affected you personally and that will stay with you as you build your professional experience.

REFERENCES

Alfes, K., Shantz, A. & Bailey, C. (2015). Enhancing volunteer engagement to achieve desirable outcomes: What can non-profit employers do? *International Journal of Voluntary and Nonprofit Organizations, 26*, 1–23. https://doi:10.1007/s11266-015-9601-3

Anderson, N., Damianakis, T., Kröger, E., Wagner, L., Dawson, D. & Binns, M. (2014). The benefits associated with volunteering among seniors: A critical review and recommendations for future research. *Psychological Bulletin.* https://doi:10.1037/a0037610

Australian Institute of Health and Welfare (AIHW) (2018). Older Australia at a Glance. Social & Economic Engagement. AIHW. www.aihw.gov.au/reports/older-people/older-australia-at-a-glance/contents/social-economic-engagement

Beyondblue Australia (2021). 3 Million Australians Are Living with Anxiety or Depression. www.beyondblue.org.au

Commonwealth of Australia (2021). Royal Commission into Aged Care Quality and Safety. Final report: Care, dignity and respect. Vol. 1, Summary and recommendations. https://agedcare.royalcommission.gov.au/sites/default/files/2021-03/final-report-volume-1_0.pdf

Darja, K. & Djurre, H. (2019) Volunteering research in Australia: A narrative review. *Australian Journal of Psychology, 71*(4), 342–60. https://doi:10.1111/ajpy.12251

Flinders University (2014). Volunteering Worth $290 Billion a Year. https://news.flinders.edu.au/blog/2014/10/31/volunteering-worth-290-billion-a-year/

Guiney, H., Keall, M. & Machado, L. (2021). Volunteering in older adulthood is associated with activity engagement and cognitive functioning. *Ageing, Neuropsychology, and Cognition, 28*(2), 253–69. https://doi:10.1080/13825585.2020.1743230

Jang, H., Tang, F., Gonzales, E., Soo Lee, Y. & Morrow-Howell, N. (2018). Formal volunteering as a protector of health in the context of social losses. *Journal of Gerontological Social Work, 61*(8), 834–48. https://doi:10.1080/01634372.2018.1476945

Lum, T. Y. & Lightfoot, E. (2005). The effects of volunteering on the physical and mental health of older people. *Research on Aging*, *27*(1), 31–55. https://doi:10.1177/0164027504271349

National Seniors Australia (2019). What Kind of Senior Surfer Are You? https://nationalseniors.com.au/members/our-generation/spring-2019/what-kind-of-senior-surfer-are-you

Nowland-Foreman, G. (2016). Outcomes, Accountability and Community & Voluntary Organisations: Holy Grail, Black Hole or Wholly Possible. Centre for Not for Profit Leadership. www.communityresearch.org.nz/wp-content/uploads/formidable/Outcomes-Accountability-and-Community-Voluntary-Organisations-G-Nowland-Foreman.pdf

Oppenheimer, M. & Warburton, J. (eds) (2014). *Volunteering in Australia*. Federation Press.

Stephens, C., Breheny, M. & Mansvelt, J. (2015). Volunteering as reciprocity:

Beneficial and harmful effects of social policies to encourage contribution in older age. *Journal of Aging Studies*, *33*(15), 22–7. https://doi:10.1016/j.jaging.2015.02.003

Stirling, C., Kilpatrick, S. & Orpin, P. (2011). A psychological contract perspective to the link between non-profit organizations' management practices and volunteer sustainability. *Human Resource Development International*, *14*(3), 321–36. https://doi:10.1080/13678868.2011.585066

Stuart, J., Kamerāde, D., Connolly, S., Ellis Paine, A., Nichols, G. & Grotz, J. (2020). The Impacts of Volunteering on the Subjective Wellbeing of Volunteers: A Rapid Evidence Assessment. Technical Report. www.volunteeringnz.org.nz/wp-content/uploads/2020_Volunteer-wellbeing-technical-report-Oct2020-a.pdf

Stuart-Hamilton, I. (2012). *The Psychology of Ageing: An introduction* (5th edn). Jessica Kingsley Publishers.

Tanner, D. (2010). *Managing the Ageing Experience: Learning from older people*. Policy Press.

Van Ingen, E. & Wilson, J. (2017). I volunteer, therefore I am? Factors affecting volunteer role identity. *Nonprofit and Voluntary Sector Quarterly*, *46*(1), 29–46. https://doi.org/10.1177/0899764016659765

Volunteering Australia (2016). State of Volunteering. www.volunteeringaustralia.org/research/stateofvolunteering/

Volunteering Australia (2020). Resources. www.volunteeringaustralia.org/resources

Warburton, J. (2012). Volunteering as a productive ageing activity: Evidence from Australia. In N. Morrow-Howell & A. C. Mui (eds). *Productive Engagement in Later Life: A global perspective*, pp. 195–206. Routledge.

9

Leisure, Sport and Recreation in the Lives of Older People

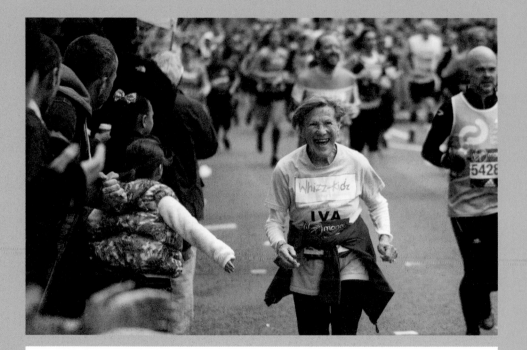

LEARNING OBJECTIVES

After reading this chapter, you will:

» examine the significance of meaningful and self-determined engagement in leisure, sport and recreation

» describe the wide variety of leisure experiences that older people can engage in, ranging from traditional activities to more contemporary activities

» explain how physically active leisure can have a positive impact on wellness, sense of identity and quality of life as a person ages

» explain how the older person is the expert on their leisure needs, so family members and/or the registered nurse or allied health professional can work with the older person and local institutions or groups to support/facilitate/enable meaningful leisure.

Introduction

The culture and environment in which people live and the lifestyles they embrace primarily through leisure can influence personal **well-being** just as much as their physiological condition (Grant & Kluge, 2012). In this chapter, leisure and **recreation** are understood as self-generated, meaningful and pleasurable engagement in physical, mental, social, emotional and/or spiritual activities or experiences that contribute to a person's health and sense of identity (Fortune & Dupuis, 2018; Kelly, 2012; Stebbins, 2012). Thus, it is the *quality and personal meaning* of the experience in the activity, not the activity *per se*, that constitutes it as leisure or recreation, with an individual's attitude, needs and lifestyle choices coming first, and dimensions of time and action second. While some older people may use leisure to pass the time, stay busy and keep their minds off losses or concerns, such as the passing away of a spouse or losses in their functional ability (Kleiber, 2016), the notion that leisure is encouraged by health professionals merely to 'pass time' with older people, manage their behaviours or increase their functioning, is outdated (Fortune & Dupuis, 2018; Dupuis et al., 2012b). For example, aged care organisations have often planned repetitive activities for older adults with the main purpose of filling in time, rather than adopting a person-centred approach to aged care. The 2018–2019 Royal Commission into Age Care Quality and Safety in Australia highlighted the importance of 'the place of the individual in the aged care system' by discussing that the new Aged Care Quality Standards represent 'a shift toward a more person-centred approach in aged care' (Commonwealth of Australia, 2019a, p. 64). The related Charter of Aged Care Rights (see Aged Care Quality and Safety Commission, 2019) 'aims to build an understanding of the rights of people receiving aged care, and to provide protections for those rights … Providers must comply with the Charter, in addition to the Standards', or sanctions will be imposed (Commonwealth of Australia, 2019a, p. 64). These standards and rights place the older person at the centre of aged care, which has implications for leisure and recreation in the lives of older Australians, and for health practitioners in aged care.

Meaningful and joyful engagement in leisure requires (and satisfies our need for) **self-determination** by enabling a sense of autonomy, competence and (at times) relatedness with significant others (Coleman & Iso-Ahola, 1993; Ryan & Deci, 2000). At the same time, leisure and recreation experiences occur in the cultural world of possibilities and challenges; this means that not everyone has the resources, ability and/or desire to remain physically, mentally or socially active in their leisure time, especially those living in or requiring the services of the aged care system. This reality must be acknowledged given that we live in a time and context where **physically active leisure** is promoted to all older people through policy, the professions, academic literature and other stakeholders. The promotion of 'keeping physically active as we age' has become a prominent feature in the media, popular press, social media and across the allied health sector in response to the COVID-19 global pandemic. For example, the Australian Physiotherapy Association, in consultation with members of the Australian Association of Gerontology, developed a 'Safe Exercise at Home' website to encourage older Australians to keep active safely at home during the pandemic restrictions, as well as support long-term exercise participation. Furthermore, many conflicting assumptions about older people, ageing and exercise are hidden in the promotion of physical activity through the **active ageing**, **successful ageing** and **healthy ageing** agendas, which have become particularly evident in health-related policy and practice since the 1990s (Dionigi, 2017; Dionigi & Gard, 2018a, 2018b; Pike, 2011; World Health Organization, 2002).

well-being
The contented feeling people have about their holistic state of health and quality of life at any given moment.

recreation
Activity that contributes to one's health and sense of identity (in contrast to traditional understandings of recreation in health-care settings, such as therapeutic recreation).

self-determination
The fulfilment of a person's psychological need for autonomy, competence and relatedness.

physically active leisure
Leisure activity that involves bodily movement.

active ageing
A program of policies and discourses that generally encourage people to remain physically, socially and mentally active as they age.

successful ageing
Ageing where the person perceives themselves as healthy, disability (if any exists) is not impeding their enjoyment of life and they are functioning at a level that enables them to be actively engaged in activities they enjoy or find fulfilling.

healthy ageing
The development of mental, social and physical well-being across the lifespan.

See Chapter 4
for definitions
and discussion of
successful ageing.

identity management
The process by which
adults negotiate and
construct a personal
and social sense of self.

Learn more
Watch Videos 1.1
and 4.1: Hear about
what older people
are engaged in
and the effect of
these activities on
their experience
of ageing. Ray and
George discuss
the significance
of leisure and
recreation
appropriate for men.

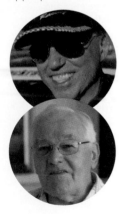

Ultimately, regardless of what agenda is being pushed in policy, in the literature or among health professionals, finding personal meaning in leisure activities is necessary if an individual's leisure experiences are to contribute to their overall health, quality of life and **identity management**. As a future health professional, you are in a prime position to place older people at the centre of their leisure decision-making processes and get to know them and their interests so that you can help them find meaning and pleasure in leisure, regardless of the type of activity. This chapter will discuss, through the use of two case studies (Iris and Lily), the meaning of leisure, sport and recreation in later life, and the types of leisure and recreation in which older people engage (with particular emphasis on physically active leisure pursuits). It will suggest some effective ways for health professionals to facilitate meaningful participation in leisure and recreation, especially as a person transitions from a highly active to less active lifestyle, and from independent living to dependent, long-term aged care living, as in the cases of Iris and Lily, respectively.

Leisure in later life in contemporary times

Iris (introduced in case study 9.1) grew up in a cultural period when understandings of ageing were predominantly associated with the acceptance of natural bodily decline (Jones & Higgs, 2010), while high levels of physical activity or sport were considered inappropriate, dangerous and unnecessary for girls, women and older people (Dionigi, 2017, 2010a; Grant, 2001). From the age of approximately 60, Iris has lived in a climate that is shaped and defined by a resistance to old age and one in which 'active ageing' is promoted in media reports, government policies, gerontology and the sports/exercise sciences (Gard et al., 2017; Gard & Dionigi, 2016; Dionigi & Gard, 2018a, 2018b; Lassen & Moreira, 2014; Moulaert & Biggs, 2013).

Today's older population is considered more active, affluent, better educated, assertive and healthier than its predecessors (Biggs, 2014; Dionigi, 2008; Gilleard & Higgs, 2013). In 2006, it was found that Australian '[m]en and women aged 65 years and over spent more time on recreation and leisure activities (6 hours and 19 minutes and 5 hours and 50 minutes a day respectively) than any of the other age groups' (ABS, 2006, p. 8). Although more recent ABS data on leisure behaviour are unavailable, the COVID-19 pandemic undoubtedly affected leisure time, practices and options for everyone. The pandemic has resulted in reduced leisure opportunities for many, particularly the most vulnerable populations, such as older people and those living in long-term aged care facilities, as well as restrictions to international and national travel due to border closures and the absence of opportunities for human connection that often occurs in social leisure spaces, such as community sport, art galleries, cafés, schools, churches, retirement homes, cinemas and so on. With regard to older people, the enforced restrictions to leisure and social contact resulted in heightened feelings of loneliness and isolation, not only among those living in aged care homes but community-dwelling older people as well. At the same time, the global pandemic gave rise to creative leisure practices of self-expression and health protection, such as people exercising at home or with an online class. The pandemic reinforced the need for self-expressive and self-determined leisure in our lives, not only in terms of helping individuals cope with the fallout of a global pandemic, but also with the absence of, and/or restrictions to, leisure highlighting the positive contribution meaningful leisure participation makes to society.

In addition, variations to the age structure, coupled with early retirement and increased affluence, means that an increasing number of people could possibly spend 20–30 years in what is known as the **Third Age** (Higgs et al., 2009; Laslett, 1989). A key feature of the Third Age is 'the effective use of leisure' and ongoing engagement in 'activity, exercise, travel, eating out, self-maintenance and self-care' (Gilleard & Higgs, 2007, p. 25). A goal of the Third Age is to delay or prevent the **Fourth Age**, which is characterised by sickness, dependency, frailty, institutionalisation and the imminence of death (Blaikie, 1999). Therefore, due to various social changes throughout the latter half of the twentieth century, the older generation (especially since the 1990s) has typically felt 'less moral prohibition against leisure' (Godbey, 1999, p. 194) and it is likely that current older individuals have acquired many leisure skills throughout their lives.

Third Age
Approximately between the ages of 65 and 80 years, following retirement, and a time when there are fewer responsibilities, coupled with greater freedom to pursue self-fulfilment.

Fourth Age
A period towards the end of life, older than 80 years, which is typically characterised by sickness, dependency, frailty and the imminence of death.

9.1 Getting to know the person: Iris' story

From the age of 60 to 85 years, Iris had developed an identity as an active older person. In her older age she had come to identify herself through the effective use of her body. Whether she realised it or not, she had followed the 'active ageing' agenda, which promotes continued engagement in physical, mental and social activities, particularly those that society deems 'productive' in terms of reducing the health-care budget and stimulating the economy through ongoing consumerism. Thus, Iris maintained her good health and independence by keeping physically and socially active as she aged, just as the media and policies surrounding her at the time had endorsed. She played golf twice a week, played cards with her girlfriends twice a week, went to the local seniors centre to eat out and socialise once a week and regularly walked to the shops or along the beach. Iris found great pleasure and meaning in these activities and she looked forward to experiencing them each week.

When aged in her seventies, Iris competed twice in the Australian **Masters Games** in golf and race walking. In these competitions Iris pushed her body to its maximum. She trained at least twice a week in the months leading up to these events, which are held every two years, and she aimed to win medals. She got a silver medal in the 70–74 years golf at one games and a gold in the 75–80 years race walking at another. At one point, there was an article about Iris in her local newspaper in which she was referred to as a 'local hero' because of her Masters Games victories. At these multi-sports events, Iris would pay for her own accommodation and travel, enjoy the nearby tourist sites and activities, and dine out for her meals. In other words, Iris was visible in the local community, she was admired on the golf course and she was valued by society because she was seen to be ageing healthily, productively and actively.

Masters Games
A multi-sport and entertainment event, such as the Australian Masters Games and World Masters Games, held at local, state, national and/or international levels for mature-aged athletes.

RYLEE A. DIONIGI

FOCUS QUESTIONS

- What were your initial reactions to and thoughts or feelings about older people competing in sport? Why did you feel this way?
- What are the benefits for Iris as a highly active person in old age?
- In what ways can physically active leisure pursuits be a form of resistance to stereotypes of ageing and a source of personal empowerment?

OPPORTUNITIES FOR PHYSICALLY ACTIVE LEISURE AND COMPETITIVE SPORT IN OLDER AGE

With increased longevity, improved health among the ageing population and more opportunities for leisure, many people are pushing the boundaries of conventional understandings of 'age-appropriate' leisure activities for an older person. According to Grant (2001, p. 777):

> Rather than being 'over the hill', more and more older people are 'taking the hill by storm' and seeking opportunities to be involved in a multitude of activities, some new and others rekindled from earlier years.

Iris did not define herself as an athlete, but she was 'a golfer'; she competed in two Australian Masters Games and her sporting and leisure experiences are representative of many older athletes described in the literature below.

Resistance and empowerment through leisure in old age

On the one hand, participation in sport (as leisure) in older age can be a personally empowering experience, particularly for older women and late-life beginners to sport like Iris. It can inspire youth, have many psychosocial benefits for participants and appears to be resisting traditional gender and/or ageing norms (Dionigi, 2016; Stone et al., 2018). The following discussion summarises the research that reports these findings. On the other hand, due to the social determinants of health, such as education, housing, healthcare, socioeconomic status and so on (see PwC Global, 2019), the promotion of sport and physical activity to older people is not straightforward and it can be highly problematic for individuals and society (see Dionigi, 2017; Dionigi & Gard, 2018b; Son & Dionigi, 2020).

PSYCHOSOCIAL BENEFITS OF SPORT PARTICIPATION

Competing in sport at an older age provides many psychosocial benefits and experiences for participants that have been summarised into four broad areas: physical and psychological health benefits (including identity management); social networks; enjoyment; and competition (Dionigi, 2006, 2016; Gayman et al., 2017; Kim et al., 2020; Stone et al., 2018). Across these general benefits of sport participation, broader issues in general and sociocultural issues specifically of mainstream sport versus alternative sports (including sport for older people), resisting and reinforcing negative stereotypes associated with ageing (such as ageing as a state of decline), and reproducing health promotion discourses all emerged as important areas requiring further research (Dionigi, 2016). With regard to multi-sport events specifically, such as the World Masters Games, qualitative research has reported outcomes in addition to the general psychosocial benefits of physical activity. Refer to Table 9.1 for a summary of some of the research on late-life sport participation.

TABLE 9.1 Outcomes of competitive sport that go beyond those gained from general physical activity

OUTCOME	STUDY PARTICIPANTS	REFERENCE
Compete against peers at an older age, travel nationally and internationally, develop ongoing friendships and regular social interaction in the form of a mega multi-sport and entertainment event	World Masters Games participants (male and female) aged 56–90 years (mean = 72 years)	Dionigi et al. (2011)
In addition to multi-faceted physical, mental and social health benefits, sport helped women overcome barriers such as disease, pain, injury and finances, and gender and age norms. It also provided them with social roles, such as being role models for other women and younger people, as well as being evangelical about exercise for older people	Women aged 70–86 years who were World Masters Games participants	Horton et al. (2018)
Competing in sport allowed for social comparison with those of a similar age and resistance to loss in performance and physical ability, as well as assigning individual blame to those less active for compromised health (with little mention of uncontrollable factors or social determinants that affect one's ageing and health)	Men (aged 70–90 years) who participated in either the 2013 or 2017 World Masters Games	Horton et al. (2019)
A unique social world of like-minded individuals, an identity as a senior athlete, demonstrated perseverance and significant effort	Senior Games' participants (men and women aged 50 years and over) who had participated in their chosen sport for 10–50 years (as a form of serious leisure)	Heo et al. (2013)
Golf is low intensity, enables fair competition (due to the handicap system) and social and community engagement, as well as time for self, and an 'opportunity to exercise without it feeling like exercise' (p. 257)	Regular golfers (male and female, aged 55–74 years) who were members of private/semi-private metropolitan and country/regional golf clubs	Stenner et al. (2016)
The choice in activities provided for fun, competition, creativity, socialising and health	North Carolina Senior Games participants (male and female) aged 50 years and over	Henderson et al. (2012)

In addition to competitive sport, the North Carolina Senior Games (see Table 9.1) offer choice in a range of physical and social activities, such as walking, line dancing and arts. The authors argue that 'the element of fun cannot be overlooked' because if people do not enjoy the activities, they are less likely to maintain involvement (Henderson et al., 2012, p. 32). This finding aligns with the main argument of this chapter: that finding meaning and pleasure in leisure experiences (regardless of the activity) in old age is central to identity management and overall well-being. In fact, Henderson and colleagues (2012) found that those who were doing more than sports at these events perceived greater outcomes. This study highlighted the potential for sport as 'one way to introduce older adults to other community options', such as the arts (see A New Approach, 2019), that may better suit their interests and needs (Henderson et al., 2012, p. 32), especially if these interests change from active to less active pursuits as one ages, as will be discussed later in this chapter in the case of Lily.

Lifelong sport versus starting sport in later life

Iris is known as a 'late bloomer' to sport (Dionigi, 2008, 2015), in the sense that she began competing later in life, which, in her case, was when she was aged in her sixties. Differences between the experiences of lifelong sport participants (sport continuers) and those who begin sport in later life (late bloomers) are emerging in the literature (see Dionigi, 2015), and gender seems to play a key role in this process (see Smith, 2016), as seen in Table 9.2.

As was shown in Iris' case, older people can establish new or alternative identities as a winner, a sports champion and/or a highly physically active and independent person – identities that were not available to older people in the first half of the twentieth century and ones that may not have been part of their youth. Women like Iris were resisting ageing and gender norms that position older women as inactive and incapable of physically demanding, competitive sport (Dionigi, 2010a; Eman, 2012; Pfister, 2012). In addition, Kirby and Kluge (2013) also described the importance of belonging to a group for women, which is similar to findings of community in other studies on middle-aged and older women in team sports (Litchfield & Dionigi, 2011, 2012) and older people in exercise programs (Dionigi & Lyons, 2010; Lyons & Dionigi, 2007). Team sports and group contexts appear to foster spaces for women to support each other on their ageing journey, especially if they are beginners to sport at an older age (Dionigi, 2016).

TABLE 9.2 Outcomes for sport continuers and sport beginners

OUTCOMES	BEGINNERS OR CONTINUERS	STUDY PARTICIPANTS	REFERENCE
Some participants, particularly women, could *become* athletes in later life.	Beginners	World Masters Games participants (male and female) aged 56–90 years (mean = 72 years)	Dionigi et al. (2011)
Sport participation helped older people manage their identity, especially women who were previously identified as a mother or wife.	Beginners	Australian Masters Games participants (male and female) aged 55–94 involved in physically intense individual and team sports	Dionigi (2010b)
Participation in sport was personally empowering.	Continuers	Female and male New Zealand Masters competitors aged in their seventies who were involved in individual sports such as swimming, croquet, badminton, tennis, bowls, athletics, cycling, golf or running	Grant (2001)
'… the women experienced cultural lag and age-related barriers to resources when playing competitive softball in late adulthood. In addition, the network of shared relationships occupied by these women had both positive and negative influences on their participation in competitive sports'	Continuers	Six competitive softball teams of women ranging from 55–79 years	Wong et al. (2019, p. 72)
Participants were willing to try something new in later life, despite the reactions of others; they highly valued being part of a team for the first time and would not have formed a team without the support of the university.	Beginners	US women who began competing in a team sport (volleyball) at age 65	Kirby & Kluge (2013)

However, beginning sport in later life can also be a daunting experience, particularly for women who have not had previous exposure to or opportunity for regular sport participation in their earlier years. For example, the women volleyball players had to overcome fears of injury, failure and lack of fitness, as well as negotiate the reactions of friends and relatives who questioned the reasoning behind their involvement in sport at an older age (Kirby & Kluge, 2013). As Griffin and Phoenix (2014, pp. 401–2) explained:

Taking up a new activity at an older age means that we inevitably bring to it a lifetime of assumptions, preconceptions, and insecurities. For policy and program developers and providers, in turn, this has implications for how we might be more sensitive to the biographical background of each potential participant going forward rather than targeting discrete, commonly reported barriers to participation.

This recommendation to take a **person-centred approach** when assisting or encouraging an older person to embark on new leisure activities is important for health professionals who are working with older people in whatever capacity. Notably, the 2018–2019 Royal Commission into Aged Care Quality and Safety in Australia highlighted the importance of a person-centred approach in the aged care context. Furthermore, in the study by Kirby and Kluge an **authentic partnership** was formed between the university, the researchers and the participants. Without this partnership the women's volleyball team would have nowhere to train, no support, no coach and no opportunity to continue playing (Kirby & Kluge, 2013). Dionigi and Lyons (2010) found a similar sense of community manifesting among older people involved in a university exercise intervention. In this study, participants felt a sense of belonging and emotional connection to the university gym environment, the university researchers and students, and the broader community of active older people. The importance of establishing authentic partnerships in the aged care context is discussed next.

> **person-centred approach**
> A focus on participant involvement in decision making about leisure activities and nurturing individuals' strengths in leisure contexts through leisure experiences.

> **authentic partnership**
> A partnership focusing on the decision-making processes of the older person, family members, health professionals and local community through joint efforts, discussion and regular critical reflection.

Authentic partnerships through leisure

Leisure plays a key role in moving towards respecting ageing as an individualised, localised process that is diverse and steeped in older people's everyday practices. Recently, there has been a shift away from the leisure intervention model, which calls for self-responsibility for health and targets individual behaviour change, to a focus more on changing policy and culture, and promoting action in the local community and in the workplace (e.g. among leisure, recreation and health professionals in aged care settings) to improve individual and population health outcomes. For example:

- Dupuis and colleagues developed an authentic partnership model (see Figure 9.1) that involves universities working with local aged care providers and older residents to focus on wellness and leisure in later life, particularly in long-term health-care settings and among people living with dementia (Dupuis, 2008; Dupuis et al., 2012b; Lopez & Dupuis, 2014).

FIGURE 9.1 Authentic partnership model

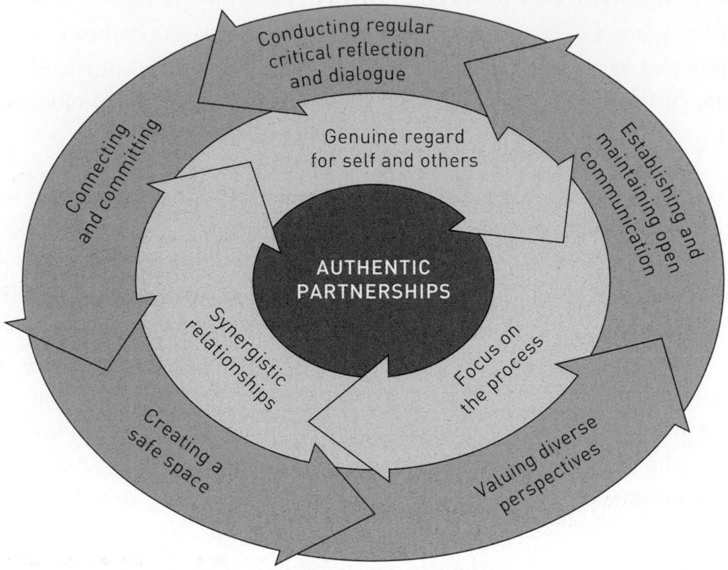

Genuine regard
for self and others

Conducting regular
critical reflection
and dialogue

Connecting
and committing

Establishing and
maintaining open
communication

AUTHENTIC
PARTNERSHIPS

Synergistic
relationships

Focus on
the process

Creating a
safe space

Valuing diverse
perspectives

Source: Dupuis et al., 2012a, p. 436.

- In 2018, Fortune and Dupuis examined the perceptions of leisure and recreational practitioners in aged care in Canada in relation to the potential for leisure to be a key contributor to a long-term care culture that focuses on humane, resident-driven and relational models of care. They found that fulfilling, participant-driven leisure enabled authentic and caring relationships to develop between residents, health staff, family members and the local community. For example, 'through leisure experiences, skills and abilities of residents, team members, and family members can be revealed, enabling team members to be known for more than their work roles, and residents to be known for more than their illness or disability' (Fortune & Dupuis, 2018, p. 339).

- Wiersma and Chesser (2012) explored how health professionals can assist older people as they transition from living independently in the community to an aged care facility, by developing a sense of community among residents and by making nursing homes/residential aged care facilities a valued part of the community.

- Miller and colleagues (2020, p. 296) examined the experiences of workers and residents in an aged care facility in Australia. The study highlighted 'the importance of authentic leadership in creating a client-centred organizational culture where "happiness" is an explicit core value. Educating and recruiting staff that share this vision, alongside reflective engagement, rituals and symbols, enabled the building of a responsive care culture that facilitated acts of "brilliance" in healthcare'.

- Genoe and Dupuis (2014) found that leisure provided a sense of normalcy for individuals with dementia (who lived in the community) by enabling them to maintain or develop their identities.

- Dionigi and colleagues (2018) seek to apply the authentic partnership approach that involves 'working with' people living with dementia as partners, rather than 'caring for' them (Dupuis et al., 2012b). Specifically, Dionigi and colleagues want to enhance the quality of life of people living with dementia in the Port Macquarie, NSW, Australia area by examining their experiences in creative and arts-based programs. Port Macquarie is one of the top ten areas with the highest prevalence rates for people living with dementia in Australia (Dementia Australia, 2014). The arts are a powerful way to transform the lives of individuals and reduce the stigma and social exclusion associated with people living with dementia (A New Approach, 2019; Clark et al., 2018; Baines, 2007; Bungay & Clift, 2010; Dupuis et al., 2016a; Dupuis et al., 2016b). Community-based, dementia-friendly arts and health programs – such as Creative Ageing Art, Hands-On-Heritage and TimeSlips Heritage – have not been formally researched, despite Port Macquarie being recognised by Dementia Australia NSW as a community taking positive steps to make it dementia friendly (Bartholomew & Moore, 2014). A free 12-week program funded by Create NSW's 'Health and Wellbeing Initiative' in response to COVID-19 called 'Treasured Stories, Poetry and Song' was designed and led by Lisa Hort in Port Macquarie in 2020. It is 'a project that brings together technology, historical images, shared moments, meaningful engagement and stimulating conversation especially designed for people living with dementia and their carer or support person' during the time of a global pandemic.

Health professionals, particularly those working within the aged care system, need to keep finding creative ways to engage or enable older people in meaningful leisure and recreation. To achieve this goal:

- First would be to embrace the psychosocial discontinuities that occur as we age, rather than fear personal change (Biggs, 2014, p. 14). That is, we must accept that ageing is a time of ongoing change and not prescribe expectations for ourselves or older people in general. As stated in a report from Australia's Royal Commission enquiry, 'Aged care must include high quality clinical and personal care, and this includes supporting emotional and psychological wellbeing throughout a person's old age' (Commonwealth of Australia, 2019b, p. 4).

- Second would be to listen to older people and allow them to express their leisure desires so that these desires can be enabled. Therefore, 'Aged care must be designed for the people it is intended to help, and based on their dignity, rights, choices, quality of life, involvement and feedback' (Commonwealth of Australia, 2019b, p. 4).

- Last, but not least, we must think about how we would like to age and ask ourselves: 'What is meaningful to me, especially as I get older?' In the aged care context, 'Every person seeking and receiving care is an individual with their own life history, and the aged care sector should recognise this. Aged care should support people to pursue and enjoy meaning and quality in life – whether they receive care at home or in a residential service' (Commonwealth of Australia, 2019b, p. 4).

In Australia, the current aged care system 'is constrained by controls on the availability of services to meet the government's fiscal risk rather than to deliver care according to need [and the system] comprises funding models that differ markedly depending on the setting in which care is delivered rather than the needs of the person receiving care' (Commonwealth of Australia, 2019b, p. 4). In other words, profit or economic concerns are being put before the needs and quality of life of the older person, their carers and families, and/or health workers. This situation must change. More broadly, in searching for 'meaning in later life that is not solely contingent upon economic materialism', Biggs (2014, p. 15) argued:

> We should, given this historic turn in age relations, see what it can tell us about the human condition, the ways we lead our lives and the kind of futures we collectively desire.

In Australia, and globally, many older people fear going into a nursing home (like Lily, in the case study below): 'Receiving aged care should not require a sacrifice of choice and control over one's own life. It is unacceptable that we have an aged care system that people are frightened to access' (Commonwealth of Australia, 2019b, p. 4).

9.2 Getting to know the person: Lily's story

Lily is 89 years old, and she is moving from independent living to a long-term residential aged care facility. In her recent past, she was highly active in ways similar to Iris; however, now she is interested in pursuing passive leisure activities, such as painting, writing and bird watching. She is fearful of this move into a nursing home, but she is also looking forward to living closer to her great grandchildren.

FOCUS QUESTIONS

- What strategies could you use to facilitate Lily's leisure interests?
- What are some ways you could facilitate leisure and interaction with Lily's family who live nearby?
- In what ways could you ease Lily's fear of moving from independent living to an aged care facility?

Leisure in residential aged care settings

The importance and experience of leisure and wellness among residents in long-term aged care settings (like Lily) and people living with dementia has become a recent focus in the literature and policy: 'A person should not have to risk losing their sense of self and be disconnected from society simply because they require care and support in older age' (Commonwealth of Australia, 2019b, p. 4). For example, Miller (2016) qualitatively examined what restricts and facilitates leisure for three men and 17 women (with an average age of 80 years) who reside in a residential aged care facility near Brisbane, Australia. The residents were involved in the following activities:

- home leisure (usually alone): television, radio, reading and working on a hobby
- 'active leisure': walking, swimming, dancing, exercises and gardening
- 'social leisure': attending organised group activities, such as arts and crafts, religious services, card games and bingo (Miller, 2016, p. 39).

Three broad themes were identified to represent 'the residents' leisure experience: (1) as a structure for living, (2) creating social connections and (3) maintain ability' (Miller, 2016, p. 35). Miller described how many residents embraced certain activities, while some withdrew and found it difficult 'to convince staff to respect their desire to be alone and not engage in activities' (p. 43). One woman expressed 'her personal dislike for the "fake jolliness" of some staff' (p. 44) and one man was angry about 'not [being] allowed to use his walker after 2 pm because staff thought he was too tired in the afternoon' (p. 44). Therefore, it is important for health professionals to respect the desired privacy and inactivity of residents' leisure choices, as well as provide social and active leisure opportunities for those who desire them. Leisure can be personal and private, particularly for those in long-term residential care settings. Likewise, in Canada, Whyte and Fortune (2017) and Fortune and Dupuis (2018, p. 340) described how 'the move away from a sole focus of leisure programming led to the creation of natural social spaces within [an aged care] home that encouraged spontaneous leisure experiences and a more enriched social environment'.

See Chapter 13 for in-depth information about dementia.

Regarding policy, the 2018–2019 Royal Commission into Aged Care Quality and Safety in Australia highlighted that, among other limitations, the current aged care system 'is focused more on the funding relationship between government and providers than the choices and the rights of the older person seeking care' (Commonwealth of Australia, 2019b, p. 2). The enquiry 'concluded that there was a need for a fundamental overhaul of the design, objectives, regulation and funding of aged care in Australia. The aged care system is in desperate need of redesign – not mere patching up' (Commonwealth of Australia, 2019b, p. 3). As pointed out at the beginning of this chapter, aged care facilities often use leisure to pass time or view it as another 'task' or activity for an older person to complete. Such an approach ignores the necessity of 'putting people at the centre' of their leisure needs and experiences to ensure they are meaningful to everyone involved. As per the Royal Commission's findings, 'Aged care should be delivered in the context of trusting, respectful and collaborative relationships between the person receiving care, their family, staff and management. Aged care should not be seen as a commodity, and success should not be measured by the mere completion of tasks' (Commonwealth of Australia, 2019b, p. 4).

OLDER PEOPLE WITH DEMENTIA AND THE ROLE OF LEISURE

In the specific context of dementia care, researchers are using innovative approaches to better understand the role of leisure in the lives of people with dementia. In Australia, the health benefits of engaging older people with dementia in arts and culture, including museums and galleries running creative programs (Clark et al., 2018), arts-based activities, the use of music and theatre in nursing homes, and incorporating 'innovative and creative design solutions and aesthetics within health settings', are enhanced social inclusion; reduced feelings of depression stress and loneliness; and increased confidence and feelings of self-worth (A New Approach, 2019, p. 49). In thinking about the future, A New Approach (2019, p. 56) asks:

How could Australia be transformed if we …
- Promoted the health benefits of arts and cultural activities to the general public in a similar vein to the promotions of physical activity (such as 'Find 30 [minutes] every day'), and developed new and innovative health programs that incorporate arts and culture in government run health care facilities?
- Invested in effective creative programs for older Australians, with the understanding that arts and culture has been shown to raise quality of life for the elderly and may play a critical role in preventing dementia?

See Chapter 13 for examples of art-based activities in residential aged care.

Learn more
Watch Video 13.1: David talks about his continued enjoyment of leisure and recreation while living with dementia.

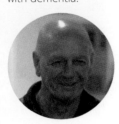

In a Canadian study by Dupuis et al., 2012c, p. 246), the participants were celebrating and living life through leisure by using art and other means such as drama to express their identity and past experiences ('Being me'), create a sense of community with others ('Being with'), have fun and feel valued ('Making a difference'), escape ('Seeking freedom') and find balance and learn new things ('Growing and developing'). The people with dementia explained to the researchers that:

> when someone is first diagnosed with a disease-causing memory loss, life is spinning, seemingly out of control. This is depicted in the image as the 'eye of the storm' in the left of the picture [referring to a piece of artwork they created for the study]. Over time, the experience grows to reveal a rich tapestry of meaningful experiences and personal understandings, often facilitated through leisure.

To highlight the significance of meaningful leisure, one participant in the Dupuis study (Dupuis et al., 2012c, p. 240 – emphasis added) said:

> Many think it is the disease [dementia] that causes us to withdraw, and to some extent I believe this is true. But, for many of us, we withdraw because we are not provided with *meaningful opportunities* [as found in leisure] that allow us to continue to experience joy, purpose and engagement in life.

FIGURE 9.2 Resident wellness model

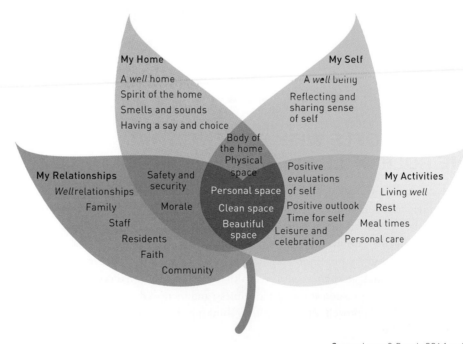

Source: Lopez & Dupuis 2014, p. 145.

Like leisure, wellness is subjective and multidimensional, and emphasises balance across the domains of wellness, such as physical, mental, social, emotional and spiritual (Lopez & Dupuis, 2014). Through an authentic partnership approach, Lopez and Dupuis created a flower (see Figure 9.2) to represent the needs and meanings of wellness among residents of an aged care facility in Canada. In their study, 'leisure was a thread found to permeate all aspects of residents' lives enabling them to meaningfully engage with others, themselves and their environment' (2014, pp. 144–5). Figure 9.2 is a resident **wellness model**:

> that emphasises the importance of my relationships, myself, my home and my activities to the wellness of LTC [long-term care] home residents and provide[s] insights into how wellness in LTC homes as well as residents' leisure can be better supported [by health professionals, staff, residents, family, community, etc.].

wellness model
A model that focuses on valuing wellness and possibilities in later life, as opposed to a disease model, which focuses on illness, dependency and decline.

Where to from here?

As a society and as health professionals we need to focus more broadly on the concepts of leisure, wellness, **ageing well** or desired ageing as defined and experienced by older people themselves. As future health professionals you can play a key role in helping older adults, of varying abilities, means and desires, to find meaning and pleasure in all/any forms of leisure, whether it be emotional, spiritual, social, mental and/or physical. That is, the goal is to support and encourage diversity and difference in leisure during old age and recognise that older people's interests, capabilities and practices can continually shift back and forth along a continuum from active to sedentary pursuits, and from solitary to social activities. To enable meaningful leisure throughout this transition, society, family members and health professionals must support and enable older adults by listening, providing, respecting and creating the conditions that allow for informed *choice*. The Royal Commission into Aged Care Quality and Safety supports this view (Commonwealth of Australia 2019b, p. 3). This inquiry noted that, over the past decade:

ageing well
The ability to maintain a sense of physical, mental and social health over time.

> … aged care has been on a path to a consumer-driven, more market-based system … The aged care sector is not, and is unlikely to ever be, a fully efficient market. The direction of current reforms puts too much faith in market forces and consumer choice as the primary driver of improvement in the aged care system. It gives insufficient attention to constraints on the availability of choice in many parts of Australia and to the supports required for people to exercise informed choice. Giving people more information to make decisions about their aged care will give them greater control, but it will only address some of the existing market imbalances.

Conclusion

Health professionals are in a prime position to place older people at the centre of their leisure decision-making processes and help individuals find meaning, identity management, wellness and pleasure in leisure, regardless of the type of activity. Consistently, Best (2010, p. 1) saw the leisure experience as an 'attempt to fulfil pleasure and desire and about the construction of an identity we feel comfortable with'. To enact these ideas, society, as a whole, must think about 'desired ageing through leisure' (from the perspective of the older person and through authentic partnerships with others such as health-care professionals) in all disciplines, work domains and policy.

Learn more
Access additional resources – such as weblinks, further readings and podcasts – to broaden your understanding of this chapter. See the Guided Tour for access details.

REVISION QUESTIONS

1   What are key features of authentic partnerships and how could this influence your practice as a health professional?

2   Why is the meaning of leisure experiences (rather than the type of leisure activity) important in later life?

3   How can you help engage an older person in meaningful leisure who 1) lives in the local community, 2) resides in an aged care facility or 3) has dementia?

4   What strategies will you employ to respect older people's privacy and choices in regard to leisure?

REFERENCES

A New Approach (2019). Transformative: Impacts of Culture and Creativity. Insight research series. Report two. Australian Academy of the Humanities.

Aged Care Quality and Safety Commission (2019). About the Aged Care Standards. Updated 20 December. www.agedcarequality.gov.au/standards/guidance-introduction

Australian Bureau of Statistics (ABS) (2006). Time Use on Recreation and Leisure Activities. Cat. no. 4173.0. ABS. www.ausstats.abs.gov.au/Ausstats/subscriber.nsf/0/91FB93C8E82F220CCA25771F0018AE29/$File/41730_2006.pdf

Baines, P. (2007). *Quality Dementia Care Nurturing the Heart: Creativity, art therapy and dementia.* Alzheimer's Australia.

Bartholomew, J. & Moore, B. (2014). A guide to becoming a dementia-friendly community. Dementia Australia. www.dementiafriendly.org.au/find-resources/guide-becoming-dementia-friendly-community

Best, S. (2010). *Leisure Studies: Themes and perspectives.* Sage.

Biggs, S. (2014). Adapting to an ageing society: The need for cultural change. *Policy Quarterly, 10*(3), 12–16.

Blaikie, A. (1999). *Ageing and Popular Culture.* Cambridge University Press.

Bungay, H. & Clift, S. (2010). Arts on prescription: A review of practice in the UK. *Perspectives in Public Health, 130*(6), 277–81.

Clark, G., Moir, E., Moonen, T., Morrissey, C. & Nunley, J. (2018). Culture, value and place. A Report for NSW Department of Planning and Environment.

Coleman, D. & Iso-Ahola, S. E. (1993). Leisure and health: The role of social support and self-determination. *Journal of Leisure Research, 25*(2), 111–28.

Commonwealth of Australia (2019a). Royal Commission into Aged Care Quality and Safety. Interim report: Neglect. Vol. 1.https://agedcare.royalcommission.gov.au/sites/default/files/2020-02/interim-report-volume-1.pdf

Commonwealth of Australia (2019b). Royal Commission into Aged Care Quality and Safety. Aged care program redesign: Services for the future. Consultation paper 1.

Dementia Australia (2014). Dementia figures support the need for creating a Dementia-Friendly Nation.

Dionigi, R. A. (2006). Competitive sport and aging: The need for qualitative sociological research. *Journal of Aging and Physical Activity, 14*(4), 365–79.

Dionigi, R. A. (2008). *Competing for Life: Older people, sport and ageing.* Verlag Dr. Müller.

Dionigi, R. A. (2010a). Older sportswomen: Personal and cultural meanings of resistance and conformity. *International Journal of Interdisciplinary Social Sciences, 5*(4), 395–408.

Dionigi, R. A. (2010b). Managing identity in later life through leisure: Interpreting the experiences of older athletes. In B. Humberstone (ed.). *Third Age and Leisure Research: Principles and practice.* Leisure Studies Association, pp. 59–80.

Dionigi, R. A. (2015). Pathways to Masters sport: Sharing stories from sport 'continuers', 'rekindlers' and 'late bloomers'. In E. Tulle & C. Phoenix (eds). *Physical Activity and Sport in Later Life: Critical approaches.* Palgrave Macmillan, pp. 54–68.

Dionigi, R. A. (2016). The competitive older athlete: A review of psychosocial and sociological issues. *Topics in Geriatric Rehabilitation, 32*(1), 55–62.

Dionigi, R. A. (2017). I would rather die than live sedentary: Is the demonization of passive leisure creating a future generation of older people who will not accept inactivity? *Topics in Geriatric Rehabilitation, 33*(3), 156–61.

Dionigi, R. A., Baker, J. & Horton, S. (2011). Older athletes' perceived benefits of competition. *International*

Journal of Sport and Society, 2(2), 17–28.

Dionigi, R. A., Black, R., Sommers, D., Hort, L. & Dupuis, S. L. (2018). Creative ageing: Evaluating dementia-friendly, arts-based programs in Port Macquarie, NSW using an authentic partnership approach. A paper presented at The 10th Annual International Arts and Health Conference: The Art of Good Health and Wellbeing, 12–15 November.

Dionigi, R. A. & Gard, M. (eds) (2018a). *Sport and Physical Activity Across the Lifespan: Critical perspectives.* Palgrave Macmillan.

Dionigi, R. A. & Gard, M. (2018b). Sport for all ages? Weighing the evidence. In R. A. Dionigi & M. Gard (eds) *Sport and Physical Activity Across the Lifespan: Critical perspectives,* Palgrave Macmillan, pp. 1–20.

Dionigi, R. A. & Lyons, K. D. (2010). Examining layers of community in leisure contexts: A case analysis of older adults in an exercise intervention. *Journal of Leisure Research*, 42(2), 317–40.

Dupuis, S. L. (2008). Leisure and ageing well. *World Leisure Journal*, 50(2), 91–107.

Dupuis, S. L., Gillies, J., Carson, J., Whyte, C., Genoe, R., Loiselle, L. & Sadler, L. (2012a). Moving beyond patient and client approaches: Mobilizing 'authentic partnerships' in dementia care, support and services. *Dementia*, 11(4), 427–52.

Dupuis, S. L., Kontos, P., Mitchell, G., Jonas-Simpson, C. & Gray, J. (2016b). 'Reclaiming citizenship through the arts'. *Dementia, 15*(3), 358–80.

Dupuis, S. L., McAiney, C.A., Fortune, D., Ploeg, J. & Witt, L. D. (2016a). Theoretical foundations guiding culture change: The work of the Partnerships in Dementia Care Alliance. *Dementia, 15*(1), 85–105.

Dupuis, S. L., Whyte, C. & Carson, J. (2012b). Leisure in long-term care settings. In H. J. Gibson & J. F. Singleton (eds). *Leisure and Aging: Theory and practice.* Human Kinetics, pp. 217–37.

Dupuis, S. L., Whyte, C., Carson, J., Genoe, R., Meshino, L. & Sadler, L. (2012c). Just dance with me: An authentic partnership approach to understanding leisure in the dementia context. *World Leisure Journal, 54*(3), 240–54.

Eman, J. (2012). The role of sports in making sense of the process of growing old. *Journal of Aging Studies, 26*(4), 467–75. https://doi:10.1016/j.jaging.2012.06.006

Fortune, D. & Dupuis, S. L. (2018). The potential for leisure to be a key contributor to long-term care culture change. *Leisure/Loisir 42*(3), 323–45. https://doi:10.1080/14927713.2018.1535277

Gard, M. & Dionigi, R. A. (2016). The world turned upside down: Sport, policy and ageing. *International Journal of Sport Policy and Politics, 8*(4), 737–44.

Gard, M., Dionigi, R. A., Horton, S., Baker, J., Weir, P. & Dionigi, C. (2017). The normalisation of sport for older people? *Annals of Leisure Research, 20*(3), 253–72.

Gayman, A. M., Fraser-Thomas, J., Dionigi, R. A., Horton, S. & Baker, J. (2017). Is sport good for older adults? A systematic review of psychosocial outcomes of older adults' sport participation. *International Review of Sport and Exercise Psychology 10*(1), 164–85.

Genoe, M. R. & Dupuis, S. L. (2014). The role of leisure within the dementia context. *Dementia*, 13(1), 33–58.

Gilleard, C. & Higgs, P. (2007). The Third Age and the Baby Boomers: Two approaches to the social structuring of later life. *International Journal of Ageing and Later Life, 2*(2), 13–30. https://doi:10.3384/ijal.1652- 8670.072213

Gilleard, C. & Higgs, P. (2013). *Ageing, Corporeality and Embodiment.* Anthem Press.

Godbey, G. (1999). *Leisure in Your life: An exploration* (4th edn). Venture Publishing.

Grant, B. C. (2001). 'You're never too old': Beliefs about physical activity and playing sport in later life. *Ageing & Society, 21*(6), 777–98. https://doi:10.1017/S0144686X01008492

Grant, B. C. & Kluge, M. A. (2012). Leisure and physical well-being. In H. J. Gibson & J. F. Singleton (eds). *Leisure and Aging: Theory and practice.* Human Kinetics, pp. 129–41.

Griffin, M. & Phoenix, C. (2014). Learning to run from narrative foreclosure: One woman's story of aging and physical activity. *Journal of Aging and Physical Activity, 22*(3), 393–404. https://doi:10.1123/japa.2012-0300

Henderson, K. A., Casper, J., Wilson, B. E. & Dern, L. (2012). Behaviors, reasons, and outcomes perceived by Senior Games participants. *Journal of Park and Recreation Administration, 30*(1), 19–35.

Heo, J., Culp, B., Yamada, N. & Won, Y. (2013). Promoting successful aging through competitive sports participation: Insights from older adults. *Qualitative Health Research, 23*(1), 105–13. https://doi:10.1177/1049732 312457247

Higgs, P., Hyde, M., Gilleard, C., Victor, C., Wiggins, R. & Jones, I. R. (2009). From passive to active consumers? Later life consumption in the UK from 1968–2005. *Sociological Review, 57*(1), 102–124.

Horton, S., Dionigi, R. A., Gard, M., Baker, J. & Weir, P. (2018). 'Don't sit back with the geraniums, get out': The complexity of older women's stories of sport participation. *Journal of Amateur Sport, 4*(1), 24–51.

Horton. S., Dionigi, R. A., Gard, M., Baker, J., Weir, P. & Deneau, J. (2019). 'You can sit in the middle or be one of the outliers': Older male athletes and the complexities of social comparison. *Frontiers in Psychology, 10,* 2617. https://doi.org/10.3389/fpsyg.2019.02617

Jones, I. R. & Higgs, P. (2010). The natural, the normal and the normative: Contested terrains in ageing and old age. *Social Science and Medicine, 71*(8), 1513–19.

Kelly, J. R. (2012). *Leisure* (4th edn). Sagamore Publishing.

Kim, A. C. H., Park, S. H., Kim, S. & Fontes-Comber, A. (2020). Psychological and social outcomes of sport participation for older adults: A systematic review. *Ageing & Society, 40*(7), 1529–49. https://doi.10.1017/S0144686X19000175

Kirby, J. B. & Kluge, M. A. (2013). Going for the gusto: Competing for the first time at age 65. *Journal of Aging and Physical Activity, 21*(3), 290–308.

Kleiber, D. A. (2016). Leisure activities in later life. In N. A. Pachana (ed.). *Encyclopedia of Geropsychology.* Springer Science Business Media, pp. 321–29.

Laslett, P. (1989). *A Fresh Map of Life: The Emergence of the Third Age.* George Weidenfeld & Nicholson.

Lassen, A. J. & Moreira, T. (2014). Unmaking old age: Political and cognitive formats of active ageing. *Journal of Aging Studies, 30*(1), 33–46. https://doi.10.1016/j.jaging.2014.03.004

Litchfield, C. & Dionigi, R. A. (2011). The meaning of sports participation in the lives of middle-aged and older women. *International Journal of Interdisciplinary Social Sciences, 6*(5), 21–36.

Litchfield, C. & Dionigi, R. A. (2012). Rituals in Australian women's veteran's field hockey. *International Journal of Sport & Society, 3*(3), 171–89.

Lopez, K. J. & Dupuis, S. L. (2014). Exploring meanings and experiences of wellness from residents living in long-term care homes. *World Leisure Journal, 56*(2), 141–50.

Lyons, K. D. & Dionigi, R. A. (2007). Transcending emotional community: A qualitative examination of older adults and Masters' sports participation. *Leisure Sciences, 29*(4), 375–89.

Miller, E. (2016). Beyond bingo: A phenomenographic exploration of leisure in aged care. *Journal of Leisure Research, 48*(1), 35–49.

Miller, E., Devlin, N., Buys, L., Donoghue, G. (2020). The happiness initiative: Changing organizational culture to make 'brilliance' mainstream in aged care. *Journal of Management and Organization, 26*(3): 296–308. https://doi:10.1017/jmo.2019.59

Moulaert, T. & Biggs, S. (2013). International and European policy on work and retirement: Reinventing critical perspectives on active ageing and mature subjectivity. *Human Relations, 66*(1), 23–43.

Pfister, G. (2012). It is never too late to win – sporting activities and performances of ageing women. *Sport in Society, 15*(3), 369 84. https://doi:10.1080/17430437.2012.653206

Pike, E. C. J. (2011). The *active aging* agenda, old folk devils and a new moral panic. *Sociology of Sport Journal, 28*(2), 209–25. http://eprints.chi.ac.uk/545/1/ActiveAgingAgenda.pdf

PwC Global (2019). The urgency of addressing social determinants of health. A PwC Health Research Institute report.

Ryan, R. M. & Deci, E. L. (2000). Self-determination theory and the facilitation of intrinsic motivation, social development, and well-being. *American Psychologist, 55,* 68–78.

Smith, M. M. (2016). I am woman, see me (sweat)!: Older women and sport. *Kinesiology Review, 5*(1), 75–80. https://doi.org/10.1123/kr.2015-0055

Son, J. & Dionigi., R. A. (2020). The complexity of sport-as-leisure in later life. In

S. Kono, K. Spracklen, A. Beniwal & P. Sharma (eds) *Positive Sociology of Leisure.* Palgrave, pp. 109–24.

Stebbins, R. A. (2012). *The Idea of Leisure: First principles.* Transaction Publishers.

Stenner, B. J., Mosewich A. D. & Buckley, J. D. (2016). An exploratory investigation into the reasons why older people play golf. *Qualitative Research in Sport, Exercise and Health, 8*(3),257–72. https://doi:10.1080/2159676X.2016.1148773

Stone, R. C., Dionigi, R. A & Baker, J. (2018). The role of sport in promoting physical activity among older people. In S. R. Nyman, A. Barker, T. Haines, K. Horton, C. Musselwhite, G. Peeters, C. R. Victor, J. K. Wolff (eds). *The Palgrave Handbook of Ageing and Physical Activity Promotion.* Palgrave Macmillan, pp. 673–91.

Whyte, C. & Fortune, D. (2017). Natural leisure spaces in long-term care homes: Challenging assumptions about successful aging through meaningful living. *Annals of Leisure Research, 20*(1), 7–22. https://doi:10.1080/11745398.2016.1175954

Wiersma, E. & Chesser, S. (2012). Bridging community and long-term care settings. In H. B. Gibson & J. F. Singleton (eds). *Leisure and Aging: Theory and Practice.* Human Kinetics, pp. 239–53.

Wong, J. D., Son, J. S., West, S. T., Naar, J. J. & Liechty, T. (2019). A life course examination of women's team sport participation in late adulthood. *Journal of Aging and Physical Activity, 27*(1), 73–82. https://doi.org/10.1123/japa.2017-0193

World Health Organization (2002). Active Ageing: A Policy Framework. A contribution of the World Health Organization to the Second United Nations World Assembly on Ageing, April. http://apps.who.int/iris/bitstream/10665/67215/1/WHO_NMH_NPH_02.8.pdf

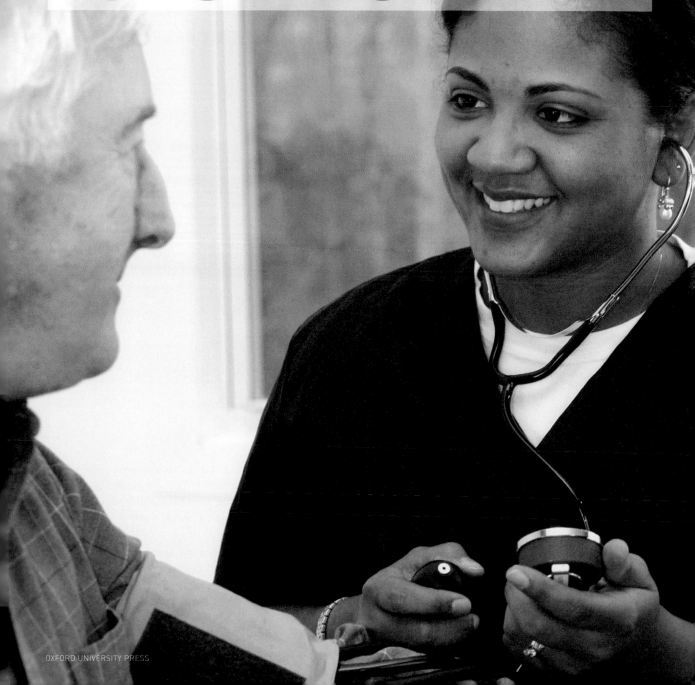

PART 3

The Clinical Aspects of Ageing and Aged Care

10 The Impact of Physiological Changes on Older People: Implications for Nursing Practice

MAREE BERNOTH AND JED MONTAYRE

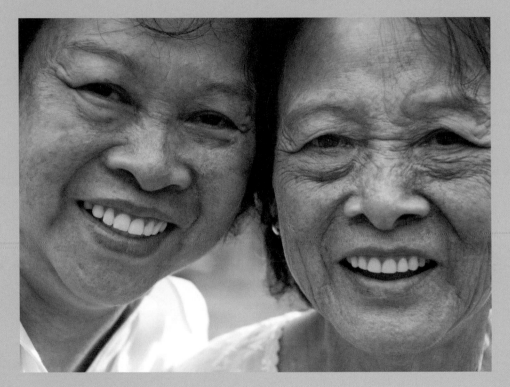

LEARNING OBJECTIVES

After reading this chapter, you will:

» determine that, although there are changes due to the ageing process, ageing is an individual experience

» identify ageing as inevitable, yet age-related changes can be retarded or accelerated by healthy lifestyle choices throughout the life span

» articulate the causes of ageing that are supported by research

» deduce that, as a result of the ageing process, the older person's ability to maintain homeostasis is impaired, making them vulnerable to trauma and disease

» determine that assessment of older people includes skilled communication and person-centredness involving family, significant others and an interdisciplinary team of health professionals.

Introduction

The focus of this chapter is the physiological changes that occur as people age. Even though the chapter is dominated by physical changes, it is acknowledged that we are complex beings with biopsychosocial, cultural and spiritual aspects that contribute to our individuality. As you learnt in Chapter 4, although changes happen as ageing occurs, when they occur and the speed with which they occur, depend on the individual. The meaning and significance of the changes are similarly individual experiences. Being aware of age-related changes enables registered nurses and other health professionals to work collaboratively with individuals in initiating programs that retard and/or prevent deterioration, pathology and trauma, and support the older person to live the life they aspire to. Knowledge of age-related changes enables astute assessment and helps with being able to differentiate between an age-related change and pathology. Age-related changes underpin different responses to the external environment and challenges to health for the older person. As this is essential knowledge for a registered nurse and other health professionals, the chapter is presented in a way that makes the information readily accessible and articulates that, although ageing is universal, it is also individual. It emphasises the significance of assessment and outlines the particular role of the registered nurse in prolonging functionality, enabling the maintenance of connections with family, friends and the community and supporting the older person to adapt to their ageing journey.

10.1 Getting to know the person: Kelly's story

Hey, Kelly here. I'm 22 years old and a second-year computer science student. I grew up in a small rural town and my parents migrated from the Philippines and are committed members of their local church. My time is usually spent gaming with mates, listening to metal and trying to fit in some uni work. I use ear buds to get the best effects from my music and to stop the complaints from people around me. I only use a bit of ice on the weekends and I'm trying to cut back on the smokes. I overdosed once. My parents had to call the paramedics and then, when I recovered, they made me go and live on campus. I make my way through the come down with energy drinks and coffee. When I need food, I hit up the local takeaway.

- To what extent is Kelly representative of everyone in Generation Z?
- What are the potential stereotypes applied to Zoomers if society in general considers Kelly typical of this age group?
- What would the attitude of health professionals be towards young adults if they perceived Kelly as typical of everyone of this age?
- As you read through the chapter, consider the implications of Kelly's lifestyle choices during the ageing process. Take the opportunity to learn about your own lifestyle choices and the implications of these on your ageing journey.

The impacts of stereotyping

stereotyping
The belief that all the members of a particular category of people are the same.

Stereotyping people based on their age has grave implications for:

- *the quality of life of the person:* stereotyping leads to failure to appreciate the person as an individual, be respectful of them as an individual and address their issues based on their assessed needs
- *their family:* it is distressing for the family to have a loved one ignored, treated disrespectfully or patronised rather than having their issues listened to and addressed
- *their community:* an unwell person cannot enjoy their place in the community, their circle of friends or their normal activities
- *service provision:* if there is a lack of astute assessment, no referrals are generated or there is inappropriate referral
- *health-care professionals:* where there is an absence of professionalism, there is little willingness to assess, collaborate with team members and refer appropriately, based on the needs and wishes of the individual.

heterogeneous
Diverse, different, varied, mixed.

If it is not appropriate or helpful to stereotype all 22 year olds, it is not appropriate or helpful to stereotype older people. People over 65 years of age make up one of the most **heterogeneous** groups in society (AIHW, 2018). While there are common physiological changes related to ageing, this process is different for each individual. Some people are old before they reach 65, and some report that they are fit and healthy into their nineties and beyond.

The World Health Organization's *World Report on Ageing and Health* (WHO, 2015a) highlighted the uniqueness of older people's needs and how every older person is different in terms of their levels of function in relation to their chronological age (see Figure 10.1). Table 10.1 outlines factors that affect ageing and contribute to making ageing an individual experience.

FIGURE 10.1 Factors for healthy ageing

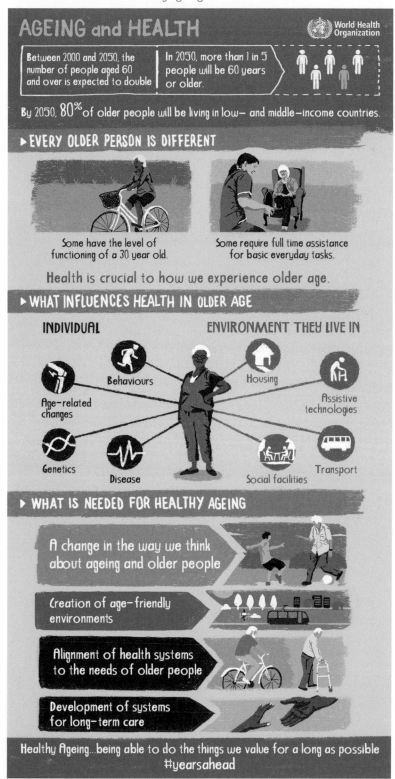

Source: WHO, 2015b.

TABLE 10.1 Factors affecting the ageing experience

FACTOR	IMPACT	CONSIDERATIONS	PREVENTION AND MONITORING STRATEGIES
Genetics	» The length of a person's life can be determined by their genetic make-up. Genes can either protect from or make a person vulnerable to conditions and diseases. » Examples: breast cancer, high cholesterol, cardiovascular disease	» Age of death of parents and grandparents » Family history of illness » Cause of death of family members	» Genetic testing and health screening are providing opportunities to be aware of genetic issues and to implement relevant monitoring and prevention programs. These include annual mammograms and preventative medications for women who have a genetic predisposition to breast cancer. » Genetic testing for the general population is becoming more affordable and accessible. » Inherent in genetic testing are many ethical dilemmas. What is the impact on the individual if they are aware they carry the APOE genes that predispose them to dementia?

Pre-conception health of both parents (Moss & Harris, 2014)	» Impact on birth outcomes and longevity	» Maternal and paternal diabetes status
		» Maternal high blood pressure
		» Maternal use of alcohol
		» Maternal depression
		» Paternal consumption of fast food
		» Maternal stress during pregnancy
			» Antenatal monitoring and support for pregnant women
			» Provision of primary healthcare for both sexes during childbearing years focusing on:
			  – mental health
			  – diabetes
			  – blood pressure
			  – reducing alcohol consumption
			  – minimising fast-food consumption
			  – health coaching for at-risk adults during child-bearing years.

Lifestyle	This includes: » smoking » obesity » lack of exercise » vaccination status » alcohol and drug abuse » frequent exposure to loud noise » hazardous occupations » ability and willingness to access health services.	» Sensitive communication skills that build rapport with the individual help to elicit this information and help change behaviours. » Often there are sensitivities and guilt in revealing these behaviours.	» Programs to educate the public about the potential outcomes from unhealthy behaviours dominate advertising space » Workplace health and safety legislation aims to prevent injury, short and long term, but consider, for example, how does a bricklayer function without bending and twisting and what are the long-term implications? » The public is being educated about harmful outcomes of behaviours, but there is limited impact and the messages have to be repeated (e.g. about exercise). » Consider: what does this means for health education and achieving behavioural change? » Research has shown that failure to exercise in the thirties and forties leads to smaller brains in the seventies and eighties, making the inactive person more vulnerable to cognitive changes than an active person (Boyle et al., 2015).

TABLE 10.1 Continued

FACTOR	IMPACT	CONSIDERATIONS	PREVENTION AND MONITORING STRATEGIES
Diseases and medications	» Chronic diseases that are not managed appropriately (such as diabetes, respiratory diseases and musculoskeletal conditions) can exacerbate age-related changes. For example, consider diabetes. This pathology exacerbates the age-related changes in the sensory system, renal system and nervous system. » An example of the impact of medications on ageing is cortico-steroids, with the changes to the endocrine system and the skeletal systems exacerbating the ageing process.	» Before undertaking an assessment, it is important to access the person's medical history and be aware of pre-existing patho-physiologies and medications. » It is also significant to enquire about the length of time the person has experienced the conditions and the time since the last medication review.	» Managing chronic conditions and ensuring medications are used therapeutically requires models of care such as interdisciplinary teams, **person-centred care** and collaborative care to achieve optimal health » Accessing government guidelines related to models of care for people with chronic diseases » Engaging with evidence-informed texts and journals to ensure currency of knowledge and skills
Psychosocial aspects	» Attitudes to ageing – the meaning and significance the person places on becoming older » Connection to family » Involvement in social networks » Status of mental health » Involvement in the community and connectedness to people » Spiritual practices of different cultural groups that allows sense of connectedness	» Involves sensitive assessment and appreciation of the person as a whole. The individual wishes of the person are appreciated in conjunction with knowledge related to mental health. » The individual's choices, such as ability to continue and practise spiritual beliefs, will enable a sense of connectedness in ageing.	» The activity theory of ageing states that a person is more likely to age in a healthy way if they remain connected to family and social groups and contribute in some way to society (Maddox, 1963). » Knowledge of and willingness to access relevant services and professionals who can provide support and implement prevention strategies are essential throughout life. » Older people are sensitive to how others in their environment perceive them. How they are spoken to and spoken about impacts their sense of self either positively or negatively. This demonstrates the significance of respectful communication.
Culture	» For example, First Nations peoples have a 6–10-year gap in longevity compared to other Australians. » Fear, ignorance, language barriers and suspicion of the purpose of services may prevent people from different cultures accessing healthcare and services that could assist them. » Services available to First Nations peoples and those from diverse cultures require culturally competent and culturally sensitive health professionals.	» What is the meaning and significance of culture for the individual? » What are the customs and norms that are meaningful? » Has the person experienced trauma and, if so, have the residual effects been addressed?	» Have culturally appropriate services been accessed? » Are interpreters needed and accessed? » Is there engagement with relevant communities? » Registered nurses need to be reflective of their own culture and the stereotypes and attitudes they hold that may affect the person they are assessing. Health professionals need to be culturally safe and culturally competent.

(Continued)

TABLE 10.1 Continued

FACTOR	IMPACT	CONSIDERATIONS	PREVENTION AND MONITORING STRATEGIES
Socioeconomic status	» It is difficult to engage in health-promoting activities if the cost is beyond what can be afforded by the individual or family (e.g. insecure housing, dental treatment). » This works in conjunction with levels of health literacy.	» Consider the cost of dental care, for example. How can a family on a low wage afford to access these services? If they want to access government services, the wait can be long. Poor dental care affects nutrition, hydration and cardiac function, and the psychosocial aspects can lead to withdrawal from social activities and depression.	» Is the individual aware of primary health-care initiatives and government support strategies? » Are people in lower socioeconomic groups aware of the importance of accessing these support strategies? » Consider the impact of COVID-19 and the socioeconomic implications of the lockdowns and inability to earn an income.
Environment	» Cramped, overcrowded and poor living conditions (inadequate ventilation and temperature control) » Accessibility to and quality of water and nutrition » Polluted air and/or water » History of working in environments that contain toxins (e.g. asbestos) » Frequent exposure to noise (e.g. the armed forces, people exposed to loud music and builders) » Exposure to the trauma of war and terrorism » Exposure to the sun and extreme climate conditions » The availability of resources that enable technology to be used properly (i.e. internet connection)	» Consider this aspect in conjunction with the cultural aspect. With a multicultural society, there are unresolved trauma issues that may resurface as the person ages and influence their mental health and behaviour. » The individual may have lived in conditions beyond their control that were/are less than optimal.	» In what environment did the person spend their childhood? » Determine their interests and professions. » What protective strategies did they use? » What screening did they engage with? » What is the person's attitude to personal protective equipment? Was it used? » Determine their skills in utilising technology that could be useful for older adults to socially participate, access telehealth services and retrieve useful health information. » There are serious issues here with climate change with increasingly challenging and uncertain living conditions across the world.
Attitudes of health professionals to working with older people	These include: » knowledge about ageing » willingness to skilfully and thoroughly assess the person and include family and/or significant others in the assessment process » willingness to collaborate with the person and their families to achieve a mutually agreed outcome.	» If a health professional deems that older people are 'bed blockers' and are costing the health system too much money, what is the chance the older person will be assessed appropriately? » Consider the outcome for an older person if the staff in the emergency department cannot differentiate between dementia and delirium.	Registered nurses and other health professionals with the attitudes, skills and knowledge to ensure all health consumers are provided with evidence-based information and care based on assessed needs, are essential in encouraging people to adopt healthy lifestyles.

person-centred care
Treatment and care provided by health services that places the person at the centre of their own care and considers the needs of the older person's carers.

- There are conditions that are beyond the control or the choices of the individual and their family. Consider climate change, socioeconomic status and mental health challenges. Are we always able to adapt and make optimal choices for our health and well-being?

- Now that you are aware of the factors that impact the experience of ageing, think about the aspects in your life that are having positive and negative effects on your own ageing. What strategies can you use to enhance your ageing experience?

- Despite public education about lifestyle choices, people continue to engage with behaviours that have a negative impact on their ageing journey. Suggest reasons why these education programs have a limited effect. What strategies would you consider to be more effective in engaging with young adults to promote healthy ageing?

FOCUS QUESTIONS

10.2 Getting to know the people: Betty's and Catherine's stories

Betty is a 68-year-old, proud Indigenous woman. Her community is Kupungarri in northern Western Australia, where she has lived all of her life. Betty has a strong sense of community and place despite the challenges that rural living entails. She has difficulty with mobility and spends most of her time at home. As a child, Betty lived with extended family in a small house and suffered numerous ear and upper respiratory tract infections. The closest GP was 50 kilometres from their home and, even when they were able to get there, Betty's mother had to endure discrimination and lack of understanding of First Nations traditions in order to get assistance for her daughter. As an adult, these experiences made Betty reluctant to seek medical assistance except from the Aboriginal Medical Service when it opened in her community in 1985. Betty's mother died at 42 years (of lung cancer) and her father at 40 years (of cardiovascular disease). Betty smokes heavily, is overweight and has diabetes, and her renal function is closely monitored. Betty is a widow, but she is supported by her four children.

Catherine is an 87-year-old woman who was born and lived all her life in a large, regional Australian city. Catherine and her family enjoy sport; Catherine taught swimming for a number of years and now enjoys watching most forms of sport on television. Catherine's mother died at 91 years of age (stroke) and her father at 75 years (of alcohol-related dementia). Widowed 30 years ago, Catherine has a strong sense of community demonstrated through years of volunteer work, attends church when she is able, meets with her group of friends at least monthly and occasionally cares for her 10-year-old great-grandson. Catherine smoked for 10 years, but ceased smoking about 20 years ago. Her health issues are that she is breathless in the mornings, fatigues easily, has hypertension and high cholesterol and she reports that her feet ache. Apart from the birth of her five children, Catherine has been hospitalised only once: for a cholecystectomy in 1993. Catherine visits her GP regularly and is assessed by the practice nurse annually.

Refer to Chapter 18 for more on chronic health and health coaching.

Refer to Chapter 3 for more on health considerations for First Nations peoples.

**FOCUS
QUESTIONS**

- Compare and contrast the factors influencing the ageing experience for each of these women.
- Consider the physical and psychosocial challenges each woman will face as she continues to age.
- What health assessments would be relevant for each of these women?
- Nominate relevant referrals to other health professionals for both Betty and Catherine.

The causes of ageing

Scientists recognise that ageing is not just related to biology. Rather, it is the complex relationship between biological, environmental and social factors. López-Otín et al. (2013) termed the concept of researching ageing as 'geroscience'. The following section outlines some recent research outcomes, followed by a table encapsulating the main causes of ageing.

In Chapters 1 and 4 of this book, you read about theories of ageing. The biomedical theories have attempted to explain why ageing happens; however, scientists are more frequently engaged in exciting research to identify what causes the process of ageing. McCay and colleagues (1939) were early researchers who used mice and rats to undertake research that linked calorie restriction with prolonged lifespan. More recently, Livingstone and her research team have identified that eating a Mediterranean diet lowers the risk of heart disease and heart attack (Livingstone et al., 2020). So, we are becoming increasingly aware that diet is a significant aspect in quality and quantity of life.

Read more about nutrition in Chapter 15.

Since scientists mapped the human genome and discovered the function of individual genes (Collins, 2003), as far as physiological ageing is concerned, there is more certainty about factors that cause ageing. Important Australian research has identified that age-related changes occur as a result of damage to chromosomes due to the shortening and eventual fraying of the telomeres (Jacobs et al., 2014). Telomeres are at the ends of each chromosome and hold together the double-stranded helix of the chromosome. As chromosomes fray, the replication of the cell is inhibited and eventually the cell dies, leading to a reduction in the number of cells in the tissues.

In 1984, Professor Elizabeth Blackburn, an Australian researcher and Nobel laureate, along with Carol Greider, discovered an enzyme called telomerase. This enzyme lengthens the telomeres which, in turn, preserves the genetic material of the cell ensuring accurate replication. A drug called TA-65 preserves telomeres; however, the challenge for scientists is that telomerase is also the enzyme that protects cancer cells, so TA-65 potentially increases vulnerability to cancer (Jacobs et al., 2014; Liebich, 2020).

Complementing Professor Blackburn's research, Professor David Sinclair has discovered a group of genes called sirtuin genes. There are seven sirtuin genes, all with different functions that protect the chromosomes, burn fat, protect the brain and prevent degenerative conditions such as Alzheimer's and Huntington's diseases. They also control how energy is stored and metabolised. Sinclair has identified a chemical found in red wine (resveratrol) that protects these genes (Sinclair & Guarente, 2014; Palliyaguru et al., 2020). Unfortunately, it takes 200 glasses of red wine to provide enough resveratrol to be effective! Research is continuing into resveratrol and the means of making it available in more effective ways than by drinking 200 glasses of red wine.

Professor Justin Cooper-White claims that there is a means of reversing ageing. His research is in the field of regenerative science and he claims the outcomes of the research will not lead to a longer life span – but rather, a prolonged health span. Cooper-White claims that body tissues are not only elastic and solid but are also like liquid, which he terms as viscoelasticity. Viscoelasticity is focused on the pushing, pulling or shearing forces that impact tissues, making them less elastic, with research investigating how the impact of these forces can be reversed (Chaudhuri et al., 2020).

Figure 10.2 encapsulates the impact of changes to physiology as we age, which are exacerbated by environmental and social factors. The outcomes of these changes are illustrated as you move across the diagram. Remember that ageing is an individual experience, with many older people continuing to adapt as they are confronted by changes and subsequently enjoying quality of life. What these changes mean is that the person is more vulnerable to disability and chronic diseases rather than disease being inevitable. Your knowledge of age-related changes means that you are equipped with information to share with any patient or client. Engaging patients/clients in conversations, using health coaching, empowers the person to make their choices about the way they wish to age.

FIGURE 10.2 A summary of age-related changes and the potential physiological outcomes

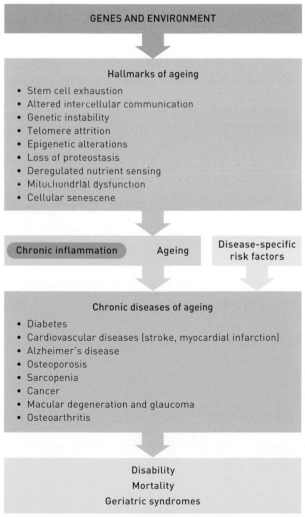

Source: Campisi et al., 2019.

Table 10.2 provides an explanation of the hallmarks of ageing articulated in Figure 10.2.

TABLE 10.2 Explaining the hallmarks of ageing

HALLMARKS OF AGEING	IMPLICATIONS
Stem cell exhaustion	Impacts on the regeneration of viable cells
Altered intercellular communication	Essential for regulation of cell growth, differential and development
Genetic instability	Impaired ability of the cell to replicate itself accurately. Increases vulnerability to tumours
Telomere attrition	Telomeres at the ends of the chromosomes fray causing the loss of genetic material and impacting viability of replication of the material in the cell
Epigenetic alterations	Impacts reliable replication of the cell, destruction of unwanted cells, cell repair and telomere structure and function
Loss of proteostasis	Breakdown of foreign materials in the cell impeded, making the cell vulnerable to infection and destruction
Mitochondrial dysfunction	Reduced energy for the cell to perform its functions
Cellular senescence	Less reliable replication of the cell and vulnerability to cancer

Source: Campisi et al., 2019.

Read Chapter 18 for more information about chronic conditions.

Using the information in Figure 10.1 and Table 10.2, you can appreciate how changes associated with ageing make the older person vulnerable to chronic diseases conditions – even multiple chronic conditions.

FOCUS QUESTIONS

- What is the impact of mitochondrial dysfunction on the heart and the implications for the individual?
- What are the implications of changes to intercellular communication in:
  - the lungs
  - the nervous system?
- Outline the impact of stem cell exhaustion on wound healing.

The role of the registered nurse

Aged care is one of the most challenging, exciting, frustrating and rewarding disciplines of nursing. The registered nurse's role in aged care encompasses technical nursing skills, critical thinking and most importantly the registered nurse's ability to empathise with older people and their families. In terms of what nurses do in aged care, Montayre and Montayre (2017) reported in their review that registered nurses undertake myriad care coordination activities while at the same time addressing non-clinical yet important tasks as part of their role (i.e. undertaking stock inventories and placing orders). The registered nurse's work in aged care is complex and requires registered nurses to understand their role.

The registered nurse can have a substantial impact on the quality of the life of older people and the life of their family if they are prepared to:

- build therapeutic rapport
- assess accurately
- identify interventions and prioritise these according to the older person's wishes
- work collaboratively with the person and the health team.

It is essential that a registered nurse is aware of age-related changes and the impact on homeostasis. These changes affect the quality of life of an older person and increase vulnerability to pathophysiology and trauma. With this awareness you can:

- appreciate the individual nature of ageing
- undertake appropriate assessments and be alerted to early signs of altered health status
- support the older person in their decision making about their health
- recognise health-related limitations to optimise the individual's participation in social activities
- offer health coaching to delay age-related changes
- refer to relevant services or health professionals where necessary
- make informed choices about your own lifestyle with the knowledge that the experience of ageing is influenced by the choices made throughout your life.

The registered nurse can make a difference by:

- working with the older person to maintain and enhance their lifestyle
- empowering the older person to live as independently as possible for as long as possible
- removing some of the challenges of caring from the family and significant others
- providing the opportunity for optimum quality of life.

An example of the complex skills of a registered nurse working with older people is encapsulated in the following scenario.

An older lady was referred to community nursing for wound care after moving from her long-term home to be closer to her daughter. When the community nurse first visited, she commented on a beautiful ceramic vase owned by the older lady. The nurse's comments elicited tears from the older woman. With sensitive questioning, she revealed that the vase contained her husband's ashes and the woman was anxious to have them interred. With the help of the community nurse, the ashes were placed in a columbarium at a local church and in the process the older woman was introduced to members of the church community. She found that, like her, some of the ladies enjoyed playing cards. So, each Wednesday after that, the older woman played cards and each Sunday she was taken to church, ensuring she was not lonely in her new environment. The community nurse continued to visit until the wound healed, confident that both physical and psychosocial needs were met.

In being sensitive to the most important issue confronting this older woman, the community nurse did far more than attend to a wound. The community nurse used communication skills, assessment skills and knowledge of the local community to facilitate a positive outcome.

You can find more information related to assessment in Chapter 11.

For older people, a small intervention can make a substantial difference to their lives. The intervention may take time to identify, but it is exquisitely satisfying for all concerned when the assessment is skilled and sensitively conducted and the intervention is mutually agreed upon. For the registered nurse, working with older people ensures that clinical skills are constantly being challenged and expanded. Issues are not always obvious, yet the satisfaction of implementing an effective strategy and witnessing the effect on the person, their family and the community is professionally and personally rewarding.

OPTIMISING CONTRIBUTION AND SOCIAL PARTICIPATION

Registered nurses play an important role in identifying the abilities and limitations of older people with regard to health. Undertaking accurate assessments and understanding age-related physiological changes facilitates planning of activities that acknowledges limitations while also optimising ability. For example, in aged care settings, if mobility is an issue for an older person, participating in active exercise activities in an indoor common area with others may not be possible. However, the activity might be appropriate in an outdoor space with enough room for mobility assistive devices. The registered nurse can create a plan of activities and discuss this with the other members of the team coordinating these activities.

In the community setting, being aware of the common barriers and facilitators to social participation in older adults is also important for registered nurses. These can include:

- age and socio-economic factors
- personal motivation and health
- accessibility, transport and neighbourhood cohesion
- pre-existing social networks.

Assessment process

Assessing an older person involves sophisticated nursing skills and sensitive interpersonal skills. An older person will not share their most intimate issues or the issues that cause them embarrassment unless there is trust established between them and the registered nurse. Trust is built through establishing rapport based on respect, with the basic premise that the nurse and the older person are both adults with the rights and responsibilities of adults. It is a partnership that is worked through together based on communication with the registered nurse willing to listen, clarify and arrive at a mutually agreeable care plan.

Older people can be intimidated by assessment tools. Multiple questions, which are often repetitive, can be confronting and confusing. They may be perceived as a test that the older person must pass so they are not referred to residential aged care. The assessment tool is perceived as a barrier to open and honest communication between the older person and the health professional. If the registered nurse is familiar with the common questions included in the assessment tools, they can have a general conversation with the older person and their family and gain the information needed throughout the conversation. Forms are then completed away from the older person.

In the community, a valuable means of assessment is to accept an older person's invitation to have a 'cuppa' together. Observing an older person prepare a cup of coffee or tea provides invaluable information about:

- eye–hand coordination
- safety
- the ability to progress logically through a task
- the contents of the refrigerator
- the contents of cupboards
- food hygiene (Baker at al., 2018).

It is also an opportunity to have a general conversation to elicit information about social circumstances, general interests, family and any topic raised by the older person. For clinically focused assessments, registered nurses should consider asking questions during a nursing assessment that enable the older person to initiate some relevant conversation. For example, when asking about sleeping patterns, instead of directly asking 'How many hours of sleep do you get each day, on average?', start by asking 'What are your usual routines before bed time?' and then follow up with 'When is your usual bed time?', continuing the conversation using the assessment framework, without intimidating the older person.

In an aged care facility setting, when undertaking assessments avoid making assumptions about the older person's abilities. It is important to collect both objective and subjective cues. For example, when assessing nutrition and food intake, consider that a lack of appetite is a combination of factors such as physiological changes and sociocultural aspects (i.e. personal food preferences). An older person may have less appetite due to personal food preferences rather than because of mouth sores or an inability to swallow.

> You can find more information related to nutrition in Chapter 15 and oral health in Chapter 16.

Another example is medication administration and swallowing. When assessing an older person's ability to swallow pills, it is important to note that some older people prefer to take medication with food (e.g. yoghurt), not because they have difficulty swallowing but because of the unpleasant taste of some medications. If we assume that there is a swallowing problem, these observations might have an impact on how food is prepared for an older person in aged care.

> You can find more information related to medication in Chapter 14.

Age-related changes to body systems

Table 10.3 outlines the age-related changes to the various body systems, the impact these changes can have on the individual, and the assessment strategies and interventions that the registered nurse can use to address these changes. The information is presented in this format to facilitate ease of reading and to understand how changes, impacts and interventions fit together.

The list of interventions is not exhaustive and can add to these as your knowledge of ageing and clinical experiences evolve.

TABLE 10.3 Age-related changes, their impact, suggested assessments and interventions

SYSTEM	AGE-RELATED CHANGE	IMPACT ON THE INDIVIDUAL	POSSIBLE ASSESSMENT	POSSIBLE INTERVENTION
Gastrointestinal system – buccal (oral) cavity	» Atrophy of the gums » Atrophy of the taste buds for sweet and salty » Reduced muscle strength around the mouth and throat » Reduced output of salivary glands, leading to a reduction in the sensation of thirst and making the older person vulnerable to infection	» Exposure of the roots of the teeth ('long in the tooth') leading to loose teeth, cavities and tooth decay » Loose dentures with accompanying ulceration » Impaired mastication of food » Reduction in the intake of foods that require chewing, e.g. apples (fibre), nuts (protein) and steak (iron) » Impairment of the initial breakdown of food, as saliva is needed to begin the digestive process » Increase in the intake of sweet and salty foods, increasing vulnerability to diabetes and hypertension » Reduction in the intake of fluids, especially water » Increased vulnerability to infections in the mouth and cardiac infection	» Look in the mouth and observe for cracked lips, dry mouth, ill-fitting dentures, missing teeth, ulceration, and a dry and furry tongue. » Smell the breath and be aware of halitosis. » Ask about changes in taste and food preferences. » Examine the toothbrush and the type of toothpaste used. » Enquire about ulceration, difficulty chewing and swallowing, and any food restrictions as a result.	» Initiate a discussion about oral health and the significance of oral health to general health. » Discuss fluid intake and negotiate ways to achieve optimal hydration. » Enquire about how oral health is maintained and collaboratively determine ways to rectify any habits that may be detrimental. » With the agreement of the older person, make a referral to an oral health therapist or dentist if necessary. » Suggest a less abrasive toothpaste or brush.
Oesophagus	» Reduced peristaltic movement because of decrease in muscle strength » Thinning of the oesophageal wall » Slower emptying of oesophagus » Reduced effectiveness of epiglottis	» Food is more difficult to swallow so the older person may avoid foods such as apples and steak. » The oesophagus may narrow and constrict. » Food is more readily aspirated into the trachea.	» Ask about foods that are avoided. » Ask about changes in food preferences. » Enquire about any episodes of choking.	» Demonstrate the optimal positioning when eating and swallowing. » Discuss food choices and options to ensure safe swallowing. » Outline strategies to relieve choking. » Refer to a dietician and speech pathologist if necessary.

TABLE 10.3 Continued

SYSTEM	AGE-RELATED CHANGE	IMPACT ON THE INDIVIDUAL	POSSIBLE ASSESSMENT	POSSIBLE INTERVENTION
Stomach	» Reduced force of gastric churning related to decreased contractility of muscles and nervous **innervations** » Increased pH (decreased acidity) of gastric enzymes » Decreased viability of the stricture at the lower cardiac stricture	» Elongated transit time of food, fluids and medications » Prone to gastric ulceration » Increased **adverse drug reactions** and interactions » Reduced appetite » Increased gastric reflux » Ulceration of lower oesophagus » Avoidance of foods that initiate reflux » Increased use of antacids » Confusion between the symptoms of a myocardial infarction (heart attack) and gastric reflux	» Assess diet and any changes in food preferences. » Undertake a medication review with particular attention to interactions and medications metabolised in the stomach. » Be alert for halitosis. » Enquire about gastric pain or burning and when it occurs. » Ask about the use of antacids or breath fresheners. » Check pulse and blood pressure to ensure the symptoms are not cardiac-related.	» Negotiate strategies with the patient and/or their family/carers. » Small frequent meals may be more conducive to effective digestion than large meals. » Discuss how and when medications are taken to ensure those that need to be accompanied by food are taken correctly.
Liver, pancreas, gall bladder	» The changes to these organs is dependent on lifestyle (high fat diet, high sugar diet and alcohol consumption), medications and diseases » Reduced liver mass and blood flow to the liver » Liver less efficient in metabolising alcohol » Changes in the composition of bile » Decreased synthesis of bile salts » Decline in pancreatic secretions	» The older person can experience more flatulence. » They may develop Type 2 diabetes. » Changes to the liver can affect medication metabolism, contributing to the increased **half-life** of drugs. » Gall stones may form, causing pain that can be difficult to localise and diagnose. » Less tolerance of fatty and spicy food	» Determine blood glucose level. » Ask about abdominal pain and where and when it occurs. » Undertake an alcohol intake assessment. » Enquire about any liver function tests that have been conducted recently.	» Implementing changed behaviours in relation to diet and alcohol consumption is challenging but if you are prepared to work collaboratively with the patient/client and within an interdisciplinary team, goals can be negotiated to achieve some changes. This takes a willingness to collaborate and patience.
Small intestine	» Reduced peristaltic movement across the organ, related to decreased muscle strength and nervous innervation » Reduced blood flow to and from the organ, reducing the uptake of nutrients	» Increased transit time » Dryer chime delivered to the large intestine » Decrease in electrolytes absorbed from the organ and distributed throughout the body, which particularly affects brain function » Reduced uptake of medications from the small intestine, which leaves free drugs within the body, increasing half-life and the chance of adverse drug reactions	» Changes to the small intestine are not obvious until there is an illness or other health challenge. » Conduct abdominal palpation to check for bloating or masses. » **Auscultate** to check for bowel sounds.	» Interventions depend on the particular problem the patient is experiencing. » After consultation with the patient a referral to a dietician may be needed.

(Continued)

TABLE 10.3 Continued

SYSTEM	AGE-RELATED CHANGE	IMPACT ON THE INDIVIDUAL	POSSIBLE ASSESSMENT	POSSIBLE INTERVENTION
Small intestine (cont.)	» Reduced metabolism of vitamins K, B1 and B12, and the absorption of calcium and iron	» Reduced vitamin K, which increases the blood clotting time and increases bruising » Reduced vitamin B and calcium affects nervous innervation and brain function » Reduced iron affects the ability of haemoglobin to carry oxygen efficiently	» Check skin for bruising. » Undertake a dietary assessment.	» Discuss with the older person any issues arising from the dietary assessment and work with them to identify strategies to address the issues.
Large intestine	» Reduced haustral churning » Slower nervous innervations across the bowel » Reduction in the intensity of peristaltic movement across the bowel » Longer transit time » Decrease in mucous secretions » Reduced blood flow to and from the bowel impeding the absorption of water » Weakness in the internal wall » Reduction in the viability of the stricture of the anus	» Increased risk of constipation and impaction » Vulnerable to dehydration » Increased concentration of medications » Straining at stool leading to haemorrhoids and bleeding » Propensity to develop **diverticula** » Reduced awareness of the need to defecate	» Enquire about bowel habits and any changes in usual routine. » Ask about the colour of faeces and the presence of blood (black stool) and/or mucus. » Ask about fluid intake. » Auscultate to check for bowel sounds.	» Ask about bowel habits. » Demonstrate the optimal positioning on the toilet for defecation. » Negotiate fluid intake. » Discuss fibre intake but be mindful that increased fibre requires increased fluids, especially the commercial fibre products. Fibre is not always recommended for patients with Parkinson's disease. » Ensure that you use language that the patient is comfortable with and understands.
Cardiovascular system *Heart*	» 35% reduction in cardiac output by 60 years » Valves become less viable » Calcified and fatty deposits in the **sinoatrial node** and through the **Purkinje fibres**, affecting the electrical conduction across the heart and the strength and rhythm of cardiac contractions » Reduced cardiac muscle viability and contractility prolonging the cardiac cycle	» Reduced perfusion of oxygenated blood to the body » Vulnerability to respiratory congestion » Less efficient blood flow through the heart » Blood pressure more difficult to regulate » Ensuring variable oxygen requirements are met becomes more difficult	» Undertake blood pressure and pulse monitoring (for rhythm, rate and strength). » Assess breathing for rate, sounds, depth and pain. » Enquire about activity levels.	» The older person feels fatigued or is easily fatigued so activities need to be staged to ensure activity but not exhaustion. » The older person is more vulnerable to injury and has elongated healing times so, in conjunction with the older person, an environmental audit is conducted and changes made to ensure optimal safety.

TABLE 10.3 Continued

SYSTEM	AGE-RELATED CHANGE	IMPACT ON THE INDIVIDUAL	POSSIBLE ASSESSMENT	POSSIBLE INTERVENTION
Cardiovascular system *Heart* (cont.)	» **Arteriosclerotic** and atherosclerotic changes to the cardiac arteries, reducing perfusion of the cardiac arteries » **Baroreceptors** and **chemoreceptors** in the aorta become less sensitive as the aorta loses elasticity » Collateral circulation gradually develops around the heart as it is challenged by age-related changes » Increase in size of the heart, beginning with the left ventricle	» Reduced perfusion of cardiac muscle with oxygenated blood » Effort required to return blood flow to the heart from the body and lungs » The ability to maintain homeostasis is reduced as the heart has less capacity to meet internal and external challenges » Vulnerability to hypertension, **transient ischaemic attacks** and stroke	» Ask about pain that could be related to the cardiovascular system (chest, shoulder, arm, jaw, on exertion). » Check warmth of peripheries. » Check pedal pulses. » Observe skin colour of legs, feet, hands, tip of the nose and lips. » Check skin integrity of the legs and arms. » Enquire about activity levels and any changes in activities related to fatigue. » Listen for abnormal lung sounds.	» Referral to health professionals (such as GP, podiatrist, occupational therapist), and home maintenance service, where appropriate.
Arteries	» Reduced strength of contractions related to changes in muscle and nervous innervations » Atherosclerotic and arteriosclerotic plaques reduce the width of the lumen and contractility of the arterial wall. » Aorta loses elasticity, affecting chemoreceptors and baroreceptors (previously discussed). » Reduced capillary blood flow » Reduced metabolism of vitamin K, increasing clotting times	» See previous section » Elongated healing times of wounds » Vulnerability to stroke » Reduced sensation in the peripheries » Breathlessness » Difficulty regulating body temperature » Difficulty managing blood pressure within acceptable levels	» Check pulses – carotid, brachial, pedal – for rhythm, rate and strength. » Monitor blood pressure. » Vulnerable to injury » Elongated healing times lead to vulnerability to infection. » Assess peripheral pain and colour – pain and pallor on elevation of the leg indicate arterial insufficiency. » Enquire about cramping.	» Protect limbs to prevent injury as healing times are prolonged. » Apply moisturising cream to **integument**. » Exercise commensurate with physical health. » Collaboratively determine a plan to promote exercise and weight loss, and manage smoking. » Refer as appropriate.

(Continued)

TABLE 10.3 Continued

SYSTEM	AGE-RELATED CHANGE	IMPACT ON THE INDIVIDUAL	POSSIBLE ASSESSMENT	POSSIBLE INTERVENTION
Veins	» Reduction in the viability of valves » Reduced venous return	» **Oedema**, venous distension and varicose veins » **Hyperpigmentation**, especially above the ankles	» Observe for oedema, venous distension and varicose veins and discolouration of the skin on the legs.	» Protect limbs from trauma. » Elevate legs to reduce oedema. » Promote leg exercises to encourage venous return. » Collaboratively determine a plan to promote exercise and weight loss, and manage smoking.
Respiratory system	» Commencing at the base of the lungs, alveoli lose elasticity and enlarge, and viability decreases. » Impaired osmotic pressure across the cell membrane impedes gas exchange and increases water retained in the alveoli. » The strength and rebound capacity of the diaphragm is affected by changes to muscle and nervous innervations. » Stiffening of the **costal cartilage** » Reduction of the cilia lining the trachea » Altered chemoreceptor function at the peripheral and central receptor sites » Reduced cardiac output leads to reduced blood flow through the lungs, further affecting gas exchange and the retention of fluids	» Fatigue » Breathlessness » Vulnerability to infection » Reduced cough response to inhaled material » Increased risk of infection and aspiration » Reduction in strength of speech » Changes to this body system are very much dependent on lifestyle choices, environmental factors and genetics » Difficulty maintaining body temperature » Difficulty adapting to changes in the internal and external environment » Difficulty in achieving maximum lung volume » Slowed response to hypoxia and hypercapnoea	» Assess breathing rate and depth. » Assess for breathlessness on exertion. » Observe for hypoxia – peripheries, tip of nose and lips. » Auscultate for breathing sounds. » Audit environment for allergens and temperature control.	» Collaborate in undertaking lifestyle choices that enhance lung health. » Demonstrate deep breathing exercises. » Protect peripheries from trauma. » Annual immunisations for pneumonia and influenza » Collaborate in developing strategies related to managing extremes in external temperature. » Discuss staging activities throughout the day. » Refer to relevant health professional: physiotherapist, GP, nurse practitioner. » Ensure any nebulised medication is being taken correctly (get the person to demonstrate their technique). » Undertake a medication review to determine any adverse drug reactions that may affect breathing, fluid retention, cardiac function.

TABLE 10.3 Continued

SYSTEM	AGE-RELATED CHANGE	IMPACT ON THE INDIVIDUAL	POSSIBLE ASSESSMENT	POSSIBLE INTERVENTION
Renal system	» Decrease in **nephrons** » Decrease in kidney size » Decrease in **glomeruli** » Reduced glomerular filtration rate » Reduced elasticity in glomeruli » Impaired osmotic pressure, reducing the efficient exchange of waste from blood to glomeruli » Reduced blood flow to the kidneys, further affecting elimination of waste and retention of electrolytes » Reduced rennin and **aldosterone** levels » Bladder atrophies » Men – prostate enlarges » Women – reduced oestrogen can lead to atrophied bladder » Urethral shortening (in women) » Decreased pelvic floor muscle tone	» Difficulty maintaining electrolyte levels especially when challenged by changes in metabolism or external temperature » Reduced ability to concentrate water and conserve sodium » Difficulty maintaining blood pressure » Difficulty with **micturition** » Decrease in **creatinine** clearance	» Assessing renal function requires sensitive communication skills as it is a source of embarrassment. » Assess for changes in toileting habits. » Monitor blood pressure. » Undertake a urinalysis. » Observe for swollen extremities. » Be aware of the smell of stale urine. » Observe clothing for urine stains. » Assess for medications excreted by the kidneys and also assess for any toxicities or other adverse drug reactions.	» Inform the older person of services available to assess and support their continence needs. This may take time as some are not confident that there are strategies to assist them, e.g. a continence clinic. » Enquire about the need for an elevated toilet seat or other related aids. » Provide information regarding government-sponsored schemes to assist with incontinence that cannot be treated. » Refer men with prostate issues appropriately. » Refer women to a women's health nurse.
Integumentary system	» Reduced subcutaneous fat » Reduced collagen » Thinning of the skin » Reduced capillary blood flow to structures such as nerve bulbs, subcutaneous glands, hair follicles, sweat glands, **melanocytes**, nails » Reduced melanocytes, turning hair grey » Reduced number of hair follicles on the head and pubic areas » Alterations in hormone balance, leading to hair growth on the face for women and in ears for men » Nails thicken and become harder as capillary blood flow is reduced.	» Wrinkles » Grey hair » Vulnerability to trauma » Prolonged wound healing times, which leads to susceptibility to infection » Reduced sensitivity to heat, cold and sources of trauma » Reduction in perspiration » Reduced elasticity related to reduction of **sebum** » Increased susceptibility to injury from pressure and trauma » Increased risk of skin tears	» Changes to the integument are the first signs of ageing and are a cause of anxiety. » Changes to the integument involve skilled observation and sensitive communication to determine the significance of the changes to the individual. » Remove patient's shoes and observe for any infections, trauma and/or maceration. » Discuss appropriate footwear.	» Protect the extremities from trauma. » Promote safe temperature regulation. Include information about managing safety on days of extreme temperature. » Encourage daily use of emollient cream to the face, legs and arms. » Encourage movement about every 20 minutes to prevent injury from pressure. » Stress the need for sun protection: UV cream, hat, long-sleeved clothing, sun glasses. » Put hat on before going outside to reduce glare and falls risk. » Skin tears and wounds need prompt attention. » Refer to podiatrist, occupational therapist and/or physiotherapist where appropriate.

(Continued)

MAREE BERNOTH AND JED MONTAYRE

TABLE 10.3 Continued

SYSTEM	AGE-RELATED CHANGE	IMPACT ON THE INDIVIDUAL	POSSIBLE ASSESSMENT	POSSIBLE INTERVENTION
Nervous system	» Increased conduction time in peripheral nerves » Prolonged reflex arc response » Processing new information can take longer. » Reduced number of nerve cells in the hippocampus » Enlarged ventricles in the brain » Calcified and fatty deposits within nerve fibres » Neurotransmitters: some become less viable, which slows the synaptic transmission and nerve responses » Loss of myelinated fibres, which leads to problems with gait and balance » Nerve cells develop pigments (lipofuscin), plaques and tangles	» Intellectual performance remains unchanged in the absence of disease but responses are slower. » In the absence of cognitive impairment, intellectual capacity is unchanged. » Recall of recent memory can take longer. » The older person is more vulnerable to injury. » Vulnerability to trips, slips and falls	» Falls assessment » Cognitive assessment » An environment assessment to reduce trauma injuries	» Never assume slow responses are evidence of dementia. » Investigate any changes in cognition to eliminate delirium. » Suggest intellectually stimulating activities such as puzzles, crosswords and social interactions. » Provide information about living safely. » Encourage involvement with programs that are designed to prevent falls, such as tai chi and yoga. » Refer to an occupational therapist for environmental assessment. » Use preferred music to stimulate memory and promote well-being.
Musculoskeletal system	» Shrinkage of the vertebral discs » Reduced bone density » Reduced calcium deposits in bones » Reduced viable muscle tissue » Skeletal muscle atrophies » Reduced ratio of neurone to muscle cells » Decreased muscle stamina and strength » Reduced costal cartilage » More rigid and less flexible ligaments, joints and tendons	» Decreased height » Vulnerable to falls » Vulnerable to breaks and fractures » Mobility becomes problematic and painful. » Joints stiffen. » Pain affects mobility and sleep. » Changes in muscle strength affect all organs in the body as outlined in other sections. » Reduced range of motion in some joints » Difficulty maintaining balance » Changes in posture » Reduced activity » More easily fatigued	» Falls assessment » Pain assessment » Bone density test » Mobility » Footwear assessment » Environmental assessment	» Discuss opportunities for exercise. » Refer to local exercise program. » Refer appropriately to podiatrist, occupational therapist and /or physiotherapist. » Address pain and any problems related to sleep deprivation. » Discuss suitability and safety aspects of footwear.

TABLE 10.3 Continued

SYSTEM	AGE-RELATED CHANGE	IMPACT ON THE INDIVIDUAL	POSSIBLE ASSESSMENT	POSSIBLE INTERVENTION
Sensory organs	» Changed structure of the **pinna** » Narrowing of auditory canal » Atrophy of **cerumen** glands » Thicker tympanic membrane » Calcification of the bone in the middle ear » Reduced hairs in cochlea that detect high-pitched sounds » Retina has less distinct margins (arcus senilis). » Yellowing of the lens » **Lacrimal** secretions decrease. » Lens is less elastic	» Problematic sound detection » Difficulty transmitting sound to the ear drum » Difficulty hearing high-pitched sounds, which can advance to sound in general » Cerumen becomes thicker » Proprioception becomes problematic, contributing to falls. » Colour perception changes. » Eyes become drier and vulnerable to infection.	» Assess pinna, inner canal and tympanic membrane. » Undertake a falls risk assessment.	» Use drops to soften and then remove excessive cerumen. » Encourage the use of drops to address dry eyes. » Discuss strategies to prevent falls. » Refer for a hearing assessment. » Provide information about the variety of devices to assist someone with a hearing or visual deficit. Focus the information on the devices to address the challenges that are affecting the quality of life and safety of the person and their family.

For definitions of bolded glossary terms in this table, please see the glossary at the back of the book.

Source: Adapted from Bullock & Hales, 2013; Lewis & Foley, 2014; Jackman et al., 2020.

Overall impact of ageing changes

Reading Table 10.3, with so many age-related changes, can be confronting, but remember that there is individuality in ageing and in the factors that affect the ageing process, as previously outlined in this chapter. The overall impact of age-related changes impact:

- homeostasis, with resultant vulnerability to pathophysiology and trauma
- atypical presentation of pathophysiology.

Let's now look at each of these briefly.

> You can find more information on assessing an older person admitted to acute care in Chapter 11 and on assessing on older person with multimorbidity in Chapter 18.

HOMEOSTASIS

Homeostasis is the ability of the internal systems of the body to maintain equilibrium despite changes in external conditions. Impaired homeostasis affects the body's ability to respond quickly to the external and internal changes required to control thermoregulation, electrolyte balance, infection and hydration, among other things (Jackman et al., 2020). The loss of physiological and functional reserves in older people means that they respond to challenges to homeostasis in an exaggerated manner. Consequently, it takes longer for the body of an older person to return to normal, emphasising the need for sensitive assessment by a registered nurse and any other health professional to provide astute and prompt interventions.

For the older person, impaired homeostasis is related to the ability to maintain:

- thermoregulation (ability to maintain body temperature)
- an acid–base balance (balance in the pH of fluids in the body)

- the conservation of water and sodium
- proprioception (awareness of body position in relation to the environment)
- elimination (ridding the body of gaseous, fluid and solid waste) (Jackman et al., 2020).

FOCUS QUESTIONS

- Review Table 10.3 and identify the age-related changes that contribute to impaired:
    - thermoregulation
    - acid–base balance
    - conservation of water and sodium
    - proprioception
    - faecal elimination
    - cognition.
- What age-related changes contribute to incontinence? What strategies can you use to assess, prevent and manage incontinence? Does continence have impacts on the older person that extend beyond the physical aspects?

ATYPICAL PRESENTATIONS

Age-related changes influence how pathophysiology presents in older people. Vague and non-specific signs and symptoms can be indicators of more insidious issues; this means that the registered nurse must have astute assessment skills if the issues confronting the older person are to be assessed accurately and resolved quickly and effectively. The term 'aypical presentations' applies when there are no signs, or unusual signs and symptoms, or not what is expected (Limpawattana et al., 2016). Failure to assess and intervene appropriately affects the quality of life of the older person and their carer/s and can result in inappropriate referral to residential aged care. There are also implications for community services and the potential cost to the health system when there are multiple admissions for the treatment of unresolved issues.

Often, there is an indication of potential underlying conditions, which requires more in-depth communication than a focus on the obvious presentation. Non-specific presentations for older people that require further assessment when any of the following common conditions are present include:

- falls
- weakness
- functional decline
- dizziness
- breathlessness
- decreased appetite
- altered continence
- pain
- changed cognition.

Any of these can indicate a serious underlying cause that requires skilled assessment and investigation. Assessment includes gathering information on onset of the signs and symptoms, including how recently they began. Is the picture presented typical of the patient and, if not, when did the signs occur? When an older person presents with changed cognition, *always assume delirium, trauma or pathophysiology* and *never* assume dementia. Table 10.4 differentiates between some atypical and typical presentations.

TABLE 10.4 Comparison of atypical and typical presentations of common pathophysiology

PATHOPHYSIOLOGY	ATYPICAL PRESENTATION	TYPICAL PRESENTATION
Infection	Afebrile A fall Altered cognition	Fever Leukocytosis
Urinary tract infection	Altered cognition Incontinence Malodourous, dark urine	Dysuria Pain on micturition Incontinence and frequency
Pneumonia	Confusion Lethargy	Shortness of breath Fever Cough
Acute abdomen	Functional decline Change in bowel habits Change in appetite Confusion	Point or rebound abdominal tenderness
Myocardial infarction	Dyspnoea Fatigue Change in functional status Nausea	Substernal chest pain Jaw and arm pain
Heart failure/pulmonary oedema	Paroxysmal dyspnoea Nocturia Sleeping changes such as using additional pillows Sleeping in a recliner	Cough Shortness of breath Oedema
Hyperthyroidism/thyrotoxicosis	Fatigue Weight loss Lethargy Confusion	Tachycardia Tremor Agitation
Depression	Somatic complaints Agitation Change in appetite Change in bowel habits	Sad mood Sleep disturbance Appetite disturbance

Source: Adapted from Vonnes & El-Rady, 2020.

> Read more about atypical presentations in Chapter 11.

Conclusion

The choices we make throughout our lives, as well as our genetic inheritance, are two factors that influence our experiences of ageing. Knowing this empowers us to make choices that will enhance our ageing. It should also motivate us to engage in any health screening we may need to ensure we enjoy the quality of life we want at every stage of life. Ageing involves changes – physical, psychosocial, spiritual and financial – but these changes are individual. As a result, we now have the most heterogeneous population of older people living in Australia of any time in history. As health professionals, we have a responsibility to be aware of age-

Learn more
Access additional resources – such as weblinks, further readings and podcasts – to broaden your understanding of this chapter. See the Guided Tour for access details.

related changes, know that the physiological changes cause pathologies to present differently and realise that we can have a positive impact on lives through therapeutic communication, skilled assessment and astute interventions, in concert with the individual and their family.

REVISION QUESTIONS

1   Review case study 10.1 related to Kelly and answer the following questions.

   a   How is the experience of ageing affected by lifestyle choices made as a young adult?

   b   What are the physical and cognitive challenges that Kelly may be confronted with in their sixties and seventies?

2   Review the age-related changes and identify those relevant to increasing the vulnerability of the older person to infections and viruses such as COVID-19 and its mutations.

3   What is the role of the health professional in protecting vulnerable older people from infection?

REFERENCES

Australian Institute of Health and Welfare (AIHW) (2018). Older Australia at a glance. www.aihw.gov.au/reports/older-people/older-australia-at-a-glance/contents/summary

Baker, S., Warburton, J., Waycott, J., Batchelor, F., Hoang, T., Dow, B., Ozanne, E. & Vetere, F. (2018). Combatting social isolation and increasing social participation of older adults through the use of technology: A systematic review of existing evidence. *Australasian Journal on Ageing, 37*(3), 184–93.

Boyle, C. P., Raji, C. A., Erickson, K, I. & Lopez, O, L. (2015). Physical activity, body mass index and brain atrophy in Alzheimer's disease. *Neurobiology of Aging, 36,* S194–S202.

Bullock, S. & Hales, M. (2013). *Principles of Pathophysiology*. Frenchs Forest.

Campisi, J., Kapahi, P., Lithgow, G. J., Melov, S., Newman, J. C. & Verdin, E. (2019). From discoveries in ageing research to therapeutics for healthy ageing. *Nature, 571*(7764), 183–92.

Chaudhuri, O., Cooper-White, J., Janmey, P. A., Mooney, D. J., & Shenoy, V. B. (2020). Effects of extracellular matrix viscoelasticity on cellular behaviour. *Nature, 584* (7822), 535–46.

Collins, F. S. (2003). Human genome project. National Human Genome Research Institute. www.genome.gov/glossary/index.cfm?id=106#human_genome_project

Jackman, C., Laging, R., Laging, B., Honan, B., Arendts, G. & Walker, K. (2020). Older person with vague symptoms in the emergency department: Where should I begin? *Emergency Medicine Australasia, 32*(1), 141–7.

Jacobs, E. G., Epel, E. S., Lin. J., Blackburn, E. H. & Rasgon, N. L. (2014). Relationship between leukocyte telomere length, telomerase activity, and hippocampal volume in early aging. *Journal of the American Medical Association Neurology, 71*(7), 921–3. https://doi:10.1001/jamaneurol.2014.870. PMID:25023551

Lewis, P. & Foley, D. (2014). *Health Assessment in Nursing* (2nd edn). Lippincott Williams & Wilkins.

Liebich, S. (2020). The cellular senescence unification model and telomerase therapy: To treat all age-related diseases. *Aging Pathobiology and Therapeutics, 2*(3), 143–54.

Limpawattana, P., Phungoen, P., Mitsungnern, T., Laosuangkoon, W. & Tansangworn, N. (2016). Atypical presentations of older adults at the emergency department and associated factors. *Archives of Gerontology and Geriatrics, 62,* 97–102.

Livingstone, K. M., Celis-Morales, C., Navas-Carretero, S., San-Cristobal, R., Forster, H., Woolhead, C., ... & Mathers, J. C. (2020). Characteristics of participants who benefit most from personalised nutrition: Findings from the pan-European Food4Me randomised controlled trial. *British Journal of Nutrition, 123*(12), 1396–405.

López-Otín, C., Blasco, M. A., Partridge, L., Serrano, M. & Kroemer, G. (2013). The hallmarks of aging. *Cell, 153*(6), 1194–217.

Maddox, G. (1963). Activity and morale: A longitudinal study of selected older adult subjects. *Society Forces, 42*(195), 195–204.

McCay, C. M., Maynard, L. A., Sperling, G. & Barnes, L. L. (1939). Retarded growth, life span, ultimate body size and age changes in the albino rat after feeding diets restricted in calories: Four figures. *The Journal of Nutrition, 18*(1), 1–13.

Montayre, J. & Montayre, J. (2017). Nursing work in long-term care: An integrative review. *Journal of Gerontological Nursing, 43*(11), 41–9.

Moss, J. L. & Harris, K. L. (2014). Impact of maternal and paternal preconception health on birth outcomes using prospective couples' data in Add Health. *Archives of Gynaecology and Obstetrics, 291*, 287–98. https://doi:10.1007/s00404-014-3521-0

Palliyaguru, D. L., Minor, R. K., Mitchell, S. J., Palacios, H. H., Licata, J. J., Ward, T. M., Abulwerdi, G., Elliott, P., Westphal, C., Ellis, J. L., Sinclair, D. A., Price, N. L., Bernier, M. & de Cabo, R. (2020). Combining a high dose of metformin with the SIRT1 activator, SRT1720, reduces life span in aged mice fed a high-fat diet. *The Journals of Gerontology: Series A, 75*(11), 2037–41.

Sinclair, D. A. & Guarente, L. (2014). Small-molecule allosteric activators of sirtuins. *Annual Review of Pharmacology and Toxicology, 54*, 363–80.

Vonnes, C. & El-Rady, R. (2020). When you hear hoof beats, look for the zebras: Atypical presentations of illness in the older adult. *The Journal for Nurse Practitioners, 17*(4), 458–61. https://doi.org/10.1016/j.nurpra.2020.10.017

World Health Organization (WHO) (2015a). World Report on Ageing and Health. WHO. https://apps.who.int/iris/handle/10665/186463

World Health Organization (WHO) (2015b). Healthy Ageing infographic. www.who.int/ageing/events/world-report-2015-launch/healthy-ageing-infographic.jpg?ua=1

11

The Older Person in Acute Care

BRIDGET HONAN AND ELYCE GREEN

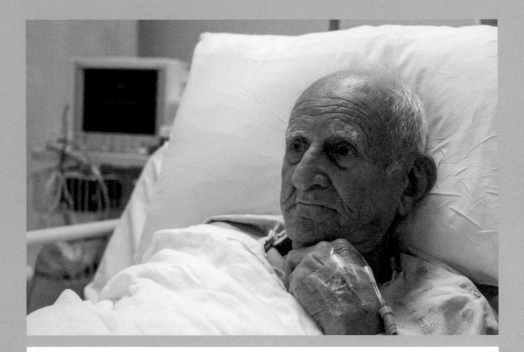

LEARNING OBJECTIVES

After reading this chapter, you will:

» reflect on how patients and families experience acute care, and how clinicians can impact their experience

» identify strategies to improve the assessment of older people in acute care, and the impact of inadequate assessment on health outcomes

» identify the key distinguishing features of delirium, dementia and depression in older people in acute care

» explain strategies to optimise medication safety for older people in acute care

» identify the role of clinicians in optimising transitions of care between home, residential aged care, hospital and palliative care.

Introduction

Older people in Australia are living longer and have a high burden of chronic diseases. People aged 65 years and older already account for one in five emergency department (ED) presentations, and nearly half of all same-day hospitalisations and overnight hospitalisations (AIHW, 2018) and this number is expected to increase in the future. It is important for clinicians to understand the attitudes, skills and knowledge required to care for older people in the **acute care** setting. Like people of any age, older people deserve high-quality person-centred care. However, there may be barriers to accessing such care due to ageism and lack of knowledge of the specific needs of older people. In this chapter, we present practical strategies for clinicians working in the acute setting to deliver high-quality, person-centred care. These strategies are based on knowledge of the clinical needs of older people and their families in this setting, and an attitude of appreciation of their experiences, including facing age-related bias.

Our goal is that the information in this chapter will inform you as you work with and support the older person when they encounter the acute care system in Australia.

acute care
Secondary healthcare where a person receives treatment for a sudden, short-term illness or exacerbation of a chronic condition.

Patient and family experience of acute care

11.1 Getting to know the person: Pauline's story

Pauline is a 75-year-old woman who was brought to the emergency department by ambulance. She is a retired teacher who normally lives alone at home, walks her dog daily and looks after her own cooking and cleaning. Her nephew, Dan, called an ambulance because he was concerned that she had been generally weak and tired for a few days, to the point where she couldn't get out of bed.

When they arrive in ED, the paramedics hand over Pauline's care to the triage nurse. Dan overhears the paramedics tell the nursing staff that Pauline is just **acopic**. The staff are rushing around and don't introduce themselves to Pauline or Dan, so they aren't sure who is looking after them. Pauline didn't bring her hearing aids and can't hear very well, especially with all staff members wearing masks, so Dan answers questions for her. He notices that different staff members are asking the same questions multiple times and worries that important information is not being handed over. When the meal tray comes around, they aren't sure whether Pauline is allowed to eat or drink, so she doesn't take anything. After eight hours in the ED, Pauline is moved to a ward bed, but she is unsure about her diagnosis or treatment plan, or how long she will be in hospital. She starts to get restless because she is anxious about her dog, who is at home alone.

acopic
A derogatory term referring to not being able to cope.

An acute illness or injury is a significant life event for an older person. An acute care encounter can be a frightening and disorienting experience and can provoke a sense of vulnerability among older people (Moons et al., 2003). Many aspects of the hospital environment, including noise, lighting and a busy atmosphere, are not ideal for effective and quality care of older adults and can impair communication (D'Avanzo et al., 2017). Staffing ratios for lower acuity patients in the acute setting may not reflect the needs of older people, leaving them with insufficient care, and clinicians may lack the knowledge to manage complex geriatric care (Hogan & Malsch, 2018).

Older people and their families value being provided with information and being able to take an active role in decision making during an acute care encounter, and expect to receive treatment that relieves symptoms (Morphet et al., 2015; Nikki et al., 2012; van Oppen et al., 2019).

FOCUS QUESTION

- What could the clinicians looking after Pauline have done differently to improve her experience?

Assessment of the older person in ED

Clinicians often perceive assessing an older person in the ED as being challenging and time-consuming. Utilising strategies to maximise the amount of information you can gather from an older person will make the assessment quicker and decrease errors, enhance safety and improve patient outcomes.

Implications for practice

Strategies to enhance assessment of older people in acute care

- Use language that is simple to understand without being colloquial or patronising. Avoid using terms of endearment (e.g. 'dear') or over-simplifying language, as this can make the older person feel disrespected and conveys the impression that the clinician assumes they are cognitively impaired (Hogan & Malsch, 2018).
- Make time to speak to the older person and give them your full attention. Clinicians are frequently interrupted in the ED and this can impair safe communication. Sharing life stories is sometimes perceived as being a waste of time in the ED but can add to your assessment as they can illustrate the values and goals of care for the older person (Hogan & Malsch, 2018).
- Demonstrate empathy by being friendly and attentive, anticipating patient needs and taking time to listen (Graham et al., 2019). Make eye contact when talking to someone (if culturally appropriate), rather than looking at a computer screen or notes (Hogan & Malsch, 2018).

- Identify hearing and visual impairments and use aids when possible. Position yourself close to the person rather than speaking to them from the end of the bed. If they wear glasses, ensure the person is wearing them and that they are clean. Ensure you have adequate lighting and a quiet space (Hogan & Malsch, 2018).
- Obtain the person's history from multiple sources. Different perspectives may be obtained from the patient, family, long-term carers, GPs, treating specialists and friends and neighbours. Some will offer background health information, details of functional decline or recent acute illness that the patient may not be aware of or may not be able to describe themselves.

MASK WEARING AND COMMUNICATION

Wearing masks and other **personal protective equipment** (PPE) is essential to prevent spread of respiratory viral disease but can impair communication between clinicians and patients. Communication breakdowns can occur because patients may not be able to hear speech, read lips or non-verbal cues or even recognise the different individuals involved in their care. Communication while wearing a mask is a rapidly evolving area of practice change. Consider some of the strategies suggested in the following Implications for practice box.

personal protective equipment
Clothing or accessories worn by a worker to protect them from hazards.

Implications for practice

Strategies to enhance communication when wearing a mask

- Minimise noise and distractions in the environment where possible.
- Introduce yourself at the beginning of each interaction including your name, role and the tasks you will perform. Some clinicians show a photo of themselves not wearing PPE to help with recognition in subsequent interactions.
- Acknowledge the issues with wearing PPE and explain why it is necessary.
- Communicate non-verbal information verbally. For example: 'I'm smiling back at you'.
- Use technology such as video calls to have important conversations, or pre-recorded videos to explain a diagnosis or management plan.
- Allocate additional time for each patient encounter.

Source: Marler & Ditton, 2020.

COMPREHENSIVE GERIATRIC ASSESSMENT

A comprehensive geriatric assessment (CGA) is used to identify and manage complex needs and barriers to functional independence in older people and is thus both diagnostic and therapeutic (Harding, 2020). Performing a CGA may reduce the risk of hospital admission and increases the likelihood of the older person being alive and community-dwelling at 12 months (Ellis et al., 2017). See Figure 11.1 for the core components included in a CGA.

FIGURE 11.1 Core components of the comprehensive geriatric assessment (CGA)

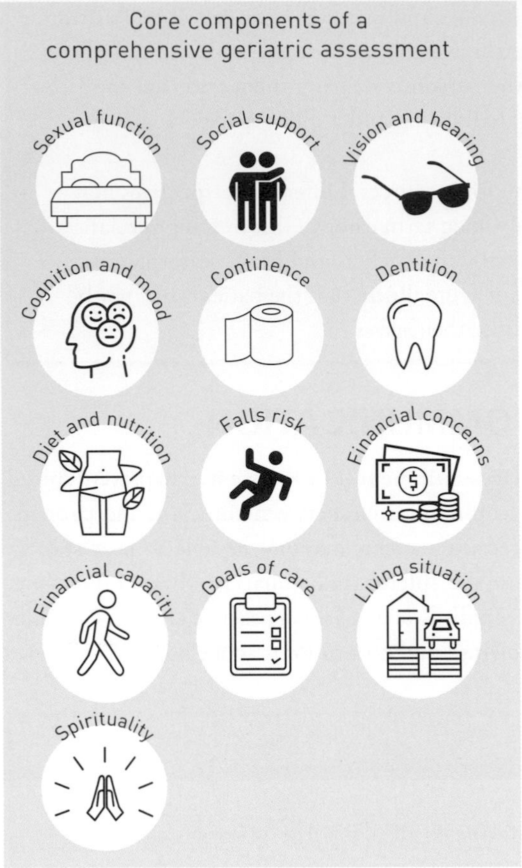

Core components of a comprehensive geriatric assessment

Sexual function · Social support · Vision and hearing · Cognition and mood · Continence · Dentition · Diet and nutrition · Falls risk · Financial concerns · Financial capacity · Goals of care · Living situation · Spirituality

Source: Adapted from Han & Grant, 2016.

Once the CGA has been completed, findings and recommendations are communicated to community teams for actioning. For example, the clinician performing the CGA may refer the older person to their GP and outpatient allied health service such as a physiotherapist, or a specialist clinic such as a falls clinic, depending on the services available in the local area. If recommending follow-up, clinicians should provide information about location and transport options for accessing the service.

The CGA may be deferred initially due to time constraints or because the person is too unwell. If not completed, this should be handed over. In many health-care services, there is a specialist team called the Aged Care Services Emergency Team (ASET), who can complete the assessment. Some emergency departments have introduced specialised models of care for older people to streamline their initial assessment and management (Wallis et al., 2018).

THE IMPACT OF INADEQUATE ASSESSMENT AND STEREOTYPING

The term 'acopia' (not being able to cope) is sometimes used to label older adults who are thought to have no acute medical problems, are suffering from functional or social problems or are considered to be an inappropriate admission (Oliver, 2008). Clinicians using this pejorative term may perceive that older people seeking acute care are an unnecessary burden on clinical load and the health service (Kee & Rippingale, 2009; Peate, 2014).

Using the label of acopia can affect the attitudes of clinicians who encounter the person and has serious negative implications for the care of the older person in the acute setting. Age-related treatment bias is well documented and the diagnosis of acopia may result in under-investigation and delays in treatment for the older person (Kee & Rippingale, 2009; Oliver, 2008). It is important to recognise that nearly all older adults labelled with acopia have another primary medical diagnosis on presentation to the acute hospital, and the risk of death during that hospital admission has been estimated at 22 per cent (Dyer et al., 2018). Furthermore, a diagnosis of acopia may also result in early and unsuitable admission to long-term care due to inappropriate decision making.

Clinicians must avoid using this prejudicial term in order to advocate for older people to receive dignified and thorough care during their acute illness or injury. Instead, clinicians should seek to identify underlying (often reversible) acute pathology and use the comprehensive geriatric assessment as a framework to individualise and optimise care for the older person in acute care.

- Why might the clinicians looking after Pauline have called her acopic?
- How might this label of acopia influence the clinicians in their assessment and management of Pauline?
- What strategies to improve communication while wearing PPE have you seen or heard about?

FOCUS QUESTIONS

ATYPICAL PRESENTATIONS

Older people with acute illness or injury can present with atypical symptoms and signs of the illness, or with vague complaints, such as confusion, weakness, fatigue or dizziness (Jackman et al., 2020). **Delirium** may be the only manifestation of serious pathology (see next section on delirium). Older people who present with non-specific complaints are more likely to be misdiagnosed, take longer to get treatment and are more likely to die within 30 days, compared to patients with classical symptoms (Nemec et al., 2010; Wachelder et al., 2017). Physiological changes associated with ageing, comorbidities and polypharmacy may mask typical presentations of conditions like acute myocardial infarction, sepsis, surgical emergencies and serious trauma. Table 11.1 describes how the usual approach to assessing conditions might differ in older people.

delirium
A sudden onset of confusion that can be resolved when the cause is identified and treated.

URINARY TRACT INFECTION

Urinary tract infection (UTI) is a common diagnosis in older people. While this condition can cause serious illness, there is increasing concern that it may be over-diagnosed (Lee et al., 2015). This means that some older people are mistakenly thought to have a UTI when in fact there is another cause for their vague or atypical symptoms. For example, cloudy or malodourous urine is not a reliable sign of UTI (Gbinigie et al., 2018). Furthermore, bedside urinalysis can also be misleading as the presence of leukocytes or nitrites in the urine could indicate asymptomatic bacteriuria rather than UTI (Nicolle et al., 2019). It is important to check current local evidence-based guidelines prior to collecting a urine sample and sending it to the lab for microscopy and culture. Inappropriate or premature diagnosis of UTI can expose the older person to unnecessary antibiotics (Burkett et al., 2019).

TABLE 11.1 Considerations during the assessment of an older person

CONDITION	ASSESSMENT CONSIDERATIONS
Acute abdominal emergencies	» Life-threatening conditions such as appendicitis, ruptured abdominal aortic aneurysm, **mesenteric ischaemia** and acute cholecystitis are frequently misdiagnosed as renal colic or functional constipation (Spangler et al., 2014) » Older people with serious abdominal pathology may have normal vital signs, a soft abdomen and no focal tenderness » Mortality is high for older patients presenting with abdominal pain (Leuthauser & McVane, 2016)
Acute myocardial infarction (AMI)	» Older patients with AMI commonly present without chest pain (Jung et al., 2017); other common symptoms of AMI include shortness of breath, dizziness, weakness and syncope (Gupta et al., 2012) » Age-related treatment bias means that older people are less likely to have a **coronary angiogram** and cardiac follow-up care after an AMI, compared to younger people (Kaura et al., 2020)
Elder abuse	» Be aware of red flags for elder abuse (see Chapter 7) » Listen to the older person, ask if they feel safe to talk and arrange for privacy if needed » Refer to social workers and/or advanced practice nurses with an understanding of elder abuse
Sepsis and infections such as urinary tract infection (UTI) and pneumonia	» Fever is absent in 30–50% of frail older adults with an infective process (Yoshikawa & Norman, 2017) » Medications (such as **beta-blockers** and **calcium channel blockers**) may mask tachycardia due to **septic shock** » An older person may experience adverse effects of hypotension due to septic shock even if they appear to have a normal blood pressure reading due to physiological changes associated with ageing and pre-existing chronic hypertension » Carefully assess for sepsis in older people who present with a vague complaint as they may not manifest the usual signs, and are at increased risk of delayed diagnosis, delayed treatment (including antibiotics) and worse outcomes (Nasa et al., 2012)
Trauma	» Age-related bias affects initial triage of older trauma patients. Older patients are less likely to be assigned a higher **triage category** than younger people, despite later being found to have major traumatic injuries (Lukin et al., 2015) » Medications (such as beta-blockers and calcium channel blockers) may mask tachycardia due to traumatic shock; a heart rate greater than 90 beats/min is associated with increased risk of mortality in elderly trauma patients, compared to 130 beats/min in younger patients (Heffernan et al., 2010) » An older person may experience adverse effects of hypotension due to septic shock even if they appear to have a normal blood pressure reading due to physiological changes associated with ageing and pre-existing chronic hypertension. A systolic blood pressure less than 110 mmHg is associated with increased risk of mortality in older trauma patients, compared to 95 mmHg in young patients (Heffernan et al., 2010) » It is important to be vigilant when assessing older patients who are injured, even if the mechanism of injury does not appear serious or they have apparently normal vital signs (Cox et al., 2014)

For definitions of bolded glossary terms in this table, please see the glossary at the back of the book.

11.2 Getting to know the person: Pauline's story

The clinicians looking after Pauline find that her vital signs are all within normal range but note that her urine is malodorous. They assume she is confused because she isn't answering their questions, but in fact she just can't hear them because she isn't wearing her hearing aids. They diagnose her with a UTI and start antibiotics.

Pauline deteriorates over a few days despite being treated with antibiotics. A registered nurse looking after Pauline performs a comprehensive geriatric assessment and realises that Pauline had been coping very well at home until this acute illness. After performing a thorough physical examination, ECG, blood tests and x-rays, the team determine that Pauline has suffered an acute myocardial infarction and start the right treatment.

- Considering age-related changes in older people, can the nurses determine that observations within normal limits provide enough information about Pauline's health status?
- What has been the impact on Pauline of the health professionals' assumptions about her condition?
- How could the delay in diagnosing Pauline have been prevented?

FOCUS QUESTIONS

Delirium

As articulated in Pauline's case study, assumptions made by nurses and other health professionals can have devastating, even fatal, impacts on an older person. As you read in the previous chapter, confusion is the age-related change that first indicates a health emergency or pathology in an older person. When an older person presents with confusion, astute assessment to differentiate between acute confusion (delirium) or dementia is imperative. Never assume confusion is dementia; failure to differentiate between delirium and dementia can have fatal consequences.

11.3 Getting to know the person: Peter's story

Peter is a Wiradjuri man from a small First Nations community approximately 300 kilometres from the nearest base hospital. He is very connected with his

 BRIDGET HONAN AND ELYCE GREEN

community and spends a lot of time with his grandchildren while his daughter and son-in-law are at work in a nearby town. His grandchildren are very active and while outside with them Peter falls and cuts his arm. Not wanting to worry his grandchildren, Peter bandages his arm and does not mention his injury.

Two days later, Peter's daughter notices that when she drops the kids off on her way to work Peter is confused about why they are there. She becomes concerned and calls an ambulance but cannot accompany him to hospital because she has to look after her children. While the paramedics are on scene they conduct a physical assessment of Peter and an environmental assessment of his home. They also collect his current medications to take with Peter to hospital.

FOCUS QUESTIONS

- Keeping in mind what you learnt in Chapter 3, what are the experiences of First Nations peoples in acute care and how could support be provided for Peter?
- Considering what you have learned about assessment of the older person in acute care, what would be your immediate concerns and areas of focus for Peter's care?

DEFINITION OF DELIRIUM

Diagnostic and Statistical Manual of Mental Disorders (DSM-5)
A manual of descriptions, symptoms and other criteria for diagnosing mental disorders.

psychomotor behaviour
Physical movements controlled by the brain.

The characteristics of delirium described in the ***Diagnostic and Statistical Manual of Mental Disorders*** **(DSM-5)** include rapid onset; fluctuation of confusion and consciousness; inability to focus, sustain or shift attention; and a change in cognition or development of a perceptual disturbance that is not attributed to dementia. Delirium can be classified as hyperactive, hypoactive or mixed, depending on **psychomotor behaviour** (Martins & Fernandes, 2012).

Although delirium is widely recognised, the pathophysiology is still not well understood and it is thought to occur due to a variety of pathogenic mechanisms (Fong et al., 2009; Oh et al., 2017). There are predisposing factors (those that make the person more vulnerable to delirium) and precipitating factors (delirium triggers). These are outlined in Table 11.2.

TABLE 11.2 Predisposing and precipitating factors for delirium

benzodiazepines
A group of drugs that depress the nervous system.

PREDISPOSING	PRECIPITATING
advanced age	concurrent illness
alcohol abuse	drugs (particularly **benzodiazepines**, narcotic analgesics and anticholinergics)
comorbid conditions (increases with severity of comorbid disease)	iatrogenic complications
dehydration and malnutrition	indwelling catheters
dementia and depression	intensive care unit admission
functional dependence	metabolic derangements
male gender	physical restraints
polypharmacy	primary neurological conditions (i.e. stroke)
visual and/or hearing impairment	surgery
	uncontrolled pain

Source: Based on the work of Martins & Fernandes, 2012; Saxena & Lawley, 2009.

The broad clinical signs and varying causes of delirium make it a complex condition to identify and treat. Older people admitted to acute care facilities are significantly more likely to experience delirium compared to people who are younger (Nguyen et al., 2020). Delirium is associated with functional decline, loss of independence, increased length of stay, institutionalisation and mortality (Fong et al., 2009; Fortini et al., 2014; Han et al., 2017; Vasilevskis et al., 2012). The experience of delirium can cause emotional distress, a disrupted sense of autonomy and perceptual disturbances (Lee-Steere et al., 2020; Weir & O'Brien, 2019). Delirium can also be a cause of distress for the older person's family (Martins et al., 2018; Partridge et al., 2019).

Delirium is often under-recognised or mistreated by clinicians (Martins & Fernandes, 2012). The complexity, prevalence and poor outcomes associated with delirium make it imperative that clinicians work as a team to standardise practices that will decrease the risk of delirium for older people in acute care.

Learn more
Watch Video 11.1 and reflect on Max's experience of delirium.

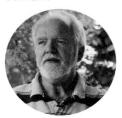

- Consider the information presented in Table 11.2. How many of these factors were present in Pauline's and Peter's cases?
- How could Peter's and Max's situations have been managed to ensure optimal outcomes?
- Reflecting on both Peter's and Max's experiences, consider the personal implications of delirium for the older person: how you would feel in this situation?

FOCUS QUESTIONS

PREVENTION OF DELIRIUM

Delirium is largely preventable (Cotton et al., 2011; Inouye, 2006) and therefore careful attention should be paid to ensure the acute care environment is focused on delirium reduction. This can be achieved using the strategies shown in the Implications for Practice box.

Implications for practice

Strategies to prevent delirium

- Keep rooms quiet, with appropriate light for the time of day and clocks and calendars for orientation.
- Encourage family visits.
- Reduce room changes.
- Ensure visual and hearing aids are available.
- Provide opportunities for early and ongoing mobilisation.
- Rationalise medications.
- Avoid physical restraints.
- Avoid benzodiazepines, anticholinergics and **psychoactive drugs**.
- Use interpreters for people from culturally and linguistically diverse backgrounds and refer to First Nations health practitioners and liaisons where appropriate.

Source: Based on the work of ACSQHC, 2016; Fong et al., 2009; Kalish et al., 2014; Traynor & Britten, 2010.

psychoactive drugs
Chemicals that affect a person's mental state.

Clinicians should build these strategies into their everyday practice so they become routine. It is important that delirium prevention is viewed as a priority that is owned by the multidisciplinary team and that all prevention strategies are multimodal in nature (Rivosecchi et al., 2015).

ASSESSMENT OF DELIRIUM

There are several tools available for the assessment of delirium. Health services should adopt a consistent approach to screening patients, particularly those who are at high risk such as older people (ACSQHC, 2016). Diagnostic tools include:

- 4AT
- the confusion assessment method (CAM) (also available in a modified version for intensive care use)
- the delirium symptom interview (DSI)
- the delirium risk assessment tool (DRAT)
- the delirium rating scale (DRS).

In addition to standardising the tool used to identify delirium, health services should have procedures that outline the regularity of delirium assessment.

The presence of delirium is an indication of an underlying issue and should never be ignored or assumed to be a normal consequence of illness or ageing (Nguyen et al., 2020). Due to the multitude of factors that can cause delirium in an older person, a thorough history and physical examination should be undertaken when delirium is identified. Clinicians should take particular notice of medications, signs of infection, changes in urination, changes in bowel habits and pain (ACSQHC, 2016).

The PINCHME mnemonic can help to recall some of the common reversible causes of delirium:

- **P**ain
- **I**nfection
- **N**utrition
- **C**onstipation
- **H**ydration
- **M**edication
- **E**nvironment.

TREATMENT OF DELIRIUM

The treatment of delirium in an older person is multimodal and must focus on maintaining safety, managing symptoms, identifying the cause and reversing the cause (where possible) (Aftab & Shah, 2017; Martins & Fernandes, 2012). These goals can only be achieved by adopting a treatment plan that focuses on person-centred care and involves a multidisciplinary team. Management strategies are shown in Figure 11.2.

FIGURE 11.2 Management of delirium symptoms

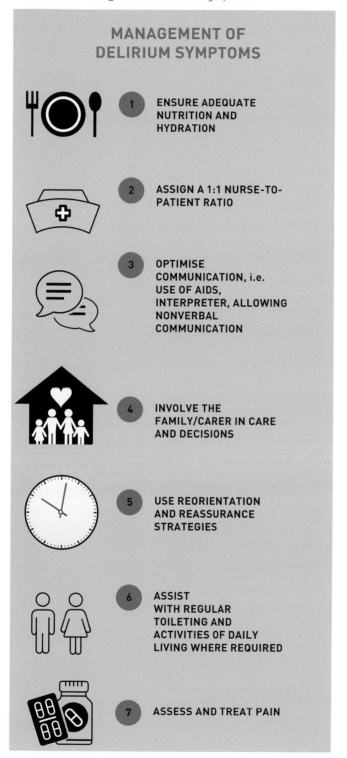

MANAGEMENT OF DELIRIUM SYMPTOMS

1. ENSURE ADEQUATE NUTRITION AND HYDRATION

2. ASSIGN A 1:1 NURSE-TO-PATIENT RATIO

3. OPTIMISE COMMUNICATION, i.e. USE OF AIDS, INTERPRETER, ALLOWING NONVERBAL COMMUNICATION

4. INVOLVE THE FAMILY/CARER IN CARE AND DECISIONS

5. USE REORIENTATION AND REASSURANCE STRATEGIES

6. ASSIST WITH REGULAR TOILETING AND ACTIVITIES OF DAILY LIVING WHERE REQUIRED

7. ASSESS AND TREAT PAIN

Source: Based on Aftab & Shah, 2017; ACSQHC, 2016.

Sedative and psychotropic medications are not useful in the treatment of delirium and should never be used for this purpose (van Velthuijsen et al., 2018; Zirker et al., 2013). Occasionally, medication may be required to manage acute severe behavioural symptoms of delirium, but this should only be used after careful consideration and with close observation.

11.4 Getting to know the person: Peter's story

Let's revisit Peter's acute care presentation. The clinician in ED responsible for his care begins a CGA and immediately notices that Peter is confused.

Due to the promptness of the clinician recognising that Peter is confused, and conducting a thorough assessment, he is able to be diagnosed with an infected arm wound and delirium. In addition to commencing antibiotics, the treating team implements several strategies to keep Peter safe, such as;

- involving a First Nations health practitioner in his care
- speaking to Peter's daughter to collect information for his health and social assessment
- providing Peter with a 1:1 nurse
- providing Peter with reorientation and assistance with activities of daily living.

Three days later, Peter is responding to antibiotics and his delirium is resolved. Several members of his family arrive and are keen to see him. The treating team has a meeting with Peter and his family about his treatment and goals of care. Peter identifies that it is his goal to be discharged home to his family as soon as possible. The treating team is able to provide him with a take-home pack of oral antibiotics and a referral to the local a First Nations medical service for follow-up review of his wound and mobility.

FOCUS QUESTIONS

- Using the PINCHME mnemonic, identify the potential causes of Peter's delirium.
- How can the registered nurse include family in determining if Peter's confusion is delirium or dementia?
- What appropriate referrals to other health professionals and services would support Peter in the short and longer term?

Delirium and dementia

You can find more information about delirium in Chapters 12 and 13.

As the incidence of dementia increases in the Australian population so too will the number of people with a diagnosis of dementia who are admitted to hospital. People with a diagnosis of dementia who are admitted to hospital are at increased risk of falls, reduced mobility, incontinence, functional decline, mortality, longer length of stay, reduced quality of life and increased likelihood of discharge to residential care (Desai et al., 2013; Fogg et al.,

2017; Sampson et al., 2014; Timmons et al., 2015). People who have a cognitive impairment and are admitted to hospital are at increased risk of developing delirium compared to those without any form of cognitive impairment (Fortini et al., 2014). The coexistence of dementia and delirium in an older person again adds a heightened level of risk as this dual diagnosis is associated with significantly higher hospital costs, increased functional decline and in-hospital mortality (Avelino-Silva et al., 2017; Fick et al., 2013; Morandi et al., 2014). **Behavioural disturbances** occur in up to 75 per cent of people with dementia who are admitted to hospital and may manifest as agitation or aggression (Sampson et al., 2014). These behavioural disturbances should not be considered normal and should instigate an investigation of possible underlying causes and screening for delirium (Aftab & Shah, 2017).

behavioural disturbances Changes in the way a person acts that are generally distressing and puts them or others at risk.

The heightened level of risk and distress for a person experiencing a dual diagnosis of dementia and delirium makes it imperative that health-care professionals implement practices that reduce the risk of delirium (such as those mentioned in the previous Implications for Practice box). Clinicians should be vigilant in screening older people with cognitive impairment for delirium to ensure that it is recognised early and treated appropriately.

PHYSICAL AND PHARMACOLOGICAL RESTRAINTS

Physical or pharmacological restraint has been described as 'dehumanising and disempowering … an affront to dignity and personal autonomy' (Commonwealth of Australia, 2019, p. 193). The use of restraints is not recommended in the treatment of delirium or dementia. Restrictive practices such as restraining a person on a chair or bed, or using sedative medication, should only be used when it is absolutely necessary to protect the person from a serious and imminent risk of harm. In older people, pharmacological sedation is high risk in the short term because of the potential for over-sedation, **respiratory depression** and hypotension (Simpkins et al., 2016).

respiratory depression Slow and ineffective breathing.

Depression

Depression is underdiagnosed in older people and can be confused as delirium or dementia (see Table 11.3). Appropriate screening is needed if an older person presents with low mood and symptoms of depression; this should be taken seriously and not be dismissed as part of ageing. Screening for depression in older people can be done using a Geriatric Depression Scale (GDS) with a comprehensive mental assessment. There are also tools that can be used to identify depression in people with a diagnosis of dementia, such as the Cornell Depression Scale (Alexopoulos et al., 1988). Table 11.3 briefly compares the three conditions, referred to as the 3 Ds (delirium, depression and dementia).

You can find more information about depression in Chapter 12.

Pain

Supporting people who experience pain is something that challenges many health professionals who struggle to alleviate the life-changing impacts this condition has on older people. As you saw in Max's video, he is experiencing chronic pain and in the following scenario, you will read about Margaret, who is trying to find meaning in pain that constantly reminds her of her terminal illness.

TABLE 11.3 Comparison of the symptoms of depression, delirium and dementia (the 3 Ds)

	DEPRESSION	DELIRIUM	DEMENTIA
Definition	A change in mood that lasts at least two weeks and includes sadness, negativity, loss of interest and pleasure, and/or decline in functioning	An acute or sudden onset of mental confusion as a result of a medical, social, and/or environmental condition	Progressive loss of brain cells resulting in decline of day-to-day cognition and functioning. A terminal condition
Duration	At least six weeks, but can last several months to years, especially if not treated	Hours to months, dependent on speed of diagnosis	Years (usually eight to 20 years)
Thinking	May be indecisive and thoughts highlight failures and a sense of hopelessness	Fluctuates between rational state and disorganised, distorted thinking with incoherent speech	Gradual loss of cognition and ability to problem solve and function independently
Mental status testing	Capable of giving correct answers; however, often may state 'I don't know'	Testing may vary from poor to good depending on time of day and fluctuation in cognition	Will attempt to answer and will not be aware of mistakes
Memory	Generally intact, though may be selective. Highlights negativity	Recent and immediate memory impaired	Inability to learn new information or to recall previously learnt information
Sleep–wake cycle	Disturbed, usually early morning awakening	Disturbed. Sleep–wake cycle is reversed (up in night, very sleepy and sometimes non-responsive during the day)	Normal to fragmented
Hallucinations and delusions	Can be present in severe depression. Themes of guilt and self-loathing	Often of a frightening or paranoid nature	Can be present. May misperceive. In Lewy Body dementia, visual hallucinations are present
Diagnosis	May deny being depressed but often exhibit anxiety. Others may notice symptoms first. Increased complaints of physical illness. Social withdrawal is common	Diagnosis based on rapid onset of fluctuating symptoms. Can be mistaken for progression of the dementia	Usually diagnosed approximately three years after onset of symptoms. Must rule out other causes of cognitive decline (e.g. depression or delirium)
Care approaches	Identify the symptoms of depression early. Help person to follow treatment plan and offer them hope	Early recognition is key. Keep person safe, find cause of the delirium and treat as quickly as possible	Maintain and enhance abilities that remain. Focus on the positive and support the lost abilities
Prognosis	Treatable and reversible condition	Treatable and reversible with early diagnosis but can lead to permanent disability or death	Progression can be slowed but not reversed
Treatment	Antidepressants, ECT, interpersonal therapy, behavioural-cognitive therapy. Assist person to improve confidence and self-esteem through conversation and activity	Treat underlying cause. Monitor response. Be alert for relapse – occurs in 90% of cases	Cholinesterase inhibitors slow the progression of some dementias. Symptomatic treatment with environmental and staff approaches

Source: Island Health Authority, 2014.

11.5 Getting to know the person: Margaret's story

Margaret is 81 years old and still independently living on her small farm in rural New South Wales. Since she lost her husband three years ago, Margaret has been running the farm with some help from her family. She is passionate about the upkeep of her garden and insistent that all her animals are well cared for, including her dog, cat, sheep, horse and birds. Unfortunately, her routine faecal occult blood test this year showed abnormalities and further investigations revealed she has **metastatic** bowel cancer. Margaret's family notice that she often grimaces when working in the garden and occasionally becomes withdrawn after a day of work in the yard. When asked if she is OK, Margaret insists she 'is not sick' and therefore does not need any analgesia. She tells her granddaughter that she believes having pain confirms that she is ill and signifies that she is less capable to work on her farm. Margaret's granddaughter has been able to convince her to come to the ED today because Margaret has severe stomach cramping. After conducting an initial assessment, you become aware that Margaret has some complex pain requirements. You retrieve some analgesia for her stomach cramps and prepare to conduct a thorough history.

metastatic cancer
When cancer cells spread from a primary tumour to another part of the body.

- What are some potential sources of pain for Margaret based on what you already know about her diagnosis, life stage and activity levels?
- What are some potential challenges you might have when conducting a thorough assessment of Margaret's pain?
- What are some strategies you can use to build rapport with Margaret to encourage her to self-report pain?

FOCUS QUESTIONS

DEFINITION OF PAIN

Pain in the older person is a complex and sometimes mysterious symptom that is complicated by the subjectivity of the experience of pain. The International Association for the Study of Pain (IASP) defines pain as 'An unpleasant sensory and emotional experience associated with, or resembling that associated with, actual or potential tissue damage' (Raja et al., 2020).

Reflecting the complexity and subjectivity of pain, the IASP also adds key notes to their definition that signify pain is a personal experience influenced by individual factors; it is not a solely physical phenomenon and can be learnt through experience. Importantly, clinicians should respect self-reported pain and be aware that the experience of pain is not dependent on a person's ability to report it.

ACUTE VERSUS CHRONIC PAIN

Acute pain is a short-lived response to an acute injury – such as trauma, surgery or other noxious stimuli – that only lasts until the injury heals (Painaustralia, 2020). Older people admitted to acute care will commonly experience some form of acute pain (Gibson & Lussier, 2012). Conversely, chronic pain is pain that persists beyond the original injury, or recurs for more than three months (Treede et al., 2019). In 2018, 1.03 million older Australians (65 years and over) were living with chronic pain, with rates almost twice as high as the working age population (Deloitte Access Economics, 2019). Therefore, acute pain in older people is often complicated by pre-existing chronic pain, which can complicate assessment and management.

DIFFERENT EXPERIENCES OF PAIN

It is important to recognise that the experience of pain varies across individuals. There is an abundance of research that shows the effects of pain varies according to emotion, activities of daily living, communication, culture and past experiences (Booker & Haedtke, 2016; Dunham et al., 2013). Furthermore, the experience of pain can have different meanings for people (Collis & Waterfield, 2015; Dunham et al., 2017). For some older people, experiencing pain is viewed as meaning they are 'sick' or not as strong as others. It may also be seen as an inevitable part of ageing. The story behind the meaning an individual gives their pain is an important consideration during assessment. Understanding the complexity of pain in older people is essential for clinicians so they can work with patients to achieve optimum outcomes. An understanding of the complex interaction between the pathophysiological, emotional and cultural elements of pain will also allow clinicians to ensure the treatment of pain is holistic and focused on improved quality of life, promoting dignity and independence where possible (Dunham et al., 2013).

The presence of pain has several implications for the older person in acute care including delayed recovery from illness, heightened immune response and delirium (Curtiss, 2010; Hall, 2016; Hwang & Platts-Mills, 2013; Hwang et al., 2010). There is an increased likelihood of adverse effects for older people who experience pain, such as falls, fatigue, decreased quality of life, depression and premature death (Blyth et al., 2007; Crowe et al., 2017; Domenichiello & Ramsden, 2019; Hall, 2016).

ASSESSMENT OF PAIN

The subjective nature of pain means it is important that clinicians work with patients in both assessment and treatment. Several methods of pain assessment have been developed for use in acute care including numerical rating scales, verbal rating scales and visual scales. Examples of such tools that have been tested for reliability and validity for use with cognitively intact and cognitively impaired verbal older adults include the Iowa Pain Thermometer, the Verbal Descriptor Scale, the Faces Pain Scale (revised) and the 0–10 numeric rating scale (Hadjistavropoulos et al., 2007; Hicks et al., 2001; Hjermstad et al., 2011). Despite the plethora of tools available, it is continually reported that older people in acute care are at a high risk of experiencing untreated or undertreated pain (Curtiss, 2010). Evidence recommends the use of a self-reported pain rating scale where possible (Curtiss, 2010). Individual health services may standardise the pain assessment tools used in their facilities, so you should investigate local policy and procedures during orientation to a new service.

Assessing someone's pain is not a simple question; it is a discussion. As a clinician, it is essential that you use your communication skills in your assessment to ascertain what the person is experiencing. This may require you to use different words to describe pain, such as 'hurt', 'sore', 'burn' or 'ache' (Curtiss, 2010). People may not immediately identify their experience with the word 'pain'. A discussion about pain is also dependent on the older person's willingness to report pain. This can be affected by the rapport they have with the clinician, and their personal beliefs about pain, stoicism, ethnicity, culture and understanding of their condition (Booker & Haedtke, 2016). Take the time to build rapport and learn about how the older person identifies and experiences pain. Don't fall into the trap of assuming that the absence of physical signs such as moaning, grimacing or a racing heart, or the ability of a patient to eat, sleep or talk, is an indication that they are not in pain (Booker & Haedtke, 2016; Curtiss, 2010).

The assessment of pain is ongoing. As has been discussed, pain in the older person can be either a constant or fragmented experience so dialogue between the clinician and the person experiencing pain should continue throughout the episode of care. You should continually reassess pain in the older person, especially if you have provided an intervention – you need to know if it worked!

Assessment of pain is also dynamic and should consider any potential painful stimuli. If an older person has pneumonia, they might not be in pain when they are talking to you, but this can escalate to severe pain on deep inspiration or during a cough. Similarly, an older person who has undergone a joint replacement might be comfortable sitting in bed, but they are unlikely to participate in physiotherapy if movement triggers pain. A thorough pain assessment that includes identification of the possible cause and/or pathophysiology of pain will allow you to better adapt to the needs of the older person and pre-empt possible painful stimuli.

PAIN IN OLDER PEOPLE EXPERIENCING DELIRIUM OR DEMENTIA

Assessing pain in people who are experiencing delirium, dementia or other pathophysiology that may impair communication can be challenging. Self-report may be possible for people with mild or moderate cognitive impairment and their ability to self-report should be tested before other methods of assessment are considered (Cornelius et al., 2017). When cognitive impairment is severe, it may not be possible for an older person to report their experience of pain. Of course, the absence of reporting does not equate to the absence of pain, and a diagnosis of dementia does not affect the somatosensory cortex of the brain, which is responsible for interpreting pain stimuli (Bjoro & Herr, 2008). In these situations, clinicians must use alternative tools to assess pain. Options for assessing pain in people with a cognitive impairment include Checklist of Nonverbal Pain Indicators (CNPI) (Lints-Martindale et al., 2012; Neville & Ostini, 2014), Pain Assessment in Advanced Dementia (PAINAD) (DeWaters et al., 2008), the Critical-Care Observation Tool (Ersek et al., 2010; Lints-Martindale et al., 2012; Neville & Ostini, 2014) and the Abbey Pain Scale (Abbey et al., 2004).

As clinicians, we have an obligation to advocate for vulnerable people. Older people who are unable to fully communicate their needs can be very vulnerable, as demonstrated by accounts of untreated pain in residents of aged care facilities (Commonwealth of Australia, 2021) and research showing that these patients may be subject to inadequate administration of analgesia

(Fry et al., 2016; Green et al., 2016). If the older person with delirium or dementia is unable to self-report pain, clinicians should use other strategies to manage pain such as:

- searching for a potential cause
- observing patient behaviours
- obtaining surrogate reports (from family members, parents or caregivers) about pain, and behaviour and activity changes
- attempt an analgesia trial (Curtiss, 2010).

Clinicians should also be aware that pain in older people with dementia and delirium can manifest in different ways, such as agitation or aggression, and a change in the behaviour of an older person with cognitive impairment should instigate a pain assessment (Koo et al., 2018).

TREATMENT OF PAIN

Treatment of pain cannot occur without accurate and ongoing assessment. Despite the complexities of acute clinical care, health-care professionals are legally, ethically and morally bound to treat pain (Denny & Guido, 2012). Clinicians should consider how their own practice influences the treatment of pain, including their communication strategies, environmental and organisational structure, personal experiences and understandings of the complex nature of pain (Gorawara-Bhat et al., 2017; Harmon et al., 2019; Manias, 2012). Pain treatment plans should be developed collaboratively between the treating clinician, the older person and, if relevant, the older person's carer or family members. Older people who have chronic or complex pain should have their pain assessed and treated by a multidisciplinary team of clinicians (Hall, 2016). It is important that treatment plans focus on both pharmacological and non-pharmacological interventions and that they are discussed with all parties before the plan is agreed upon (Harmon et al., 2019).

Non-pharmacological interventions may include the use of hot/cold packs, gentle exercise, physiotherapy, relaxation and music (Cornelius et al., 2017). These interventions are highly dependent on the cause of pain and the individual's preference. Pharmacological interventions for pain are discussed in Chapter 14, but it is important that the prescribing clinician takes into consideration any allergies, medication interactions, combining multimodal analgesia, administration route, time of onset, half-life, and kidney and liver function, as well as the older person's medication preference (Cornelius et al., 2017).

Another under-utilised option for pain management is injecting local anaesthetic in order to provide a **nerve block**. For example, a fascia iliaca nerve block is a technique that is very effective in treating pain associated with a hip fracture that involves injecting local anaesthetic into the groin. This procedure can easily and safely be performed in the emergency department, ward or even pre-hospital, and is within the scope of practice of paramedics, registered nurses and doctors who have undergone appropriate training and credentialing (Honan et al., 2020).

nerve block
Injecting medication around a specific nerve to stop a person feeling pain.

For more information on pharmacology, see Chapter 14.

11.6 Getting to know the person: Margaret's story

Let's revisit Margaret's story and reflect on the ways her pain could be appropriately assessed and managed. Being a proud, independent woman, Margaret is uncomfortable discussing illness, pain or any ailment that might impact her work on the farm. Building a rapport with Margaret is essential as she will not self-report her pain unless she feels comfortable about discussing it. This may take time and it is important to engage in the conversation. Margaret will need to be educated on the importance of pain management, and this should be contextualised for her in relation to her goals (being able to work in the garden, remain independent, etc.). Involving a multidisciplinary team is also essential for helping Margaret make a pain-management plan that is holistic. Margaret may be more comfortable with non-pharmacological options for analgesia so these could be incorporated in her pain-management plan. Most importantly, the pain-management plan must be designed in consultation with Margaret and consider her preferences. If she is not involved and does not agree with the plan you can guarantee those scripts won't be filled!

Medications

Adverse drug reactions are a significant health issue for older people in the acute care setting (Alhawassi et al., 2014; Mettälä & Vaherkoski, 2014). Up to 30 per cent of all hospital admissions in people aged 65 years and over in Australia are estimated to be medication related (Roughead et al., 2013). Acute illness or injury is frequently compounded by inaccurate medication histories on presentation, prescribing and administration errors, and poor documentation and handover on discharge (Roughead et al., 2016).

Implications for practice

Recommended strategies to optimise medication safety for older people during an acute care encounter

- Utilise a multidisciplinary team to make medication care plans, which should include hospital and primary health-care doctors, nurses and pharmacists.
- Perform a thorough medication reconciliation (including prescribed medications, over-the-counter medications and alternative therapies) on admission or handover if it cannot be completed.
- Review whether any long-term medications can be safely stopped. This is called deprescribing.

- Avoid potentially inappropriate medications. The American Geriatric Society provides guidance on how this can be achieved using the Beers Criteria for Potentially Inappropriate Medication Use in Older Adults. These are medications that should be avoided in older people because of the increased risk of adverse effects. For example, first-generation antihistamines should be avoided in older people due to the risk of anti-cholinergic side effects such as confusion, constipation and urinary retention (Fick et al., 2019).
- Minimise interruptions during medication administration. Interruptions have been shown to increase the risk of medication errors significantly.
- Ensure medications are given on time. Some conditions will worsen dramatically if a medication is delayed or forgotten. For example, delaying medications by more than one hour can cause patients with Parkinson's disease to experience worsening tremors, increased rigidity, loss of balance, confusion, agitation and difficulty communicating.

Source: Based on the work of Khalil et al., 2020.

High-risk medications are medications that have an increased risk of causing significant patient harm or death if they are misused or used in error. Although this is true of any age group, older people are at increased risk due to physiological and anatomical changes associated with ageing (as described in Chapter 10), and increased likelihood of polypharmacy. In the acute care setting in Australia, the APINCH acronym is widely used to identify high-risk medications (ACSQHC, 2019). Table 11.4 outlines the reasons why some categories of high-risk medication are particularly significant for older people in acute care.

TABLE 11.4 High-risk medications identified by APINCH

		HIGH-RISK MEDICATION CATEGORY	ADVERSE EFFECTS
A		Antibiotics	Nephrotoxicity causing renal failure and **ototoxicity** causing deafness
P		Potassium and other electrolytes	Arrhythmias leading to cardiac arrest
I		Insulin	Hypoglycaemia leading to coma
N		Narcotics and sedatives	Respiratory depression and **apnoea**
C		Chemotherapy agents	Haematological problems and **neurotoxicity**
H		Heparin and anticoagulants	Internal bleeding (e.g. in the head, gut or joints) either spontaneously or after a minor injury

Source: Based on the work of ACSQHC, 2019.

ototoxicity
Damage to the inner ear caused by chemicals.

apnoea
When someone stops breathing.

neurotoxicity
Nervous system problems occurring from exposure to chemicals.

- Reflect on the importance of your current or future role in ensuring safe prescription, administration and monitoring of medications. How this looks will depend on your discipline area. For some it will be ensuring an appropriate assessment and plan has been developed; for others it may mean taking notice of changes in an older person's condition and raising concerns with other members of the multidisciplinary team. What are three things you could do as a clinician to increase medication safety?

FOCUS QUESTION

The patient journey

11.7 Getting to know the person: Graham's story

Graham is a 72-year-old man and is a retired plumber with a wife, two grown-up children and five grandchildren. He has a history of Parkinson's disease and lives in a residential aged care facility. He enjoys chatting to family and carers. He requires two assistants to get in and out of his wheelchair and move around in the chair. His wife Lynne lives nearby and visits daily. On one of her visits, she notices that Graham appears short of breath and has a productive cough. The carers at the facility call an ambulance to take him to ED for assessment. The paramedics ensure they take a handover from the carers, including Graham's medication list and his advance care plan.

Transitions of care occur when an older person moves between their home, hospital and subacute health-care facilities. Older people who were living in their own home prior to hospitalisation may require additional support and community-based services in order to return home after an acute encounter or may transition to a residential aged care facility or palliative care facility. Older people who are already living in residential aged care have particular risk factors and needs associated with transfer to and from an acute care encounter.

During 2018–2019, 37 per cent of aged care facility residents presented to an ED at least once (Commonwealth of Australia, 2020). Frail older residents of aged care facilities are at increased risk of an unplanned transfer to hospital if they come from a facility with poor staff-to-resident ratios, a lower proportion of senior staff or a lack of access to primary health care and specialist geriatricians (Dwyer et al., 2015). Residents who undergo an unplanned transfer to hospital will potentially be subjected to multiple handovers during transfer by emergency ambulance, a prolonged ED stay spanning multiple staff shifts, and referral to a ward. At every handover, there is potential for loss of information that could adversely impact the older person's care. It is important to provide communication and documentation to ensure high-quality and safe handovers (Morphet et al., 2014). Key information that should accompany the resident when transitioning between home and hospital include:

- reason for transfer
- past medical history

For more information on family relationships and carers, see Chapter 5.

- current medications
- cognitive function
- advance care directive
- contact details for carers and other clinicians involved in the care of the older person (Griffiths et al., 2014).

11.8 Getting to know the person: Graham's story

By the time Graham arrives at the hospital and is seen by a registered nurse, he has missed a dose of his regular anti-Parkinsonian medication. This leaves him frozen stiff, unable to move, confused and unable to talk. Fortunately, the paramedics who transported Graham have brought the medication list with them. When they realise that Graham has missed a dose of his anti-Parkinsonian medication, they arrange for the right medication to be given and he recovers from the **akinetic** crisis.

Graham is diagnosed with pneumonia and is treated with oral antibiotics. He does not require oxygen or an intravenous drip.

akinetic
The loss of the normal ability to move the muscles.

FOCUS QUESTIONS

- Could the deterioration in Graham's condition have been prevented?
- What are some of the benefits and risks of being admitted to hospital for Graham?

ADVERSE EFFECTS OF HOSPITALISATION

Most older people who are brought to the ED will be admitted to hospital (Dwyer et al., 2014). However, hospital is not a benign environment for frail older persons, who are at risk of a high rate of complications associated with hospital admission including delirium, **pressure sores** and **hospital-acquired infections** (Southerland et al., 2019). Some older people may choose to decline hospital-based investigations (such as a CT scan) or treatment (such as an invasive surgery). Avoiding hospital-based care may improve an older person's quality of life by helping them maintain autonomy and allowing them to spend more time in their own environment with family and friends. When a person is unable to make health-care decisions for themselves – due to dementia, for example – health-care providers may rely on advance care directives and surrogate decision makers, such as family members, to help decide what investigations and treatment the person would choose for themselves. This process of weighing up health-care options based on the individual's own values and goals of care is called shared decision making and is a powerful tool in delivering person-centred care (Bunn et al., 2018; Muthalagappan et al., 2013).

pressure sores
Wounds caused by prolonged periods of pressure on a part of the body.

hospital-acquired infections
When bacteria or viruses get into the body because of medical treatments.

Imagine you go to a store to buy a new laptop. You ask the sales assistant, 'What's the best laptop?' If she just told you to buy Laptop A, you would have no knowledge or understanding of why it was the best laptop. But if you decided to do all the research yourself, you might spend hours on the internet learning all about the hundreds of different laptop specifications available, which could become overwhelming and not help you make a decision.

Another approach would be to follow a shared decision-making model. The sales assistant would check your needs and preferences by asking, 'What programs will you be using? What battery life do you need? How much do you want to spend?' This would take into consideration your personal values in choosing the best laptop for you.

Similarly, if older people were given the opportunity to consider their values and goals, this could be helpful in deciding what treatments might be best for them.

It is important for clinicians to understand the potential complications and limitations of acute admission for the older patient and to help identify the older person's values and goals in order to provide person-centred care.

TRANSITION TO COMMUNITY SERVICES

During an acute care encounter, the treating team should assess the functional status and needs of the older person to inform discharge planning and prevent post-discharge complications such as falls and unplanned readmission (Gupta et al., 2019; Southerland et al., 2019). Table 11.5 outlines the important things to consider prior to discharging an older person from hospital.

TABLE 11.5 Discharge considerations

ASPECTS FOR REVIEW	SPECIFIC ASSESSMENTS TO BE CHECKED
Cognition	Changes in mental status have resolved
Ambulation	Older person can mobilise safely and at baseline
Level of care	Carer is available and able to provide the level of care needed
Abuse	No concerns about abuse or neglect on screening
Medications	Medications have been reviewed for potential drug interactions and adverse effects. Instructions for administration have been provided in written form and the patient/carer can correctly articulate the medication schedule
Discharge instructions	Older person and carer understand discharge instructions including home care advice, when to return and follow-up
Patient/family concerns	Any concerns raised by the older person and carers have been addressed
Communication with GP and allied health	Discharge plan has been discussed with patient's GP and other health-care providers

Post-discharge, older people may require assistance with housekeeping, allied health and therapy services, transport and meal delivery. They may be eligible for a government-assisted program such as the Commonwealth Home Care Packages Program. However, many older people who have been assessed as eligible for care are not able to access a package in a timely way, with average waiting time exceeding a year (Commonwealth of Australia, 2021). Other programs exist to support discharge from acute care, such as the transition care program, where an older person can access short-term residential care while recovering from an acute illness or injury.

11.9 Getting to know the person: Graham's story

Graham's team organise his discharge home to the residential care facility. The pharmacist makes a list of all of Graham's medications, including what they are for and when to take them, and sends a copy to the residential care facility and to Graham's GP. The treating team talk to Graham's wife Lynne and answer all her questions about his illness and the expected recovery. They also ring the residential care facility and hand over to the registered nurse, including an update on Graham's care needs during this acute illness.

FOCUS QUESTIONS

- What aspects of discharge planning for Graham were managed well?
- Are there any outstanding issues that haven't been addressed?

Learn more
Watch Video 7.1: Mardi discusses finding a suitable residential aged care facility for her grandmother.

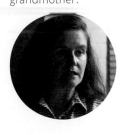

Learn more
Watch Video 11.2: This case study features Denise and her experiences of palliative care.

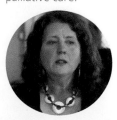

TRANSITION TO RESIDENTIAL AGED CARE

Nearly all older people who were living at home prior to hospitalisation can return home without needing to go into residential aged care (Commonwealth of Australia, 2020). If an older person is identified as having increased care needs, they will be referred for a comprehensive assessment with the Aged Care Assessment Team (ACAT) assessor in order to determine whether they are eligible for a home care package, respite (short-term) care or permanent placement in residential aged care. The assessment process and decision to accept a higher level of care can cause worries about loss of independence, loss of health and well-being, and financial concerns for the older person, their family, friends and carers. They may require assistance and support to understand the financial costs associated with residential aged care and choosing the right facility. The support of the ASET nurse, the discharge planner and the social worker is invaluable in assisting the family and the older person through this confronting time. The experiences of older rural people and their families searching for suitable aged care services and accommodation can be a traumatic and emotional experience associated with difficulty finding suitable facilities, as well as joy and satisfaction when there is a positive outcome (Bernoth et al., 2012).

TRANSITION TO PALLIATIVE CARE

Up to 34 per cent of older people admitted from residential aged care will die in hospital during an acute admission (Dwyer et al., 2014). For some, this occurs suddenly in the context of an acute illness or injury, whereas others have experienced slow decline over time due to terminal illness, organ failure or frailty. Health-care professionals working in the acute care setting should recognise signs of decline and identify when the goal of care for an older person is palliative. Many hospitals have specialist palliative care teams, often including a palliative care nurse practitioner, who can provide further assessment and management. Ideally, an older person who is receiving palliative care should not remain on an acute care ward, but instead should be moved to a more appropriate setting such as a palliative care ward or hospice.

For more information on preparing for the end of life, see Chapter 19.

Conclusion

In this chapter, case studies have been used to illustrate some of the experiences of older people in acute care. After reading the chapter, you can appreciate that clinicians have a significant role in providing care that enhances the quality of life of older people. It is very satisfying professionally to contribute to positive outcomes. Our skills and knowledge are constantly challenged by aspects of aged care such as atypical presentations, caring for people with delirium and dementia in the acute care setting, and providing optimal pain relief. All of this makes aged care an important and dynamic area of healthcare.

Learn more
Access additional resources – such as weblinks, further readings and podcasts – to broaden your understanding of this chapter. See the Guided Tour for access details.

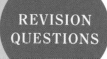

REVISION QUESTIONS

1 In each of the case studies in this chapter, what are some of the barriers and facilitators to providing person-centred care?

2 What knowledge, skills and attitudes do you already have, and what will you need to develop, in order to be an effective clinician caring for older people in the acute care setting?

3 How is caring for an older person in the acute setting similar to and different from caring for people from younger age groups?

REFERENCES

Abbey, J., Piller, N., Bellis, A. D., Esterman, A., Parker, D., Giles, L. & Lowcay, B. (2004). The Abbey pain scale: A 1-minute numerical indicator for people with end-stage dementia. *International Journal of Palliative Nursing, 10*(1), 6–13. https://doi.org/10.12968/ijpn.2004.10.1.12013

Aftab, A. & Shah, A. A. (2017). Behavioral emergencies: Special considerations in the geriatric psychiatric patient. *Psychiatric Clinics of North America, 40*(3), 449–62. https://doi.org/10.1016/j.psc.2017.05.010

Alexopoulos, G. S., Abrams, R. C., Young, R. C. & Shamoian, C. A. (1988). Cornell scale for depression in dementia. *Biological Psychiatry,*

23(3), 271–84. https://doi.org/10.1016/0006-3223(88)90038-8

Alhawassi, T. M., Krass, I., Bajorek, B. & Pont, L. G. (2014). A systematic review of the prevalence and risk factors for adverse drug reactions in the elderly in the acute care setting. *Clinical Interventions in Aging, 9*, 2079–86. https://doi.org/10.2147/CIA.S71178

Australian Commission on Safety and Quality in Health Care (ACSQHC) (2016). *Delirium clinical care standard*. www.safetyandquality.gov.au/our-work/clinical-care-standards/delirium-clinical-care-standard

Australian Commission on Safety and Quality in Health Care (ACSQHC) (2019). *APINCH classification of high risk medicines*. www.

safetyandquality.gov.au/our-work/medication-safety/high-risk-medicines/apinchs-classification-high-risk-medicines

Australian Institute of Health and Welfare (AIHW) (2018). Older Australia at a Glance. People at Risk of Homelessness. AIHW. www.aihw.gov.au/reports/older-people/older-australia-at-a-glance/contents/diverse-groups-of-older-australians/people-at-risk-of-homelessness

Avelino-Silva, T. J., Campora, F., Curiati, J. A. E. & Jacob-Filho, W. (2017). Association between delirium superimposed on dementia and mortality in hospitalized older adults: A prospective cohort study. *PLoS Medicine, 14*(3), 1–18. https://doi.

org/10.1371/journal.
pmed.1002264

Bernoth, M. A., Dietsch, E. &
Davies, C. (2012). Forced
into exile: The traumatising
impact of rural aged care
service inaccessibility. *Rural
and Remote Health, 12*(1),
1–9.

Bjoro, K. & Herr, K. (2008).
Assessment of pain in the
nonverbal or cognitively
impaired older adult.
*Clinics in Geriatric
Medicine, 24*(2), 237–62.
https://doi.org/10.1016/j.
cger.2007.12.001

Blyth, F. M., Macfarlane, G. J. &
Nicholas, M. K. (2007). The
contribution of psychosocial
factors to the development
of chronic pain: The key
to better outcomes for
patients? *PAIN, 129*(1), 8–11.
https://doi.org/10.1016/j.
pain.2007.03.009

Booker, S. Q. & Haedtke, C.
(2016). Assessing pain in
nonverbal older adults.
Nursing, 46(5), 66–9.
https://doi.org/10.1097/01.
NURSE.0000480619.
08039.50

Bunn, F., Goodman, C., Russell,
B., Wilson, P., Manthorpe,
J., Rait, G., Hodkinson, I.
& Durand, M. A. (2018).
Supporting shared decision
making for older people with
multiple health and social
care needs: A realist synthesis.
BMC Geriatrics, 18(1), 1–16.
https://doi.org/10.1186/
s12877-018-0853-9

Burkett, E., Carpenter, C. R.,
Arendts, G., Hullick, C.,
Paterson, D. L. & Caterino,
J. M. (2019). Diagnosis
of urinary tract infection
in older persons in the
emergency department:
To pee or not to pee, that
is the question. *Emergency
Medicine Australasia,
31*(5), 856–2. https://
doi.org/10.1111/1742-
6723.13376

Collis, D. & Waterfield, J. (2015).
The understanding of pain
by older adults who consider
themselves to have aged
successfully. *Musculoskeletal
Care, 13*(1), 19–30. https://
doi.org/10.1002/msc.1083

Commonwealth of Australia
(2019). Royal Commission
into Aged Care Quality
and Safety. Interim report:
Neglect. Vol. 1. https://
agedcare.royalcommission.
gov.au/sites/default/
files/2020-02/interim-report-
volume-1.pdf

Commonwealth of Australia
(2020). Royal Commission
into Aged Care Quality
and Safety. Hospitalisations
in Australian aged care:
2014/15–2018/19. https://
agedcare.royalcommission.
gov.au/sites/default/
files/2021-02/research-paper-
18-hospitalisations-australian-
aged-care.pdf

Commonwealth of Australia
(2021). Royal Commission
into Aged Care Quality and
Safety. Final report: Care,
dignity and respect. https://
agedcare.royalcommission.
gov.au/sites/default/
files/2021-03/final-report-
volume-1_0.pdf

Cornelius, R., Herr, K. A.,
Gordon, D. B. & Kretzer,
K. (2017). Evidence-
based practice guideline:
Acute pain management
in older adults. *Journal
of Gerontological Nursing,
43*(2), 18–27. https://doi.
org/10.3928/00989134-
20170111-08

Cotton, D., Taichman, D.,
Williams, S. & Marcantonio,
E. R. (2011). Delirium.
*Annals of Internal Medicine,
154*(11). https://doi.
org/10.7326/0003-4819-154-
11-201106070-01006

Cox, S., Morrison, C., Cameron,
P. & Smith, K. (2014).
Advancing age and trauma:
Triage destination compliance
and mortality in Victoria,
Australia. *Injury, 45*(9),
1312–19. https://doi.org/
https://doi.org/10.1016/j.
injury.2014.02.028

Crowe, M., Jordan, J., Gillon,
D., McCall, C., Frampton,
C. & Jamieson, H. (2017).
The prevalence of pain and its
relationship to falls, fatigue,
and depression in a cohort
of older people living in
the community. *Journal of
Advanced Nursing, 73*(11),

2642–51. https://doi.org/
https://doi.org/10.1111/
jan.13328

Curtiss, C. P. (2010). Challenges in
pain assessment in cognitively
intact and cognitively
impaired older adults with
cancer. *Oncology Nursing
Forum, 37*(5), 7–16. https://
doi.org/10.1188/10.ONF.
S1.7-16

D'Avanzo, B., Shaw, R., Riva,
S., Apostolo, J., Bobrowicz-
Campos, E., Kurpas, D.,
Bujnowska, M. & Holland,
C. (2017). Stakeholders'
views and experiences of
care and interventions for
addressing frailty and pre-
frailty: A meta-synthesis of
qualitative evidence. *PLoS
ONE, 12*(7), e0180127.
https://doi.org/10.1371/
journal.pone.0180127

Deloitte Access Economics
(2019). *The cost of pain in
Australia*. www.painaustralia.
org.au/static/uploads/
files/the-cost-of-pain-in-
australia-final-report-12mar-
wfxbrfyboams.pdf

Denny, D. L. & Guido, G. W.
(2012). Undertreatment
of pain in older adults: An
application of beneficence.
Nursing Ethics, 19(6),
800–9. https://doi.
org/10.1177/0969733301
2447015

Desai, S., Chau, T., & George,
L. (2013). Intensive Care
Unit Delirium. *Critical Care
Nursing Quarterly, 36*(4),
370-389.

DeWaters, T., Faut-Callahan, M.,
McCann, J. J., Paice, J. A.,
Fogg, L., Hollinger-Smith,
L., Sikorski, K. & Stanaitis,
H. (2008). Comparison of
self-reported pain and the
painad scale in hospitalized
cognitively impaired and
intact older adults after hip
fracture surgery. *Orthopaedic
Nursing, 27*(1), 21–8.

Dixon, M. (2021). Assessment
and management of older
patients with delirium in
acute settings. *Nursing Older
People, 33*(1). https://doi.
org/10.7748/nop.2018.e969

Domenichiello, A. F. & Ramsden,
C. E. (2019). The silent
epidemic of chronic pain

in older adults. *Progress in Neuro-Psychopharmacology and Biological Psychiatry, 93*(January), 284–90. doi.org/10.1016/j.pnpbp.2019.04.006

Dunham, M., Allmark, P. & Collins, K. (2017). Older people's experiences of cancer pain: A qualitative study. *Nursing Older People, 29*(6), 28–32. https://doi.org/10.7748/nop.2017.e943

Dunham, M., Ingleton, C., Ryan, T. & Gott, M. (2013). A narrative literature review of older people's cancer pain experience. *Journal of Clinical Nursing, 22*(15–16), 2100–13. https://doi.org/10.1111/jocn.12106

Dwyer, R., Gabbe, B., Stoelwinder, J. U. J., Lowthian, J., Gabbe, B. & Lowthian, J. (2014). A systematic review of outcomes following emergency transfer to hospital for residents of aged care facilities. *Age and Ageing, 16*(7), 759–66.

Dwyer, R., Stoelwinder, J., Gabbe, B. & Lowthian, J. (2015). Unplanned transfer to emergency departments for frail elderly residents of aged care facilities: A review of patient and organizational factors. *Journal of the American Medical Directors Association, 16*(7), 551–62. https://doi.org/10.1016/j.jamda.2015.03.007

Dyer, A. H., Ryan, D. & O'Callaghan, S. (2018). 'Acopia' and 'inability to cope' remain unhelpful and pejorative labels for complexity in older adults presenting to the acute hospital. *Age and Ageing, 47*(3), 488. https://doi.org/10.1093/ageing/afy013

Ellis, G., Gardner, M., Tsiachristas, A., Langhorne, P., Burke, O., Harwood, R. H., Conroy, S. P., Kircher, T., Somme, D., Saltvedt, I., Wald, H., O'Neill, D., Robinson, D. & Shepperd, S. (2017). Comprehensive geriatric assessment for older adults admitted to hospital. *Cochrane Database of Systematic Reviews.* https://

doi.org/10.1002/14651858.CD006211.pub3

Ersek, M., Herr, K., Neradilek, M. B., Buck, H. G. & Black, B. (2010). Comparing the psychometric properties of the Checklist of Nonverbal Pain Behaviors (CNPI) and the Pain Assessment in Advanced Dementia (PAIN-AD) Instruments. *Pain Medicine, 11*(3), 395–404. https://doi.org/10.1111/j.1526-4637.2009.00787.x

Fick, D. M., Semla, T. P., Steinman, M., Beizer, J., Brandt, N., Dombrowski, R., DuBeau, C. E., Pezzullo, L., Epplin, J. J., Flanagan, N., Morden, E., Hanlon, J., Hollmann, P., Laird, R., Linnebur, S. & Sandhu, S. (2019). American Geriatrics Society 2019 updated AGS Beers Criteria® for potentially inappropriate medication use in older adults. *Journal of the American Geriatrics Society, 67*(4), 674–94. https://doi.org/10.1111/jgs.15767

Fick, D. M., Steis, M. R., Waller, J. L. & Inouye, S. K. (2013). Delirium superimposed on dementia is associated with prolonged length of stay and poor outcomes in hospitalized older adults. *Journal of Hospital Medicine, 8*(9), 500–5. https://doi.org/10.1002/jhm.2077

Fogg, C., Meredith, P., Bridges, J., Gould, G. P. & Griffiths, P. (2017). The relationship between cognitive impairment, mortality and discharge characteristics in a large cohort of older adults with unscheduled admissions to an acute hospital: A retrospective observational study. *Age and Ageing, 46*(5), 794–801. https://doi.org/10.1093/ageing/afx022

Fong, T. G., Tulebaev, S. R. & Inouye, S. K. (2009). Delirium in elderly adults: Diagnosis, prevention and treatment. *Nature reviews. Neurology, 5*(4), 210–20. https://doi.org/10.1038/nrneurol.2009.24

Fortini, A., Morettini, A., Tavernese, G., Facchini, S., Tofani, L. & Pazzi, M.

(2014). Delirium in elderly patients hospitalized in internal medicine wards. *Internal and Emergency Medicine, 9*(4), 435–41. https://doi.org/10.1007/s11739-013-0968-0

Fry, M., Chenoweth, L. & Arendts, G. (2016). Assessment and management of acute pain in the older person with cognitive impairment: A qualitative study. *International Emergency Nursing, 24*, 54–60. https://doi.org/10.1016/j.ienj.2015.06.003

Gbinigie, O. A., Ordóñez-Mena, J. M., Fanshawe, T. R., Plüddemann, A. & Heneghan, C. (2018). Diagnostic value of symptoms and signs for identifying urinary tract infection in older adult outpatients: Systematic review and meta-analysis. *Journal of Infection, 77*(5), 379–90. https://doi.org/10.1016/j.jinf.2018.06.012

Gibson, S. J. & Lussier, D. (2012). Prevalence and relevance of pain in older persons. *Pain Medicine, 13*(2), S23–S26. https://doi.org/10.1111/j.1526-4637.2012.01349.x

Gorawara-Bhat, R., Wong, A., Dale, W. & Hogan, T. (2017). Nurses' perceptions of pain management for older-patients in the Emergency Department: A qualitative study. *Patient Education and Counseling, 100*(2), 231–41. https://doi.org/10.1016/j.pec.2016.08.019

Graham, B., Endacott, R., Smith, J. E. & Latour, J. M. (2019). 'They do not care how much you know until they know how much you care': A qualitative meta-synthesis of patient experience in the emergency department. *Emergency Medicine Journal, 36*(6), 355–63. https://doi.org/10.1136/emermed-2018-208156

Green, E., Bernoth, M. & Nielsen, S. (2016). Do nurses in acute care settings administer PRN analgesics equally to patients with dementia compared to patients without dementia? *Collegian, 23*(2), 233–9. https://doi.org/10.1016/j.colegn.2015.01.003

Griffiths, D., Morphet, J., Innes, K., Crawford, K. & Williams, A. (2014). Communication between residential aged care facilities and the emergency department: A review of the literature. *International Journal of Nursing Studies, 51*(11), 1517–23. https://doi.org/10.1016/j.ijnurstu.2014.06.002

Gupta, B. P., Huddleston, J. M., Kirkland, L. L., Huddleston, P. M., Larson, D. R., Gullerud, R. E., Burton, M. C., Rihal, C. S. & Wright, R. S. (2012). Clinical presentation and outcome of perioperative myocardial infarction in the very elderly following hip fracture surgery. *Journal of Hospital Medicine, 7*(9), 713–16. doi.org/https://doi.org/10.1002/jhm.1967

Gupta, S., Perry, J. A. & Kozar, R. (2019). Transitions of care in geriatric medicine. *Clinics in Geriatric Medicine, 35*(1), 45–52. https://doi.org/10.1016/j.cger.2018.08.005

Hadjistavropoulos, T., Herr, K., Turk, D. C., Fine, P. G., Dworkin, R. H., Helme, R., Jackson, K., Parmelee, P. A., Rudy, T. E., Beattie, B., Chibnall, J. T., Craig, K. D., Ferrell, B., Ferrell, B., Fillingim, R. B., Gagliese, L., Gallagher, R., Gibson, S. J., Harrison, E. L., … Williams, J. (2007). An interdisciplinary expert consensus statement on assessment of pain in older persons. *The Clinical Journal of Pain, 23*, S1–S43.

Hall, T. (2016). Management of persistent pain in older people. *Journal of Pharmacy Practice and Research, 46*(1), 60–7. https://doi.org/10.1002/jppr.1194

Han, B. & Grant, C. (2016). A short mnemonic to support the comprehensive geriatric assessment model. *Emergency Nurse, 24*(6), 18–22. https://doi.org/10.7748/en.2016.e1554

Han, J. H., Vasilevskis, E. E., Chandrasekhar, R., Liu, X., Schnelle, J. F., Dittus, R. S. & Ely, E. W. (2017). Delirium in the Emergency Department and Its Extension into Hospitalization (DELINEATE) Study: Effect on 6-month function and cognition. *Journal of the American Geriatrics Society, 65*(6), 1333–8. https://doi.org/10.1111/jgs.14824

Harding, S. (2020). Comprehensive geriatric assessment in the emergency department. *Age and Ageing, 49*(6), 936–8. https://doi.org/10.1093/ageing/afaa059

Harmon, J., Summons, P. & Higgins, I. (2019). Experiences of the older hospitalised person on nursing pain care: An ethnographic insight. *Journal of Clinical Nursing, 28*(23–4), 4447–59. https://doi.org/10.1111/jocn.15029

Heffernan, D. S., Thakkar, R. K., Monaghan, S. F., Ravindran, R., Adams, C. A., Kozloff, M. S., Gregg, S. C., Connolly, M. D., MacHan, J. T. & Cioffi, W. G. (2010). Normal presenting vital signs are unreliable in geriatric blunt trauma victims. *Journal of Trauma – Injury, Infection and Critical Care, 69*(4), 813–18. https://doi.org/10.1097/TA.0b013e3181f41af8

Hicks, C. L., von Baeyer, C. L., Spafford, P. A., van Korlaar, I. & Goodenough, B. (2001). The Faces Pain Scale – Revised: toward a common metric in pediatric pain measurement. *PAIN, 93*(2), 173–83. https://doi.org/10.1016/S0304-3959(01)00314-1

Hjermstad, M. J., Fayers, P. M., Haugen, D. F., Caraceni, A., Hanks, G. W., Loge, J. H., Fainsinger, R., Aass, N. & Kaasa, S. (2011). Studies comparing numerical rating scales, verbal rating scales, and visual analogue scales for assessment of pain intensity in adults: A systematic literature review. *Journal of Pain and Symptom Management, 41*(6), 1073–93. https://doi.org/10.1016/j.jpainsymman.2010.08.016

Hogan, T. M. & Malsch, A. (2018). Communication strategies for better care of older individuals in the Emergency Department. *Clinics in Geriatric Medicine, 34*(3), 387–97. https://doi.org/10.1016/j.cger.2018.04.004

Honan, B., Davoren, M., Preddy, J. & Danieletto, S. (2020). Hip fracture pain management in a regional Australian emergency department: A retrospective descriptive study. *Australasian Emergency Care, 23*(4), 221–4. https://doi.org/https://doi.org/10.1016/j.auec.2020.04.001

Hwang, U. & Platts-Mills, T. F. (2013). Acute pain management in older adults in the emergency department. *Clinics in Geriatric Medicine, 29*(1), 151–64. https://doi.org/10.1016/j.cger.2012.10.006

Hwang, U., Richardson, L. D., Harris, B. & Morrison, R. S. (2010). The quality of emergency department pain care for older adult patients. *Journal of the American Geriatrics Society, 58*(11), 2122–8. https://doi.org/10.1111/j.1532-5415.2010.03152.x

Inouye, S. K. (2006). Delirium in older persons. *New England Journal of Medicine, 354*(11), 1157–65. https://doi.org/10.1056/NEJMra052321

Island Health Authority (2014). Comparison of Depression, Delirium and Dementia. www.islandhealth.ca/sites/default/files/2018-05/delirium-3d-difference.pdf

Jackman, C., Laging, R., Laging, B., Honan, B., Arendts, G. & Walker, K. (2020). Older person with vague symptoms in the emergency department: Where should I begin? *EMA – Emergency Medicine Australasia, 32*(1), 141–7. https://doi.org/10.1111/1742-6723.13433

Jung, Y. J., Yoon, J. L., Kim, H. S., Lee, A. Y., Kim, M. Y. & Cho, J. J. (2017). Atypical clinical presentation of geriatric syndrome in elderly patients with pneumonia or coronary artery disease. *Annals of Geriatric Medicine and Research, 21*(4), 158–63. https://doi.org/10.4235/agmr.2017.21.4.158

Kalish, V. B., Gillham, J. E. & Unwin, B. K. (2014). Delirium in older persons: Evaluation and management. *American Family Physician, 90*(3), 150–8.

Kaura, A., Sterne, J. A. C., Trickey, A., Abbott, S., Mulla, A., Glampson, B., Panoulas, V., Davies, J., Woods, K., Omigie, J., Shah, A. D., Channon, K. M., Weber, J. N., Thursz, M. R., Elliott, P., Hemingway, H., Williams, B., Asselbergs, F. W., O'Sullivan, M., … Mayet, J. (2020). Invasive versus non-invasive management of older patients with non-ST elevation myocardial infarction (SENIOR-NSTEMI): A cohort study based on routine clinical data. *The Lancet, 396*(10251), 623–34. https://doi.org/10.1016/s0140-6736(20)30930-2

Kee, K. & Rippingale, C. (2009). The prevalence and characteristic of patients with acopia. *Age and Ageing, 38*(1), 100–3. https://doi.org/10.1093/ageing/afn238

Khalil, H., Kynoch, K. & Hines, S. (2020). Interventions to ensure medication safety in acute care: An umbrella review. *International Journal of Evidence-Based Healthcare, 18*(2), 188–211. https://doi.org/10.1097/XEB.0000000000000232

Koo, V., Jin, S., Wan, B. A., Ahrari, S., Lam, H., Rowbottom, L., Chow, S., Chow, R., Chow, E. & Deangelis, C. (2018). Pain management in older adults with dementia: A selective review. *Journal of Pain Management, 11*(4), 333–44.

Lee, M. J., Kim, M., Kim, N. H., Kim, C. J., Song, K. H., Choe, P. G., Park, W. B., Bang, J. H., Kim, E. S., Park, S. W., Kim, N. J., Oh, M. D. & Kim, H. B. (2015). Why

is asymptomatic bacteriuria overtreated?: A tertiary care institutional survey of resident physicians. *BMC Infectious Diseases, 15*(1), 1–8. https://doi.org/10.1186/s12879-015-1044-3

Lee-Steere, K., Liddle, J., Mudge, A., Bennett, S., McRae, P. & Barrimore, S. E. (2020). 'You've got to keep moving, keep going': Understanding older patients' experiences and perceptions of delirium and nonpharmacological delirium prevention strategies in the acute hospital setting. *Journal of Clinical Nursing, 29*(13–14), 2363–77. https://doi.org/10.1111/jocn.15248

Leuthauser, A. & McVane, B. (2016). Abdominal pain in the geriatric patient. *Emergency Medicine Clinics, 34*(2), 363–75. https://doi.org/10.1016/j.emc.2015.12.009

Lints-Martindale, A. C., Hadjistavropoulos, T., Lix, L. M. & Thorpe, I. (2012). A comparative investigation of observational pain assessment tools for older adults with dementia. *The Clinical Journal of Pain, 28*(3), 226–37.

Lukin, W., Greenslade, J. H., Chu, K., Lang, J. & Brown, A. F. T. (2015). Triaging older major trauma patients in the emergency department: An observational study. *Emergency Medicine Journal, 32*(4), 281–86. https://doi.org/10.1136/emermed-2013-203191

Manias, E. (2012). Complexities of pain assessment and management in hospitalised older people: A qualitative observation and interview study. *International Journal of Nursing Studies, 49*(10), 1243–54. https://doi.org/10.1016/j.ijnurstu.2012.05.002

Marler, H. & Ditton, A. (2020). 'I'm smiling back at you': Exploring the impact of mask wearing on communication in healthcare. *International Journal of Language & Communication Disorders, 56*(1), 205–14.

Martins, S. & Fernandes, L.

(2012). Delirium in elderly people: A review. *Frontiers in Neurology, 3*, 1–12. https://doi.org/10.3389/fneur.2012.00101

Martins, S., Pinho, E., Correia, R., Moreira, E., Lopes, L., Paiva, J. A., Azevedo, L. & Fernandes, L. (2018). What effect does delirium have on family and nurses of older adult patients? *Aging and Mental Health, 22*(7), 903–11. https://doi.org/10.1080/13607863.2017.1393794

Metsälä, E. & Vaherkoski, U. (2014). Medication errors in elderly acute care – a systematic review. *Scandinavian Journal of Caring Sciences, 28*(1), 12–28. https://doi.org/10.1111/scs.12034

Moons, P., Arnauts, H. & Delooz, H. H. (2003). Nursing issues in care for the elderly in the emergency department: An overview of the literature. *Accident and Emergency Nursing, 11*(2), 112–20. https://doi.org/10.1016/S0965-2302(02)00163-7

Morandi, A., Davis, D., Fick, D. M., Turco, R., Boustani, M., Lucchi, E., Guerini, F., Morghen, S., Torpilliesi, T., Gentile, S., MacLullich, A. M., Trabucchi, M. & Bellelli, G. (2014). Delirium superimposed on dementia strongly predicts worse outcomes in older rehabilitation inpatients. *Journal of the American Medical Directors Association, 15*(5), 349–54. https://doi.org/10.1016/j.jamda.2013.12.084

Morphet, J., Decker, K., Crawford, K., Innes, K., Williams, A. F. & Griffiths, D. (2015). Aged care residents in the emergency department: The experiences of relatives. *Journal of Clinical Nursing, 24*(23–24), 3647–53. https://doi.org/10.1111/jocn.12954

Morphet, J., Griffiths, D. L., Innes, K., Crawford, K., Crow, S. & Williams, A. (2014). Shortfalls in residents' transfer documentation:

Challenges for emergency department staff. *Australasian Emergency Nursing Journal, 17*(3), 98–105. https://doi.org/10.1016/j.aenj.2014.03.004

Muthalagappan, S., Johansson, L., Kong, W. M. & Brown, E. A. (2013). Dialysis or conservative care for frail older patients: Ethics of shared decision-making. *Nephrology Dialysis Transplantation, 28*(11), 2717–22. https://doi.org/10.1093/ndt/gft245

Nasa, P., Juneja, D. & Singh, O. (2012). Severe sepsis and septic shock in the elderly: An overview. *World Journal of Critical Care Medicine, 1*(1), 23–30. https://doi.org/10.5492/wjccm.v1.i1.23

Nemec, M., Koller, M. T., Nickel, C. H., Maile, S., Winterhalder, C., Karrer, C., Laifer, G. & Bingisser, R. (2010). Patients presenting to the emergency department with non-specific complaints: The Basel Non-specific Complaints (BANC) Study. *Academic Emergency Medicine, 17*(3), 284–92. https://doi.org/10.1111/j.1553-2712.2009.00658.x

Neville, C. & Ostini, R. (2014). A psychometric evaluation of three pain rating scales for people with moderate to severe dementia. *Pain Management Nursing, 15*(4), 798–806. https://doi.org/10.1016/j.pmn.2013.08.001

Nguyen, T. H., Atayee, R. S., Derry, K. L., Hirst, J., Biondo, A. & Edmonds, K. P. (2020). Characteristics of Hospitalized Patients Screening Positive for Delirium. *American Journal of Hospice and Palliative Medicine, 37*(2), 142–8. https://doi.org/10.1177/1049909119867046

Nicolle, L. E., Gupta, K., Bradley, S. F., Colgan, R., DeMuri, G. P., Drekonja, D., Eckert, L. O., Geerlings, S. E., Köves, B., Hooton, T. M., Juthani-Mehta, M., Knight, S. L., Saint, S., Schaeffer, A. J., Trautner, B., Wullt, B. & Siemieniuk, R. (2019). Clinical practice guideline for the management of asymptomatic bacteriuria: 2019 update by the Infectious Diseases Society of America. *Clinical Infectious Diseases, 68*(10), E83–E110. https://doi.org/10.1093/cid/ciy1121

Nikki, L., Lepistö, S. & Paavilainen, E. (2012). Experiences of family members of elderly patients in the emergency department: A qualitative study. *International Emergency Nursing, 20*(4), 193–200. https://doi.org/10.1016/j.ienj.2012.08.003

Oh, E. S., Fong, T. G., Hshieh, T. T. & Inouye, S. K. (2017). Delirium in older persons: Advances in diagnosis and treatment. *JAMA, 318*(12), 1161–74. https://doi.org/10.1001/jama.2017.12067

Oliver, D. (2008). 'Acopia' and 'social admission' are not diagnoses: Why older people deserve better. *Journal of the Royal Society of Medicine, 101*(4), 168–74. https://doi.org/10.1258/jrsm.2008.080017

Painaustralia (2020). What is Pain? www.painaustralia.org.au/about-pain/painaustralia-what-is-pain

Partridge, J. S. L., Crichton, S., Biswell, E., Harari, D., Martin, F. C. & Dhesi, J. K. (2019). Measuring the distress related to delirium in older surgical patients and their relatives. *International Journal of Geriatric Psychiatry, 34*(7), 1070–7. https://doi.org/10.1002/gps.5110

Peate, I. (2014). An unprofessional and unhelpful label. *British Journal of Nursing, 23*(6), 301. https://doi.org/10.12968/bjon.2014.23.6.301

Raja, S. N., Carr, D. B., Cohen, M., Finnerup, N. B., Flor, H., Gibson, S., Keefe, F. J., Mogil, J. S., Ringkamp, M., Sluka, K. A., Song, X.-J., Stevens, B., Sullivan, M. D., Tutelman, P. R., Ushida, T. & Vader, K. (2020). The revised International Association for the Study of Pain definition of pain: Concepts, challenges, and compromises. *PAIN, 161*(9), 1976–82.

Rivosecchi, R. M., Smithburger, P. L., Svec, S., Campbell, S. & Kane-Gill, S. L. (2015). Nonpharmacological interventions to prevent delirium: An evidence-based systematic review. *Critical Care Nurse, 35*(1), 39–49. https://doi.org/10.4037/ccn2015423

Roughead, E. E., Semple, S. J. & Rosenfeld, E. (2013). Literature Review: Medication Safety in Australia. www.safetyandquality.gov.au/publications-and-resources/resource-library/literature-review-medication-safety-australia

Roughead, E. E., Semple, S. J. & Rosenfeld, E. (2016). The extent of medication errors and adverse drug reactions throughout the patient journey in acute care in Australia. *International Journal of Evidence-Based Healthcare, 14*(3), 113–22. https://doi.org/10.1097/XEB.0000000000000075

Sampson, E. L., White, N., Leurent, B., Scott, S., Lord, K., Round, J. & Jones, L. (2014). Behavioural and psychiatric symptoms in people with dementia admitted to the acute hospital: Prospective cohort study. *British Journal of Psychiatry, 205*(3), 189–96. https://doi.org/10.1192/bjp.bp.113.130948

Saxena, S. & Lawley, D. (2009). Delirium in the elderly: A clinical review. *Postgraduate Medical Journal, 85*(1006), 405–13. https://doi.org/10.1136/pgmj.2008.072025

Simpkins, D., Peisah, C. & Boyatzis, I. (2016). Behavioral emergency in the elderly: A descriptive study of patients referred to an Aggression Response Team in an acute hospital. *Clinical Interventions in Aging, 11*, 1559–65. https://doi.org/10.2147/CIA.S116376

Southerland, L. T., Pearson, S., Hullick, C., Carpenter, C. R. & Arendts, G. (2019). Safe to send home? Discharge risk assessment in the emergency department. *Emergency Medicine Australasia, 31*(2), 266–70. https://doi.org/10.1111/1742-6723.13250

Spangler, R., Van Pham, T., Khoujah, D. & Martinez, J. P. (2014). Abdominal emergencies in the geriatric patient. *International Journal of Emergency Medicine, 7*(1), 43. https://doi.org/10.1186/s12245-014-0043-2

Timmons, S., Manning, E., Barrett, A., Brady, N. M., Browne, V., O'Shea, E., Molloy, D. W., O'Regan, N. A., Trawley, S., Cahill, S., O'Sullivan, K., Woods, N., Meagher, D., Ni Chorcorain, A. M. & Linehan, J. G. (2015). Dementia in older people admitted to hospital: A regional multi-hospital observational study of prevalence, associations and case recognition. *Age Ageing, 44*(6), 993–9. https://doi.org/10.1093/ageing/afv131

Traynor, V. & Britten, N. (2010). Delirium Care Pathways: Final report. NSW Health and Health Care of Older Australian Standing Committee. https://ro.uow.edu.au/smhpapers/3221

Treede, R. D., Rief, W., Barke, A., Aziz, Q., Bennett, M. I., Benoliel, R., Cohen, M., Evers, S., Finnerup, N. B., First, M. B., Giamberardino, M. A., Kaasa, S., Korwisi, B., Kosek, E., Lavand'homme, P., Nicholas, M., Perrot, S., Scholz, J., Schug, S. … Wang, S.-J. (2019). Chronic pain as a symptom or a disease: The IASP Classification of Chronic Pain for the *International Classification of Diseases (ICD-11). PAIN, 160*(1), 19–27. https://doi.org/10.1097/j.pain.0000000000001384

van Oppen, J. D., Keillor, L., Mitchell, Á., Coats, T. J. & Conroy, S. P. (2019). What older people want from emergency care: A systematic review. *Emergency Medicine Journal, 36*(12), 754–61. https://doi.org/10.1136/emermed-2019-208589

van Velthuijsen, E. L., Zwakhalen, S. M. G., Mulder, W. J., Verhey, F. R. J. & Kempen, G. I. J. M. (2018). Detection and management of hyperactive and hypoactive delirium in older patients during hospitalization: A retrospective cohort study evaluating daily practice. *International Journal of Geriatric Psychiatry, 33*(11), 1521–9. https://doi.org/10.1002/gps.4690

Vasilevskis, E. E., Han, J. H., Hughes, C. G. & Ely, E. W. (2012). Epidemiology and risk factors for delirium across hospital settings. *Best Practice & Research: Clinical Anaesthesiology, 26*(3), 277–87. https://doi.org/10.1016/j.bpa.2012.07.003

Wachelder, J. J. H., Stassen, P. M., Hubens, L. P. A. M., Brouns, S. H. A., Lambooij, S. L. E., Dieleman, J. P. & Haak, H. R. (2017). Elderly emergency patients presenting with non-specific complaints: Characteristics and outcomes. *PLoS ONE, 12*(11), 1–12. https://doi.org/10.1371/journal.pone.0188954

Wallis, M., Marsden, E., Taylor, A., Craswell, A., Broadbent, M., Barnett, A., Nguyen, K.-H., Johnston, C., Glenwright, A. & Crilly, J. (2018). The Geriatric Emergency Department Intervention model of care: A pragmatic trial. *BMC Geriatrics, 18*(1), 1–9. https://doi.org/10.1186/s12877-018-0992-z

Weir, E. & O'Brien, A. J. (2019). Don't go there – It's not a nice place: Older adults' experiences of delirium. *International Journal of Mental Health Nursing, 28*(2), 582–91. https://doi.org/10.1111/inm.12563

Yoshikawa, T. T. & Norman, D. C. (2017). Geriatric infectious diseases: Current concepts on diagnosis and management. *Journal of the American Geriatrics Society, 65*(3), 631–41. https://doi.org/10.1111/jgs.14731

Zirker, W., Dorokhine, I., Knapp, C. M., Patel, N. & Musuku, M. (2013). Haloperidol overdosing in the treatment of agitated hospitalized older people with delirium: A retrospective chart review from a community teaching hospital. *Drugs and Aging, 30*(8), 639–44. https://doi.org/10.1007/s40266-013-0087-7

12 Maintaining Mental Health through the Ageing Experience

PETER SANTANGELO AND JOHN DOBROHOTOFF

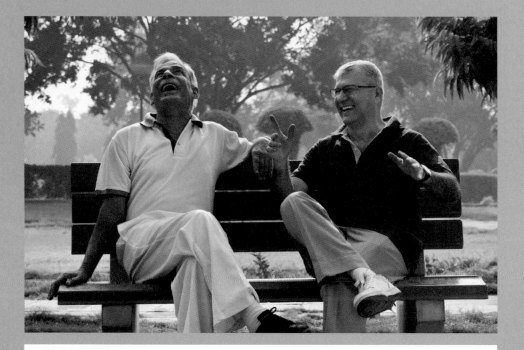

LEARNING OBJECTIVES

After reading this chapter, you will:

» implement skilled and sensitive communication strategies as the basis for astute assessment of older people

» explain how evidence-based assessment can facilitate the effectiveness of treatment

» identify that the common comorbid mental illnesses in older adults are anxiety and depression

» conclude that interdisciplinary approaches increase the ability to provide the older adult with holistic and person-centred care

» differentiate between depression, anxiety, delirium and dementia, which all share similar symptoms.

Introduction

For a novice health professional, or even for an experienced practitioner, the issues around mental health care can seem complex and unfamiliar, or even confusing. Specialist psychiatric and mental health consultation may be of assistance to you in evaluating what appropriate care can be provided. Nevertheless, you will also have acquired your own skills of observation, engagement, assessment and evidence-based decision making, which will help you recognise and manage the mental health issues that present.

Throughout this chapter, we will encourage you to broaden your perspective of mental health in older people, including and beyond biomedical considerations alone – seeing the person before the diagnosis and including their perspective of their health issues in your assessment and management of them. It is sometimes difficult to fully appreciate the perspective of an older person when you have not had that lived experience yourself, so their assistance is invaluable.

As well as information about mental health, we have included two comparative case studies for some detailed analysis. Also, along the way, we have included some points for reflection, and focus questions that may prompt your thinking to a broader level.

Mental health of older people: a global perspective

Maintaining mental health is essential for overall good health in older people. According to the World Health Organization (WHO), mental health is an integral part of health and well-being: 'Health is a state of complete physical, mental and social well-being and not merely the absence of disease or infirmity' (WHO, 2013, p. 7). It further declares that the determinants of mental health and mental disorders 'include not only individual attributes such as the ability to manage one's thoughts, emotions and behaviours and interactions with others, but also social, cultural, economic, political and environmental factors such as national policies, social protection, living standards, working conditions, and community social supports' (WHO, 2013, p. 7).

WHO also identifies vulnerable groups potentially at higher risk of experiencing mental health problems, which includes older people. With a globally ageing population, WHO estimates that, for adults aged 60 years and over, mental and neurological disorders account for 6.6 per cent of the total disability for this age group, with about 15 per cent suffering from a mental disorder. Three other assertations made by WHO are that:

- substance abuse problems among older people are often overlooked or misdiagnosed
- mental health problems are under-identified by health-care professionals and older people themselves
- the stigma surrounding these conditions makes people reluctant to seek help.

While most older people have good mental health, many are at risk of developing mental disorders, neurological disorders or substance use problems and other health conditions, any of which can result in significant loss in capacities and decline in functional ability. Older people are also exposed to other psychological risks such as bereavement and a drop in socioeconomic status. In addition, current evidence suggests that one in six older people experience elder abuse. Elder abuse can lead not only to physical injuries, but also to serious, sometimes long-lasting, psychological consequences, including depression and anxiety. Furthermore, as people age, they are more likely to experience several conditions at the same time (WHO, 2017).

ageist attitude
An attitude, based on the age of the person, that fails to respect the uniqueness of the individual and instead stereotypes older people as all being the same.

polypharmacy
The use of more than five medications, often with medications prescribed to address the side effects of other pharmaceutical products.

Therefore, maintaining mental health in older age involves other issues that include the impact of managing the needs of an increasing population on health-care demands, the effect of **ageist attitudes** on health-care delivery, the complex effects of **polypharmacy** on older people and the physiological complexities of ageing. An approach to care for older people needs to acknowledge these special circumstances and utilise multidisciplinary and collaborative services that encompass not only assessment, diagnosis and intervention based on scientifically based medical knowledge (biomedical), but also other factors such as their social, cultural and psychological circumstances and current state (psychosocial). The emphasis, too, should be on the whole spectrum of health-care delivery, which includes a continuum from prevention to early intervention, treatment in the community, primary health and hospital settings – all underpinned by a health-promotion agenda.

An Australian context

Contrary to commonly held beliefs or stereotypes, most older people have good mental health. While the prevalence of mental health disorders tends to decrease with age, there are certain sub-groups of the older population that are at higher risk. These groups include people in hospital and supported accommodation, people with dementia and older carers (AIHW, 2018).

It is thought that between 10 and 15 per cent of older people experience depression and about 10 per cent experience anxiety (NARI, 2009). Rates of depression among people living in residential aged care are believed to be much higher, at around 35 per cent (Amare et al., 2020).

A survey of community-dwelling Australians aged 65–85 years found that 8 per cent had experienced an affective disorder, 10 per cent an anxiety disorder and 12 per cent a substance use disorder at some point in their life. Findings showed that in the 12 months prior to the survey, participants met criteria in the following percentages: 2 per cent for mood disorders, 4 per cent for anxiety and 1 per cent for substance abuse. The survey also found that the presence of a physical disorder, a disability and greater treatment service use were associated with any mental disorder in the past 12 months (Sunderland et al., 2015).

It is important to remember, however, that it is *not* normal for older people to suffer with depression, anxiety, acute confusion or dementia. As in younger people, older people continue to respond to treatment and generally do well if they develop mental health problems.

Unfortunately, despite recent advances in our understanding of mental health, there remain common myths that depression or cognitive impairment is inevitable as we age. Such beliefs or attitudes can be 'ageist' in nature.

Loss of independence and freedom, and a restriction to participating in ordinary community life can affect anyone's mental outlook. The restrictions related to the COVID-19 pandemic are a good example.

- What must it be like for older people who experience these restrictions?

- Can you provide examples from your own experience that can help you imagine this?

FOCUS QUESTIONS

The Royal Australian and New Zealand College of Psychiatrists (RANZCP) (2015) reinforces that most older people have neither a mental illness nor dementia. However, if they do have a mental illness, they are likely to also have significant social and physical health problems (see Miriam's story in this chapter). Therefore, there is a risk that symptoms of treatable mental illness may be wrongly attributed to the irreversible effects of ageing or to physical or environmental changes. While mental illness occurs in older people, it is often unrecognised by individuals, family and health-care professionals and consequently there is a tendency not to refer enough older people with mental illness for specialised psychiatric treatment.

12.1 Getting to know the person: Miriam's story

Miriam is a 78-year-old lady who presented to her GP with weight loss and in generally poor condition and admitted to an inadequate diet. Her GP arranged for her to receive Meals on Wheels and when the first meal was delivered it was discovered that Miriam's house was neglected and in disarray and that she was clearly not functioning. As a result, her GP referred her for a specialist mental health assessment during which she was diagnosed with acute major depression. She was treated with antidepressant medication and given personal and social supports until she was able to resume healthy independent living.

- How common do you think this may be in the community?
- What other issues could have been considered on the initial presentation?

FOCUS QUESTIONS

An ageing population means there is an increasing number of older people with both existing and newly emerging mental illness. Miriam's story is a common example of an older person who manages well for a period of time and then can't anymore without support. The RANZCP lists several important points about older people and mental illness:
- Such illnesses include depression, anxiety disorders, schizophrenia and other psychotic illnesses, bipolar disorder, alcohol and substance misuse disorders and dementia.

- The presentation of depression alters with age, but the incidence and prevalence remain significant and similar to early life when all depressive conditions are included.
- A disproportionate number will also have cognitive impairment or dementia, which may present earlier in life, but the prevalence of which increases exponentially with age.
- There are increasing numbers of people for whom the mental health services that are provided for younger people may not be appropriate. So, services specially catering for older people need to be employed.
- Increasing numbers of very old men, who have among the highest risk for suicide, will suicide.
- Increasing numbers of people live in residential aged care facilities, where there are unacceptably high rates of depression and other mental illness with often inadequate treatment, and neglect (Commonwealth of Australia, 2021).
- There are, without action or government intervention, increasing numbers of older people exposed to excessive prescription of psychotropic medications.
- There are increasing numbers of older carers who themselves are at significantly increased risk of depression and excess mortality.

Maintaining mental health is a significant aspect of good overall health in older people. Some people may enter their older years having experienced mental health issues either intermittently or as an enduring issue in their earlier life. Others may experience mental health issues as older people for the first time. Be aware that presentations of mental health issues vary and they are less defined than physical illnesses. Multiple causes of mental health issues involving physical, psychological, social and cultural determinants, either as single factors or as interacting factors, adds a layer of complexity to understanding them. Therefore, especially developed skills are required to assess and care for people with such issues.

Approaches to mental health care delivery

In this section, we cover approaches to the delivery of mental health care and, as you have read in other chapters of this book, the focus is always on the person who is in need of our support.

PERSON-CENTRED RECOVERY-FOCUSED CARE

An approach to care for older people should be recovery focused, person centred and biopsychosocial in nature. Interventions such as talking therapies, supportive care including that from **peer workers**, and attention to physical health, delivered in collaboration with the older person and their family and/or carers, are as important as pharmacological and other physical treatments.

peer workers
People who, through their unique and valuable experiences, harness the lived experience of mental ill-health and recovery to support others and foster hope.

While there is no single definition of recovery, central to recovery paradigms are the promotion of hope, self-determination and management, empowerment and advocacy. Underpinning this is a notion of a 'person's right to full inclusion and to a meaningful life of their choosing, free of stigma and discrimination' (Australian Health Ministers' Advisory Council, 2013, pp. 16–17).

Leamy et al. (2011) developed a conceptual framework for personal recovery in mental health and outlined the recovery process as five categories by using the acronym CHIME. It is described as follows:

- *Connectedness* – incorporating relationships and support from others and support groups as well as peer support and being part of the community

- *Hope* – including optimism about the future. This encompasses belief in the possibility of recovery, motivation to change, hope-inspiring relationships, positive thinking, valuing success and having dreams and aspirations

- *Identity* – important elements of this are rebuilding and redefining a sense of identity and overcoming stigma

- *Meaning* – in life, the experience of mental illness in social roles and goals, spirituality and rebuilding life, and enhancing its quality

- *Empowerment* – with a focus on strengths, personal responsibility and control over life.

Personal recovery is much broader than clinical recovery. While recovery is unique to the individual it is likely to involve some or all the domains of a meaningful life, including the person's values, goals and needs. It can be achieved by genuinely empowering individuals, which includes encouraging real choices by people and engendering hope in the belief that problems are solvable rather than permanent. This is divergent from an 'illness' approach to care where professional expertise takes prominence.

One of the principal domains of the recovery model is a holistic approach, a concept that acknowledges, in human terms, that people are complex and individual beings. Therefore, each needs to be viewed as a whole consisting of interacting parts and address a range of factors. These include social determinants that impact on the well-being and social inclusion of people experiencing mental health issues and their families such as:

- housing
- education
- employment, income and socio-economic hardship
- isolation and geographic distance
- relationships and social connectedness
- personal safety and trauma
- stigma and discrimination (Australian Health Ministers' Advisory Council, 2013, p. 26).

In a contemporary mental health service context, the concept of 'holism' has broadened to embrace the paradigm of recovery approaches to care. This perspective drives practice that seeks solutions in the broadest way, facilitating the range of resources required to achieve resolution of a person's needs through negotiation and collaboration with them.

BIOPSYCHOSOCIAL APPROACH USING A MULTI-DISCIPLINARY TEAM

The most common specialist health professionals providing direct mental health services are psychiatrists, psychologists, social workers, occupational therapists and mental health nurses. Each has specific qualifications that define their scope of practice and orientation to mental health care, bringing discrete perceptions, knowledge, skill and experience. The care of an older person with mental health issues is not necessarily confined to these health professionals as other skills may be required. For example, a physiotherapist, exercise physiologist, speech pathologist, dietician, pharmacist or general practitioner may be needed to provide strategies to overcome the disruptions to normal activities of daily living to which the older person may be vulnerable, thereby enhancing their participation and quality of life; this will ultimately also enhance their mental health. Most importantly in mental health care delivery, there is a growing emphasis on support from persons with lived experience of mental health issues and peer workers, with an increasing formal peer workforce of such workers.

Each clinical presentation must be assessed on the specific needs of the individual concerned, acknowledging physical, social, mental and spiritual health as interdependent factors that maintain good health overall.

Personal stories of mental health presentations and care

In this chapter, personal stories are used to demonstrate the complexity faced when assessing and supporting older people with mental health issues. It is not possible to outline the full spectrum of mental health issues affecting older people, but the two following case studies will help stimulate thinking about principles of care that may be applied across several case examples, as well as encourage exploration beyond issues represented here. Resources are suggested to guide this exploratory process. The case studies offer some insight into the knowledge, assessments and strategies that can be applied by health professionals in their practice.

12.2 Getting to know the person: Keith's story

Keith is a 73-year-old man living alone in a mobile home village in a regional Australian town.

He visits his GP wanting something to help him sleep, which has been a problem for him over the past three months or so. He normally sees his GP for treatment of hypertension, but not regularly, so this visit is unusual.

A couple of years before Keith retired as an accountant, he lost money through some poor investments during the Global Financial Crisis. Soon after he retired (about eight years ago) his wife left him. As a self-funded retiree, he is worried he will soon run out of money and he is also concerned that he may have given his former clients poor financial advice and is fearful they might sue him.

He has been quite involved in a Pentecostal church but has stopped attending, feeling a lack of confidence driving the 20 kilometres to Sunday services. Other church members have offered to come and pick him up, but he feels this would be too much of a burden to them, as they are also older people.

He has two children but not much contact with them as they have criticised him for not looking after his health or preparing properly for retirement and they don't like his repeated attempts urging them to join the church.

About a year ago he had decided to resume work. With his professional background in financial management, and pastoral care in the church, he decided to set up his own business as a life coach and had printed some business cards and advertising material, but this venture was unsuccessful.

He has few friends outside the church, and none live close by, nor does he mix with others in the village. One of his neighbours complained that he has left too much leaf litter on his roof and around his mobile home, and that Keith is causing a fire hazard as the village backs onto a nature reserve. He is not sure if he should get up on his roof to clean it.

On further questioning he feels that his memory is not as good as it used to be. He has trouble concentrating; he does not see much future for himself and feels his life is not worth living. He has not thought about suicide because of his religious beliefs. He lacks energy, his motivation is low and feels he's a failure. His appetite has been poor and while he has lost 5 kilograms over the last six months, he remains obese. He eats a lot of tinned food such as baked beans and soups. Otherwise, his diet is mostly potatoes, biscuits, toast and Weet-Bix. He rarely eats vegetables as 'they go off before I use them'. He drinks one or two glasses of wine each night.

His mother and sister both suffered with some sort of mental disorder, but he does not know many details. His mother was in a psychiatric hospital for eight months towards the end of her life and had electro-convulsive therapy (ECT). She did not fully recover and ended up in an aged care facility. He thinks she might have had post-natal depression earlier in life, but she became reclusive in middle age and rarely went outside the home. He is not too sure about his sister's problems. She's on some medication but she's fairly private. They might see each other every couple of years.

- From Keith's account in this case study, what do you consider are the issues requiring attention in terms of physical, cognitive, emotional and other life issues?

- Can you identify symptoms that may require medical/other health professional assessment and follow-up? What are they and who do you consider may provide the best assistance? Provide a rationale for your response.

- How would you prioritise Keith's issues, focusing on keeping him safe and well?

FOCUS QUESTIONS

Mental health care delivery: a four-stage approach

We will describe mental health care delivery using the case studies of Keith and Emily (discussed later in the chapter) to illustrate each stage. The stages involve engagement, assessment, intervention and evaluation of the care delivered.

STAGE ONE: ENGAGING AND DEVELOPING RAPPORT

In this section, we guide you through the skills you need to develop to build a rapport with older people and engage them in meaningful conversations that focus on recovery.

Access to care

Older adults such as Keith who present to their GP with mental health issues for the first time tend to have a higher level of complexity than younger adults who are making their first presentation. This complexity can confound clinicians in terms of what support can be offered in the short, medium and long term. While treatment for mental health issues generally requires specialist training, there are a few brief and low-risk interventions that can be provided by multidisciplinary health professionals in primary and other health-care settings.

Building a therapeutic alliance

Therapeutic communication skills in the context of a strong therapeutic relationship can support a person to promote their own resourcefulness. While the life experiences of older adults bring complexity to the experience of mental health issues, they can also bring resilience through long-term experience of dealing with life's challenges. These strengths need to be understood and developed through a therapeutic relationship.

Mental health issues are often associated with social stigma and older people may not be used to talking about their emotional experiences. For example, the perceived or conveyed authority of the clinician may discourage Keith from disagreeing with the clinician's understanding of his experiences. The health professional needs to be aware of these social factors and power imbalances and focus on generating a rapport with Keith in a collaborative and trusting relationship that will be essential to facilitate the assessment and treatment processes.

The first stage of developing engagement is to generate a rapport with Keith. Start by:

- explaining your role
- explaining why you are meeting with him
- explaining how you fit into the wider team of people that he has seen or may provide care
- informing him that your encounter with him is confidential but with some limitations – for example, if he discloses that he is at risk of harming himself or someone else, this information may have to be shared to protect him or others
- respecting his dignity and gaining his consent to assess him
- using easy-to-understand language and avoiding using health or medical jargon
- employing active and reflective listening; ask open-ended questions and, when you get stuck, reflect on what has been said to you to show that you understand what is being said and that you are actively listening. Reflective listening acknowledges not only the content of Keith's response but also the emotion or feeling that goes along with it
- validating Keith's feelings – that is, accepting his emotional reaction to his situation without judgment, demonstrating acceptance and encouraging further communication.

EXAMPLE DIALOGUE

Health professional: Hi Keith, it's nice to meet you. My name is David and I'm the mental health nurse. Your GP suggested to check out how you were managing at the moment and if there is some support our service may be able to offer you. Did you have any trouble getting here this morning?

Keith: Well, I haven't been driving much lately so it was a bit stressful not having been here before and not knowing what to expect.

Health professional: I'm glad you were able to make it even though it was stressful for you. Our service helps people sort out and manage any issues they may be having with their mental health, such as things that may be creating some anxiety or unhappiness. Can you tell me what has been happening to you that you may need some help with in understanding better or sorting out?

This question is designed to build rapport by showing interest in Keith, but also to seek information about his concerns as he sees them.

Keith: I went to my GP because I wasn't sleeping well and after talking to him realised there were a number of things I was worried about.

Health professional: So, there were other things than your sleeping problem that were concerning you. What were some of those things?

The nurse starts with topics that provide important information about Keith's context, but are relatively low risk in terms of the stigma surrounding mental health.

- What skills did the health professional use here to generate rapport?
- How was reflective listening and/or validation used in this dialogue?

FOCUS QUESTIONS

STAGE TWO: ASSESSMENT

The following section is significant as it outlines the assessment process, which is essential for determining the issues and then identifying optimal management strategies.

Factors to consider in the initial clinical interview

A mental health assessment is dependent upon building a rapport with the older person using effective and sensitive communication. Principles necessary for building a rapport and establishing a therapeutic relationship are outlined below and supported by examples of dialogue.

Presenting problem

Once an initial rapport is developed and established towards a therapeutic relationship, the health professional should seek information on the presenting problem using open-ended questions – that is, questions that require more than a 'yes' or 'no' answer. Information sought should include:

- the *nature* of the presenting problem
- when the *onset* of issues or symptoms occurred
- the *frequency*, *intensity* and *duration* of the issues or symptoms

- what makes the issues or symptoms *better* or *worse*
- when and *under what circumstances* they are most noticeable.

....

EXAMPLE DIALOGUE

Here are some examples of open-ended questions that a health professional might ask Keith:

'So, Keith, I understand that things have been stressful recently. Please tell me a little more about that.'

'What has your mood been like this last week? Please rate it out of 10, zero being having no stress and 10 being the worst ever. What makes it better or worse?'

'What effect do these issues have on your everyday life?'

'How long have these issues been affecting you in a way you are not happy with?'

....

FOCUS QUESTION
- What is the benefit of using an open-ended question when completing an assessment?

Considering and assessing Keith's issues

Presenting problems may be taken at face value, but consideration also needs to be given to any underlying issues that may inform your assessment more fully, so that you can determine the issues that may require intervention and by whom. These could be symptoms of a pathological process (either physical or psychiatric) or a reaction to other life issues. Table 12.1 outlines the main problems that Keith has identified.

Keith describes feeling 'worried' and there are several things that may be underlying this feeling. He may be experiencing symptoms of anxiety and depression, which are common mental illnesses. The treating team needs to determine what are the main issues, whether there are other processes occurring, such as dementia, and how best to work with him.

However, Keith's experience of depression is different from that of younger adults and, while he may be at lower statistical risk of depression when compared to other age groups, it is important to investigate why he has presented to his GP with symptoms that could be from anxiety and/or depression when this appears to be out of character for him. In addition, Keith's symptoms may be of greater concern for the GP when compared to a younger adult presenting with anxiety, as older adults experience greater functional impairment than younger adults. This means that Keith's anxiety may be more likely to interfere with his quality of life, and his ability to go about his day-to-day life, when compared to younger adults.

FOCUS QUESTION
- For each of the issues in the left-hand column of Table 12.1, write down all the possible underlying causes you can think of that may contribute to that issue in the middle column. Then think about what you may need to ask to either verify or exclude the possible cause to guide your thinking about what additional information you require to complete your assessment (Column 3).

TABLE 12.1 Issues for consideration in assessing Keith's presenting problems

ISSUES DESCRIBED AS PROBLEMS FOR KEITH	WHAT COULD BE THE UNDERLYING CAUSE?	WHAT MORE INFORMATION IS NEEDED TO UNDERSTAND THIS BETTER?
Difficulty in sleeping		
Reluctance to seek help regularly for his health issues		
Concerns about his financial future		
Fearful of repercussions from his past professional life		
Apparent social isolation		
Loss of confidence in driving		
Estranged relationship with his children		
Some difficulty in decision making		
Self-perceived memory deterioration		
Feels life is not worth living		
Lacking in energy and motivation		
Poor appetite		
Poor diet		
Alcohol intake		
Lack of social contact		
Emotionally avoidant and becoming isolative		

Mental health assessment

Assessment is about finding out what health and mental health issues may require some intervention or support. Learning about the person's biographical and health history is important to understand the context of their current health status. It provides an insight into the person's past and present health behaviours and other biopsychosocial, spiritual and cultural factors that influence the way they think about and behave towards their own health (Shea, 2017).

Issues for consideration in a thorough mental health assessment are:

1   Significant background history, including:
  - past psychiatric and medical history
  - family developmental history
  - medications and allergies
  - drug and alcohol use
  - psychosocial issues – for example, living situation and finances

PETER SANTANGELO AND JOHN DOBROHOTOFF

- occurrence of abuse and trauma – considering the person's strengths in dealing with these as well as their negative impact on their life and health.

2   Cognitive functioning:

- Distinguishing dementia from delirium. In contrast to delirium, dementia:

  » is a form of chronic and progressive cognitive impairment occurring over a period of months to years

  » is characterised by a cognitive decline from a previous level of performance in one or more cognitive domains, most commonly including memory impairment

  » can affect a range of abilities, from an inability to perform cognitive functions to impairments that may not necessarily interfere with capacity for independence in everyday activities but may require compensatory strategies, or greater effort, to perform them.

- Distinguishing delirium and dementia from other mental health issues. Symptoms of delirium and dementia that can be mistaken for primary mental health problems include:

  » hallucinations

  » delusions

  » mood disturbances

  » agitation

  » apathy

  » disinhibition

  » sleep disturbances (APA, 2013).

On the other hand, depression and other mental health problems can cause significant impairment that can be mistaken for delirium or dementia. And to further complicate the picture, it is common to have more than one of these conditions present at the same time.

Specific cognitive tests may need to be employed to ascertain the current status of cognitive functioning.

> Dementia is covered more fully in Chapter 13.

12.3 Getting to know the person: Emily's story

Emily is a 67-year-old woman who is well known to her GP. She lives in a retirement village in an outer suburb of a major capital city. She moved there about four months ago after selling the family home following the death of her husband, after a short illness, 18 months ago.

Emily has two daughters and a son. Her son lives nearby, one daughter lives in a regional area about three hours' drive away and her other daughter lives interstate.

Emily has had long-term contact with her local doctor, who has been involved with maintenance treatment with antidepressant medication for her depression spanning the past 25 years. In that time, she has had two admissions to hospital when her depression became disabling to a point where she could not be managed at home: once about 25 years ago and again eight years ago following the death of her parents. Emily was the principal support person for them over the three years prior to their death, which occurred within six months of each other.

Her last admission was of five weeks' duration, in which time she was successfully treated with antidepressant medication – although she was somewhat slow to respond and electro-convulsive therapy (ECT) was considered. However, she slowly improved.

Over the past three months, her son noticed she has become increasingly withdrawn, less active, has lost about five kilograms in weight and was looking rather thin and gaunt. She had not been deliberately dieting but had lost interest in food. When he visited her recently, her son was concerned that she was very low in her mood and expressed thoughts of 'life being worthless' and that there was 'not much point to her existence'. She was also tired during the day as she had been waking each morning at about 3 am and not able to get back to sleep. Her son was alerted, through his experience of his mother's depression, that this indicated a decline in her mental state. He contacted her local doctor, who referred her for assessment with a public health psychiatrist. A diagnosis of a relapse of major depressive disorder was confirmed and a review of, and increase in, her anti-depressant medication was initiated.

Her son agreed to have her stay at his house over the next few weeks to provide support and monitoring of her recovery with an understanding that if her condition deteriorated and required greater levels of supervision, a hospital admission would be arranged. The mental health service also assigned a mental health nurse to visit weekly and monitor her mental state.

- Considering her history and current presentation, how do Emily's current mental health issues differ from Keith's? Cite some examples.
- What are the similarities in their current mental health issues?

FOCUS QUESTIONS

Examining a person's mental state

Assessment of specific mental health issues is made through the mental state examination (MSE). See Table 12.2. Its purpose is to obtain a comprehensive cross-section of the person's mental state at the time of the assessment. Combined with other historical and assessed information, it provides the clinician the opportunity to formulate an informed diagnosis required for coherent treatment planning.

The information is collected using direct and focused questions, observation and interpretation of these data. It is a structured way of observing and describing the person's current state of mind using the domains of their appearance, attitude, behaviour, mood and affect, speech, thought process, thought content, perception, cognition, and insight and judgment. The MSE should not be confused with the Mini-Mental State Examination (see Chapter 13), which is one of many available brief screening tests for dementia.

PETER SANTANGELO AND JOHN DOBROHOTOFF

TABLE 12.2 Mental state examination

Appearance	A person's appearance can provide useful clues about their quality of self-care, lifestyle and daily living skills. A description can include any distinctive features, clothing, grooming and hygiene.
Behaviour and attitude	As well as describing what a person looks like, attention should also be paid to behaviours, described as non-verbal communication, which can reveal much about the person's emotional state and attitude. Indicators include facial expression, body language and gestures, posture, eye contact, response to the assessment itself, rapport and social engagement, level of arousal (calm or agitated), anxious or aggressive behaviour, under- or over-activity and any unusual features such as tremors or slowed, repetitive or involuntary movements. Can the person hear well and attend to the interview? Or are they distracted and drifting off to sleep? Can they sustain their attention and for how long?
Mood and affect	'Affect' refers to immediate expressions of emotions while 'mood' refers to emotional experience over a longer period of time. A common analogy is that of the weather (affect) and the season (mood). Affect can reflect happiness (ecstatic, elevated, lowered, depressed), anxiety or irritability. Affect can be expressed as ranging from being restricted to blunted, flat or expansive. It can also be appropriate, inappropriate or incongruous, and may be stable or labile (fluctuating).
Speech	Speech should be described in terms of its rate, volume, tone, quantity, ease of conversation and how well organised or coherent it is. Does the person stay on topic or frequently switch topics? Is the content of their speech appropriate to the situation? A depressed person may speak softly and slowly or even become mute due to the level of depression. A manic person may speak at a loud or rapid pace that is difficult to interrupt. An anxious person may present excessive detail in an overinclusive manner.
Thought form and process	This refers to the formation of coherent thoughts and is inferred through speech and expression of ideas (relevance, coherence and flow, vagueness, nonsense words, pressured).
Thought content	This includes what is in the person's thinking (delusions, overvalued ideas, preoccupations, depressive thoughts, suicidal or homicidal, obsessions, anxiety, phobias).
Perception	This includes hallucinations, which are perceptual disturbances related to any of the person's five senses, the most common of which are auditory hallucinations. It also includes illusion (the perception of things as different from the usual but accepting that they are not real or perceived differently by others) or dissociative symptoms (derealisation and depersonalisation).
Cognition	This refers to the person's current capacity to process information and is important because it is often sensitive to mental health problems. Its components include: » level of consciousness » orientation to reality (time, place and person) » memory function (short-term memory, and memory for recent and remote information and events) » literacy and arithmetic skills » visuospatial processing (e.g. copying a diagram or drawing a bicycle) » attention and concentration (e.g. counting backwards by sevens from 100) » general knowledge » language (naming objects, following instructions) » ability to deal with abstract concepts (e.g. describing conceptual similarity between two things).
Insight and judgment	Insight involves acknowledgment of a possible mental health problem, understanding potential treatment options and the ability to identify possible pathological events such as hallucinations. 'Judgment' refers to a person's problem-solving ability and can be evaluated by exploring their decision making or posing a practical dilemma for them to resolve.

Source: adapted from House, 2014; Royal Children's Hospital Melbourne, n.d.

FOCUS QUESTIONS

- What domains in the MSE relate to Keith and Emily? List these for each and provide your rationale for this selection.

- Who else would you include in your discussions about the outcome of the assessment?

- When would a reassessment be performed?

Risk of suicide

We need to identify factors that may indicate Keith's or Emily's risk of suicide. Their experience of disruption to their mental health means that they may be at risk of suicide, yet we need to look at individual factors that may increase the risk.

In Australia, suicide rates for males are higher than those for females across all age groups. Although males are more likely to die by suicide, females are more likely to attempt suicide than males and are hospitalised for intentional self-harm twice as frequently (AIHW, 2019).

• What information do Keith and Emily disclose that suggests they may be at risk of suicide? **FOCUS QUESTION**

EXAMPLE DIALOGUE

Health professional: 'How do you see your future?'
Keith: 'Really, I don't see much future for myself.'
Health professional: 'Do you sometimes feel your life is not worth living?'
Keith: 'Well, it's not and I can't see it getting any better.'
Health professional: 'Have you had thoughts of doing away with yourself?'
Keith: 'Sometimes I feel I'd rather kill myself.'
Health professional: 'Have you thought of ways of doing that?'
Keith: 'I guess it's crossed my mind; I think I'd be too chicken to do anything.'

• Do your attitudes and perception influence your willingness to explore self-destructive behaviours in others? For example, what thoughts and feelings do you experience when you think about asking a person about their suicidal thoughts? **FOCUS QUESTION**

To assess Keith's and Emily's current vulnerability to suicidal behaviour, we also need to know if they have a history of suicide attempts. If so, it needs to be determined *what led up to each attempt, whether it was planned, what method was used* and *whether the attempt had been preceded by using drugs or alcohol.*

Protective factors, as well as risk factors, also need to be explored. For example, in terms of support from interpersonal relationships:

• What family or friends are engaged with them?

• Where are their sources of strength? Identify the personal strengths they have displayed in the past that have been effective.

• Who helps them with their activities of daily living?

• Who do they talk to on the phone?

Organisations providing mental health and well-being support include Suicide Prevention Australia, Lifeline and Beyond Blue.

There is also growing evidence that 'safety planning' is an effective suicide preventative strategy that can be employed by professional and non-professional people alike (Stanley et al., 2020; Stanley et al., 2018; Stanley et al., 2016). Beyond Blue and the Zero Suicide Institute of Australasia have some excellent video resources on safety planning.

Interdisciplinary assessment

Both Keith and Emily have been seen by a GP, who needs to decide on whether their assessment and treatment should involve a specialist service. The key determinants of this should be:

- the risk to their personal safety or that of others
- any significant functional impairment and need for specialist diagnosis and intervention
- evidence of a dementia process in the absence of delirium.

Older adults may be seen in a variety of health contexts, and this involves several different specialist mental health professionals who have an interest in understanding their experiences of anxiety and low mood. Each mental health professional may have a view about what has caused an older person's mental health issues, and what treatment is needed, based on their own training in mental health. The team working with them need to work cohesively, deciding what role each team member will take in the assessment and treatment process. Keith and Emily should be informed of who they will meet and when, and what their role is. The information gathered should be shared and discussed as a team and shared with Keith and Emily in a collaborative way that establishes a therapeutic partnership led by them.

It is essential that the health professionals caring for them do not make assumptions that relegate their distinctive experience to that of other older adults that they have seen. Furthermore, the assessment is an opportunity to engage therapeutically with them and destigmatise their experience of mental health issues. Assessment can take place through clinical interviews and other specific assessment measures, being clear about who is coordinating that care so that there is minimal duplication and no gaps in the assessment process.

Specialist assessment: diagnosis of mental disorders

Diagnosis of mental disorders is generally conducted by a psychiatrist or GP. The role of these medical practitioners is to gather a relevant history of symptoms and mental state examination to support the determination of a diagnosis. The assessed symptoms are then used as key points in determining a care plan for intervention.

In Australia, diagnosing mental disorders is guided by recognised systems of classification of diseases, such as:

- *The Diagnostic and Statistical Manual of Mental Disorders*, fifth edition (DSM-5) (APA, 2013)
- the *International Classification of Diseases* (ICD-11) (WHO, 2019).

Classification systems are intended to facilitate an objective assessment of symptom presentations in a variety of clinical settings. They contain diagnostic criteria and codes for a broad range of mental disorders and describe the features of each that distinguishes them from one another. However, there is inevitably some overlap of diagnoses. It reflects the complexity that is ever present in the identification and treatment of mental disorders.

Additional assessment measures

As a team, deciding on the appropriate treatment involves quantifying the level of mental health disorder the person is experiencing. Assessment measures should not be used alone, but rather as an adjunct to clinical interviews with the person. Measures should be appropriate, based on the person's cultural and spiritual background and may need to be read aloud to enable older adult to complete them if they have sensory impairments or literacy skill issues.

- *Depression* – the Geriatric Depression Scale (Yesavage et al., 1983) is a 15-item scale that assesses depression in older adults. It has been validated with older adults in Australasia.

- *Anxiety* – the Geriatric Anxiety Inventory (Pachana et al., 2007) is a 20-item self-reporting measure of anxiety developed for older adults. It has been validated with older adults in Australasia.

- *Cognitive screening* – it is essential that older adults are screened for cognitive functioning prior to generating a treatment plan. This should be undertaken following a discussion with the wider team to ensure the best approach is taken for the person, using the appropriate screening measure. The Addenbrookes Cognitive Examination is a well-validated measure for use in Australia and New Zealand (Strauss et al., 2012).

Psychiatric comorbidity

Anxiety and depression often coexist. Even when older people present with prominent anxiety symptoms, it can be that they are experiencing an underlying depressive disorder. It is not always straightforward, and attention needs to be paid to understanding the individual's experience of their problems and how they are manifested and dealt with emotionally.

Table 12.3 links Keith's and Emily's issues with those identified in the DSM-5 as being symptoms of anxiety and depressive disorders.

TABLE 12.3 Summary of characteristics of anxiety and depression in relation to Keith's and Emily's presentation and history

CHARACTERISTICS OF ANXIETY AND DEPRESSION	KEITH'S SYMPTOMS FROM CASE STUDY	EMILY'S SYMPTOMS FROM CASE STUDY	DSM-5 SYMPTOMS OF GENERALISED ANXIETY DISORDER	DSM-5 SYMPTOMS OF MAJOR DEPRESSIVE DISORDER
Cognitive (thoughts)	» Complaints of memory loss » Rumination » Thoughts of suicide » Worry about finances, health, family, driving	Expressed thoughts of 'life being worthless' and that there was 'not much point to [her] existence'	» Excessive anxiety and worry about a range of events or activities » Difficulty concentrating or mind going blank	» Feelings of worthlessness or excessive or inappropriate guilt » Diminished ability to think or concentrate » Recurrent thoughts of death (not just fear of dying), recurrent suicidal ideation, suicide attempt or plan to commit suicide
Behaviour	» Avoiding driving » Lying awake at night » Unable to complete plans » Social withdrawal	» Increasingly withdrawn » Less active » Tired during the day	» Sleep disturbances (difficulty falling asleep or returning to sleep when waking up) » Restlessness or feeling keyed up or on edge	» Appears tearful » Insomnia or hypersomnia » Psychomotor agitation or retardation nearly every day

(Continued)

TABLE 12.3 Continued

CHARACTERISTICS OF ANXIETY AND DEPRESSION	KEITH'S SYMPTOMS FROM CASE STUDY	EMILY'S SYMPTOMS FROM CASE STUDY	DSM-5 SYMPTOMS OF GENERALISED ANXIETY DISORDER	DSM-5 SYMPTOMS OF MAJOR DEPRESSIVE DISORDER
Emotions	Distressed and perplexed, particularly in situations where he does not feel in control	Very low in mood	» Excessive anxiety » Irritability	» Depressed mood most of the day, nearly every day (sad, empty, hopeless) » Diminished interest or pleasure in all, or almost all, activities most of the day, nearly every day
Physiological sensations	Lack of energy	» Lost 5 kilograms in weight » Looking rather thin and gaunt » Lost interest in food » Waking each morning at about 3 am and not able to get back to sleep	» Muscle tension » Easily fatigued	» Significant weight loss when not dieting, or weight gain (5% within a month), or decrease or increase in appetite nearly every day » Fatigue or loss of energy nearly every day

Factors contributing to anxiety and depression in older adults

Considering Keith's and Emily's stories, imagine what life was like for them in their younger years and contrast that to now and the significant physical, emotional, cognitive, social and financial changes since that time. These changes may positively or negatively affect their self-esteem, depending on how they interpret their meaning for themselves and their future.

Cohort factors

The generation in which older adults were born contained different sociohistorical and cultural contexts, and this in turn shapes their personality, cognitive abilities, ways of being in the world and, ultimately, their experiences of mental illness (Knight & Poon, 2008). Keith's generational experiences have shaped his world view. His involvement with the church, for example, may influence his whole philosophy on life and the change that he feels is within his power to change. For Emily, the loss of both her parents and husband may confront her with issues around her own mortality.

Loss of identity

Keith was a successful financial provider for his family, and he is from a generation where 'being a man' means to work, to provide practical support for the family, and to be strong both physically and emotionally. A large part of Keith's identity developed through his professional career and involvement with the church, and his current lack of engagement in these are two major areas of loss for him. His third area of importance is being part of his family – the loss of a lifetime partner through divorce and the loss of contact with his children.

Emily's long-term experience with significant mental health issues and the stigma surrounding that may well influence how she sees herself as a capable and contributing person. The health professional needs to understand how people reconcile these situations, ask them what their current role is and consider how this can be enhanced.

Cognitive experiences

Older adults have a number of processes that affect their cognitive experiences of anxiety and depression. In the absence of dementia, intelligence, as it relates to acquired knowledge (crystallised intelligence), only shows a mild decline because of ageing (Salthouse, 2004). Knight and Poon (2008) suggested that clinicians working with older adults can capitalise on their wealth of life experience to help them in embracing changes in life and solve problems.

On the other hand, normal ageing also brings a significantly slower ability to process information (processing speed), as well as difficulty remembering information and processing it to produce a result (working memory) (Salthouse, 2004). Furthermore, older adults have difficulty screening out non-important information or distractions to enable them to focus on essential information (selective attention) (Knight & Poon, 2008). This means that older adults may have difficulty following complex verbal information in the presence of background noise.

Emotional experiences

Older adults experience a greater complexity of emotions compared to younger adults. However, their ability to recognise and respond to these may be impaired by their tendency to suppress negative emotions (Ready et al., 2008) and 'get on with things'. So, it should not be assumed that older people understand mental health issues in the same way as younger people.

Stoicism

Older adults experience a high level of stigma when discussing issues relating to mental health. Older adults in today's world lived through periods of time where institutionalisation for mental illnesses was common, and mental illness was experienced as shameful and not talked about. Furthermore, emotional experiences were not readily talked about, and pushed aside to 'get on with things'. Considering this, older adults may readily identify *others* as experiencing problems with anxiety and depression, but strongly deny that possibility for themselves. Older people may have less knowledge of mental illness compared to younger people, and consequently experience greater shame and stigmatisation (Knight & Poon, 2008). A gentle approach that seeks to understand experiences and not label them as 'anxiety' or 'depression' is likely to yield more information and develop a stronger rapport than a direct approach in the initial stages of assessment.

> Read more about the significance of culture to mental health in Chapters 3 and 6.

Learn more
Watch Video 6.1: Preet discusses how feeling cut off from her culture has affected her mental health.

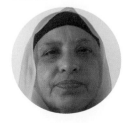

Culture

Both Keith and Emily are from a Western culture and so are likely to view the mind and body as separate, and that the person is separate from their social and spiritual contexts (Knight & Poon, 2008). This is in contrast to people whose culture and history is integral to identity, such as First Nations peoples. It is therefore essential that we ask and listen to Keith, Emily and any other older person we are assessing – that is, what they understand about the origins of their anxiety and depression, which includes the meaning of culture and the impact of their cultural history – and match this to their treatment and to their needs.

Manifestations of anxiety

As people get older, it may be expected that they will worry somewhat about health, finances and family. However, what people worry about is less important than *how* they worry. For example, is worry persistent and pervasive and perceived as out of their control? Worry that interferes with daily life and is perceived as uncontrollable is more problematic than worry that is channelled into productive activities that can allow the person to function in their activities of daily living. Keith's and Emily's topics of worry are unique to their life situation and are unlikely to be the same as those of their older adult friends and acquaintances.

Therefore, knowing the effect that the worry has on the person (e.g. loss of sleep, or withdrawal from or restriction of social activities) is much more important than focusing on each worry individually and trying to reassure the person.

FOCUS QUESTIONS

- What are some problems you may encounter when assessing and offering treatment to an older adult who is highly anxious or depressed?
- How do you begin to engage with a person of a different generation from you?
- How might physiological changes manifest as other issues?
- What can you look for or enquire about when attempting to understand the underlying emotions of a person?
- How can your language reflect sensitivity and respect for people who may have difficulty identifying with certain health issues?
- How can you go about understanding the specific culture and spirituality of a person and the impact that these have on their thinking and beliefs?
- What issues do you need to consider in order to see the distinctive and individual meaning behind a person's symptoms or behaviour?

STAGE THREE: INTERVENTIONS AND COLLABORATIVE CARE PLANNING

The following section explains evidence-based interventions that support older people experiencing mental health challenges. It also articulates the significance of teams working together to provide optimal support.

Generic interventions

Following a collaborative assessment with Keith and Emily, we should reflect to them what we consider to be the primary issues, and check if these also match their understanding. This is the starting point for negotiating some mutually agreed goals.

Goal setting

Identify what the person wants help with. It is very easy to see opportunities to help a person by imposing our perceptions and ideas on them, rather than facilitating them finding their own way. For example, Keith is keen to establish some meaningful work for himself and the clinician seeing him may feel that he would benefit from directing his efforts towards what he is familiar with – that is, work in the financial management area. However, if that is not Keith's goal, and he is more frustrated with his lack of sleep, we should negotiate starting with sleep and perhaps offer to help him with his future work goals but move on if it is not in his plan. It is important not to move forward until you have a clear picture that the person is invested in and take ownership of the proposed goals.

- What is likely to happen if a person agrees to a goal that they are not invested in?

- Think about a time when someone you knew well thought they were helping you by suggesting to you what they thought was a good idea, but not what you wanted to do. What happened? How did you feel? How can you generalise this in relation to Keith or Emily?

FOCUS QUESTIONS

SMART goal setting

A guide to successful goal setting is the SMART goals (Doran, 1981). They are:

- *Specific* – target a specific area for improvement.

- *Measurable* – how will I know if I have progressed?

- *Achievable* – is this a goal that can be attained?

- *Realistic* – is this appropriate and achievable given the resources I have?

- *Time-bound* – when can I expect to know if I have achieved my goal? When do I hope to have this done?

Psychoeducation

As the name suggests, psychoeducation is about providing information to the person regarding the mental health issues they are experiencing from what is known about them from a professional and health perspective. Such information includes what is known about the cause and course of such issues and what can be expected in terms of treatment and recovery. The health professional needs to bear in mind that such information is generic in nature – that is, it's based on evidence from a number of case studies or research. However, for information to be useful to the person, it needs to be relayed in a way that is targeted to their individual experience of these mental health issues and the specific impact on them and their lives. Jargon terms should be avoided and, instead, cues from the person about their experience, using their terms for such issues, is preferable.

In Keith's case, this involves describing the nature of his issues as coming from his life issues and as being expressed via depression and anxiety. It provides him with information about what he can expect and what he can do to help himself as well as what other help may be available from professional or other services. Part of psychoeducation includes the way he is using alcohol – for example, how it may be helpful in the short term, but that there are long-term consequences. He also needs information about the role alcohol plays in his wakefulness and subsequent fatigue.

> Consider the concept of health coaching, discussed in Chapter 18, and the importance of family and support people, covered in Chapter 5.

For Emily, information about the effects of medication on symptoms of depression can convey confidence in her eventual recovery and help monitor improvements along the way for her and her family. Similarly, encouraging a healthy diet and some moderate exercise provides other ways of improving her overall health.

Care must be taken in providing psychoeducation in a non-judgmental manner and always collaboratively with the older person and their significant partner or other supports. The focus, in providing information, is to enhance healthy choices for recovery.

Specific interdisciplinary intervention for mental health issues

Before moving into any treatment regimen for older adults, it is essential that there is a clear understanding of the problem, what causes it and what keeps it going. Moving too quickly into treatment without this understanding may arrest the patient's therapeutic progress and result in reassessment.

Table 12.4 outlines interventions for the mental health issues we have discussed.

TABLE 12.4 Interventions for anxiety and depression

BRIEF ANXIETY TREATMENTS	BRIEF DEPRESSION TREATMENTS
» Sleep hygiene » Relaxation » Problem solving (if solvable) » Distraction (use sparingly) » Medication	» Sleep hygiene » Behavioural activation » Re-engagement in activities previously enjoyed » Activity scheduling » Problem solving » Distraction (use sparingly) » Medication

The following points of discussion expand on these interventions.

Medication

Read more about medications in Chapter 14.

Older adults have a different physiological make-up from younger adults. Considering this, it is reasonable to expect that older adults may have a different response to medications compared to younger adults. Psychoactive medications should be used sparingly and titrated very slowly, with careful monitoring of side effects and adverse effects. Medication should be used cautiously and be provided alongside behavioural and psychosocial interventions.

Behavioural interventions

Encourage the older person to engage in activities that provide a sense of accomplishment or have previously been enjoyable. These must be small enough steps that the person can achieve them and get a sense of progression.

Keith appears to be experiencing difficulties with initiating activities and is overwhelmed at the prospect of attending activities that he used to enjoy. We should explore with Keith what gets in the way. It is likely that he looks at the activity in its entirety as being overwhelming, and then feels deterred from starting. However, if the activity is broken down into a series of tasks, these are individual problems that can be solved through achievable smaller steps. So, for Keith, who may want to secure some more certain income for himself into the future, individual steps could include planning a budget of what income he may need, exploring job advertisements that may suit his needs and temperament, and working out a back-up plan in case his attempts to secure work are not successful, being mindful that these need to be done at his own pace and within his capacity.

EXAMPLE DIALOGUE

Here are some examples of questions a health professional might ask Keith:

- 'What have you stopped doing that you used to like?'

- 'What do you enjoy doing?'

Activity scheduling

Encourage the person to prepare a daily and weekly schedule of activities as this will give them something regular that they can look forward to, and help them experience enjoyment from both the activity and the anticipation. Again, it is important to match the level of detail and planning with their ability. For example, Emily could schedule regular visits from her daughter, or participate in shopping or other family activities. Writing this in a calendar enables her to see what is coming up and problem-solve any issues that may arise.

Emotional interventions

Emotional interventions involve supporting the older person while they are learning to tolerate feelings of sadness and anxiety and learning that these come and go. Mental health education should *normalise* the experience of anxiety as being part of life, and make it an important function in enabling the older person to be ready to cope with potentially negative or dangerous events. Sadness is a natural response to something that we perceive as uncontrollable, or a loss, or personal setback. It signals a reduction in activity so that mourning can take place and resources can be gathered and has a social cue eliciting help from others. Anxiety and depression become problematic when these emotions become overwhelming, intense and at times crippling. Talking therapies such as counselling and psychotherapy are indicated here.

Cognitive interventions

Cognitive behavioural therapy (CBT) is an evidence-based treatment for a range of mental illnesses including depression and anxiety. The underlying premise of CBT is that mental illness originates from a combination of biological and psychological factors. Psychological factors include irrational thoughts and beliefs. Therapeutic change comes from modifying thoughts and behaviours to change or alleviate emotions (Beck, 2011). CBT must be delivered by clinicians who have specialised training in CBT and mental health.

Problem solving is a structured method of assisting a person to independently resolve any number of issues that may arise. This differs from CBT as it does not require specialist training and is unlikely to interfere with psychotherapeutic interventions. Problem solving is a constructive thought process that focuses on how to effectively deal with a problem at hand, identifying the problem clearly and then evaluating possible solutions, and developing a plan of action.

Worry involves imagining the worst-case scenario and thinking about all the possible problems. People often mistakenly believe that when they are worrying, they are problem solving. For example, 'My phone bill is due, and I don't know how I can pay it' is a solvable problem, even though it may be causing anxiety, whereas 'I might be in a car accident' is a worry that cannot be problem solved, and distraction techniques should be used.

Problem solving involves four basic steps:

1 *Defining the problem* – ensure the problem is specific and clear.

2 *Generating alternatives* – identify all the possible solutions to the problem.

3 *Evaluating and selecting alternatives* – the health professional would discuss with the person which are the better options and help them to weigh up the relative merits of each. Further investigation may be needed to clarify the options available.

4 *Implementing solutions* – the person chooses the best option and then goes about acting it out.

The goal here is to help the person and their family learn the process of problem solving and become proficient at it, *not* to make them rely on the health professional to coach them each time.

STAGE FOUR: EVALUATING THE EFFECTIVENESS OF THE INTERVENTION

Recording the goals and interventions that have been agreed on accurately and specifically is crucial in evaluating their effectiveness. The clearer these are understood by both the health professional and the person they are working with, the greater the chance of their achievement.

This requires the health professional to continually check with the person whether the agreed strategies are progressing as intended or expected, and if so, what factors have contributed to that and how to proceed for further improvement. If not, then a review of where they have been ineffective can be discussed and alternative strategies employed if necessary. The aim is to foster a collaborative approach that identifies health-enhancing goals to which both the health professional and the person contribute. Encouraging as equal as possible input from both parties is helpful in balancing the dialogue and facilitating a sense of mutual respect.

For example, at each visit, ask Emily what she feels has gone well that week, and what has not. Ask her to rate her mood from 0 to 10, and what she thinks needs to happen to move her closer to a better score. For example, ask, 'What would it take to move you from a 5 to a 6?' The use of a validated measure such as the Outcome Rating Scale (ORS) (Miller et al., 2003) can be a simple and meaningful way for the clinician and Emily to evaluate her progress across several domains, including interpersonal, social, personal and overall well-being.

Learn more
Access additional resources – such as weblinks, further readings and podcasts – to broaden your understanding of this chapter. See the Guided Tour for access details.

Conclusion

Understanding and dealing with mental health issues can be complex and challenging. Unlike physical conditions, they are more difficult to define diagnostically and very rarely involve a single treatment. Because causes of disruption to a person's mental health are multifactorial, any intervention requires a diverse range of skills and professional perspectives. Therefore, the principles of person-centred care and collaborative partnerships with service users and their carers, incorporating notions of recovery and holistic care, become extremely important.

It can be argued that ageing can make the process of maintaining mental health in older adults challenging. Keith's and Emily's stories have attempted to illustrate these complexities and challenges in a manner that can assist you, as a health professional, to explore common aspects that need to be confronted to provide the most appropriate, respectful and healing care possible. Their stories explore only a narrow example of mental health disorders, but they outline some generic considerations in assessment and intervention that can facilitate understanding and insight into other presentations of mental health issues.

This chapter should not be read in isolation. Mental health is interactive and interdependent with the other aspects of caring for older people's health as outlined in other chapters of this book.

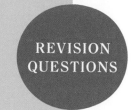

REVISION QUESTIONS

1   Discuss how older age can influence mental health. Consider the physical, social, spiritual and cultural aspects of ageing.

2   Outline the skills required by a health professional to determine what mental health issues require specialist intervention.

3   Identify the skills you already have and those you need to develop to interact with and assess an older person with compromised mental health.

REFERENCES

Amare, A. T., Caughey, G. E., Whitehead, C., Lang, C.E., Bray, S. C., Corlis, M., Visvanathan, R., Wesselingh, S. & Inacia, M. C. (2020). The prevalence, trends and determinants of mental health disorders in older Australians living in permanent residential aged care: Implications for policy and quality of aged care services. *Australian & New Zealand Journal of Psychiatry, 54*(12).

American Psychiatric Association (APA) (2013). *Diagnostic and Statistical Manual of Mental Disorders* (5th edn). American Psychiatric Publishing.

Australian Health Ministers' Advisory Council (2013). A National Framework for Recovery-Oriented Mental Health Services: Policy and Theory. Commonwealth of Australia.

Australian Institute of Health and Welfare (AIHW) (2018). Older Australia at a Glance. www.aihw.gov.au/reports/older-people/older-australia-at-a-glance/contents/service-use/mental-health

Australian Institute of Health and Welfare (AIHW) (2019). Suicide and Self-Harm Monitoring. www.aihw.gov.au/suicide-self-harm-monitoring/data/deaths-by-suicide-in-australia/suicide-deaths-over-time

Beck, J. S. (2011). *Cognitive Behavior Therapy: Basics and Beyond*. Guilford Press.

Commonwealth of Australia (2021). Royal Commission into Aged Care Quality and Safety. Final report: Care, dignity and respect. Vol. 1, Summary and recommendations. https://agedcare.royalcommission.gov.au/sites/default/files/2021-03/final-report-volume-1_0.pdf

Doran, G.,T. (1981). There's a S.M.A.R.T. way to write management's goals and objectives. *Management Review, 70*(11), 35–6.

House, R. M. (2014). The Mental Status Examination. www.brown.edu/Courses/BI_278/Other/Clerkship/Didactics/Readings/THE%20MENTAL%20STATUS%20EXAMINATION.pdf

Knight, B. G. & Poon, C. Y. M. (2008). The socio-cultural context in understanding older adults: Contextual adult lifespan theory for adapting psychotherapy. In R. Woods & L. Clare (eds). *Handbook of the Clinical Psychology of Ageing*. Wiley, pp. 439–56.

Leamy, M., Bird, V., Le Boutillier, C., Williams, J. & Slade, M. (2011). Conceptual framework for personal recovery in mental health: Systematic review and narrative synthesis. *The British Journal of Psychiatry, 199*, 445–52. https://doi:101192/bjp.bp.110.083733

Miller, S. D., Duncan, B., Brown, J., Sparks, J. & Claud, D. (2003). The outcome rating scale: A preliminary study of the reliability, validity, and feasibility of a brief visual analog measure. *Journal of Brief Therapy, 2*(2), 91–100.

National Ageing Research Institute (NARI) (2009). Depression in Older Age: A Scoping Study. Final Report, September. www.beyondblue.org.au/docs/default-source/research-project-files/bw0143---nari-2009-full-report---minus-appendices.pdf?sfvrsn=1f53b1e9_4

Pachana, N., A., Byrne, G., J., Siddle, H., Koloski, N., Harley, E. & Arnold, E. (2007). Development and validation of the Geriatric Anxiety Inventory. *International Psychogeriatrics, 19*(1), 103–114. https://doi:10.1017/S1041610206003504

Ready, R., E., Carvalho, J., O. & Weinberger, M., I. (2008). Emotional complexity in younger, midlife, and older adults. *Psychology and Aging, 23*(4), 928–33. https://doi:10.1037/a0014003

Royal Australian and New Zealand College of Psychiatrists (RANZCP) (2015). Psychiatry Services for Older People: A Report on Current Issues and Evidence. www.ranzcp.org/files/resources/reports/psychiatry-services-for-older-people.aspx

Royal Children's Hospital Melbourne. (n.d.) *Mental State Examination*. www.rch.org.au/clinicalguide/guideline_index/Mental_State_Examination

Salthouse, T. A. (2004). What and when of cognitive aging. *Current Directions in Psychological Science, 13*(4), 140–4.

Shea, S. (2017). *Psychiatric Interviewing: The Art of Understanding: A Practical Guide for Psychiatrists, Psychologists, Counsellors, Social Workers, Nurses and other Mental Health Professionals* (3rd edn). Elsevier.

Stanley, B., Brown, G. K., Brenner, L. A., Galfalvy, H. C., Currier, G. W., Knox, K. L., Chaudhury, S. R., Bush, A. L. & Green, K. L. (2018). Comparison of the safety planning intervention with follow-up vs usual care of suicidal patients treated in the emergency department. *JAMA Psychiatry, 75*(9).

Stanley, B., Chaudhury, S. R., Chesin, M., Pontoski, K., Mahler Bush, A., Knox, K. L. & Brown, G. K. (2016). An emergency department intervention and follow-up to reduce suicide risk in the VA: Acceptability and effectiveness. *Psychiatric Services, 67*(6).

Stanley, I. H., Hom, M. A., Sachs-Ericsson, N. J., Gallyer, A. J. & Joiner, T. E. (2020). Pilot randomized clinical trial of a lethal means safety intervention for young adults with firearm familiarity at risk for suicide. *Journal of Consulting and Clinical Psychology, 88*(4), 372–83. http://dx.doi.org/10.1037/ccp0000481

Strauss, H., M., Leathem, J., Humphries, S. & Podd, J. (2012). The use of brief screening instruments for age-related cognitive impairment in New Zealand. *New Zealand Journal of Psychology, 41*(2), 11–20.

Sunderland, M., Anderson, T. M., Sachdev, P. S., Titov, N. & Andrews, G. (2015). Lifetime and current prevalence of common DSM-IV mental disorders, their demographic correlates, and association with service utilisation and disability in older Australian adults. *Australian and New Zealand Journal of Psychiatry, 49*(2), 145–55.

World Health Organization (WHO) (2013). *Mental Health Action Plan 2013–2020*. www.who.int/publications/i/item/9789241506021

World Health Organization (WHO) (2017). Mental Health of Older Adults. www.who.int/news-room/fact-sheets/detail/mental-health-of-older-adults

World Health Organization (WHO) (2019). International Classification of Diseases and Related Health Problems (ICD-11). www.who.int/standards/classifications/classification-of-diseases

Yesavage, J. A., Brink, T., Rose, T. L., Lum, O., Huang, V., Adey, M. & Leirer, V. O. (1983). Development and validation of a geriatric depression screening scale: A preliminary report. *Journal of Psychiatric Research, 17*(1), 37–49.

13 Dementia

MARGUERITE BRAMBLE AND KATHRYN LITTLE

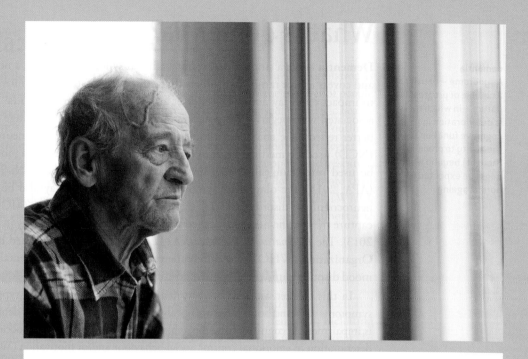

LEARNING OBJECTIVES

After reading this chapter, you will:

» differentiate between the various types of dementia, and the associated physiological, cognitive and behavioural changes

» discuss the latest evidence associated with the dementia spectrum, risk factors, differential diagnosis and best practice care

» consider the major aspects of holistic assessment and person-centred care for a person with dementia in collaboration with their family

» articulate the psychosocial benefits of innovative approaches to dementia care, such as artistic and creative initiatives

» reflect on dementia within the framework of spirituality, palliative care and end-of-life care.

OLDER PEOPLE FROM CULTURALLY AND LINGUISTICALLY DIVERSE BACKGROUNDS (CALD)

In Australia, one in three older people are from culturally and linguistically diverse (CALD) backgrounds (AIHW, 2018). Statistics regarding dementia and prevalence in CALD populations is sparse in Australia and research underpinning this data has been found to under-represent persons from a CALD background (Goeman et al., 2016; Low et al., 2019), meaning that results may not be indicative of the true nature of the dementia spectrum in this population.

One study examining dementia incidence and support among CALD populations in Australia reports significant barriers in accessing health-care services (Goeman et al., 2016). Several of these are language, navigation of the health-care service systems and limited culture-specific services and supports. Previously, there have been limited appropriate assessment tools that can hamper early diagnosis and implementation of health-care support for First Nations peoples and CALD communities.

In recent years, several organisations have recognised these barriers, with many resources developed to improve and educate health professionals, carers, and individuals diagnosed with dementia. The National Ageing Research Institute (NARI) has conducted a review of current practice and guidelines in dementia assessment services for CALD clients and has included several tip sheets specifically designed for individuals from CALD backgrounds. Identification of modified assessment tools and culturally appropriate resources are included with a modified Kimberley Indigenous Cognitive Assessment tool for regional and urban areas (KICA-COG) (NARI, 2020). The Rowland Universal Dementia Assessment Scale (RUDAS) is another screening tool that was designed to reduce differences in cultural learning and language when conducting cognitive screening (see Table 13.3 later in this chapter for a summary of screening tools for dementia).

The role of primary health services in dementia care

Primary healthcare has a vital role in providing dementia care and education in communities across Australia. Dementia-friendly communities can address the stigma associated with the condition, and timely diagnosis enables individuals to plan for their future, access services for support to remain in their homes, if desired, and build a care plan with health-care providers that gives them information and choices. However, as described by the Australian National Framework for Action on Dementia (2015–2019), under-diagnosis and under-disclosure of dementia in Australia is widespread with around 50 per cent of cases of early dementia not detected on initial contact with primary health providers (Australian Government Department of Health, 2014). These figures give rise to the need for multidisciplinary approaches to best-practice dementia education, recognition and care, and a focus on the individual's unique experience of cognitive change seen within the context of delivering person-centred, integrated care (see the section later in this chapter, 'Best-practice dementia care').

In 2016, the Australian Government developed the Aged Care Roadmap to support people with different needs and dementia (Aged Care Sector Committee, 2016). The aim of the roadmap is to promote evidence-based dementia care with a consumer-directed care philosophy. In its interim report, the Royal Commission identified gaps in specified targets to improve data on dementia diagnosis, with less than 50 per cent of the Organisation for Economic Cooperation and Development (OECD) countries having a rate of recorded dementia diagnosis (OECD, 2018).

13.2 Getting to know the person: Rose's story

Catherine, who lives close by, visits Rose regularly but is disheartened by her mother's obvious sadness, loss of appetite and physical decline. Despite John's death five years previously, Rose appears to still be mourning and has lost interest in both her physical appearance and the activities she so loved. Despite protestations from Rose, Catherine decides it is time for her to visit her GP the next week. During that week, Catherine visits daily and notices several changes in Rose, including some forgetfulness, lack of motivation to take care of herself and occasional outbursts of anger.

- What might be the causes of Rose's lack of motivation, forgetfulness and occasional bursts of anger?
- What reasons could there be for Rose's sadness, loss of appetite and physical decline?

FOCUS QUESTIONS

The dementia spectrum

The dementia spectrum covers a range of disorders, with up to 100 types now identified. The four main dementia types – Alzheimer's disease, vascular dementia, Lewy body dementia and frontotemporal dementia – account for around 90 per cent of those diagnosed. Alzheimer's disease and vascular dementia are the two most common types, and frequently present together (Power et al., 2018). Frontotemporal dementia and Lewy body dementia are the next most common types. Differentiating between the physiological changes in the brain due to the ageing process and those associated with individual disorders can be difficult for health professionals (Power et al., 2018). Although terminology and classification updates for neurocognitive disorders have given clarity to differences and diagnoses of the many dementia types, the difficulty remains in the prediction of symptoms, the order in which they present and the rate of progression between individuals (Public Health Agency of Canada, 2019). Figure 13.1 provides an overview of dementia types and global prevalence.

Variables associated with genetics, lifestyle choices, life experiences, education levels, comorbidities and environmental factors all coexist to individually define each person's unique experience with dementia. The pathology of dementia may be present years or decades before its clinical presentation, so acknowledgment of signs of cognitive decline can inform our understanding of pre-clinical dementia and prevention (Irwin et al., 2018). Furthermore, the pathology of dementia can be present in older people with normal cognitive function

FIGURE 13.1 Overview of dementia types

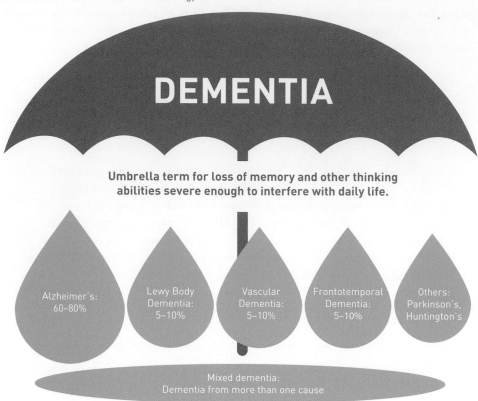

Source: Alzheimer's Association, 2020.

with the presence of plaques and tangles normally attributable to Alzheimer's disease only evident at post mortem (Fillit et al., 2017, p. 542).

Current evidence suggests that a traditional approach of 'ruling out' or excluding dementia disorders in the quest for a diagnosis can impinge on the person's functional abilities and quality of life (Fillit et al., 2017). This will be discussed further in the section 'Best-practice dementia care'.

Table 13.1 lists the major types of dementia, their prevalence, pathology and basic manifestations. The purpose of the table is to present an overview of each dementia type's prevalence, sub-types, pathophysiology and progression. Each major dementia type is also discussed in more detail in the following sections.

TABLE 13.1 Overview of dementia types

TYPE OF DEMENTIA	SUB-TYPES	SIGNS AND SYMPTOMS OVERVIEW	LINKS AND PROGRESSION
Alzheimer's dementia (AD)	Sporadic Most common (after 65 years) Familial (onset in 40s to 50s)	Cascade of Processes: deposits inside and outside brain cells causing cell death and brain shrinkage	80% of people with AD will have VD pathologies too Symptoms and progression vary with individuals (3–20-year span)

TABLE 13.1 Continued

TYPE OF DEMENTIA	SUB-TYPES	SIGNS AND SYMPTOMS OVERVIEW	LINKS AND PROGRESSION
Vascular dementia (VD)	Post-stroke Multi-infarct (most common) Subcortical (Binswanger's disease) Ischemic Can embrace many syndromes	Non-cognitive symptoms: depression, anxiety, psychosis Less memory deficit, but higher executive function deficit and depression than AD	May be preventable Variable disease progression, rapid onset or gradual Normally more rapid decline than AD
Lewy body dementia (LBD)	Collections of proteins that develop inside nerve cells	Fluctuating cognition Gait disturbance Bradykinesia and Rigidity Visual hallucinations	Linked to Parkinson's disease Dangerous sensitivity to neuroleptic meds Progression can be more rapid than Alzheimer's disease
Frontotemporal lobar dementia (FTLD)	Behavioural variant (bvFTD) Primary Progressive Aphasia (PPA): semantic variant and non-fluent/ agrammatic variant	Personality and behaviour changes Isolated and severe progressive language impairment	Strong genetic component, also included in younger onset dementia syndromes
Mixed dementias	More than one type of dementia is present Diagnosis on autopsy, individual pathologies (Power et al., 2018)	Abnormal brain changes linked to a combination of plaque deposits, blood vessel damage and Lewy body dementia	Approximate number of cases unknown and prognosis not determined
Young-onset dementia	Can include AD or FTLD Can result from traumatic brain injuries	Personality changes Difficulty undertaking previously familiar tasks Unable to competently fulfill employment responsibilities	Family history Brain trauma – accidents and sporting related Rapid deterioration Unemployment Socioeconomic issues for the family Impacts on children and partner
Parkinson's disease dementia (PDD)	Results from the loss of dopamine in the brain (involved in the control of voluntary movements)	Impairments in attention, executive function and visuospatial function Language well preserved	Insidious onset Variable progression rates
Alcohol-related dementia	Wernicke's encephalopathy Korsakoff's syndrome Wernicke-Korsakoff syndrome Alcoholic dementia	Caused by a combination toxic effect of alcohol on nerve cells, vitamin B1 deficiency and head injury	Wernicke's: sudden onset Korsakoff's: gradual onset
Huntington's disease dementia	Inherited disorder caused by defective gene Characterised by twisting or jerking movements	Caused by single defective gene on chromosome 4 Dominant trait	Progressive disease that is eventually accompanied by dementia
Creutzfeldt-Jakob disease (CJD) dementia	Sporadic CJD Hereditary CJD Acquired CJD	Known as transmissible spongiform encephalopathies (TSE) Caused by prion diseases Causes 'sponge-like' holes in brain tissue	Rapidly progressive (1 year) Similar symptoms to AD and Huntington's, but unique brain changes seen only on autopsy

Source: compiled from Fillit et al., 2017; Alzheimer's Association, 2020.

MARGUERITE BRAMBLE AND KATHRYN LITTLE

Types of dementia

Dementia is an umbrella term for several diseases that are mostly progressive, affect cognitive abilities and behaviour, and interfere significantly with a person's ability to maintain activities of daily living.

ALZHEIMER'S DEMENTIA (AD)

Alzheimer's disease accounts for approximately 80 per cent of neurocognitive disorders, and age is the greatest risk factor (Dementia Australia, 2020c). It is a progressive disease with two main neurological pathologies. The first is comprised of extracellular deposits of a protein called beta-amyloid – or A-beta – that clump together to form amyloid plaques, which prevent signals from being transferred between neurons in the brain, eventually leading to nerve cell death. Amyloid plaque deposits begin a cascade of pathophysiological processes that cause inflammation, alter homeostasis and result in nerve-cell damage and synaptic loss (Fillit et al., 2017). The second pathology involves protein tangles called tau, or neurofibrillary tangles. The tau proteins' normal function is to provide a base for materials to be transported to brain cells to maintain life. Abnormalities occur when the proteins collapse and twist, forming tangles that stop vital nutrients and energy reaching cells and causing cell death. It is currently estimated that 5 per cent of all cases have younger onset Alzheimer's disease (Dementia Australia, 2020a).

Infiltration of plaques and tangles into areas of the brain can occur up to 15 years prior to presentation of clinical symptoms and initially involve areas of the brain concerned with learning, memory, thinking and planning (see Figure 13.2). It is characterised by atrophy in the entorhinal cortex (medial temporal lobe; see Figure 13.2) and hippocampus, and as the disease progresses it spreads to large areas of the neocortex (Fillit et al., 2017). People with a mild form of Alzheimer's disease are unable to learn and retain verbal information (Fillit et al., 2017). Other early impairments include loss of episodic memory, complex attention and organisational skills. Language abilities can be impacted in the normal ageing process and are often referred to as 'senior moments'. However, in early Alzheimer's, inability to recall words can be an indicator

FIGURE 13.2 Anatomy of the brain, including entorhinal and neocortex, and associated cerebral functions

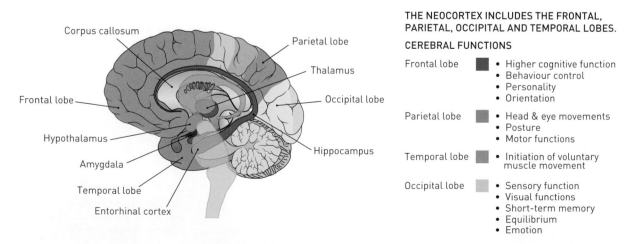

of the disease. Disease progression varies from person to person, and late-stage AD sees the person require full care with complete dependence for all activities of daily living.

Figure 13.2 shows the basic anatomy of the brain and the location of the entorhinal cortex and hippocampus, parts of the brain essential in the formation of memories. As more nerve cells are impacted and eventually die, other areas of the brain are affected and brain tissue begins to shrink.

As the disease becomes more widespread, functions and abilities are lost, impacting language, visuospatial abilities, attention, judgment and aspects of behaviour. These changes are evidenced by difficulty with 'word finding', wandering, decision making, completing daily activities such as dressing, and fluctuations in mood and apathy. Symptoms can be exacerbated by illness, change of environment, pain and time of day (Dementia Australia, 2020c).

Recent research suggests that the progression of dementia is more closely linked to the number of neurofibrillary tangles and synapses lost rather than the toxic effects of beta-amyloid on the brain, as previously believed (Fillit et al., 2017, p. 542; Dementia Australia, 2020c; DeTure & Dickson, 2019). Evidence also suggests a strong link between frailty and Alzheimer's incidence, particularly mild cognitive impairment. This has a bearing on current trends in dementia statistics, confirming that dementia is more apparent as we age and live longer.

VASCULAR DEMENTIA (VD)

Vascular dementia is the second most common cause of dementia and accounts for 15 to 20 per cent of all cases (Dementia Australia, 2020b). It is the broad term given for dementia associated with decreased blood flow to brain tissue primarily caused by cerebrovascular disease. The effect on the brain is dependent on the size and location of reduced blood flow, and the progression of vascular dementia is generally more rapid than Alzheimer's dementia (Dementia Australia, 2020b).

Varied mechanisms – such as single infarctions, multiple infarctions, hypoperfusion, haemorrhage, white matter lesions and lesions that are present with other brain disorders – can cause interruptions to cerebral blood flow (Fillit et al., 2017, p. 556). VD is sometimes classified as small or large vessel disease with small vessel disease being more common. Examples include microbleeds and white matter lesions. Symptoms can mimic those of stroke and may include difficulty walking (apraxia), problems related to speech (aphasia), difficulty recognising objects (agnosia) and numbness or paralysis. The '7As' of dementia will be discussed later in the chapter (see Table 13.2).

Age and education are two main factors that have been shown to influence the incidence of dementia in persons with VD. Other factors that can increase the risk of VD include hypertension, smoking, diabetes, high cholesterol, evidence of previous vessel disease and mild strokes (Dementia Australia, 2020b). Early diagnosis is highly desirable to prevent further infarcts and to address lifestyle choices that may improve health outcomes. Alzheimer's dementia and vascular dementia often coexist; this will be discussed later in the chapter under the heading 'Mixed dementias'.

LEWY BODY DEMENTIA (LBD)

Lewy body dementia accounts for 5 to 10 per cent of all dementia types and is caused by the abnormal accumulation of a protein called alpha-synuclein in nerve cells, which results in nerve cell degeneration and is thought to cause cell death (Alzheimer's Association, 2020).

The exact mechanisms that cause a clumping of this protein are still not fully understood. These protein deposits became known as Lewy bodies after the physician who discovered them in the early 1900s. The presence of the protein clumps causes nerve cells to be less effective and eventually die and is closely associated with Parkinson's disease. In contrast to Parkinson's disease dementia, Lewy bodies can be found scattered around the cerebral cortex, while in Parkinson's disease they are normally located in the substantia nigra in the midbrain (Fillit et al., 2017, p. 102). Chemicals within the brain are also impacted, causing widespread damage to areas that are affected – for example, acetylcholine and dopamine. Dopamine has an essential role in sleep, mood, movement and cognition (National Institute on Ageing, 2018). Although symptoms vary, there is normally a change in cognitive function, concentration span, movement, development of hallucinations and disturbance in REM sleep. Other symptoms of agitation, anxiety, apathy, delusions and paranoia may also be seen and worsen as the disease progresses. Impacts on the autonomic nervous system can include issues with blood pressure, dizziness, fainting, sensitivity to heat and cold, incontinence and constipation (National Institute on Aging, 2018).

FRONTOTEMPORAL LOBAR DEMENTIA (FTLD)

In frontotemporal lobar dementia (FTLD), progressive disease in nerve cells of the frontal and temporal lobes results in significant alteration in function in areas of the brain involved in higher functioning tasks related to behaviours and personality (see Figure 13.2). The frontal lobe is involved in higher cognitive functioning, concentration, mood, planning, judgment, emotional expression, creativity and inhibition. The temporal lobe is involved with encoding memory and auditory processing and to a lesser extent language, emotion and equilibrium. FTLD accounts for 5 to 10 per cent of all dementia diagnoses (Dementia Australia, 2020c). It is also referred to as younger onset dementia, with age of onset ranging from the late twenties to the eighties, but primarily occurs in the 45-to-65-year age range (Alzheimer's Association, 2020; Fillit et al., 2017). FTLD has been previously known as Pick's disease, named after the neurologist Arnold Pick, approximately 100 years ago (Fillit et al., 2017).

Differential diagnosis between FTLD and behavioural disorders characterised by schizophrenia can be challenging and should be supported by interdisciplinary assessment and evaluation of pathophysiology (Cipriani et al., 2020). The symptoms of FTLD are broad and unique to each person, depending on the specific pathological alteration in nerve cells. FTLD is separated into the following types: behaviour variant frontotemporal dementia (bvFTD) and primary progressive aphasia (PPA). Primary progressive aphasia is then separated into two groups: semantic variant (inability to understand or form words) and nonfluent/agrammatic variant (difficulties with speaking) (Fillit et al., 2017). Accurate assessment and screening are valuable in diagnosis and management. The pathway outlined in Figure 13.3 later in the chapter can assist and guide practitioners when there is diagnostic uncertainty and rare types of frontal features that require specialist consultation.

MIXED DEMENTIAS

There are no definitive numbers or percentages for this type of dementia although it is believed to be far more common than previously thought. The mixed intricacies of Alzheimer's dementia and vascular dementia are thought to account for most dementia cases in older adults in the community (Fillit et al., 2017, p. 560). In most cases the abnormal deposits associated with

Alzheimer's dementia dwell with the blood vessel damage associated with vascular dementia (Alzheimer's Association, 2020). Recent evidence suggests that the pathologies of vascular dementia facilitate disease in Alzheimer's dementia and vice versa (Fillit et al., 2017, p. 560). Lewy body dementia can also be included in mixed dementia cases and is currently the second most common after AD and VD coexistence (Alzheimer's Association, 2020). Mixed dementias remain difficult to accurately diagnose, and autopsy results indicate that brain changes can be attributable to all three dementia types (Alzheimer's Association, 2020). The symptoms of mixed dementia are extremely varied, again dependent on the areas of the brain affected.

YOUNGER ONSET DEMENTIA

Dementia diagnosed in people under the age of 65 years of age is commonly referred to as younger onset dementia (Alzheimer's Association, 2020). Younger onset dementia includes traumatic brain injury. For dementia diagnosed earlier in life it can be attributable, but not limited, to brain injuries associated with trauma, Alzheimer's disease, frontotemporal lobe dementia, alcohol abuse and HIV. Symptoms of dementia can differ in younger people compared to older people with the same disease (Alzheimer's Society, 2021). A diagnosis of younger onset Alzheimer's disease is usually associated with an atypical form of Alzheimer's disease – for example, posterior cortical atrophy (PCA), which results in difficulties understanding visual information. A diagnosis in earlier years, when people can be in full-time employment and have responsibilities with raising families, requires a more specific set of interventions and support services. This trend has been highlighted by Dementia Australia in relation to the Royal Commission into Aged Care Quality and Safety, where several recommendations were made to improve service pathways, improve education of staff and look at accommodation needs that were more designed towards the needs of the younger person with dementia (Dementia Australia, 2020a).

PARKINSON'S DISEASE DEMENTIA (PDD)

Parkinson's disease dementia is characterised by abnormal deposits of the protein alpha-synuclein, also known as Lewy bodies (Alzheimer's Association, 2020). Parkinson's disease, Lewy body dementia (LBD) and Parkinson's disease dementia (PDD) are thought to be linked due to similar changes in the brain. The plaques and tangles associated with Alzheimer's disease can also be found in people who have PDD and LBD, complicating the pathologies further (Alzheimer's Association, 2020).

It is estimated that 50 to 80 per cent of those diagnosed with Parkinson's disease will experience dementia and that specific factors at the time of diagnosis can increase the risk of developing dementia (Alzheimer's Association, 2020). These include older age, mild cognitive impairment (MCI) and motor symptoms that are severe. Symptoms associated with PPD include changes in memory and concentration, muffled speech, delusions and hallucinations, depression, irritability and sleep disturbances (daytime drowsiness and rapid eye movement sleep disorder) (Alzheimer's Association, 2020).

CREUTZFELDT-JAKOB DISEASE (CJD) DEMENTIA

Creutzfeldt-Jakob disease is a degenerative neurocognitive disorder that can cause dementia; it progresses rapidly and affects approximately one in one million people worldwide (Alzheimer's Association, 2020). The disease is not fully understood; however, it is thought to be caused by prion proteins that develop into abnormal folds within the brain. There are three main types: sporadic Creutzfeldt-Jakob disease, familial Creutzfeldt-Jakob disease and acquired Creutzfeldt-Jakob disease (Alzheimer's Association, 2020). Diagnosis is most commonly based on rapid symptom development. The symptoms experienced can vary greatly among individuals, and some common symptoms include agitation, apathy, depression, disorientation, motor disturbances and visual changes (Alzheimer's Association, 2020).

ALCOHOL-RELATED DEMENTIA

Alcohol-related dementia is a severe side effect of excessive alcohol use and has been labelled as a '21st-century silent epidemic' by some (Listabarth et al., 2020). The mechanism of cognitive decline is believed to be associated with one or a combination of thiamine deficiency, dietary problems, ethanol neurotoxic effects and ethanol-induced inflammation causing damage to myelin sheaths (Listabarth et al., 2020). Other factors include alcohol-related cerebrovascular disease and head traumas associated with episodes of intoxication. Side effects are commonly associated with memory and learning new information. Alcohol-related dementias include Korsakoff syndrome, Wernicke encephalopathy and Wernicke-Korsakoff syndrome.

HUNTINGTON'S DISEASE DEMENTIA

Huntington's disease is a genetic neurodegenerative disease caused by a single defective gene on chromosome 4 causing increased accumulation of the huntingtin protein (Alzheimer's Association, 2020). Presently, the exact mechanism of brain atrophy causing cognitive degeneration is poorly understood and the rate of progression and age of onset vary widely among those diagnosed. Huntington's disease causes brain changes that commonly result in abnormal involuntary movements, neuropsychiatric symptoms, alteration in thinking and reasoning skills, and the development of dementia (Martinez-Horta et al., 2020). Recent evidence suggests that in the early stages of the disease severe cognitive impairment can occur, and physiological changes can be detected up to 15 years before symptoms occur and a diagnosis is made (Martinez-Horta et al., 2020). Currently there is no cure; however, there are treatments available to help manage symptoms.

13.3 Getting to know the person: Rose's story

Rose's GP has not seen her for six months and is surprised by her physical decline as well as the change in her overall demeanour. The GP is aware that Rose had suffered from bouts of depression after losing her husband, and at times self-medicated with alcohol. Although Rose was outgoing when her husband was alive, she has withdrawn from socialising with their friendship group, preferring to spend most of her time at home alone. Occasionally, on Sundays she joins Catherine and her family for an evening meal. Catherine expresses her concerns that Rose may be showing signs of dementia and asks the GP to clarify if this could be the cause.

- Which of Rose's symptoms would suggest she may be developing Alzheimer's or another type of dementia?
- What approach might the GP consider when differentiating between a diagnosis of dementia and depression?

FOCUS QUESTIONS

Dementia care in today's world

There is much scope to improve the quality of life for people with dementia, their families and their carers by managing symptoms and providing a supportive environment.

BEST-PRACTICE DEMENTIA CARE

Government policies and research outcomes are causing many changes in aged care in general and with dementia care in particular. You may feel there is too much to learn as a health professional when you are supporting people with dementia and their carers. This section of the chapter provides contemporary information that you need to consider as you develop your knowledge and skills. This information also supports you to work within government guidelines so that your practice is safe both for you and those you are working with.

The Aged Care Quality and Safety Commission, the regulator for aged care services, published the new quality standards in 2018 with the aim of providing a framework for improving clinical governance and quality of care and services against a more evidence-based, best-practice framework (Aged Care Quality and Safety Commission, 2020). In principle, the new standards centre on consumer dignity and choice with very clear links to **person-centred care**. The quality standards are made up of eight individual standards:

1 Dignity and choice
2 Ongoing assessment and planning with consumers
3 Personal and clinical care
4 Services and support for daily living
5 Organisational service environment
6 Feedback and complaints
7 Human resources
8 Organisational governance (Aged Care Quality and Safety Commission, 2020).

The Royal Commission into Aged Care Quality and Safety (Commonwealth of Australia, 2021) has identified areas of concern around dementia care with recommendations geared to focus on enablement, dignity and respect, choice and person-centred care (Commonwealth of Australia, 2021). Holistic and person-centred care will be discussed later in the chapter.

person-centred care
Treatment and care provided by health services that places the person at the centre of their own care and considers the needs of the older person's carers.

NON-MODIFIABLE AND MODIFIABLE RISK FACTORS AND DEMENTIA

Risk factors for dementia can be classified as non-modifiable and modifiable. Non-modifiable factors include age, gender, ethnicity and family history. Major modifiable risks are those associated with early identification and management of conditions associated with lifestyle choices. Examples include Type 2 diabetes, smoking, excessive alcohol intake, obesity, high cholesterol diets, hypertension, cognitive inactivity, depression and low educational attainment (WHO, 2021). The dementia spectrum is associated with several risk factors; however, this discussion will focus on several of the common types: Alzheimer's dementia, vascular dementia and mixed dementia.

Interest in the overlap or combination of associated risks is increasing, with recent research focusing on frailty, chronic disease, air pollution, sleep disorders, stress, traumatic brain injury, and their relationship to dementia **aetiology** (Livingstone et al., 2020). As discussed previously, the importance of primary health initiatives is valuable, given that currently 40 per cent of global dementias may be delayed or prevented as they are due to modifiable factors (Livingstone et al., 2020).

aetiology
The cause or set of causes, or manner of a disease or condition.

Age is the strongest non-modifiable risk factor, with the risk of developing AD or VD doubling every five years after the age of 65 (Alzheimer's Society, 2016). For most of the dementias, both males and females have some risk. Women are more likely to develop AD (Alzheimer's Society, 2016) even considering women tend to live longer than men. Men are at higher risk of VD due to the association of heart disease and stroke (Dementia Australia, 2020b). The role of genetics is not fully understood; however, some inherited genes can directly cause dementia while others have been identified that affect a person's risk of developing dementia. Genes known to have a familial link are those associated with early onset dementia (before the age of 60) and FTLD. Inheriting variants of the gene lipoprotein E (APOE) increase the risk of developing AD (Alzheimer's Society, 2016).

Many of these risk factors overlap and impact the individual in various life stages – for example, hypertension and Type 2 diabetes commonly occur in mid-life around the ages of 40 to 64 years and are known to increase an individual's risk of stroke, which in turn can result in vascular dementia (WHO, 2017). Smoking can increase the risk of developing AD by 45 per cent in comparison to non-smokers.

Psychological stress may increase the risk of dementia through its effect on cardiovascular diseases, or through other pathways such as depression and post-traumatic stress disorder (PTSD) (Nabe-Nielsen et al., 2019).

Contemporary studies have shown that combining modifiable risk with an understanding of protective factors such as physical exercise, cognitive training and diet, can maintain and improve cognitive capacity in older people (Kulmala et al., 2018). Protective factors, specifically cognitive reserve, in the form of relationship networks, social engagement, leisure pursuits and educational level have been shown to lower the risk of dementia (Silva et al., 2019).

The WHO (2017) developed guidelines on risk reduction of cognitive decline and dementia that highlight a public health response which also correlates with the Global Action Plan, 2017–s2025 (WHO, 2017).

SOCIAL DETERMINANTS OF AGEING AND DEMENTIA

Continuing education to higher levels beyond the age of 16 has been discussed as a way of reducing the risk of dementia in later life (Alzheimer's Society, 2016). There is also a relationship between social disadvantage, social determinants of health and living at home in the later stages of dementia (Harrison et al., 2019). Living alone has been associated with the development of dementia for older people with mild cognitive impairment (MCI) and should therefore be considered in holistic assessment (Grande et al., 2018).

DEPRESSION AND DEMENTIA

Opinions vary on whether depression is a risk factor or an early symptom of dementia. There is evidence to suggest that older men with a history of depression are at increased risk of developing dementia, but that this risk is non-modifiable (Almeida et al., 2017). Alzheimer's Society (2016) discusses possible links with dementia among those people who have experienced depression in middle age.

For more information on delirium, dementia and depression, see Chapters 11 and 12.

ENVIRONMENTAL AND GEOGRAPHICAL FACTORS FOR DEMENTIA

Exposure to exhaust fumes from living near busy roads (within 50 metres) has been found to increase the risk of dementia compared to living more than 200 metres away (Alzheimer's Society, 2021). Air pollution has also been identified as neurotoxic to the brain and reducing cerebral blood flow. A systematic review of environmental risk factors for dementia in 2016 (Killin et al., 2016) determined that there was moderate evidence for air pollution, electromagnetic fields, vitamin D deficiency and environmental tobacco being related to dementia risk.

13.4 Getting to know the person: Rose's story

Previously, the GP had prescribed antidepressants for Rose to reduce her symptoms of depression and anxiety. However, Rose had so far declined to use them. Other medications prescribed were a Ventolin inhaler (prn) for smoking-induced asthma,

Panadol osteo for chronic leg and hip pain and Atorvastatin for high cholesterol. Rose is not very forthcoming when asked questions by the GP, seemingly unable to remember events even from a week ago. Fortunately, Catherine is present to provide some background about Rose's deteriorating state and the need for some support services for Rose. The GP explains to Catherine that there could be a number of predisposing factors influencing Rose's current state of health and that he would commence the process of holistic assessment, including referrals to a psycho-geriatrician and an aged care assessment team assessment.

FOCUS QUESTIONS

- Is Rose just depressed or might she have dementia? What factors in Rose's assessment will the GP review when assessing her prior to a diagnosis of dementia?
- What are some of the non-modifiable and modifiable risk factors for Rose?

SEEKING A DIAGNOSIS OF DEMENTIA

A diagnosis of dementia is life changing for both the person with the condition and their family. However, with good planning, treatment and support a person can live well with dementia. The symptoms of dementia may be observed by families for up to three years before diagnosis. The observed factors can be addressed by you as either registered nurses or other health professionals with a primary-health-care focus so that they are reported and not dismissed as a 'normal part of ageing'. Rather than a single test, a dementia diagnostic pathway can help the multidisciplinary team to build a process towards a definitive diagnosis.

For family members of people who have dementia, your role is to ensure access to information about the condition and its progression that is commensurate with the family member's language and culture. Incomplete knowledge without understanding of the impact of dementia can have dire consequences for all concerned (Andrews et al., 2015). It is important that nurses and other members of the interdisciplinary team take this into account and ensure that family members and the person themselves are provided with information that is positive and appropriate to their needs (Alzheimer's Australia, 2015). While most people consider memory loss as the key feature of dementia, this is simplistic and memory loss will vary depending on the type and person. A person may exhibit any combination of the symptoms listed in Table 13.2.

TABLE 13.2 The 7 As of dementia

FEATURE	DESCRIPTION	IMPACTS
Amnesia	Difficulty remembering. Short-term or working memory (memory that helps you function day-to-day) is usually affected first.	May ask the same questions repeatedly, which can cause anxiety and stress. Lives in the present but recalls information from the past. Can cause anxious behaviour.
Agnosia	Being unable to recognise people, objects, places or activities using the five senses: touch, taste, sight, smell and hearing.	Difficulty understanding common objects or people. Can present as confusion. Can lead to altered behaviours and interactions.

TABLE 13.2 Continued

FEATURE	DESCRIPTION	IMPACTS
Aphasia	Difficulties with speech, writing, listening and understanding words.	Can struggle to find words and may replace one word for another. May have difficulty following conversations.
Apraxia	How the body relates to the space it fills and the space around it is called 'praxis'. Apraxia impacts purposeful movement and recognition of orientation.	Can cause problems with gait, balance and coordination. May have difficulty using common objects like feeding implements, toothbrush or writing tools.
Altered perception	This is seen in difficulties interpreting sensory signals that the environment is giving: altered depth perception, visual distortions and tactile perception.	Alterations in movement and gait; impacts ability to freely mobilise. May cause misperceptions of objects and illicit fearful behaviours (e.g. shadows cast on walls or the ground).
Anosognosia	The person does not have an understanding of their loss of ability to recall things, or of their own cognitive changes.	Unable to recall that they need assistance with some tasks, which may cause issues with personal safety. Common in temporo-parietal pathologies.
Apathy	Not commonly acknowledged as a symptom, a person with dementia may lose their drive and initiative and the ability to start activities such as feeding or dressing.	Difficulty initiating tasks and conversation. Can be engaged by caregiver. Can be interpreted as depression.

Source: compiled from Puxty et al., 2009; Fillit et al., 2017.

The information in Table 13.2 assists the health-care team in identifying symptoms and just as importantly gives clarity to individual abilities that are less obvious, giving clinicians the ability to identify areas of enablement that can be encouraged and developed.

13.5 Getting to know the person: Rose's story

The GP completes a physical assessment of Rose, and orders a full blood investigation and a medication review. It is clear to the GP that Rose is dehydrated, has signs of a urinary tract infection, appears confused and is slurring her words. He asks for the primary health nurse to complete a cognitive screening assessment as well as a Geriatric Depression Scale so that a baseline level of cognitive function can be established. In consultation with Rose and Catherine, the GP also refers Rose to a psychologist, recommending six visits as part of developing a mental health plan. The GP asks Catherine to start the process of organising some support services at home for Rose, including cleaning and Meals on Wheels.

**FOCUS
QUESTIONS**

- Were there any preventative measures that could have been initiated to prevent Rose's deterioration and depression following the death of her husband?
- What physiological factors are contributing to Rose's deteriorating state?
- What is the value of timely referral to allied health professionals such as psychologists?
- Why is a pathway for diagnosis significant in Rose's case?

HOLISTIC ASSESSMENT AND CARE PLANNING IN PRIMARY CARE

The aim of holistic assessment is to gather comprehensive information about the person presenting with altered cognition. The focus is on changed behaviour, functional capacity, psychosocial issues and relevant medical conditions to allow for a diagnosis of dementia to be made and to exclude other possible causes. Most people with dementia are diagnosed when living at home, therefore using a dementia screening, assessment and support pathway through a team approach is beneficial to the person with dementia and their family (Alzheimer's Australia, 2015; Morgan et al., 2019; NIHCE (UK), 2018). Because dementia is a chronic progressive condition, history of lifestyle over time may provide keys to the type of impairment present and the lifelong coping abilities a person has that will assist in providing a strengths-based care plan (Alzheimer's Australia, 2015; Moyle et al., 2014).

In Australia, the shift in improving best-practice dementia care is to integrate state- and Commonwealth-funded care services that cross the boundaries between primary, community, hospital, social and aged care. The aim of this integrated approach is to provide screening and assessment pathways that support the existence and extent of cognitive impairment prior to definitive diagnosis (Alzheimer's Australia, 2015). The following steps present a framework for supporting primary-health-care nurses and GPs to assist in timely diagnosis and an evidence-based practice improvement approach to support people living with dementia and their carers (Alzheimer's Australia, 2015).

- *Step 1 – Building dementia knowledge in primary care.* Health professionals working in primary care settings can identify early signs of cognitive impairment and raise initial concerns. Information can be provided at this stage about dementia prevention strategies, including lifestyle factors related to health, diet and exercise, maintaining a healthy heart, mentally challenging your brain and enjoying social activities. Cognitive screening can then be undertaken (Alzheimer's Australia, 2015).
- *Step 2 – Building a process towards dementia diagnosis.* There is no single process or test that will definitively diagnose dementia. Cognitive screening and assessment can take time and can take place over several appointments, either with a GP, nurse practitioner or other members of the multidisciplinary team. The aim of assessment is to gather sufficient information about changed behaviours, functional capacity, psychosocial issues and relevant medical conditions to allow for a diagnosis to be made and to exclude other possible causes, such as delirium or depression. Assessment can include a physical examination, functional assessment, emotional and social needs assessment, carer burden assessment and mental health assessment (Alzheimer's Australia, 2015).

A collaborative, interdisciplinary approach can support achievement of a more comprehensive assessment, combined with a dementia diagnostic pathway (see Figure 13.3).

At this stage, referral to specialists such as psycho-geriatricians and psychiatrists would address the issue of diagnostic uncertainty, given the complexity across the spectrum. Specialists can provide an extra layer of expertise for patients under 65 years old, those with rare frontal type features or early onset hallucinations, and where there are concerns about competency (Alzheimer's Australia, 2015).

- *Step 3 – Building an approach to dementia support.* We know that a diagnosis of dementia is life changing for the person and their family. It is preferable that a diagnosis is disclosed to the patient by someone who is familiar or who can put the person at ease (a GP, nurse or allied health professional) and is accompanied by written information. Treatment options and commencement of treatment should also occur at this time. With good planning, treatment and collaborative support a person can live well post-diagnosis. A person-centred, strengths-based approach ensures individual support needs are met to maintain well-being and independence for as long as possible living in the community (Alzheimer's Australia, 2015; Moyle et al., 2014).

- *Step 4 – Building sustainable dementia practice.* There is increasing evidence that in primary care a collaborative, multidisciplinary dementia practice model promotes opportunities for greater detection, diagnosis and support of people living with dementia, their families and carers. At this stage following diagnosis, it is expected that a holistic care plan will include counselling support and other multidisciplinary support strategies,

FIGURE 13.3 A dementia screening, assessment and support pathway

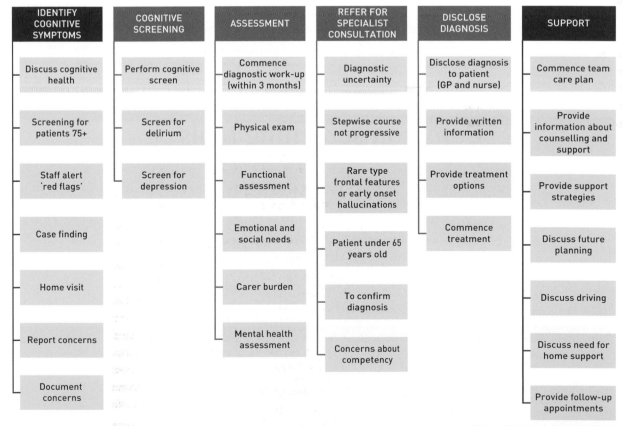

Source: Alzheimer's Australia, 2015.

 MARGUERITE BRAMBLE AND KATHRYN LITTLE

such as those provided by allied health professionals. In the early stages, monitoring of driving and other risky activities will be part of the care plan (Alzheimer's Australia, 2015). Figure 13.3 presents a helpful tool to guide the multidisciplinary team in working together within their scope of practice to achieve best-practice dementia care (Alzheimer's Australia, 2015).

13.6 Getting to know the person: Rose's story

Once the ACAT assessment is completed it is decided that Rose is eligible for support services at home. Rose seems to appreciate the support and company provided from the support care workers, who visit her twice a week. However, she is having increasing difficulty walking and cannot recognise the plants in her garden unless Catherine names them for her. She seems much happier in herself and enjoys the time with her psychologist. Catherine visits twice a week and there are regular outings with the family. Rose also has regular appointments with the primary care nurse for ongoing screening and assessment.

FOCUS QUESTIONS

- What symptoms of dementia would you consider when reading case study 13.6?
- What screening tools would the primary care nurse use to assess Rose's cognitive function?

Common screening tools

As noted in previous sections, there is no single tool you can use to ascertain a diagnosis of dementia. Cognitive screening aims to identify the presence and extent of cognitive impairment and establish a baseline level of cognitive function. Screening also provides valuable information to assist in ruling out other treatable neurocognitive disorders and should be used in conjunction with other assessments. These tools are summarised in Table 13.3 together with a description and the most appropriate application/setting of the relevant tool.

TABLE 13.3 Common screening tools for dementia

SCREENING TOOL	DESCRIPTION	APPLICATION/SETTING
Standardised Mini-Mental State Examination (MMSE)	The most widely used assessment tool, it is scored out of 30, assesses global cognition, orientation, recall, language and attention. Can be completed in 5–10 minutes. A score below 24 suggests a change in neurocognitive status.	Used in a variety of environments by physicians, GPs, nurses and formal carers. Recommended in acute care, primary health, community and residential care settings (Dementia Australia, 2020c).

TABLE 13.3 Continued

SCREENING TOOL	DESCRIPTION	APPLICATION/SETTING
Modified Mini-Mental State Examination (3MS)	This is an extended version of the MMSE and is highly recommended. It tests multiple domains: orientation, attention, memory, visuoconstructional skills, language and executive function. A validated tool that accurately identifies between dementia and mild cognitive impairment.	Used in acute, primary health, community and residential care settings. Conducted by health-care professionals
General Practitioner Assessment of Cognition (GPCOG)	Involves two parts: cognition test and if results not clear then an interview with family or carer. Takes less than 4 minutes to attend and includes the clock drawing test.	Tool for general practitioners to use in primary health settings; research states it is as effective as the MMSE in primary care settings (Dementia Australia, 2020c).
Kimberly Indigenous Cognitive Assessment (KICA-cog)	An assessment tool for First Nations Australians aged 45 years and older. Comprises 18 questions and takes 25–30 minutes to administer. Specifically designed for First Nations Australians in rural and remote regions.	Specifically for rural and remote settings and conducted by health professionals.
Kimberly Indigenous Cognitive Assessment: urban and rural areas (Modified KICA or mKICA)	Assessment tool for First Nations Australians aged 45 years and older. Comprises 18 questions and takes 25–30 minutes to administer.	Currently being redesigned for First Nations populations in urban areas in Australia.
Rowland Universal Dementia Assessment Scale (RUDAS)	Scored out of 30, short cognitive screening tool taking approximately 10 minutes to conduct. Shown to be sensitive to dementia regardless of language or level of education.	Recommended for those from culturally and linguistically diverse backgrounds.
Addenbrooke's Cognitive Examination-III (ACE-III)	Recommended when shorter assessments are inconclusive; specifically useful in differential diagnosis between Alzheimer's, frontotemporal and Parkinson's dementias. The test takes 15–20 minutes and focuses on domains of function.	Australian version available. Settings where the person can concentrate and not feel overwhelmed. Ideal for home environment.
Montreal Cognitive Assessment (MoCA)	Designed to detect mild cognitive impairment, but sensitive to dementia. Is highly recommended and has been modified into other versions for the visually impaired and those with limited years of education or who are illiterate.	
Informant Questionnaire on Cognitive Decline in the Elderly (IQCODE)	Can be used as a supplement to cognitive testing. Both long and short versions exist.	Can be conducted by health-care professional or can be completed by the informant or carer. Available in multiple languages.
Frontal Assessment Battery (FAB)	Valid in distinguishing FTLD from Alzheimer's type dementia with mild dementia. Scored out of 18; scores below 12 indicative of impaired executive function.	Can be utilised at the bedside or in primary health.
Psychogeriatric Assessment Scale-Cognitive Decline Scale (PAS-CDS)	Tracks changes over time; most notably can accurately distinguish persons with dementia from those with depression. Assesses using a scale rather than categories.	Extensive training not required for using this tool. Suitable to assess cognition in people in residential care facilities. Made up of two sections: subject and informant interview.

(Continued)

MARGUERITE BRAMBLE AND KATHRYN LITTLE

TABLE 13.3 Continued

SCREENING TOOL	DESCRIPTION	APPLICATION/SETTING
Ascertain Dementia 8 (AD8)	Brief informant interview designed to differentiate between normal ageing and dementia. Takes less than 5 minutes to complete.	Used by health-care professionals; adopted in some emergency departments. Has been adapted for multiple languages.
Clock drawing	Assesses multiple cognitive domains, often incorporated into other screening tests. Can be scored as correctly drawn or incorrectly drawn (abnormal) Usually takes 1–2 minutes to complete.	Minimal training required to administer the test. Recommended as a supplementary test of frontal abilities.

Source: compiled from Dementia Australia, 2020c; Fillit et al., 2017.

Other assessment tools that are used to establish an alteration in cognitive status across acute, residential and primary care settings include the psychogeriatric assessment scale (PAS), confusion assessment method (CAM), delirium risk assessment tool (DRAT) and geriatric depression scale. These tools can be used for initial screening or to supplement existing information. They are easy to use and can be undertaken by a wide range of health-care staff.

It is possible for a person to present very well for a brief test and still have significant cognitive impairment. Preserving dignity is essential as the individual may be embarrassed or fearful of being judged if testing shows literacy or memory issues. As previously mentioned, there is value in the primary health team being involved in this process due to established rapport and familiarity with the individual and their circumstances. Planning at this time enables the person to be involved in and direct their care using a person-centred approach.

13.7 Getting to know the person: Rose's story

At the next consultation with the GP the following week, the results of the cognitive screening tests and investigations are discussed with Rose and Catherine. The GP informs them that, although the picture is complicated by Rose's periods of depression, dementia is possible. For the next three months, Catherine does her best to provide meals, visit her mother at least twice a week and take her to the psychologist for her regular visits. One day she arrives to find Rose in a distressed state, unable to move from where she has fallen in the bathroom. She rings for an ambulance and Rose is taken to hospital. Fortunately, Rose has not sustained a fracture, but she is admitted overnight for observation for concussion.

FOCUS QUESTIONS

- What are some of the assessment results that would indicate likely dementia?
- What aspects of the case study provide cues about the type of dementia Rose is likely to be presenting with?

Person-centred care and the therapeutic response

When the therapeutic response to the person being assessed considers both neurological and social-psychological factors, clinicians and health professionals are working from a person-centred care approach (Kitwood, 1997). As identified in the overview of dementia types in Table 13.1 earlier in this chapter, dementia encompasses a number of conditions associated with neurological decline, with impairment ranging from memory loss to changes in behaviour and personality, difficulty recognising objects and understanding or expressing language, difficulties with speech and impaired judgment, and visual and auditory hallucinations (Moyle et al., 2014). The picture for each person with dementia is complex and multidimensional and requires a multidisciplinary health professional focus on person-centred care and individual personhood (Kitwood, 1997; Moyle et al., 2014).

Brooker (2007) developed the acronym VIPS to help explain the four main concepts of person-centred care beyond simply 'individual' care. These are:

V – a **value** base that asserts the value of all humans, no matter their age or cognitive ability

I – an **individualised** approach, which recognises the person as a unique human

P – understanding of the world from the perspective of the **person** being cared for

S – encouraging a **social** environment that supports the person's individualised needs (Brooker, 2007, p. 27).

Personhood and the notion of self-identity

The concept of **personhood** leads us into each person's unique therapeutic space: 'into a way of being in which emotion and feeling are given a much larger place' (Kitwood, 1997, p. 8). It also opens the door to the notion of self-identity, in which the importance of our ability to think, to remember and to make rational choices as a basic criterion of personhood is recognised (Fuchs, 2020). Kitwood (1997, p. 8) argued that personhood accords people with dementia with an ethical status that offers them absolute value and therefore an obligation 'to treat each other with deep respect'. He then argued that through good communication, or as he termed it, 'positive people work', a person with dementia's condition and sense of self-identity may improve. Calling a person by their name, affirming their views and encouraging people to explore activities they enjoy are forms of positive people work that can engender a person-centred approach to care. For health professionals in all practice settings, care that is truly person-centred, that understands the person's needs and values, is integral to providing best practice care (Alzheimer's Australia, 2015; Moyle et al., 2014).

personhood
The standing or status bestowed on a human being.

MARGUERITE BRAMBLE AND KATHRYN LITTLE

13.8 Getting to know the person: Rose's story

Following further assessment in hospital, Rose is diagnosed with vascular dementia, possibly with some overlying Alzheimer's. A case conference is organised with Rose's family and the GP, primary nurse, sociologist and psychologist to discuss her diagnosis. The aged care assessment team is also included to discuss her discharge home. At the case conference, the team asks about Rose's social and psychological history, her relationship with her family and other personal factors that may impact her recovery.

Rose and her family feel some relief about the future after her diagnosis at the interdisciplinary case conference. Rose's general demeanour also starts to improve now that she has some benefit from the psychologist visits and regular interaction with a support worker, who also organises for her to visit her beloved garden club. With help at home and regular visits from community-based care, Rose looks forward to her weekly outings and looking after her garden.

FOCUS QUESTIONS

- What services are available to provide person-centred care for Rose and her family?
- What other psychosocial supports can be provided to ensure Rose has access to therapeutic and spiritual support?

How, then, does the experience of dementia affect an individual's sense of self and personal identity over time, particularly in the later stages? Juliette Brown (2017) considers this question by examining the experiential self, where 'persons are continually coming into being – that is, undergoing generation – in the course of life itself' rather than being set on a predetermined downward trajectory (Brown, 2017, p. 1006). If the diagnosis of dementia sets a course of change and loss, with an inevitable dependency, a sense of shame often develops. This sense is tied to our notion of value and society's notion of dependence as a deeply negative concept, overriding any sense of spiritual worth and compounded by stigma (Brown, 2017). Instead of isolating people with dementia from society and working from a 'narrative of decline' there is increasing understanding that honest communication, counselling and fostering a **gerotranscendence** narrative for people with dementia and their families can promote self-esteem and produce positive change and even joy in people's lives (Jeffers et al., 2020). As a consequence, in the context of **iterative personhood**, people with dementia can show a remarkable ability to live fulfilling lives without the distressing behavioural and psychological symptoms commonly associated with dementia (Brown, 2017).

Fazio et al. (2018, p. S18) make six practice recommendations for person-centred care:

1   Know the person living with dementia.

2   Recognise and accept the person's reality.

gerotranscendence
Described as not just a continuation of the activity patterns and values of mid life, but rather a transformation characterised by new ways of understanding life, activities, oneself and others.

iterative personhood
The practice of building, refining and improving personhood over time.

3 Identify and support ongoing opportunities for meaningful engagement.

4 Build and nurture authentic, caring relationships.

5 Create and maintain a supportive community for individuals, families and staff.

6 Evaluate care practices regularly and make appropriate changes.

These recommendations are supported by the Royal Commission's final report tabled in Parliament in February 2021 (Commonwealth of Australia, 2021).

Person-centred care and the family caregiver

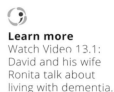

Learn more
Watch Video 13.1:
David and his wife
Ronita talk about
living with dementia.

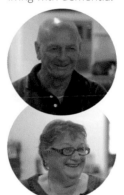

For community-dwelling people with dementia, the family caregiver is crucial to enhancing their ability to 'live well', as framed by measures of subjective well-being and quality of life (Quinn et al., 2019). However, as a person's dementia progresses and it becomes very challenging to care for them at home, signs of caregiver burden are more likely to emerge, such as depression; disturbed sleep; social isolation; poor physical health; and feelings of anger, guilt, grief, anxiety, hopelessness and helplessness (Bramble et al., 2009).

There is increasing recognition that family caregivers can experience positive consequences of caring for a loved one if well supported, and that this will positively influence the well-being of the person with dementia (Quinn et al., 2019). Other factors that influence the experience of being a caregiver are cultural influences, the nature of the illness and other family supports (Moyle et al., 2014). Health professionals can build on these positive aspects of caring by identifying strengths in providing support through maintaining a supportive community for individuals, families and staff (Fazio et al., 2018).

13.9 Getting to know the person: Rose's story

The benefits of a person-centred approach are obvious for Rose, as she takes more joy in her daily life. However, follow-up screening identifies further cognitive and functional decline. Both Catherine and Michael spend dedicated time ensuring Rose is surrounded by family and friends when possible. She spends some time walking to visit friends and to go to the shops. Six months later Rose, is admitted to residential care after having increasing difficulties managing at home alone and becoming increasingly frail. Catherine and Michael were becoming more concerned for their mother's safety at home after a series of falls and another visit to hospital. Although frail, Rose is still able to contribute to her plan of care on admission and talk about her unique interests, such as gardening and music.

MARGUERITE BRAMBLE AND KATHRYN LITTLE

FOCUS QUESTIONS

- What are some of the ways to reduce the grief associated with admission to residential care?
- When is the best time to start talking about palliative care and advance care plans?
- How can health-care staff gently go about assisting the person with dementia to complete activities of daily living without diminishing their dignity or independence?

Admission to residential care

The transition from home to residential care is often a major stressful event for the person with dementia and their family. Not only is there associated grief and loss, but also the notions of autonomy, family support and engaging in personally meaningful activity to support quality of life (Bramble et al., 2009; Davison et al., 2019). While family members are often relieved that their relative can receive a higher level of care, they describe feeling highly distressed themselves by the transition process, which for some is accompanied by conflict in their relationship with their relative (Bramble et al., 2009). While person-centred care is now part of policy and practice, evidence suggests that this approach has little effect on rates of depression during the transition to residential care (Chenoweth et al., 2019; Davison et al., 2019). Nevertheless, there is still minimal evidence to inform care interventions for people with dementia living at home in the community, or how such alternatives might impact quality of life for those who choose to stay at home (Harrison et al., 2019).

You can find more information about family and caring in Chapter 5.

Behavioural and psychological symptoms of dementia and psychotropic medication

Behavioural and psychological symptoms of dementia (BPSD) most often occur because of unmet needs. It is thought that one in five people with mid-stage dementia who mostly reside in residential aged care facilities experience symptoms of dementia-related agitation, presenting as verbal aggression, destructive and resistive behaviour, pacing and repetitive questioning and motor behaviour (Moyle et al., 2017). A lack of stimulation can be particularly detrimental to people with dementia, as it influences mood and increases loneliness and agitation (Moyle et al., 2018). Historically, psychotropic medication has been the first line of treatment for alleviating BPSD. However, considering the limited efficacy and potentially harmful side effects of pharmacological approaches, psychosocial approaches are now advocated as the primary treatment for the symptomatic benefit of BPSD (Moyle et al., 2018). Companion animal robots such as Paro may be one means of helping some people with dementia to gain comfort and improve their quality of life (Moyle et al., 2018).

psychotropic agent
Any drug capable of affecting the mind, emotions and behaviour.

Psychotropic agents are defined as medications prescribed under the classification of antipsychotics, antidepressants and/or anxiolytic/hypnotics (predominantly benzodiazepines) (Westbury et al., 2018). Antipsychotic medications are most often used in residential aged care to manage BPSD, despite the limited evidence of effectiveness and only a modest response (Westbury et al., 2018).

You can find more information on pharmacology and psychotropic medications in Chapter 14.

Creative therapies for people with dementia

Creative therapies such as art, dance, music and drama provide an opportunity for people with dementia to explore their potential for self-expression through activities they enjoy. Anywhere they can utilise residual skills will improve their self-esteem and confidence. Being and creating with others enhances engagement and communication opportunities and helps ameliorate the sense of loneliness and isolation (Brown et al., 2020). The National Institute for Health and Care Excellence (NIHCE) has identified the need for residents to have meaningful activity in care settings – particularly residents with dementia (Broome et al., 2019). Research currently suggests that participation in creative activities assists in cultivating successful ageing by facilitating purpose and meaningfulness (Yekanians et al., 2019). Studies gathering evidence on art appreciation found that participants with dementia responded to art according to their aesthetic preference, and that maintaining artistic approaches to healthcare has a range of beneficial outcomes for patients (Rylatt, 2012).

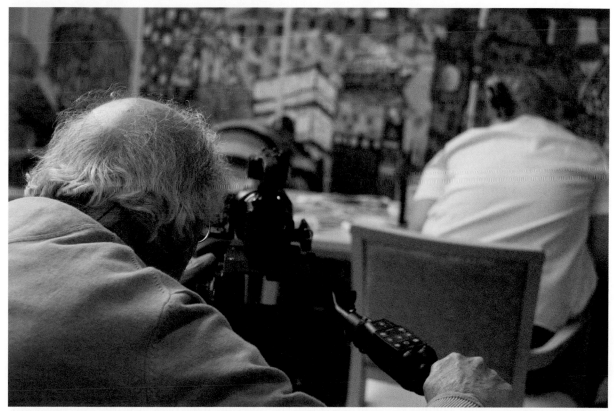

Source: Three Films by Three Thumbs Productions.

There is value in including multiple genres to accommodate the unique talents of individuals in creative pursuits. Evidence also suggests a coming together of care workers and creative educators to improve and add valuable input into the experience with their unique knowledge of residents and their preferences (Yekanians et al., 2019). Future study to improve therapeutic communication and delivery of dementia care with empathy using enhanced study design and measurement is needed (Brown et al., 2019).

MARGUERITE BRAMBLE AND KATHRYN LITTLE

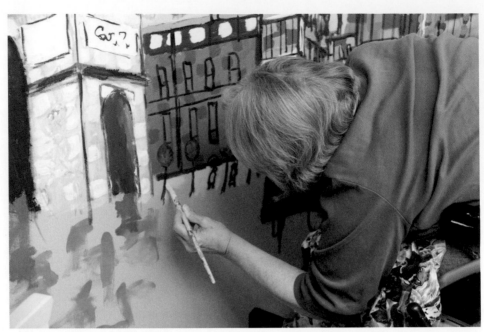

Source: Three Films by Three Thumbs Productions.

Capacity, dignity of choice and end-of-life care

On a policy level there are now legal acknowledgments of the human rights entitlements of people with dementia and their role in society (Bosco et al., 2019). For people with early stage dementia there is the opportunity to complete an advance care plan, as a dementia diagnosis does not automatically result in diminished capacity (Moyle et al., 2014). In terms of selfhood and social positioning, decision-making ability can be complex, and it is crucial that health professionals and families consider contextual dimensions surrounding a decision to maintain respect for the person's autonomy (Viaña et al., 2020).

End-of-life care for people with dementia is increasingly important because of the increasing numbers, mainly in residential and acute care (Trinh et al., 2019). However, families and caregivers continue to report a lack of attention to spiritual care and the impact of complicated grief and chronic sorrow as end of life is reached (Durepos et al., 2017; Moyle et al., 2014). Research on spiritual aspects of palliative care and dementia is relatively limited, focusing mostly on residential settings and end of life, rather than what is needed at the time of diagnosis (Palmer et al., 2020). There is increasing acknowledgment of the need to advocate for direct spiritual counselling or guidance for people with dementia and their families earlier in the trajectory, within the framework of person-centredness and individuality (Palmer et al., 2020; Toivonen et al., 2018).

You can find more information related to palliative care in Chapter 19.

Conclusion

In this chapter, the multiple aspects of dementia as a neurocognitive condition are discussed, with reference to the various types and associated physiological, cognitive and behavioural changes. The information provided is a starting point. You will need to read further and access other resources. To be effective in working with people with dementia, your knowledge will need to remain current. As health professionals, it is our responsibility to ensure we keep abreast of research outcomes and even become involved in research projects to address the challenges dementia presents. New therapeutic approaches, medications and models of care continue to evolve, such as the psychosocial benefits of artistic and creative initiatives we have included here. Always be aware of, and sensitive to, the individuality of the experience of dementia and the significance of respecting the capacity and dignity of choice at all stages of each person's journey through dementia.

Learn more
Access additional resources – such as weblinks, further readings and podcasts – to broaden your understanding of this chapter. See the Guided Tour for access details.

REVISION QUESTIONS

1 Compare and contrast the causes of Alzheimer's dementia and vascular dementia. What are the differences and similarities?

2 Identify how the health professional can reduce the risk of both types of dementia. What are the modifiable risk factors that you might educate people of any age about?

3 Outline how you would initiate assessment of a person who may have dementia and identify who you would include in the assessment process. Which communication style would you use? How would you incorporate all aspects of personhood?

4 Review the models of care discussed in this chapter and identify those that resonate with you and your professional practice. Which would be on your 'can do' list and which on your 'not me' list of professional practices?

REFERENCES

Aged Care Quality and Safety Commission (ACQSC) (2020). Aged Care Quality Standards fact sheet. Australian Government. www.agedcarequality.gov.au/resources/aged-care-quality-standards

Aged Care Sector Committee (2016). Aged Care Roadmap. www.health.gov.au/resources/publications/aged-care-roadmap

Aldus, C., Arthur, A., Dennington-Price, A., Millac, P., Richmond, P. & Dening T, e. a. (2020). Undiagnosed dementia in primary care: A record linkage study. *Health Services and Delivery Research*, 8(20). https://doi:10.3310/hsdr08200

Almeida, O. P., Hankey, G. J., Yeap, B. B., Golledge, J. & Flicker, L. (2017). Depression as a modifiable factor to decrease the risk of dementia.

Translational Psychiatry, 7(5), E1117. https://doi:10.1038/tp.2017.90

Alzheimer's Association (2020). Types of Dementia. www.alz.org/alzheimers-dementia/what-is-dementia/types-of-dementia

Alzheimer's Australia (2015). Four Steps to Building Dementia Practice in Primary Care. Alzheimer's Australia Victoria. www.dementialearning.org.au

Alzheimer's Society (2016). Risk Factors for Dementia. www.alzheimers.org.uk/sites/default/files/pdf/factsheet_risk_factors_for_dementia.pdf

Alzheimer's Society (2021). Air Pollution and Dementia. www.alzheimers.org.uk/about-dementia/risk-factors-and-prevention/air-pollution-and-dementia

American Psychiatric Association (APA) (2013). *Diagnostic and Statistical Manual of*

Mental Disorders (5th edn). https://doi.org/10.1176/appi.books.9780890425596

Andrews, S., McInerney, F., Toye, C., Parkinson, C- A. & Robinson, A. (2015). Knowledge of dementia: Do family members understand dementia as a terminal condition? *Dementia*, 1–20. https://doi:10.1177/1471301215605630

Australian Bureau of Statistics (ABS) (2020). Causes of Death, Australia. www.abs.gov.au/statistics/health/causes-death/causes-death-australia/latest-release

Australian Government Department of Health (2014). National Framework for Action on Dementia 2015–2019. www.health.gov.au/resources/publications/national-framework-for-action-on-dementia-2015-2019

Australian Institute of Health and Welfare (AIHW) (2018). Older Australia at a Glance. People at Risk of Homelessness. AIHW. www.aihw.gov.au/reports/older-people/older-australia-at-a-glance/contents/diverse-groups-of-older-australians/people-at-risk-of-homelessness

Australian Institute of Health and Welfare (AIHW) (2020). Dementia Data Gaps and Opportunities. Cat. no. AGE 105. AIHW, p. 96.

Bosco, A., Schneider, J., Coleston-Shields, D., Higgs, P. & Orrell, M. (2019). The social construction of dementia: Systematic review and metacognitive model of enculturation. *Maturitas, 120*, 12–22. https://doi.org/10.1016/j.maturitas.2018.11.009

Bramble, M., Moyle, W. & McAllister, M. (2009). Seeking connection: Family care experiences following long-term dementia care placement. *Journal of Clinical Nursing, 18*(22), 3118–25. https://doi:10.1111/j.1365-2702.2009.02878.x

Brooker, D. (2007). *Person Centred Dementia Care: Making Services Better.* Jessica Kinglsey Publications.

Broome, E., Dening, T. & Schneider, J. (2019). Facilitating Imagine Arts in residential care homes: The artists' perspectives. *Arts & Health, 11*(1), 54–66. https://doi:10.1080/17533015.2017.1413399

Brown, E., Agronin, M. & Stein, B. (2019). Interventions to enhance empathy and person-centered care for individuals with dementia: A systematic review. *Research in Gerontological Nursing, 13*(3), 158–68. https://doi.org/10.3928/19404921-20191028-01

Brown, J. (2017). Self and identity over time: Dementia. *Journal of Evaluation in Clinical Practice, 23*(5): 1006–12.

Brown, M., Mitchell, B., Quinn, S., Boyd, A. & Tolson, D. (2020). Meaningful activity

in advanced dementia. *Nursing Older People.* https://doi:10.7748/nop.2020.e1171

Chenoweth, L., Stein-Parbury, J., Lapkin, S., Wang, A., Liu, Z. & Williams, A. (2019). Effects of person-centered care at the organisational-level for people with dementia. A systematic review. *PLOS ONE, 14*(2), e0212686. https://doi:10.1371/journal.pone.0212686

Cipriani, G., Danti, S., Nuti, A., Di Fiorino, M. & Cammisuli, D. M. (2020). Is that schizophrenia or frontotemporal dementia? Supporting clinicians in making the right diagnosis. *Acta Neurologica Belgica.* https://doi:10.1007/s13760-020-01352-z

Commonwealth of Australia (2021). Royal Commission into Aged Care Quality and Safety. Final report: Care, dignity and respect. Vol. 1, Summary and recommendations. https://agedcare.royalcommission.gov.au/sites/default/files/2021-03/final-report-volume-1_0.pdf

Davison, T. E., Camões-Costa, V. & Clark, A. (2019). Adjusting to life in a residential aged care facility: Perspectives of people with dementia, family members and facility care staff. *Journal of Clinical Nursing, 28*(21–2), 3901–13. https://doi:10.1111/jocn.14978

Dementia Australia (2020a). Royal Commission into Aged Care Quality and Safety: People with Younger Onset Dementia in the Aged Care System. www.dementia.org.au/sites/default/files/2020-07/Dementia-Australia-submission-on-younger-onset-dementia.pdf

Dementia Australia (2020b). Vascular Dementia. www.dementia.org.au/about-dementia/types-of-dementia/vascular-dementia

Dementia Australia (2020c). Alzheimer's Disease. www.dementia.org.au/about-dementia/types-of-dementia/alzheimers-disease

Dementia Australia (2021). Dementia Statistics. www.dementia.org.au/statistics

DeTure, M. & Dickson, D. (2019) The Neuropathological diagnosis of Alzheimer's Disease. *Molecular Neurodegeneration 14*, 32. https://doi.org/10.1186/s13024-019-0333-5

Durepos, P., Wickson-Griffiths, A., Hazzan, A., Kaasalainen, S., Vastis, V., Battistella, L. & Papaioannou, A. (2017). Assessing palliative care content in dementia care guidelines: A systematic review. *Journal of Pain and Symptom Management, 53*(4), 804–13. https://doi.org/10.1016/j.jpainsymman.2016.10.368

Dyer, S., Gnanamanickam, E., Liu, E., Whitehead, C. & Crotty, M. (2018). Diagnosis of dementia in residential aged care settings in Australia: An opportunity for improvements in quality of care? *Australasian Journal on Ageing, 37*(4), E155–E158. https://doi.org/10.1111/ajag.12580

Fazio, S., Pace, D., Flinner, J. & Kallmyer, B. (2018). Fundamentals of person-centred care for individuals with dementia. *The Gerontologist, 58*(Supplement 1). https://academic.oup.com/gerontologist/article/58/suppl_1/S10/4816735

Fillit, H., Rockwood, K. & Young, J. (2017). *Brocklehurst's Textbook of Geriatric Medicine and Gerontology* (8th edn). Elsevier.

Flicker, L. & Holdsworth, K. (2014). First Nations People and Dementia: A Review of the Research. A Report for Alzheimer's Australia.

Fuchs, T. (2020). Embodiment and personal identity in dementia. *Medicine, Health Care and Philosophy, 23*(4), 665–76. https://doi:10.1007/s11019-020-09973-0

Goeman, D., King, J. & Koch, S. (2016). Development of a model of dementia support and pathway for culturally and linguistically diverse communities using co-creation and participatory action research. *BMJ Open, 6*(12), E013064. https://doi:10.1136/bmjopen-2016-013064

Grande, G., Vetrano, D. L., Cova, I., Pomati, S., Mattavelli, D., Maggiore, L., … Rizzuto, D. (2018). Living alone and dementia incidence: a clinical-based study in people with mild cognitive impairment. *Journal of Geriatric Psychiatry and Neurology, 31*(3), 107–13. https://doi:10.1177/0891988718774425

Harrison, K. L., Ritchie, C. S., Patel, K., Hunt, L. J., Covinsky, K. E., Yaffe, K. & Smith, A. K. (2019). Care settings and clinical characteristics of older adults with moderately severe dementia. *Journal of the American Geriatrics Society, 67*(9), 1907–12. https://doi:10.1111/jgs.16054

Irwin, K., Sexton, C., Daniel, T., Lawlor, B. & Naci, L. (2018). Healthy aging and dementia: Two roads diverging in midlife? *Frontiers in Neuroscience, 10*(275). https://dx.doi.org/10.3389%2Ffnagi.2018.00275

Jeffers, S., Hill, R., Krumholz, M. & Winston-Proctor, C. (2020). Themes of gerotranscendence in narrative identity within structured life review. *GeroPsych, 33*(2), 77–84. https://doi:10.1024/1662-9647/a000235

Killin, L. O. J., Starr, J. M., Shiue, I. J. & Russ, T. C. (2016). Environmental risk factors for dementia: A systematic review. *BMC Geriatrics, 16*, 175. https://doi.org/10.1186/s12877-016-0342-y

Kitwood, T. (1997). *Dementia Reconsidered: The Person Comes First*. Open University Press.

Kulmala, J., Ngandu, T. & Kivipelto, M. (2018). Prevention matters: Time for global action and effective implementation. *Journal of Alzheimer's Disease, 64*, S191–S198. https://doi:10.3233/JAD-179919

Listabarth, S., König, D., Vyssoki, B. & Hametner, S. (2020). Does thiamine protect the brain from iron overload and alcohol-related dementia? *Alzheimer's & Dementia, 16*(11), 1591–5. https://doi.org/10.1002/alz.12146

Livingstone, K. M., Celis-Morales, C., Navas-Carretero, S., San-Cristobal, R., Forster, H., Woolhead, C., ... & Mathers, J. C. (2020). Characteristics of participants who benefit most from personalised nutrition: Findings from the pan-European Food4Me randomised controlled trial. *British Journal of Nutrition, 123*(12), 1396–405.

Low, L., Barcenilla-Wong, A. & Brijnath, B. (2019). Including ethnic and cultural diversity in dementia research. *Medical Journal of Australia*. https://doi:10.5694/mja2.50353

Martinez-Horta, S., Sampedro, F., Horta-Barba, A., Perez-Perez, J., Pagonabarraga, J., Gomez-Anson, B. & Kulisevsky, J. (2020). Structural brain correlates of dementia in Huntington's disease. *NeuroImage: Clinical, 28*, 102415. https://doi.org/10.1016/j.nicl.2020.102415

Morgan, D., Kosteniuk, J., Seitz, D., O'Connell, M., Kirk, A., Stewart, N., … Sauter, K. (2019). A five-step approach for developing and implementing a Rural Primary Health Care Model for Dementia: A community–academic partnership. *Primary Health Care Research & Development, 20*, E29. https://doi:10.1017/S1463423618000968

Moyle, W., Bramble, M., Jones, C. & Murfield, J. (2017). 'She had a smile on her face as wide as the great Australian bite': A qualitative examination of family perceptions of a therapeutic robot and a plush toy. *The Gerontologist, 59*(1), 177–85. https://doi.org/10.1093/geront/gnx180

Moyle, W., Bramble, M., Jones, C. & Murfield, J. (2018). Care staff perceptions of a social robot called Paro and a look-alike plush toy: A descriptive qualitative approach. *Aging & Mental Health, 22*(3), 330–5. https://doi:10.1080/13607863.2016.1262820

Moyle, W., Parker, D. & Bramble, M. (2014). *Care of Older Adults: A strengths based approach*. Cambridge University Press.

Nabe-Nielsen, K., Rod, N. H., Hansen, Å. M., Prescott, E., Grynderup, M. B., Islamoska, S., … Westendorp, R. G. J. (2019). Perceived stress and dementia: Results from the Copenhagen city heart study. *Aging & Mental Health*, 1–9. https://doi:10.1080/13607863.2019.1625304

National Ageing Research Institute (NARI) (2020). Indigenous Cognitive Assessment: Regional and Urban KICA. www.nari.net.au/indigenous-cognitive-assessment

National Institute for Health and Care Excellence (NIHCE) (UK) (2018). Dementia: Assessment, Management and Support for People Living with Dementia and Their Carers. www.nice.org.uk/guidance/ng97

National Institute on Ageing (2018). What is Lewy Body Dementia? Causes, Symptoms, and Treatments. www.nia.nih.gov/health/what-lewy-body-dementia

OECD (2018). Renewing Priority for Dementia: Where Do We Stand? https://www.oecd.org/health/health-systems/Renewing-priority-for-dementia-Where-do-we-stand-2018.pdf

Palmer, J., Smith, A., Paasche-Orlow, R. & Fitchett, G. (2020). Research literature on the intersection of dementia, spirituality, and palliative care: A scoping review. *Journal of Pain and Symptom Management, 60*(1), 116–34. https://doi.org/10.1016/j.jpainsymman.2019.12.369

Power, M. C., Mormino, E., Soldan, A., James, B. D., Yu, L., Armstrong, N. M., … Schneider, J. (2018).

Combined neuropathological pathways account for age-related risk of dementia. *Annals of Neurology, 84*(1), 10–22. https://doi:10.1002/ana.25246

Public Health Agency of Canada (2019). A Dementia Strategy for Canada. www.canada.ca/en/public-health/services/publications/diseases-conditions/dementia-strategy.html

Puxty, J., Abbott- McNeil, D. & Murphy, S. (2009). Brain and Behaviour: The 7 A's of Dementia. Centre for Studies in Aging & Health. www.agefriendlyontario.ca/file/1440download?token=wRZ8WPuU

Quinn, C., Nelis, S. M., Martyr, A., Morris, R. G., Victor, C. & Clare, L. (2019). Caregiver influences on 'living well' for people with dementia: Findings from the IDEAL study. *Aging & Mental Health*, 1–9. https://doi:10.1080/13607863.2019.1602590

Radford, K., Mack, H. A., Draper, B., Chalkley, S., Daylight, G., Cumming, R., … Broe, G. A. (2015). Prevalence of dementia in urban and regional Aboriginal Australians. *Alzheimer's & Dementia, 11*(3), 271–9, https://doi.org/10.1016/j.jalz.2014.03.007

Rylatt, P. (2012). The benefits of creative therapy for people with dementia. *Nursing Standard, 26*(33), 42–7.

Silva, M., Loures, C., Alves, L., et al. (2019). Alzheimer's disease: Risk factors and potentially protective measures. *Journal of Biomedical Science, 26.* https://doi.org/10.1186/s12929-019-0524-y

Toivonen, K., Charalambous, A. & Suhonen, R. (2018). Supporting spirituality in the care of older people living with dementia: A hermeneutic phenomenological inquiry into nurses' experiences. *Scandinavian Journal of Caring Sciences, 32*(2), 880–8. https://doi:10.1111/scs.12519

Trinh, E., Lee, A. & Kim, K. (2019). End-of-life care of persons with Alzheimer Disease: An update for clinicians. *American Journal of Hospice and Palliative Medicine®, 37*(4), 314–17. https://doi:10.1177/1049909119885881

Viaña, J., McInerney, F. & Brodaty, H. (2020). Beyond cognition: Psychological and social transformations in people living with dementia and relevance for decision-making capacity and opportunity. *The American Journal of Bioethics, 20*(8), 101–4. https://doi:10.1080/15265161.2020.1781960

Westbury, J., Gee, P., Ling, T., Kitsos, A. & Peterson, G. (2018). More action needed: Psychotropic prescribing in Australian residential aged care. *Australian & New Zealand Journal of Psychiatry, 53*(2), 136–47. https://doi:10.1177/0004867418758919

World Health Organization (WHO) (2017). Global Action Plan on the Public Health Response to Dementia 2017–2025. WHO. www.who.int/publications/i/item/global-action-plan-on-the-public-health-response-to-dementia-2017---2025

World Health Organization (WHO) (2018). International Classification of Diseases (ICD-11).

World Health Organization (WHO) (2021). Dementia: Key Facts. www.who.int/news-room/fact-sheets/detail/dementia

Yekanians, S., Bramble, M., Randell-Moon, H. & Moran, J. (2019). Co creating and innovating in residential care: Three films by Three Thumb Productions. Paper presented at the Australian Association of Gerontology, Sydney. ALX.

14 Pharmacology

MAREE BERNOTH, PHILLIP EBBS AND MEGAN DANIEL

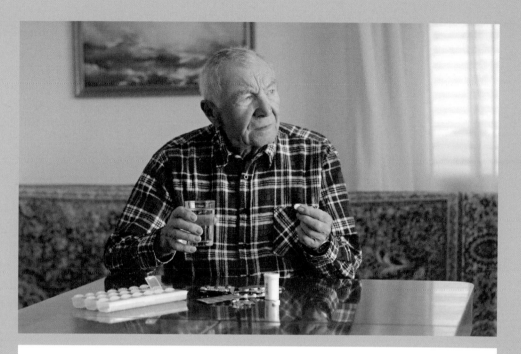

LEARNING OBJECTIVES

After reading this chapter, you will:

» discuss common medication safety issues that relate to the care of older people

» critically discuss the environmental, health-care and personal factors that commonly influence the safe and effective use of medicines by older people, including polypharmacy

» describe the foundational concepts of pharmacokinetics, and how these practically relate to health professionals' care of older people

» describe how foundational concepts in pharmacodynamics relate to older people's safe and effective use of medications

» identify the clinical signs of common adverse effects, adverse drug reactions, and allergic and allergic-like drug reactions that may present in older people.

Introduction

This chapter brings to life a topic that many health-care professionals and students find complex and challenging – that is, the topic of applied pharmacology. Many pharmacology chapters provide extensive scientific information about how medicines interact with the body, and then attempt to apply this knowledge to common pathophysiology and clinical presentations. This chapter takes a different approach. We illustrate the practical circumstances, problems, presentations and even clinical dilemmas faced by modern health-care professionals when dealing with medicines, and then use these realistic examples as a basis to explore the underpinning science and concepts of pharmacology. We do this in an iterative way throughout the chapter so as not to lose sight of what is at the very heart of our health-care professions, which is to deliver safe and high-quality care to people.

In this chapter, we focus on the aspects of pharmacology that will support safe and effective use of medicines among older people across our communities through the use of case studies.

14.1 Getting to know the person: Alex's story

It's late in the evening at Burleigh Hospital, a small facility known for the excellent rehabilitation care it provides to older patients following hip and knee surgery. You've worked here for five years and you love it – you enjoy making a difference in patients' lives, you find it satisfying to help patients regain their quality of life after surgery, and you love the comradery and friendships you have built with other health-care professionals at this small hospital.

Alex is one of your patients who has been making good progress in rehabilitation over recent weeks. However, Alex vomited after a meal this afternoon, which was quite unusual for her. After talking with Alex, a decision was made with the health-care team to observe her for the next few hours to see if the vomiting resolved by itself. Unfortunately, the vomiting has not resolved and it is getting to the stage where the on-call doctor needs to be contacted so that medications can be ordered for Alex.

The on-call doctor is subsequently contacted by one of your colleagues, and the drug metoclopramide (a relatively safe and very common anti-emetic) is ordered. Like most health professionals, you know what type of drug metoclopramide is and have a broad appreciation of how it may work. You are worried, however, that this may not be a safe medication for Alex.

FOCUS QUESTIONS

- In your health profession, do you have a role in identifying medication safety issues?
- For what reasons might you be aware of a potential medication safety issue when other health-care professionals are not?
- Would the medication ordered cause you to have concerns for Alex?

Why is pharmacology important?

Why should all health-care professionals have a basic theoretical and practical knowledge of medicines? After all, not all health-care professionals administer medicines, fewer health-care professionals prescribe medicines, still fewer dispense medications, and no health-care professional acts without some form of oversight and regulation when dealing with medicines.

One might ask, should nurses not simply comply with the medication order provided by the nurse practitioner or doctor? Should paramedics not simply follow the emergency clinical guidelines that are used in their jurisdiction? Should physiotherapists, speech pathologists and occupational therapists not be concerned with the non-pharmacological aspects of care, leaving consideration of medications to other professions? Similar questions could be asked of chiropractors, dentists, medical radiation practitioners, psychologists and many other health-care professions who deal with older people. Yet the simple answer to these questions is 'no'.

When caring for older people, modern health-care professionals cannot afford to be uninformed about medicines any more than they can afford to be unaware of the patients' circumstances at home, changes at work and within their social settings, or changes in their physical environment. The use of medicines is so common among older people, and the effects of medicines can be so substantial on various aspects of an older person's life, that it is simply not reasonable for modern health-care professionals to be uneducated about the basics of pharmacology.

Furthermore, the dynamic and sometimes unpredictable nature of modern life means that mistakes and unexpected developments may occur that risk compromising the safety or effectiveness of a medication being taken by an older person. For this reason, all health-care professionals have a role to play in working with ageing people whose quality of life and well-being may be affected by medications.

Quality care should enhance the older person's health and well-being and avoid reasonably preventable harm. However, the Royal Commission into Aged Care Quality and Safety in Australia has shown that the routine care of older people, particularly in residential aged care, often does not meet these expectations. A number of the commissioner's recommendations to address substandard care specifically focus on improving medication safety. In particular, better medication management, monitoring and review systems and a reduction in the inappropriate prescription of chemical restraints are warranted (Commonwealth of Australia, 2021). These findings reinforce that we have a vital role to play in preventing potential harms caused by medicines, just as we have a responsibility to ensure the care we provide is informed by a basic knowledge of medicines, their intended effects and their common risks.

Implications for practice

As a health-care professional, you have a positive role to play in ensuring the safe and effective use of medicines by:
* identifying mistakes that sometimes occur when medications are ordered, prescribed, dispensed or administered

MAREE BERNOTH, PHILLIP EBBS AND MEGAN DANIEL

- identifying concerns that the older person has about when to take a medication, the effects of a medication and where to get further information about a medication
- monitoring the older person for unexpected changes in their condition that may be caused by medications, or that may require current medicines to be reviewed
- supporting and communicating to ensure that the use of medicines aligns with the older person's goals for their own health and well-being.

<table>
<tr><td>FOCUS
QUESTION</td><td>• Access the competencies and codes that govern your health discipline. Which of these relates to your role as a health professional in relation to medication management and administration?</td></tr>
</table>

Over the remaining sections of this chapter, we will examine the common issues of medication safety among older people and then explore the main branches of pharmacology (pharmacokinetics and pharmacodynamics) to gain a basic understanding of how medications work, how easily therapeutic medications can cause adverse effects in the older people we care for, and importantly, what presentations might alert us to a medication safety issue.

MEDICATION SAFETY

Medicines have revolutionised healthcare over the past 100 years, providing innumerable benefits to humankind, whether by improving the longevity or quality of life, providing the alleviation of pain or discomfort, or providing vaccinations and cures for many illnesses. The impact of medicines on the modern health-care setting is truly remarkable. Yet as health-care professionals, we must also be aware of the significant risks and burdens presented by medicines. This is because – notwithstanding their remarkable benefits – the mistakes, misuse and unintended effects of medicines have also been responsible for countless deaths, preventable disability, lifelong pain and other suffering. When medication errors occur, the family, carers and health-care professionals involved will also experience understandable distress.

Medications represent a remarkable element of modern healthcare, but they come with risks. It is for this reason that all health-care professionals have important roles to play in monitoring, supporting and communicating with older people to ensure the safe and effective use of medications.

<table>
<tr><td>FOCUS
QUESTIONS</td><td>• Access the Australian Commission on Safety and Quality in Health Care website: 'Medication Safety in Australia'. Identify the guidelines that relate to your profession and area of practice.
• After reading the guidelines, refer to case study 14.1. What is your professional responsibility to ensure Alex is safe with regard to his medications?</td></tr>
</table>

Medications and the older person

Healthy, active, desired ageing is the process of feeling good about ourselves, maintaining positive attitudes and keeping fit and healthy as we get older. It is maintaining an active body and mind and continuing to have a meaningful engagement with life. As our population ages, nurses and other health professionals will have the opportunity to support people in the ageing process and to help them to maintain health and quality of life as they adapt to becoming older. As previously explained in this chapter, part of that support will centre on the use of medicines (prescribed or self-accessed) that the older person chooses to utilise. However, to ensure safe and optimal use of medications, the registered nurse and other health professionals must have knowledge of physiological age-related changes, the way the changes affect medications (**pharmacokinetics**), the actions of medications on the older body (**pharmacodynamics**), the impact of using multiple medications (**polypharmacy**) and the vulnerability of older people to **adverse drug reactions (ADRs)**.

Physiological age-related changes

Ageing-related physiological changes affect the way drugs are ingested, absorbed, distributed, metabolised and excreted. Chapter 10 introduced these changes, and of particular relevance to pharmacology are the changes to the gastrointestinal, integumentary, renal and cardiovascular systems. Yet, before any medication is taken, the older person has to access the medication and understand why they are taking the drug, how to take it, when to take it, the possible adverse reactions and then what to do if they have any ADRs. So, the process of attaining a therapeutic drug level is complex.

Ensuring medications are used therapeutically requires models of care such as interdisciplinary teams, person-centred care and collaborative care to achieve optimal health for the older person. Reference to these essential concepts will inform the discussion throughout this chapter, as they are foundational to the ways in which nurses and other health-care professionals advocate for the older person.

Pharmacokinetics

Pharmacokinetics is the process of drug movement to achieve drug action, or how a drug is altered as it travels through the body via four phases (ADME):

- **A**bsorption
- **D**istribution
- **M**etabolism
- **E**xcretion (Kim & Parish, 2021).

Normal age-related physiological changes can have a significant impact on the older body's ability to process and clear drugs efficiently and, with a subsequent predisposition for prolonged duration of drugs within the body, the older person is at increased risk of ADRs. ADRs can be regarded as untoward drug effects (unintended and occurring at normal dose) that may reflect the drug's action in other body tissues, causing mild

Read more about healthy ageing in Chapter 4. See Chapter 10 for more about age-related physiological changes.

pharmacokinetics
The process of drug movement to achieve drug action, or how a drug is altered as it travels through the body.

pharmacodynamics
The study of the way a drug affects the body: a primary (desired) or secondary (desired or undesired) physiological effect, or both.

polypharmacy
The use of more than five medications, often with medications prescribed to address the side effects of the other pharmaceutical products.

adverse drug reaction (ADR)
An untoward drug effect (unintended and occurring at normal dose) that may reflect the drug's action in other body tissues, causing mild to severe side effects, including toxicities, allergic reactions and idiosyncratic side effects.

 MAREE BERNOTH, PHILLIP EBBS AND MEGAN DANIEL

toxicity
Where the blood drug level exceeds the maximum therapeutic range and a harmful and unintended response to the drug results.

idiosyncratic
A rare and unpredictable adverse drug reaction that is specific to the individual (e.g. anaphylaxis); such a reaction is not related to the known pharmacological properties of the drug and does not suggest a dose–response relationship.

pinocytosis
The process by which a cell carries a drug across its membrane by engulfing the drug particles.

bioavailability
The percentage of the administered dose of the unchanged drug that reaches the systemic circulation; for intravenous drugs, it is 100 per cent as the drug is administered directly into the circulatory system.

to severe side effects, including **toxicities**, allergic reactions and **idiosyncratic** reactions (McCuistion et al., 2020).

Looking more closely at the normal age-related changes that affect each of these phases will assist you to understand why drug processing and clearance is altered in older people. Health professionals need to be able to draw on a sound knowledge of pharmacokinetics and pharmacodynamics when assessing for possible ADRs (McCuistion et al., 2020).

ABSORPTION

Absorption refers to the processes by which the drug enters the bloodstream (Bories et al., 2021). A drug can be administered via several routes, with the time for the drug to enter the systemic circulation varying between routes. For example, intravenous drug delivery is instantaneous, but drugs administered by other routes will take longer to reach the bloodstream.

Some of the physiological changes that affect drug absorption in older people are related to two of the body's most extensive surface areas: the gastrointestinal tract (GIT) and the skin. Most drugs, however, are administered orally. The absorption of oral medicines is the movement of drug particles from the GIT to body fluids – passively, actively or via **pinocytosis** – with the mechanism of movement influencing **bioavailability** (McCuistion et al., 2020).

Changes that affect the GIT include reduced blood flow, reduced gastric secretions, prolonged gastric emptying and decreased GIT motility (McCuistion et al., 2020). These changes can result in a longer transit time for food, fluids and medications, increased ADRs and interactions, gastric ulceration and increased use of antacids. Reduction in the intensity of peristaltic movement across the bowel also prolongs medication transit time, potentially increasing the concentrations of some medications and the likelihood of dehydration and constipation.

The site of absorption for most drugs is the small intestine (Burchum & Rosenthal, 2021). Some drugs are protected by an enteric coating so that the active component of the drug is not deactivated by exposure to stomach acids before it reaches the duodenum. However, alterations to gastric pH (acidity) and prolonged gastric emptying associated with ageing might result in the erosion of this enteric coating before the drug has left the stomach, potentially altering the drug's composition and influencing bioavailability. Although the rate of absorption of oral medications is not considered to be significantly altered by normal age-related changes to the stomach, the tendency for older people to use antacids to alleviate symptoms of gastric reflux can raise gastric pH (lower acidity, particularly through altered magnesium levels) and this can block or slow the absorption of certain medications (McCuistion et al., 2020). Examples are digoxin and angiotensin-converting enzyme (ACE) inhibitors such as enalapril (El Hussein et al., 2020). Proton pump inhibitors can also alter gastric pH, thereby affecting drug absorption (El Hussein et al., 2020).

Changes to appetite also have implications for drugs that need to be taken with food in order to achieve optimal absorption (e.g. some antibiotics). Malouh and colleagues (2020) acknowledge that swallowing difficulties arising from pre-existing conditions such as Parkinson's disease or stroke might result in the need to prescribe an oral medication as a syrup. Knowledge of these factors helps nurses understand the need to undertake a thorough medication review with particular attention to potential interactions for medications absorbed via the GIT.

Changes that affect the skin are related to structural changes (resulting in thinning) and alterations to underlying perfusion. These changes include decreased peripheral blood flow and decreased skin hydration (Vonnes & El-Rady, 2021). Altered perfusion and hydration in the skin mean that the uptake of topical medications might be slower, which has implications for drugs such as glyceryl trinitrate patches and transdermal fentanyl, which are intended to provide a sustained effect (Mion & Sandhu, 2016).

The route of administration of a drug is therefore relevant to the process of absorption. This is because some routes of administration (such as the intravenous route) allow a drug to directly enter the bloodstream, while other routes of administration (such as the oral administration of a tablet) rely on the body's physiological processes to help move the drug into the bloodstream. In Table 14.1 we summarise the common routes of drug administration.

TABLE 14.1 Common routes of administration

ROUTE OF ADMINISTRATION	DESCRIPTION
Per Oral (PO)	Swallowed/ingested and absorbed through the gastrointestinal tract
Rectal	Inserted into the anus and absorbed through the colon
Subcutaneous (SC)	Injected under the skin and absorbed through the subcutis
Intranasal/inhaled/ nebulised	Inhaled, usually as a mist, and absorbed via the nasal cavity or lungs
Intramuscular (IM)	Injected into and absorbed through muscle tissue
Sublingual	Dissolved and absorbed under the tongue
Intravenous (IV)	Injected into a vein, absorbed directly into the bloodstream

- What are the age-related changes that impact each mode of administration?
- How can you tailor your practice with the administration of medication to ensure safe, pain-free and optimum use of the drug for an older person?

FOCUS QUESTIONS

DISTRIBUTION

Distribution refers to the processes by which the drug becomes available to the target site of action (e.g. body fluids and tissues). It is influenced by blood flow, the drug's affinity to the particular tissue and protein-binding effects (McCuistion et al., 2020).

Changes that influence drug distribution include less efficiency due to reduced cardiac output, altered body composition and reduced plasma proteins. Lean body mass and total body water both decrease as a person ages, while body fat increases (Vonnes & El-Rady, 2021). This means that volumes of drug distribution are altered. As some drugs are lipophilic and some are hydrophilic, these changes to the older person's body composition will affect their distribution, with potentially unpredictable effects. For example, hydrophilic drugs such as digoxin, atenolol and aminoglycosides could become more concentrated because of the smaller volume of total body water (Greenblatt et al., 2020). Conversely, the increase in total body fat will see an increase in the volume of distribution of lipophilic drugs such as diazepam (Greenblatt et al., 2020).

As drugs are distributed in the plasma, many are bound to varying degrees with protein (mostly albumin). It is the portion of bound drug that is inactive because it is not available to receptors (McCuistion et al., 2020).

Drug binding is competitive, which can increase the chances of drug toxicity in older people who might not be able to produce sufficient plasma proteins (Kaufman, 2015, p. 200). Reduced drug-binding capacity is clinically significant for protein-binding drugs such as phenytoin and warfarin (Roberti et al., 2020). Older adults who are malnourished have even fewer proteins available for drug binding, which makes them more vulnerable to developing toxicities due to increased free concentration of the drug (McCuistion et al., 2020).

14.2 Getting to know the person: Pradesh's story

In addition to suffering poor circulation in his feet due to diabetes, Pradesh, an 80-year-old man, developed a badly infected toe and was administered an intravenous antibiotic to treat this infection. The antibiotic is slowly infused into Pradesh's bloodstream, and from there is distributed throughout Pradesh's body. This results in the antibiotic treating the infected toe, as well as having other effects (positive and negative) on Pradesh's well-being.

Three days after Pradesh received intravenous antibiotics for his infected toe, he is pleased to report that his toe is looking a lot better. However, since having the antibiotics, Pradesh has also suffered persistent bouts of diarrhoea. He reports being otherwise physically well but is distressed because he does not know why he has diarrhoea, or how long it will last.

biotransformation
The process by which the body breaks down and converts a drug into an inactive metabolite, a more potent active metabolite or a less active metabolite.

FOCUS QUESTIONS

- Why might Pradesh have been administered an intravenous antibiotic as opposed to a course of antibiotic tablets?
- Is it safe to assume diarrhoea is related to the antibiotic?
- What are the implications of diarrhoea for an older person?

METABOLISM

'Metabolism' refers to the processes by which the body inactivates or **biotransforms** drugs. In other words, drugs are altered, primarily by the liver, giving rise to inactive **metabolites** or water-soluble **substrates** for excretion (McCuistion et al., 2020).

In an older person, drug metabolism is slower due to reduced blood flow in the liver, a decrease in the size and number of hepatocytes and potentially reduced enzyme production. As liver mass is smaller, altered enzyme production can affect the liver's ability to clear drugs efficiently (Munsterman, 2020). This means the predictability of drug effects will be altered due to increased bioavailability. There is also the potential for more unbound (active) drug to be circulating in the body due to reduced albumin production by the liver (Kaufman, 2015).

metabolite
The intermediate or end product of the breakdown of chemicals in the body.

substrate
The natural environment in which an organism lives.

Reduced hepatic blood flow occurs as a result of reduced cardiac output (Munsterman, 2020). As the rate of hepatic clearance is related to hepatic blood flow, drugs that normally have a high hepatic clearance could become problematic. This is clinically significant for drugs such as morphine, propranolol and verapamil (Roberti et al., 2020).

First-pass metabolism occurs when the drug goes to the liver first to be metabolised. This affects most drugs taken orally. Certain medicines such as glyceryl trinitrate would be lost at first-pass metabolism if taken orally, so an alternative route such as a sublingual or transdermal patch is used in order to optimise the drug's benefit (Bryant et al., 2019).

EXCRETION

'Excretion' refers to the processes by which the drug (or its metabolites) is eliminated from the body. The main route of drug excretion is via the kidneys as urine, but drugs can also be eliminated in bile, faeces, breath and sweat (McCuistion et al., 2020).

Renal excretion is slower in an older person due to reduced renal blood flow and a reduced number of functioning nephrons. Renal blood flow is slower due to reduced cardiac output, so the rate at which the older person's kidneys can filter the blood is delayed. The **glomerular filtration rate (GFR)** starts to decline from about 40 years of age, with an approximate reduction of 45 per cent by 85 years of age (Oster & Oster, 2015). Combined with the reduction in renal mass due to a decrease in the number of nephrons, reduced GFR can lead to drug accumulation, increased serum creatinine and reduced urine creatinine clearance (McCuistion et al., 2020). This means that drugs with a prolonged **half-life** (e.g. digoxin and warfarin) will stay in the older person's body longer, with the risk of cumulative effects (McCuistion et al., 2020).

glomerular filtration rate (GFR)
A measure used to check how well the kidneys are working.

half-life
The time the body takes to excrete half of the dose of a drug.

Older people consume the majority of the population's prescribed medications. In addition, they are known to use a range of **over-the-counter** preparations likely to have some sort of interaction with their prescribed medications (Barry & Hughes, 2021). In many cases, the client's doctor might not have been informed of the concomitant over-the-counter use (Per et al., 2019). When the potential for drug-to-drug interactions remains 'hidden', the monitoring of cumulative side effects or ADRs is not as vigilant, simply because the health professional might not have pre-empted them.

over-the-counter
Substances purchased by the person, without requiring a prescription, from pharmacies, supermarkets, health-food shops and herbalists.

We also know that even in the absence of renal disease, GFR declines in the older person due to normal ageing. If we understand this, we can appreciate that processing multiple medicines is likely to be a challenge to the older person's body. In one way, it can be viewed as older people needing to rely on proportionately less of the organ capacity of a younger person to try to eliminate proportionately more drugs than a younger counterpart.

This is important to recognise for renally excreted drugs such as digoxin. Even though digoxin is prescribed at a lower dose for older people, given the fact that it has a long half-life, even if it is taken exactly as prescribed, there is still a strong potential for toxicity, simply related to the normal decline in GFR. This means that nurses need to be extremely vigilant in monitoring for signs and symptoms of digoxin toxicity and ensuring that digoxin serum levels are regularly checked and doses adjusted (Burchum & Rosenthal, 2021).

To summarise this section, the main ageing-related physiological changes that impact on pharmacokinetics are:

- progressive decrease in total body water and lean body mass and an increase in body fat, which alters the volume of distribution for medicines

- reduction in blood flow and liver size, which can prolong the rate of clearance in medicines that normally rely on a high hepatic extraction rate
- reduction in renal blood flow and kidney mass, which leads to a decline in total clearance for renally excreted drugs such as digoxin, gentamicin and lithium.

Pharmacodynamics

Pharmacodynamics is the study of the way a drug affects the body in terms of a primary (desired) or secondary (desired or undesired) physiological effect, or both (McCuistion et al., 2020). Pharmacodynamics represents the interactions between a drug and its molecular target and the pharmacological result achieved, be that therapeutic or adverse (Bryant et al., 2019). In other words, pharmacodynamics describes what drugs do to the body and how they do it, given the interaction of drug molecules with their target receptors or cells and their biochemical and physiological effects. Adverse responses can be interactions with other medications, side effects, allergic reactions or idiosyncratic reactions.

Pharmacodynamic responses are less predictable in the older person's body, and certain classes of drugs are more likely than others to be associated with ADRs. These include vasodilators, antihypertensives, benzodiazepines, antipsychotics, anticoagulants, anticonvulsants, non-steroidal anti-inflammatories (NSAIDs), opioids and diuretics (Manias et al., 2021).

These particular drug classes are of concern either due to their sedative or blood-pressure-lowering effects or because they increase bleeding tendencies. Even two medications to treat the one comorbid condition, such as cardiac failure, can predispose the older person to falls. Combined with the anticoagulant warfarin, the outcome could be serious bleeding.

As the body ages, there are changes to receptor sensitivity at target sites, which can result in either reduced effectiveness of the drug or increased sensitivity, leading to more side effects, drug–drug interactions or drug–disease interactions (Barber & Robertson, 2020). This means that the effects of some drugs could be less than desired for therapeutic action, while others could be exaggerated (Barber & Robertson, 2020).

A progressive decline in **homeostatic mechanisms** in older people means they can be more sensitive to the effects of some medicines, leading to stronger pharmacodynamic responses and a higher incidence and intensity of ADRs. Examples of the augmented effects of medicines in older people include:

- **orthostatic hypotension** in response to medicines that lower blood pressure
- **hypovolaemia**, dehydration and electrolyte disturbances in response to diuretics
- bleeding complications with oral **anticoagulants**
- **hypoglycaemia** with anti-diabetic medicines
- **gastrointestinal** ulceration with non-steroidal anti-inflammatory drugs (Barber & Robertson, 2020).

A strong pharmacological knowledge base underpins the nurse's ability to monitor medications, safely administer prescribed medications to pre-empt drug–drug interactions, monitor for side effects and provide education about individual drugs and their effects to clients and carers. This knowledge also helps direct the focus towards more astute assessment of the older person and the effects of the prescribed and over-the-counter agents they are taking, how well they understand the place of each medication within their overall health plan and whether adherence and/or ADRs are issues requiring further review.

homeostatic mechanism
A feedback (loop) mechanism involving organs, glands, tissues and cells that respond to changes in the internal and external environment to enable the body to function at an optimum steady state by regulating body temperature, water balance, acid–base balance, blood pressure, blood glucose and gas concentrations.

orthostatic hypotension
A drop in blood pressure when standing.

hypovolaemia
Low fluid levels in the body.

anticoagulant
Medication that thins the blood and makes a person vulnerable to bleeding.

hypoglycaemia
Low blood sugar level.

gastrointestinal
Related to the digestive system.

Specific types of drugs have implications for central nervous system functioning, so they can affect the older person's level of awareness, cognition and safety. Medications that can cause effects to the brain and nervous system include:

- antidepressants
- antiepileptics
- antipsychotics
- anxiolytics
- opioid analgesics
- sedatives (ACSQHC, 2021).

Medications can also cause **anticholinergic** effects in older people. Common groups of drugs with this effect include:

- antidepressants such as amitriptyline and paroxetine
- antipsychotics such as chlorpromazine and trifluoperazine
- drugs for urinary incontinence such as oxybutynin
- antihistamines such as chlorpheniramine
- atenolol, frusemide and nifedipine for cardiac conditions
- opioids such as codeine
- beclomethasone for asthma
- carbamazepine, an anticonvulsant
- beta blockers such as timolol eye drops for glaucoma
- the anticoagulant warfarin (Kim & Parish, 2021).

Anticholinergic effects can result in:

- drowsiness
- confusion
- memory problems
- dry mouth
- constipation
- blurred vision
- dizziness
- urinary retention (Kim & Parish, 2021).

anticholinergic
An agent that causes the loss of water in the body.

These effects can place a significant burden on the individual, causing functional decline and impaired cognition, which compromises not only their safety, but also their quality of life.

Chatterjee and colleagues (2021) outline non-prescription drugs that can also cause anticholinergic effects. These include:

- antihistamines
- cough and cold medicines
- medicines for bowel and stomach cramps
- medicines for nausea and travel sickness
- medicines for urinary incontinence.

Anticholinergic effects are compounded if a prescribed medication is taken in conjunction with a non-prescribed medication that also has an anticholinergic effect (Coupland et al., 2019).

Nurses need to be alert for any medication or non-prescription preparation with anticholinergic effects that an older person is taking because of the effects on cognition and safety. Any older person presenting as confused, or after a fall or trauma, must have a medication review.

Taking just two medications with anticholinergic effects has been found to treble the risk of death in people over the age of 65 years (Ruxton et al., 2015). For this reason, registered nurses and other health professionals need to be aware of the anticholinergic burden of all medications that an older person might be taking (including over-the-counter agents) and advocate on their behalf if necessary. However, this can happen only when a review of the older person's medications is performed regularly – at least every six months – or if there are any signs of adverse reactions, including delirium.

Nurses play a key role in ensuring that medication reviews are not only scheduled but also actually implemented, as many factors can affect the older person's capacity and/or motivation to keep medical appointments. For this reason, nurses are encouraged to ascertain all of the older person's prescribed and over-the-counter medications at every single home visit (McCuistion et al., 2020) and to vigilantly monitor the older person for signs of ADRs, including anticholinergic effects (Pont et al., 2015). This provides another level of pre-emptive monitoring so that the need for more urgent review of the person's medication (and the person themselves) is instigated between scheduled review appointments, as determined by the nurse's assessment.

The previous discussion has provided a summary of the main ageing-related physiological changes that can affect pharmacokinetic and pharmacodynamic processes in the older person. You are encouraged to revisit Chapter 10 and reflect on the ways in which you in your health-care profession could utilise this knowledge in order to help minimise ADRs and to predict undesirable pharmacodynamic responses in the older person.

14.3 Getting to know the person: Hazel's story

Hazel is an 87-year-old woman who lives independently in her own home and continues to safely drive her car. Hazel had remained well thorough her life and disliked taking any medications, even rejecting paracetamol for pain in favour of a hot pack for any joint pain she may have occasionally experienced. She was previously a very active member of the community and is visited often by her family and friends.

Over a period of a few months, Hazel became increasingly breathless in the mornings and tired easily. Her GP referred Hazel to a cardiologist, who diagnosed cardiac **amyloidosis**, prescribed medications and organised for regular appointments to monitor her condition. After some weeks, Hazel's family noticed that she was becoming confused, was repeating information and forgetting significant dates. The assumption was that Hazel's cardiac condition was causing the deterioration of cognition. The family organised for the community nurse to visit and assess Hazel's medications.

amyloidosis
A condition caused by the deposit of abnormal proteins in the muscle of the heart impacting cardiac muscle contraction.

The community nurse asked Hazel to show them the medications and Hazel got a number of boxes and bottles from the cupboard.

Hazel shared with the community nurse, the medications she was taking and when she was taking each of them:

MEDICATION	STRENGTH	FREQUENCY
Minax	100 mgs	Mane
Pradaxa	110 mgs	Mane
Lanoxin	62.5 mcgs	Not certain as Hazel combined this drug and Lasix in one container
Lasix	40 mgs	Not certain as above
Presolol	100 mgs	BD
Spiractin	25 mgs	Nocte

The medications were those prescribed by the cardiologist, but were not taken when prescribed.

The nurse noticed that the Lanoxin and Lasix were in the same container. When she asked Hazel about different-coloured medications in the one container, Hazel replied the names looked the same, so they were tipped into the one container.

- What are the indications for each of the medications Hazel is prescribed?
- Which medications have similar side effects and so present a polypharmacy risk to Hazel?
- What are the potential interactions of these medications?
- What are the main ADRs Hazel is vulnerable to with these medications?
- What are the implications for Hazel taking the medications incorrectly?

FOCUS QUESTIONS

Polypharmacy

Hazel is taking more than five prescribed medications per day. This is typically regarded as polypharmacy, and her risk of experiencing ADRs and the development of geriatric syndrome (cognitive impairment, delirium, falls, frailty, urinary incontinence and weight loss) are greatly increased as a result (Kim & Parish, 2021). Taking multiple medicines can also contribute to medicine errors or misadventures. The more prescription, non-prescription (over the counter), complementary/supplementary and/or traditional medicines an older person takes, the more likely they are to experience medicine problems.

According to Page et al. (2019), 36.1 per cent of older Australians – or 935 240 people – take at least five medications a day. Multiple medications have physical, social and financial implications for the person, as well as higher risk of mistakes in dosage and timing (ACSQHC, 2021). The issues associated with not adequately supporting the older person

 MAREE BERNOTH, PHILLIP EBBS AND MEGAN DANIEL

with medication information (including not providing the information in a way that the person can understand) and simplified regimens give way to adherence problems and an increased risk of ADRs. ADRs are the cause of 20 to 30 per cent of hospitalisation for people 65 years and older in Australia (Li et al., 2021) and are largely preventable.

This highlights the need for health professionals to support the safe and effective use of polypharmacy by older people self-managing medication regimens in the community. Nurses in particular need to be able to facilitate accurate information and strategies in order to increase client and carer health literacy regarding medications (Page et al., 2019).

FOCUS QUESTIONS

- How would you communicate with Hazel to assist her to understand her medications and when they should be taken?

- What could you do to help Hazel to take her medications so they have a therapeutic effect?

- How could you further explore any issues with understanding medication safety so that Hazel is empowered to make informed decisions regarding her medications?

- What could you do to help ensure that both prescribed and over-the-counter medicines are routinely reviewed, and any issues quickly resolved?

Use of non-pharmacological medicines and therapies

Research suggests that half of the older Australian population uses medicines or therapies that are not part of their prescribed (conventional) health-care plans (Barry & Hughes, 2021). This is in part related to traditional practices that are inherent to the older person's particular culture, and also to the fact that dietary supplements, generally considered 'natural' and inexpensive (compared to the cost of prescribed medicines), are easily self-accessed from pharmacies and supermarkets and incorporated into the older person's everyday living. The terms 'complementary medicine' or 'alternative medicine' (CAM) are often used interchangeably with 'traditional medicine' in some countries.

CONSIDERATIONS WHEN A PERSON IS USING NON-PRESCRIPTION MEDICATION

Knowing the pharmacokinetic and pharmacodynamic interactions associated with commonly used CAMs helps to identify the risk of CAM–drug interactions. Information on CAM interactions is not readily provided by the manufacturers, but evidence is available by way of case reports, independent research and web-based resources. Accessing such information can help make the interactions of CAMs with prescribed medicines more predictable, and therefore more preventable (Avila et al., 2020).

Resources for health professionals include online subscription databases that contain comprehensive complementary medicine–drug interaction checkers. One example is the Natural Medicines database.

Pain management

This section is initially based on several of the video case studies. Before commencing this section on analgesia, watch:

- Video 7.1: the video of Mardi and listen to her grandmother's experience of pain

- Video 11.1: Max's video and the way he manages his pain to enable you to engage with the issue of pain and the ways some older people attempt to manage their pain

- Video 11.2: Denise's interview, which has input related to the distraction of music but the outcome when inappropriate music is used.

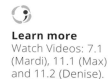

Learn more
Watch Videos: 7.1 (Mardi), 11.1 (Max) and 11.2 (Denise).

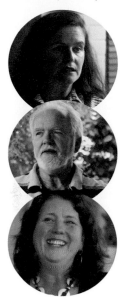

All of these case studies demonstrate the significance of knowing the person, their history and what is important to them, and then show how to work with them to initiate strategies that suit the person. Ask about pain, assess for pain, observe for cues of pain and communicate with the person, their family and carers, and the health-care team. Then be prepared to advocate on the person's behalf for pain relief.

In Australia, the prevalence of pain in older people is estimated to be up to 40 per cent for those dwelling in the community and up to 80 per cent for frail older people in residential aged care facilities (Pain Australia, 2021). Living with pain on a daily basis has significant implications for quality of life as it can affect mood, libido, appetite, sleep, functional ability and socialisation.

The assessment of pain in older people is complicated by a number of known barriers related to the knowledge and attitudes of clients and health professionals and also the progressively diminishing ability of the client with dementia to verbalise their pain and to advocate for themselves in attaining pain relief. The impact of attitudes held by clients, carers and health professionals – that pain is to be expected as a 'normal' part of ageing – can have a marked influence on the older person's decision to report pain and the health professional's decision to proactively assess it (Lane & Smith, 2018). Clients and carers who value stoicism are less likely to report pain, despite it potentially being an important component of a condition that could require urgent investigation and treatment. Failure by nurses to ask about the presence and severity of pain can hinder accurate pain assessment. Accurate pain assessment enables the nurse to initiate nursing interventions such as hot or cold packs, relaxation or whatever strategy the person identified was helpful to them. It is also the nurse's role to advocate on behalf of the person, which may involve communicating with a medical officer for analgesics, or an allied health professional such as a physiotherapist to instigate non-pharmacological pain relief measures. Ongoing assessment and evaluation of pain relief interventions is required to ensure optimal comfort for the older person.

Communication issues that arise as language is progressively lost in clients with dementia also undermine pain assessment and documentation. Health professionals who lack specific knowledge of pain and dementia are more likely to assume that if the older person does not articulate that they have pain, then it is not present. It is imperative that nurses and carers are taught how to recognise the behavioural cues that indicate pain, and to act on these to advocate pain relief for the person with dementia. Nurses need to select appropriate assessment tools such as the Abbey Pain Scale and include family members or carers in the pain assessment process, as they are more familiar with the older person and have a greater understanding of what the changes in behaviour potentially indicate in the individual client (Parkman et al., 2021).

    MAREE BERNOTH, PHILLIP EBBS AND MEGAN DANIEL

As prescribed medications are the mainstay of pain management, the need to balance polypharmacy risks against the harmful effects of unrelieved pain is also an issue for older people. Not all analgesics provide pain relief for all kinds of pain, so prescribing needs to be selective. For example, anticonvulsants and tricyclic antidepressants (as opposed to paracetamol and NSAIDs) would usually be prescribed for a neuropathic pain condition such as shingles, yet the sedative effects of these medications can increase the risk of falls and functional decline in older people (Pickering et al., 2016).

Non-pharmacological interventions are also important to incorporate within a person's pain management plan as they help reduce the burden of polypharmacy and can help people develop a sense of control by promoting sleep and relaxation, stimulating endorphins and/or lifting mood. However, the importance of providing basic nursing care cannot be understated. It is essential to ensure in all encounters with the person that their dignity is maintained and that they are comfortably positioned, well nourished, well hydrated and being cared for with empathy and respect (McCuistion et al., 2020).

> See Chapter 11 for more information on pain assessment and pain management.

<table>
<tr><td>

FOCUS QUESTIONS

</td><td>

- Had you considered that older people may use illegal drugs for recreational or therapeutic purposes?
- How would you raise these possibilities with an older person?
- Would it be significant to ask about alcohol use when doing a medication audit?
- In the case of Mardi's grandmother, what pain-relief strategies would you use in residential aged care to address her pain?

</td></tr>
</table>

Learn more
Watch Video 11.1: Max talks about his hospital experience.

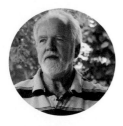

CASCADES OF MEDICATION USE

Max's experience of ageing demonstrates how one condition can affect many body systems and begin a cascade of medication use. His initial health issue was arthritis, which was affecting his ability to play sport, an activity that kept him fit and was also an important opportunity to socialise with his friends; he wanted to maintain his fitness and social contact. Table 14.2 is a list of prescribed medications and other substances Max used to manage his pain and the side effects they caused. So it is not enough for a health professional to suggest or prescribe analgesia; follow-up is required to determine the individual response to the medication, the impact the medication has on the person's life and the need for collaborations in finding interventions that suit the individual.

TABLE 14.2 The list of medications Max used to manage his pain

DRUG	ACTION	IMPLICATION FOR THE PERSON	ADVERSE EFFECT	OUTCOME
MARIJUANA	Hallucinogenic	Alleviated the pain so he could sleep	Impaired cognition, affected ability to work	Ceased
PANADOL OSTEO	Analgesic	Mild pain relief	Insufficient to facilitate a good night's sleep	Continued
PANADEINE FORTE	Strong analgesic	Facilitated sufficient analgesia to enable some sleep	Nausea, constipation, clouded consciousness	Used prn (as needed)
TEMAZEPAM	Hypnotic	Assisted with sleep	Difficulty waking, clouded consciousness	Ceased

TABLE 14.2 Continued

DRUG	ACTION	IMPLICATION FOR THE PERSON	ADVERSE EFFECT	OUTCOME
CORTISONE	Immuno- suppressant	Treatment for bronchiolitis obliterans	Delirium, water retention, diabetes	Gradually weaned off the medication over two years
METFORMIN	Hypoglycaemic	Treatment for diabetes	GI upset, lactic acidosis, impaired renal function	Continued
ZOLOFT	Antidepressant	Treatment for depression	Decreased libido	Ceased

Source: Medication actions are from MIMS Online, 2016.

In his video case study, Max acknowledges that he found little relief in the analgesia he was prescribed and reverted to other means of pain relief such as music and physical activity. His strong family relationships and spiritual beliefs also enable him to manage his pain.

The use of complementary therapies and other strategies that suit the older person is an opportunity for the nurse to provide holistic care and empower people to actively participate in their care and recovery. Holistic care seeks to treat the whole individual, as opposed to treating symptoms exclusively, and recognises the role of the mind, body and spirit in the healing process (Murgia et al., 2020). Mind–body medicine practices concentrate on the influence of the mind over bodily functions and symptoms: meditation, yoga, tai chi and guided imagery are a few examples. Simple interventions such as music therapy or foot and hand massage have been found to be inexpensive, effective and low-risk interventions to help reduce postoperative pain. The advantage of using non-pharmacological therapies such as these in order to promote relaxation and reduce anxiety is that the opioid requirements necessary to achieve adequate analgesia following surgery might be reduced in some individuals.

Learn more
Watch Video 1.1: Listen to Ray discuss the strategies that he and the men in OMNI use to prevent and manage depression.

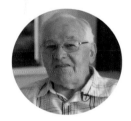

Conclusion

This chapter has discussed the potential impact of multiple medication use on healthy ageing and considered the role of the registered nurse and other health professionals in supporting older people to maintain quality of life, despite needing drug treatment in order to manage comorbid conditions. In particular, this chapter has reinforced the following:

- The use of multiple medications can be both a necessity related to ageing and associated comorbidities and a burden in relation to ADRs arising from altered pharmacokinetic and pharmacodynamic mechanisms, polypharmacy and issues affecting adherence (including under-treatment).
- Comprehensive assessment is a necessary undertaking in order to promote healthy ageing. Taking a thorough medication history, assessing for medication adherence, determining a client's understanding about their medications and monitoring for ADRs are all important aspects of comprehensive assessment.
- Advocating regular medication reviews and simplified medication regimens is an essential part of maintaining the older person's health and wellness, and is aimed at reducing the functional decline and/or cognitive disturbances often associated with polypharmacy.

There is a fine balance to be struck between achieving safe use of medications within the often-complicated medication regimens needed to manage comorbid conditions and

See Chapter 11 for more information on analgesia.

For more information on communicating with older people, see Chapters 3, 12 and 19.

See Chapter 18 for information on health coaching.

MAREE BERNOTH, PHILLIP EBBS AND MEGAN DANIEL

Learn more
Access additional resources – such as weblinks, further readings and podcasts – to broaden your understanding of this chapter. See the Guided Tour for access details.

not being physically, cognitively, psychologically and/or socially restrained by any ensuing ADRs. Part of your role as a health-care professional is to assist the older person to negotiate this balance through assessment of the individual and appropriate support through education, referral and monitoring. This is achieved when the older person sets the goals for treatment in line with their personal preferences and values and is supported in this endeavour by all members of the interdisciplinary team. This is the hallmark of person-centred care and the foundation from which healthy ageing can be successfully promoted and realised.

REVISION QUESTIONS

1   What are some of the most common medication safety issues you need to be aware of when you are working with older people?

2   What are some of the environmental, health-care and personal factors that commonly influence the safe and effective use of medicines by older people? Did you include factors of polypharmacy?

3   How does pharmacokinetics practically relate to your care of older people who are prescribed multiple medications?

4   How do age-related changes impact pharmacodynamics and the effective use of medications?

5   What are the considerations when assessing an older person's ability to manage their medications?

REFERENCES

Australian Commission on Safety and Quality in Health Care (ACSQHC) (2021). APINCH classification of high risk medicines. www. safetyandquality.gov.au/ our-work/medication-safety/ high-risk-medicines/apinchs-classification-high-risk-medicines

Avila, C., Grace, S. & Bradbury, J. (2020). How do patients integrate complementary medicine with mainstream healthcare? A survey of patients' perspectives. *Complementary Therapies in Medicine, 49,* 102317.

Barber, P. & Robertson, D. (2020). *Essentials of Pharmacology for Nurses* (4th edn). McGraw-Hill Education.

Barry, H. E. & Hughes, C. M. (2021). An update on medication use in older adults: A narrative review. *Current Epidemiology Reports,* 1–8.

Bories, M., Bouzillé, G., Cuggia, M. & Le Corre, P. (2021). Drug–drug interactions in elderly patients with potentially inappropriate medications in primary care, nursing home and hospital settings: A systematic review and a preliminary study. *Pharmaceutics, 13*(2), 266.

Bryant, B., Knights, K., Rowland, A. & Darroch, S. (2019). *Pharmacology for Health Professionals* (5th edn). Elsevier.

Burchum, J. & Rosenthal, L. (2021). *Lehne's Pharmacology for Nursing Care E-Book.* Elsevier Health Sciences.

Chatterjee, S., Walker, D., Kimura, T. & Aparasu, R. R. (2021). Prevalence and factors associated with cumulative anticholinergic burden among older long-stay nursing home residents with overactive bladder. *Drugs & Aging, 38*(4), 311–26.

Commonwealth of Australia (2021). Royal Commission into Aged Care Quality and Safety. Final report: Care, dignity and respect. Vol. 2, The current system. https:// agedcare.royalcommission. gov.au/sites/default/ files/2021-03/final-report-volume-1_0.pdf

Coupland, C. A., Hill, T., Dening, T., Morriss, R., Moore, M. & Hippisley-Cox, J. (2019). Anticholinergic drug exposure and the risk of dementia: A nested case-control study. *JAMA Internal Medicine, 179*(8), 1084–93.

El Hussein, M. T., Blayney, S. & Clark, N. (2020). ABCs of heart failure management: A guide for nurse practitioners. *The Journal for Nurse Practitioners, 16*(4), 243–8.

Greenblatt, D., Harmatz, J. S. & Shader, R. L. (2020). Diazepam in the elderly: Looking back, ahead, and at the evidence. *Journal of Clinical Psychopharmacology*, *40*(3).

Kaufman, G. (2015). Multiple medicines: The issues surrounding polypharmacy. *Nursing and Residential Care*, *17*(4), 198–203.

Kim, J., & Parish, A. L. (2021). Nursing: Polypharmacy and medication management in older adults. *Clinics in Integrated Care*, *8*, 100070.

Lane, P. & Smith, D. (2018). Culture, ageing and the construction of pain. *Geriatrics*, *3*(3), 40.

Li, R., Curtis, K., Zaidi, S. T. R., Van, C., Thomson, A. & Castelino, R. (2021). Prevalence, characteristics and reporting of adverse drug reactions in an Australian hospital: A retrospective review of hospital admissions due to adverse drug reactions. *Expert Opinion on Drug Safety*, (just accepted).

Malouh, M. A., Cichero, J. A., Manrique, Y. J., Crino, L., Lau, E. T., Nissen, L. M. & Steadman, K. J. (2020). Are medication swallowing lubricants suitable for use in dysphagia? Consistency, viscosity, texture, and application of the international dysphagia diet standardization initiative (IDDSI) framework. *Pharmaceutics*, *12*(10), 924.

Manias, E., Kabir, M. Z. & Maier, A. B. (2021). Inappropriate medications and physical function: A systematic review. *Therapeutic Advances in Drug Safety*, *12*, 20420986211030371.

McCuistion, L. E., Yeager, J. J., Winton, M. B. & DiMaggio, K. (2020). *Pharmacology-e-book: A Patient-Centered Nursing Process Approach*. Elsevier Health Sciences.

MIMS Online. (2016). www.mims.com.au/index.php/products/mims-online

Mion, L. C. & Sandhu, S. K. (2016). Adverse drug events in older hospitalized adults: Implications for nursing practice. *Geriatric Nursing*, *37*(2), 153–5.

Munsterman, E. (2020). Our aging patients: Are we prepared? *Gastroenterology Nursing*, *43*(4), 320–1.

Murgia, C., Notarnicola, I., Rocco, G. & Stievano, A. (2020). Spirituality in nursing: A concept analysis. *Nursing Ethics*, *27*(5), 1327–43.

Oster, K. A. & Oster, C. A. (2015). Special needs population: Care of the geriatric patient population in the perioperative setting. Association of Perioperative Registered Nurses, *AORN Journal*, *101*(4), 444–56.

Page, A. T., Falster, M. O., Litchfield, M., Pearson, S. A. & Etherton-Beer, C. (2019). Polypharmacy among older Australians, 2006–2017: A population-based study. *Medical Journal of Australia*, *211*(2), 71–5.

Pain Australia (2021). Aged care in pain. www.safetyandquality.gov.au/our-work/medication-safety/high-risk-medicines/apinchs-classification-high-risk-medicines

Parkman, S., Mastel-Smith, B., McGuire, A. & Duke, G. (2021). Insights to identifying and managing pain in persons with dementia in long-term care: A mixed methods study comparing the Abbey pain scale and pain assessment in advanced dementia scale. *Journal of Gerontological Nursing*, *47*(2), 21–30.

Per, B. L., Taylor, A. W. & Gill, T. K. (2019). Prescription medicines, over-the-counter medicines and complementary and alternative medicines use: A comparison between baby boomers and older South Australians. *AIMS Public Health*, *6*(4), 380.

Pickering, G., Marcoux, M., Chapiro, S., David, L., Rat, P., Michel, M., Bertrand, I., Voute, M. & Wary, B. (2016). An algorithm for neuropathic pain management in older people. *Drugs & Aging*, *33*(8), 575–83.

Pont, L. G., Nielen, J. T., McLachlan, A. J., Gnjidic, D., Chan, L., Cumming, R. G. & Taxis, K. (2015). Measuring anticholinergic drug exposure in older community-dwelling Australian men: A comparison of four different measures. *British Journal of Clinical Pharmacology*, *80*(5), 1169–75.

Roberti, R., Palleria, C., Nesci, V., Tallarico, M., Di Bonaventura, C., Irelli, E. C., Morano, A., De Sarro, G., Russo, E. & Citraro, R. (2020). Pharmacokinetic considerations about antiseizure medications in the elderly. *Expert Opinion on Drug Metabolism & Toxicology*, *16*(10), 983–95.

Ruxton, K., Woodman, R. J. & Mangoni, A. A. (2015). Drugs with anticholinergic effects and cognitive impairment, falls and all-cause mortality in older adults: A systematic review and meta-analysis. *British Journal of Clinical Pharmacology*, *80*(2), 209–20.

Vonnes, C. & El-Rady, R. (2021). When you hear hoof beats, look for the zebras: Atypical presentation of illness in the older adult. *The Journal for Nurse Practitioners*, *17*(4), 458–61.

15 Optimal Nutrition and Hydration

MARISSA SAMUELSON AND RUTH CRAWFORD

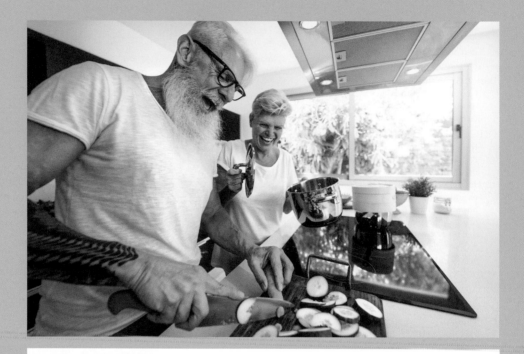

LEARNING OBJECTIVES

After reading this chapter, you will:

- » conclude that nutrition and hydration are more complex aspects of health than people expect

- » explain how maintaining optimal nutrition and hydration for older people involves more than physical aspects of eating

- » describe how diet has a significant impact on optimal health and disease prevention

- » provide examples of supplements and complementary medicines interacting with prescribed medications

- » report the particular nutrition and hydration needs of people with dementia

- » describe the role of the dietitian and understand when to refer an individual for further dietary advice.

Introduction

The question of 'the best diet' to follow to ensure good health and healthy ageing is one of continual interest and debate, not only in academic fields of research, but also in popular and social media. While the proliferation of views on healthy eating and wellness places a well-deserved spotlight on the importance of eating well, it can also lead to an increasing complexity of messages (and misinformation) being sent to consumers and uncertainty about what eating choices to make.

This chapter provides a broad view of the evidence relating to healthy ageing and nutrition in both wellness and ill health, as well as practical strategies for working with older people to improve their overall nutritional health and well-being. We maintain a focus on informed choices and enjoyment of food for optimal quality of life, and helping the reader to apply this evidence to their own unique circumstances or to inform **evidence-based practice**.

Ageing reflects all the changes that happen to a person throughout their life. Individuals can differ significantly with respect to how quickly cells age, so there is no 'one-size-fits-all' approach to dietary advice and healthy ageing. The effects of ageing are very individual, so when supporting people as they age it is appropriate to use a person-centred approach – one that places the needs and wishes of the ageing person in the centre of all care delivery (McCance et al., 2011). Personalisation, when it comes to nutrition, is the role of the dietitian (read more about this later in the chapter).

Healthy ageing, according to Shlisky and colleagues (2017), is not just about living for longer but also about increasing 'healthy active years of life'. Further, not only should we aim to minimise any decline, but we should also challenge the idea that to decline is part of normal ageing. The National Institute on Aging (2006, para. 3) notes that 'some changes that we have long thought of as normal aging can be, in fact, the signs of a potential disease'.

> **evidence-based practice**
> An approach to practice that encourages practitioners to combine research evidence with their own growing understanding and the knowledge of the unique context within which they are working.

- Review Chapter 10. What are the physiological age-related changes that affect nutrition and hydration?

FOCUS QUESTION

Further, the determinants of health extend beyond those related to the individual, and incorporate broader social, cultural, environmental and political factors that are often outside the control of the individual, but considerably more powerful in terms of their influence (Tylka et al., 2014). Nutrition and hydration are complex aspects of health, and maintaining optimal nutrition and hydration therefore involves more than physical aspects. Understanding the person and the unique circumstances that influence their food habits and nutritional status is more meaningful than simply considering their current age and physical state.

The complex range of factors that may influence a person's food and nutrition status are summarised in Table 15.1. It is important to note that these influences may not necessarily always be negative or insurmountable. Vesnaver and colleagues (2012, p. 730) found that many older people demonstrated 'dietary resilience' in the face of these challenges and were able to maintain a healthy diet by 'prioritising eating well, doing whatever it takes to keep eating well, being able to do it yourself and getting help when you need it'.

TABLE 15.1 Factors that may influence a person's food and nutrition status

INFLUENCE	EXAMPLE
Economic	Food budget
	Cost of additional services (such as Meals on Wheels)
	Cost of transport
	Cost of cooking equipment and maintenance of kitchen facilities
Environmental	Proximity to shops
	Availability (and cost) of food delivery services
	Advertising
	Social media and the internet
	Influence of others' opinions about food and nutrition (e.g. health professionals, family members and friends)
	Storage and cooking facilities
Sociocultural	Family structure
	Role in the family
	Living circumstances (e.g. at home or in residential aged care)
	Traditions, values, habits and beliefs (including cultural, social and religious)
	Access to/participation in social activities
	Social support systems
Psychological	Impact of life events such as retirement and bereavement
	Mental health and illness (e.g. depression)
Biomedical	Disease
	Drug-nutrient interactions
	Polypharmacy
	Changes in sensory, immune and gastrointestinal tract function
	Dentition and oral health
	Mobility and exercise
	Balance, strength and endurance

Source: adapted from Bernstein & Munoz, 2012; Mueller, 2015; Shlisky et al., 2017.

Factors that affect nutrition and hydration for older people are illustrated throughout this chapter through Dulcie and John's story.

15.1 Getting to know the couple: Dulcie and John's story

Dulcie migrated to Australia from Italy with her family after World War II in 1952. Her father found work on the Snowy Mountains Hydro Electric Scheme and they settled in the small country town of Cooma.

In her early twenties, Dulcie met and married John, who was a schoolteacher. They welcomed four children over the next decade and John soon became the principal of the local school. Family time while the kids were growing up was usually spent cheering on the kids playing sport and entertaining friends. Dulcie was a nurturer at heart and loved preparing a tasty and nourishing meal for her family and friends to enjoy. Her mother and grandmother had passed down their family recipes to Dulcie and she treasured sharing them with her own children. Their meals were rich with fresh vegetables and fruit from their backyard garden and the house was usually filled with the delicious aromas of home cooking. Cooking from fresh ingredients was very important to Dulcie, given her family background of Type 2 diabetes and John's high cholesterol.

Once the children had grown up and left home, and John had retired from his job, Dulcie and John settled into a comfortable routine in their family home. They were on the pension and tried hard to stick to their budget when they did their weekly grocery shop together. Dulcie's skills as a cook came in handy in thinking up good budget recipes. Dulcie enjoyed her sewing group and John volunteered with the local Rotary organisation. They were both avid readers and Dulcie did regular crosswords, as she had read somewhere it keeps the brain working well.

FOCUS QUESTION

- What are some of the key factors that might influence Dulcie and John's food and nutrition habits at this stage of their lives?

Let's take a closer look at some of the key concerns for Dulcie and John at this life stage and consider what foods and nutrients might be helpful for them to include in their diet.

Healthy diet recommendations

The Australian Dietary Guidelines (NHMRC, 2013) are evidence based and describe a healthy dietary pattern for achieving good health and well-being as well as reducing the risk of diet-related chronic diseases. Your usual diet, which is what you eat most of the time, is what influences your health. The guidelines emphasise plant foods such as vegetables, including legumes, wholegrain cereals, nuts, seeds, fruit and healthy oils. They also include meat and dairy, or the plant alternatives that provide some of the same nutrients. Eating a wide variety of foods from all the foods groups should enable you to meet your nutrition requirements. And let's not forget that food should be fun and enjoyed – so there is room in the guidelines for some **discretionary choices**. You can have that glass of wine with dinner or a piece of chocolate. Processed foods tend to be higher in energy, salt, added sugar and saturated fats and low in other nutrients. Many of the health problems in Australia now stem from not consuming enough of the core food groups, particularly vegetables, fruit and whole grains, so focusing on these foods first will help promote good health. An important caveat about the guidelines is that they do not apply to frail older people. When getting close to end of life, some weight loss may be normal and eating what is desirable is more important for quality of life.

Key nutrients considered important for healthy ageing, as well as some thoughts on energy balance, are summarised in Table 15.2. Other important nutrients, including fibre

discretionary choices
Foods that contain large amounts of fat, sugar, sodium or alcohol, and as a result may also be high in calories and lack important nutrients.

You will find more about end-of-life care in Chapter 19.

and fluid, are covered in later sections. The column on the left lists the recommended nutrients for optimum health and potential roles of the nutrient in the body. The middle column contains information that can be shared with older people (and that you can use for your own good health). References are provided in the right-hand column if you would like to read more. It is important to realise that our understanding of nutrition science continues to deepen, so this is a summary of current and emerging evidence about the relationship between nutrients and health, but it won't be the end of the story. Further, individual requirements for nutrients vary, so it is important for each person to discuss their requirements with a dietitian based on a thorough assessment of nutritional status and needs. While you read this table, keep in mind that foods and nutrients should always be considered in the context of the broader diet. In this table we are referring to the role of nutrients in foods, not in supplemental form.

sarcopenia
Commonly recognised as a loss of muscle mass, and therefore decline in function and strength.

TABLE 15.2 Healthy diet recommendations

RECOMMENDATION	PRACTICAL FOOD ADVICE	REFERENCES
Protein *Maintaining muscle mass, bone mass and a range of other structural and functional components of the body. In particular, protein plays an important role in preventing* **sarcopenia**.	Good food sources include meat, poultry, fish, eggs, dairy, grains, legumes and nuts. One way of ensuring adequate protein intake is to include a protein food at each meal and snack.	Whitney et al. (2017) Cruz-Jentoft et al. (2020) Dolan & Sale (2019) Donaldson et al. (2018) Ganapathy & Nieves (2020) Mossavagh & Vatanparast (2017)
Energy balance	Make sure the person's individual needs for energy and protein are met while they are also getting enough nutrients. If the person is a healthy weight, it is best to focus on nutrient-dense foods from the five food groups. If the person is underweight, at risk of malnutrition or needs to gain weight or muscle mass, they may need to increase their energy and protein intake. Foods that are high in energy and protein tend to be those that fit into the discretionary choices food group in the Australian Guide to Healthy Eating. Good choices from this group include ice-cream, custard and other milk-based desserts, which will provide this extra energy, as well as other nutrients such as protein and calcium.	Wellman & Kamp (2012) NHMRC (2013)
Antioxidants (vitamins E, C and beta-carotene), various phytochemicals *Immune function* *Brain function* *Reducing macular degeneration*	Good food sources include a variety of different coloured vegetables and fruits, as well as wholegrains and nuts.	Whitney et al. (2017) Kalache et al. (2019) Das et al. (2020)
Omega 3 fats *Reducing inflammation* *Mood, cognition* *Reducing macular degeneration* *Maintaining muscle mass*	Good food sources include vegetable oils (canola and flaxseed), walnuts, mackerel, salmon and sardines.	Whitney et al. (2017) Wilkes & Rennie (2009) Holland et al. (2020) Ganapathy & Nieves (2020) Chapman et al. (2019) Cruz-Jentoft et al. (2020)

TABLE 15.2 Continued

RECOMMENDATION	PRACTICAL FOOD ADVICE	REFERENCES
Vitamin B12, folate and vitamin K *Neurological function (vitamin B12)* *Cognitive and heart function (folate)* *Bone health, blood clotting, cognition (vitamin K)*	Good food sources of B12 include all animal foods and fortified products such as breakfast cereals. Good food sources of folate include fortified cereals (e.g. breakfast cereals); vegetables, especially green leafy ones (e.g. spinach, asparagus); lentils; and juice. Good food sources of vitamin K include green leafy vegetables, liver and milk. Vitamin K is also made by bacteria in the intestine.	Whitney et al. (2017) Craenen et al. (2020) Mossavagh & Vatanparast (2017) Alisi et al. (2019)
Vitamin D *Bone strength* *Immune function*	Exposure to sunlight helps the body produce Vitamin D (15 minutes daily is recommended). Good food sources include fortified foods (e.g. margarine, milk), red meat, eggs, liver and sardines.	Whitney et al. (2017) Kalache et al. (2019) Ferreira et al. (2020) Ganapathy & Nieves (2020) Mossavagh & Vatanparast (2017) Martens et al. (2020) Cruz-Jentoft et al. (2020)
Calcium *Bone strength* *Immune function*	Good food sources include animal dairy and calcium-fortified soy products, green leafy vegetables, nuts and seeds, and fish with bones (e.g. sardines).	Whitney et al. (2017) Mossavagh & Vatanparast (2017)
Zinc *Immune function*	Good food sources include high-protein foods (meat, poultry, fish, dairy, grains, legumes and nuts).	Whitney et al. (2017) Das et al. (2020)
Magnesium *Energy production* *Muscle contraction* *Immune function* *Healthy bones*	Good food sources include unprocessed plant foods such as fruits and vegetables, nuts, whole grains, beans and seeds.	Barbagallo et al. (2021)
Sodium	A low-sodium diet is recommended for good heart health and potentially bone health. While it is useful to cut down on added salt to cooking and to the plate at the dinner table, most of the sodium in most people's diets comes from processed foods. Encouraging people to choose low or reduced sodium/salt versions of processed foods (such as biscuits or cheese) and using herbs and spices instead of salt during cooking is helpful.	Fatahi et al. (2018) Whitney et al. (2017)

PREVENTION OF CHRONIC ILLNESS

What we eat plays a significant role in the development of many chronic illnesses, and unfortunately older adults are at higher risk of developing these illnesses. This increased risk is more likely to be the result of poor behaviours such as smoking, inactivity and poor diet quality than ageing per se (Shlisky et al., 2017). Research investigating the influence of food and nutrition on development and prevention of chronic illness is a relatively young field. Much of the research conducted in this area focuses on intake of individual nutrients and foods. For example, recent research has shown there may be an association between increased consumption of ultra-processed foods and a range of chronic illnesses, including cardiovascular disease and cancer, as well as depression and higher all-cause mortality (Elizabeth et al., 2020; Pagliai et al., 2021). Ultra-processed foods are foods that have undergone significant processing, including the addition of several chemicals to increase their palatability (Monteiro et al., 2019). Examples include soft drinks, packaged snacks and breakfast cereals. Of relevance to older adults is the association between processed food intake and **frailty**, possibly due to the likelihood of processed foods displacing other more nutritious foods in the diet (Dorrington et al., 2020).

One of the limitations of this kind of research is that it does not always take into account that we do not eat nutrients or foods alone, but rather we follow a complex pattern of eating composed of a combination of foods as meals and snacks (Fardet & Boirie, 2014). One particular pattern of eating of interest in contemporary research is the **Mediterranean diet** and its impact on prevention of a wide range of diseases. There is strong evidence that those who followed this pattern of eating were less at risk of disease such as cardiovascular disease, coronary heart disease, cancer, neurodegenerative disease and diabetes (Dinu et al., 2018) as well as macular degeneration (Chapman et al., 2019). The authors acknowledge that further research, however, is needed to explore the relationship between eating patterns such as the Mediterranean diet and prevention and development of chronic disease, particularly given that there is no 'one' Mediterranean diet.

Overall, evidence to date suggests that it is a plant-based diet that will deliver the most health benefits and reduce the risk of many chronic diseases (Clinton et al., 2020). This does not have to mean people need to completely exclude all animal foods, such as in the case of vegetarianism or veganism. For example, Dulcie's focus on fruits, vegetables and grains will very likely be of great benefit to her and her family's nutritional health, due to its optimal fatty acid profile (low saturated fat with a greater emphasis on unsaturated fat and adequate carbohydrate). Paying attention to dietary quality – that is, ensuring nutrient adequacy and variety in foods being consumed – is likely to be associated with better health outcomes over the life span (Miller et al., 2020). A simple way to gauge diet quality is to compare how many serves of each of the five food groups are consumed compared to what is recommended by the Australian Dietary Guidelines for a person's age and gender. Note that these guidelines do not apply to frail older people.

Experts in most nations use nutrition research to develop evidence-based dietary reference standards and food guidance systems to form the basis of advice to healthy individuals regarding a healthy diet. In Australia, the Nutrient Reference Values developed by the NHMRC, Department of Health and Ageing and the New Zealand Ministry of Health (2006) are the most current dietary reference standards used to provide guidance regarding nutrient requirements. The *Australian Dietary Guidelines* and the *Australian Guide to Healthy Eating* (NHMRC, 2013) provide practical guidance regarding appropriate intake of different food groups.

MAINTAINING SENSORY, BRAIN AND IMMUNE FUNCTION

As people age, they may experience changes to their sensory, brain and immune function. Sensory aspects of food and eating are very important to Dulcie and her family, and as a couple, Dulcie and John value staying healthy to engage in their hobbies, time with

frailty
Clinically defined as three or more of the following: weight loss, fatigue, weakness, slow walking speed and less activity.

Mediterranean diet
A dietary pattern where plant foods (such as fruit, vegetables, grains, legumes, nuts and seeds) make up the majority of the daily diet, with animal foods (such as dairy, fish, eggs and poultry) consumed in lesser quantities. Wine (consumed at meals in low to moderate amounts) and olive oil are also key components of the diet and fruit is a typical finish to a meal.

their family and in serving their broader community. Key nutrients that may be important to help maintain these bodily functions, as well as good food sources of each nutrient, are listed in Table 15.2 earlier in this chapter. It is important to note that research investigating the impact of nutrition on these body functions is not conclusive, but there is promising evidence emerging in a number of areas, such as a reduced risk of developing Alzheimer's disease in those following a Mediterranean diet (Charlton, 2015). Consuming a balanced diet that is consistent with the Australian Guide to Healthy Eating and correcting any nutritional deficiencies is considered best practice with respect to ensuring a healthy functioning immune system (Calder et al., 2020; Naja & Hamadeh, 2020).

THE MICROBIOME AND HEALTH

A promising area of research is in the exploration of how the health of the trillions of micro-organisms that live in our gastrointestinal system, specifically those in the large bowel (colon), impacts ageing and health outcomes. Scientists have known for a long time that these clever micro-organisms are essential for our bowel to function properly. However, it is now becoming clear that their impact extends well beyond the bowel to other parts and systems within the body, including the brain (Klimova et al., 2020) and immune system (Valdés-Ramos et al., 2010). We also know that the diversity of these micro-organisms declines with age, possibly because of the decline in immune function, leading to inflammation in the gut, leading to increased chance of disorders such as irritable bowel syndrome, diabetes, allergy and heart disease (Kumar et al., 2016). Emerging research also suggests links between gut microbiome with ageing and frailty, given the impact the microbiome has on a number of factors that can lead to frailty, such as inflammation, sarcopenia, insulin resistance and reduced muscle strength (Piggott & Tuddenham, 2020). Diet has a major impact on our microbiome, with plant-based diets likely being most beneficial. However, exact dietary recommendations to cultivate a healthy microbiome have not yet been identified (Kumar et al., 2016; Willis & Slavin, 2020). Other factors – such as genetics, intake of ultra processed foods, physical activity, environmental location and disease – are likely to influence the microbiome as well (Flanagan et al., 2020; Martinez & Campos, 2020).

15.2 Getting to know the couple: Dulcie and John's story

Dulcie and John often spent sunny afternoons walking their dog in the park or tending to their well-loved vegetable and herb garden. They often joked that they should sell their home-grown food because foods from the shop just didn't taste like they used to. Dulcie also worried that they weren't getting enough nutrients from foods from the shop, so she and John took a multivitamin each day to stave off any colds and flu and keep their immune systems functioning well. Dulcie still loved to cook and had recently expanded her repertoire to include homemade pies and cakes.

- What aspects of Dulcie and John's eating habits would you encourage them to continue?
- Are there any issues that may arise in the future as this couple ages? Consider their appreciation of home-grown produce.
- Why might food from the shops taste different?
- What conversations would you initiate with this couple to enhance their nutrition status?

MEDICATIONS

You will find more information about CAMs and medication interactions in Chapter 14.

There are many potential drug–nutrient interactions, including with complementary and alternative medicines, that need to be considered and should be discussed with your doctor or pharmacist.

SUPPLEMENTS

The use of supplements to obtain enough nutrients is a common practice. However, it is important to note that research investigating whether supplementation of vitamins and minerals has health benefits has varying results.

Research into supplementation to improve cognitive function or prevent cancer has found no conclusive evidence and there can actually be adverse effects of supplementation rather than benefit for people with conditions such as Alzheimer's disease (Bernstein & Munoz, 2012; Shlisky et al., 2017; Clinton et al., 2020). The immune system is negatively affected by deficiencies of vitamins and minerals, such as vitamin D, but the evidence for benefits of supplementation in those who are not deficient is unclear (Shlisky et al., 2017; Martens et al., 2020; Wu et al., 2019). In these cases, more research is needed before supplementation can be routinely recommended.

There are other situations where supplementation may be of great benefit. For example, vitamin D supplementation can be very important to help reduce the risk of fractures and falls (Renehan et al., 2012). This may be quite relevant for people who have difficulty moving around and therefore don't spend much time outside. While focusing on foods to obtain nutrients is best, supplementation may also be of benefit when a person is struggling to eat well (Bernstein & Munoz, 2012). In any case, it's always important to refer to a dietitian and GP for further investigation and advice regarding nutrition supplements.

15.3 Getting to know the couple: Dulcie and John's story

Dulcie and John eventually decided that their family home was becoming too large to manage and they moved into a lifestyle village. A few months after they moved, John had a stroke. Because the stroke left John with swallowing difficulties, the speech pathologist in his rehabilitation program had placed him on a puree diet with thickened drinks. Both John and Dulcie struggled to come to terms with this major change in the foods John could eat. He really disliked the texture of the drinks he was given and longed for a normal cup of tea. He was also placed on the medication warfarin.

Previously, John was taking a multi-vitamin that was potentially unnecessary if he was eating enough and including a variety of foods from the five food groups (unless he had a diagnosed deficiency). Now that he has difficulty swallowing, John has started to limit his intake of some foods, especially those that are harder to chew, such as meat. This has led to unintentional weight loss, a key sign that he should be referred for nutrition assessment and nutrition support, which may include nutrition supplements.

- What are some other signs or red flags that could indicate referral for nutrition assessment is warranted?

FOCUS QUESTION

An ageing population means that older people may spend time in hospital and some will live out their lives in residential aged care. In long-term aged care, food does not just contribute to the physical and functional well-being of residents but also to quality of life (Bartl & Bunney, 2015). Bernoth and colleagues (2013, p. 2) argued that the significance of the 'meaning, memories and traditions' of food is greatly increased for these people, and therefore the importance of providing food that has personal meaning as well as aiming to reduce the incidence of **malnutrition** is imperative.

Good nutrition for older people who are in hospital or aged care should:

- include choices that reflect the person's usual habits and preferences, and respect cultural and religious beliefs
- be flexible and adaptable as a person's needs change
- involve eating in dining rooms or with others
- include a balance between food safety (older people are more vulnerable) and quality of life.

It is very important to remember that the *Aged Care Act 1997* (Cth) outlines a charter of care recipients' rights and responsibilities that includes:

- to accept personal responsibility for his or her own actions and choices, even though these may involve an element of risk, because the care recipient has the right to accept the risk and not to have the risk used as a ground for preventing or restricting his or her actions and choices
- to maintain control over, and to continue making decisions about, the personal aspects of his or her daily life, financial affairs and possessions (DSS, 2014).

Unfortunately, protein-energy malnutrition is common in aged care in Australia and has been estimated to affect as many as 68 per cent of residents (Iuliano et al., 2017). A recent systematic review of longitudinal studies found there were a number of factors that increased an older person's risk of becoming malnourished, including age itself, frailty in

malnutrition
The intake of too little or too much energy, protein or other nutrients, causing negative changes in body weight, muscle and fat mass, functionality and wellness.

MARISSA SAMUELSON AND RUTH CRAWFORD

institutionalised individuals, taking many medications, general health decline (including physical and cognitive decline), presence of medical conditions (Parkinson's disease, constipation and dementia), being dependent on another person to eat, loss of interest in life, poor appetite and difficulties in swallowing (Fávaro-Moreira et al., 2016). Institutionalisation was identified as a risk factor on its own, and the latest Royal Commission into Aged Care Quality and Safety has focused on malnutrition in institutions (more on this below).

If a person's intake starts to decline, it may be preferable to consider adding protein and energy in the form of additional foods or enriching existing meals and snacks, before offering commercial oral nutrition supplements (Baldwin & Weekes, 2011; Johnson et al., 2009). For people with increased nutrition needs, try offering larger food serves or seconds; for those with poor appetites, food can be fortified (Bartl & Bunney, 2015). A recent recommendation from the World Health Organization (WHO) is for all older persons at risk of malnutrition to be assessed individually to determine their nutrition needs, and to consider adding ready-to-eat, nutritionally fortified foods as well as encouraging social dining to improve nutritional status (WHO, 2019).

Strategies for doing so include:

- offering preferred or favourite foods, desserts and nutritious mid-meal snacks in larger portions if tolerated and if appetite is not diminished
- fortifying foods, if poor appetite is a problem, with high-energy additions – such as butter, margarine or oil; cream or sour cream; grated cheese; and sugar or honey – or mixing into the food either milk powder or supplements.

15.4 Getting to know the person: John's story

After rehab, John came home to the lifestyle village with Dulcie, but it quickly became too much for Dulcie to look after him, so he moved into a residential aged care facility. Dulcie expects he will be well looked after there, but unfortunately, he is not assured of getting the nutrition care he needs in aged care.

FOCUS QUESTION

- What might be some of the changes Dulcie and John could expect to face in terms of their food and nutrition choices given John's move into aged care?

RESIDENTIAL AGED CARE

The Royal Commission into Aged Care Quality and Safety (RCACQS) has shone the light on a system that fails to meet the needs of many of our vulnerable older people, particularly when it comes to food and nutrition. Even though we would like to think we can stay at home as we get older, we often can't. And if we do go into aged care, we expect that we are going to be looked after. Unfortunately, the Royal Commission found that not all facilities provide the standard of care expected and that the food provided, and the food environment in aged care facilities, is often not good enough. This finding confirmed what many of us have witnessed when working in the sector. The Royal Commission's interim report listed as a major quality and safety issue the 'dreadful food, nutrition and hydration' (Commonwealth of Australia, 2019, p. 6) and the final report identified four quality and safety areas requiring immediate attention, of which food and nutrition was listed first (Commonwealth of Australia, 2021a, p. 92).

The Royal Commission was told that an estimated 22 to 50 per cent of people in residential aged care are malnourished. This increases to 68 per cent when those at risk of malnutrition are also counted (Iuliano et al., 2017). Dehydration and malnutrition can contribute to the rapid decline of people in aged care. Prior to the Royal Commission, food was the number one issue complained about to the aged care complaints commissioner. During the Royal Commission, more than half of the issues raised in the online submissions were about substandard care, and of those 25 per cent were about nutrition and malnourishment. Something as simple as placing drinks out of reach of a person with limited mobility, or lack of assistance at mealtimes resulting in uneaten meals, when repeated day after day, becomes 'neglect' (Commonwealth of Australia, 2021a, p. 11).

Food is such an important part of people's lives, it makes sense they will be upset when the food is bland (Commonwealth of Australia, 2021b, p. 63) and cold (Commonwealth of Australia, 2021a, p. 150). People value mealtimes, and food provides so much more than a plate of nutrition. Mealtimes should be enjoyable and an opportunity to connect and communicate with others. Dining environments need to be positive and stimulate the senses, and residents need to be included in meal and menu planning so that familiar and culturally appropriate choices are offered. Enjoyable dining experiences encourage people to eat more. Further, 'Mealtime experiences can make up 70 per cent of the waking hours of an aged care resident's day and the majority of their social interaction. They directly influence the person's quality of life' (Commonwealth of Australia, 2019, p. 26).

People in aged care need to have a say in what food is served, and the quality of food needs to be assured. It is pleasing to see that the Royal Commission's final report identifies choice for people receiving aged care as a key foundation of future systems. Similarly, it recommends an immediate increase to the 'basic daily fee' of $10/person/day with the directive to specifically address nutritional requirements of aged care residents (Commonwealth of Australia, 2021a, p. 92). The average amount being spent on food was reported as $6.08 per resident per day for all three meals and snacks (Hugo et al., 2018). No wonder the food is dreadful! While increasing the amount spent on food is important, the report falls short by not recommending minimum appropriate staffing and support for residents during mealtimes. You can serve the best food, but if it is on trays out of reach, or if residents need support and encouragement to eat it, then without the staff to do so, the virtually untouched food will still end up in the bins.

TAKING CARE OF THE CARER

As a carer, Dulcie was finding it hard to eat well. When so much energy is being put into caring for someone else, people may experience challenges in obtaining adequate nutrition across the spectrum of buying, storing, preparing and eating foods.

15.5 Getting to know the person: Dulcie's story

When John was in the rehab hospital, Dulcie continued to cook for him and would catch the bus to bring picnic baskets of food each day to his room for them to share – anything to help him enjoy his food. The other residents of the village rallied around Dulcie, realising that while she was tireless in making sure John ate as well as possible, she did not always think of her own needs and was starting to lose weight. Her appetite was often not the best. After a long day sitting with John, she often came home to steaming casseroles or freshly baked cakes on her doorstep.

The following are useful tips you could give carers to help them look after themselves while looking after others. Encourage the person to:

- maintain the pleasure of eating and eat with others when they can
- eat a variety of foods
- have a list of simple, quick, nutritional meals on hand, such as eggs on toast (jazz it up with a bit of relish or some fresh tomato and a sprinkle of cheese), baked beans on toast (add a swirl of sweet chilli sauce and some grated cheese) or a humble Aussie meat pie
- keep a supply of nourishing fluids on hand to replace a meal sometimes (see the section on hydration)
- keep a supply of pre-prepared meals in the freezer (either from leftovers or bought meals) (Renehan et al., 2012).

If fatigue or loss of appetite is an issue for carers, they can be encouraged to:

- eat small amounts more often, which may help them to obtain adequate nutrients over the day
- stay active to help stimulate appetite
- prepare familiar foods in familiar ways
- eat when hungry
- keep nourishing fluids or desserts on hand such as fruit and yoghurt
- eat softer foods that do not require as much effort to chew
- try having a pre-dinner drink to get digestive juices flowing.

An important part of ensuring that nutritional intervention or advice provided to older people is appropriate (or even warranted) is getting to know a person beyond the medical notes and physical data. We need to understand what food means to a person from a social, cultural and psychological perspective. A collaborative approach to decision making about dietary change requires the practitioner to first facilitate a discussion about these influences on dietary habits and what may make a difference to the person's preferences and ability to make change (Samuelson, 2013). Some questions that you could use to help guide conversations with older people include:

- How important is changing your eating habits at the moment? Are there other concerns you have that I could possibly help address?

- What ideas do you have for changing the foods you eat?
- Do you enjoy cooking? What sorts of meals do you like to cook?
- How would you feel about exploring options to eat meals with other people?
- Is there anything stopping you eating the sorts of foods or meals you would like to eat?

- Think about some practical strategies to help Dulcie meet her own nutritional needs while she is focusing on meeting John's needs.

FOCUS QUESTION

Maintaining a healthy weight, adequate muscle mass and bone strength

Loss of muscle mass (sarcopenia), weight and bone mass can in turn lead to a range of health concerns, most notably malnutrition, increased falls risk, impaired healing of wounds and impaired immunity (Bernstein & Munoz, 2012; Renehan et al., 2012, p. 10). This can lead to difficulties in obtaining, preparing and consuming food. As a result, people can get trapped in a vicious circle that leads to further loss of weight, muscle mass and bone strength. Dulcie is currently at risk of falling into this cycle.

Another concern that relates to nutrition is the issue of being overweight. First, we need to acknowledge that the reduction in lean body mass, which is part of normal ageing, leads to a reduction in metabolic rate and makes it more likely that you will gain body fat as you age. As a consequence, for a couple of decades now it has been acknowledged that optimal BMI for older people is a bit higher at 22–27 kg/m² (Sampson, 2009).

It is also important to note that, while being overweight can be of concern in terms of increased risk of chronic illness and cognitive decline, there is some evidence that being overweight may not increase the risk of death compared to those who are a healthy weight (Cheng et al., 2016). While research into the area is continuing, it is possible that there may be some individuals who are in the overweight or obese BMI category who are more metabolically healthy than others (meaning they are less likely to develop Type 2 diabetes or cardiovascular disease) (Cheng et al., 2016; Magkos, 2019). Magkos (2019) argues that based on this, goals relating to behaviour change such as improved physical activity and diet quality are more appropriate goals than weight loss. Further, weight loss in older people can lead to loss of muscle mass (which may or may not be accompanied by loss of fat mass) and therefore affect the person's ability to function well on a daily basis (Bernstein & Munoz, 2012; Renehan et al., 2012), meaning frailty can coexist with being over the healthy weight range (Shlisky et al., 2017). It is therefore important that individuals are assessed by a health professional (such as a dietitian) to ensure that any weight loss or gain goals and interventions are appropriate (Bernstein & Munoz, 2012).

Key nutrients that may be important to help maintain these functions include protein, vitamin D, calcium and sodium. Energy balance is also important to consider. More information about energy and these nutrients, including good food sources of each nutrient, are listed in Table 15.2 earlier in this chapter. It is also recommended to keep participating

MARISSA SAMUELSON AND RUTH CRAWFORD

in a variety of physical activities such as walking for aerobic fitness, yoga for flexibility, and balance and strength training. Regular exercise and strength training are the only way to slow the age-related loss of muscle mass, with authors of a recent review concluding that while there is promise, there are no clear dietary interventions that would provide additional benefit over and above exercise to address sarcopenia (Cruz-Jentoft et al., 2020) or frailty (O'Connell et al., 2020). Without exercise, people will lose 50 per cent of their muscle between the ages of 50 and 80 years (Faulkner et al., 2007). Strength training will also assist with maintaining bone strength. Reduced muscle mass and frailty reduce a person's capacity to recover from illness and to maintain their independence.

15.6 Getting to know the person: Dulcie's story

Sadly, John declined quickly after the stroke and passed away. To support her while she grieved, Dulcie's daughter invited her to stay with her and her family for a few months. Dulcie enjoyed the chance to keep cooking for her family and encouraged her grandchildren to join her in the kitchen. However, when it was time for Dulcie to return home, she struggled to adjust her lifelong cooking and shopping habits – now it was just her, and she was used to cooking large meals. Mealtimes were quiet and simple, when they had once been raucous and busy. The familiar and loved rituals of planning what to eat each day, shopping for ingredients, then preparing, serving and enjoying the meal now seemed like an elaborate and taxing chore. In addition, Dulcie could not drive so it was a challenge to get to the shops to buy her groceries. In the past, Dulcie would have chastised any of her family members that a cup of tea with Vegemite on toast was not a healthy, balanced meal, but nowadays it was a common item on her menu. Her neighbours regularly tried to tempt her to share a meal with them, but Dulcie did not want to be a burden or sadden her friends with her grief. She found herself spending more and more time inside.

Most people would agree that there is much more to food and eating than the health and physical aspects. Food and eating have complex and unique social, cultural and psychological connotations for every one of us and have a significant impact on our quality of life (Bernstein & Munoz, 2012). Where we eat, who we eat with, and what foods we see as acceptable or desirable are often determined by our social connections, cultural backgrounds and feelings or state of mind. People may have limited budgets for food, lack transport to get to the shops to buy food or lack the skills to cook meals (Bernstein & Munoz, 2012).

FOCUS QUESTIONS

- How would you initiate a conversation with Dulcie about her nutrition now that she is alone? What factors might increase her risk of food insecurity?
- How would you work with Dulcie in determining ways for her to maintain optimal nutrition?

15.7 Getting to know the person: Dulcie's story

Over time, Dulcie's family start noticing a few worrying changes in her behaviour. She starts forgetting family events, forgets where she is at times and has trouble remembering family members' names. After a trip to the doctor, Dulcie is diagnosed with the early stages of dementia and moves in with her family permanently.

A person with dementia may forget how to chew and swallow. Loss of appetite, loss of memory and problems with judgment can cause difficulties with food, eating and getting the right nutrition, so it is important to rule out other causes of loss of appetite, such as being unwell or mental health problems. If a person or carer is looking after someone with dementia, it can be challenging and mealtimes can become stressful. Maintaining a person's dignity and as much independence as possible while consuming a varied diet will enhance their quality of life.

Maintaining good oral health

Over the past few decades, the oral health of Australians has improved and there has been a decrease in edentulism (loss of teeth) in older people. However, due to older Australians keeping their natural teeth longer, there has been an increase in **periodontal disease** and tooth decay in this population. The population with the poorest oral health in Australia is older people in residential aged care facilities (Mariño et al., 2015).

Maintaining a healthy body weight is an important factor in oral health. Malnourished people have fewer teeth and reduced chewing ability compared to those with normal nutritional status (Samnieng et al., 2011) and adults who are obese may be more likely to develop periodontal disease (Chaffee & Weston, 2010). A recent review conducted by O'Connor and colleagues (2020) highlighted the importance of good diet quality in reducing the risk of periodontal disease. However, there is still a need for further research in this area.

periodontal disease
Inflammation of the gums (gingivae) and damage to the bone that anchors teeth in the jaws; also called 'gum disease'.

You will find more information about oral health in Chapter 16.

Hydration

Even though nutrition and hydration are intertwined, to assist you with understanding the significance of each, we have covered the two separately. Before commencing this section of the chapter, revise the age-related changes in Chapter 10 and identify any that may affect maintaining hydration for the older person.

The body is more than 50 per cent water, so for it to work properly it is important to keep it well hydrated; this is particularly important for older people and during illness. Dehydration can contribute to constipation, confusion and dizziness, which further affect homeostasis in the older person and have serious consequences for their quality of life, their independence and their health. Dehydration in older people is a risk factor for delirium, so be careful not to pass off this symptom as dementia (Popkin et al., 2010).

There are mixed views in the literature regarding whether increasing fluid intake can prevent the recurrence of urinary tract infections (UTIs) and kidney stones (Perrier et al., 2021; Scott et al., 2020; Zeng et al., 2020). Nevertheless, unless an individual requires reduced fluid intake for medical reasons, it is undoubtedly important to ensure adequate hydration, particularly given the tendency for fluid intake to decline with older age (as described below).

This section addresses some of the common questions people have about fluids.

FLUID REQUIREMENTS

Fluid needs are likely to be highly individualised, but the colour of urine can assist with monitoring hydration levels. Urine should be pale yellow or clear when sufficient fluid is consumed, whereas urine will be dark yellow when inadequate fluid is consumed (Desbrow & Irwin, 2019). Urine colour charts can be used to assess urine colour and hydration status. Cleveland Clinic has produced a useful infographic of urine colours that you can find on its website.

Incontinence occurs when a person accidently or involuntarily leaks urine (or faeces). As a person gets older, this is more common for a number of reasons, including changes to kidney function, blood flow and muscle strength. Medications and illness can also cause incontinence.

Implications for practice

1   Encourage the person to sip on drinks all day. Armstrong (2005) found that once people rated feeling from 'a little thirsty' to 'moderately thirsty' they were already mildly dehydrated. As people get older, they report having reduced thirst and **hypodypsia** relative to younger people (Popkin et al., 2010).

2   Provide easy access for the person to glasses or bottles of water and place these in a number of locations, so they can sip them regularly. Adding a squeeze of lemon or lime, cubes of frozen fruit juice or herbs such as mint might also encourage people to drink more fluid.

3   Remind the person that hot water drinks such as tea count too. Coffee can also count if consumed in recommended amounts.

4   Mineral or soda water are acceptable (note that in Australia most mineral waters have low sodium, but check labels to be sure if there is a need to minimise sodium intake).

5   Encourage the person to alternate alcoholic with non-alcoholic drinks, preferably water.

6   Encourage the person to have a full glass of water rather than just a few sips when swallowing medications.

7   For people with dementia, offer drinks regularly and prompt them to drink. Verbal prompting of nursing home residents and giving their preferred beverages are effective methods for increasing fluid intake to rehydrate, but they rely on adequate staffing or caregiver presence (Dietitians of Canada, 2015).

hypodypsia
Age-related blunting of the thirst response to dehydration.

Role of accredited practising dietitians and when to refer

Simple screening tools are available for all health professionals to use to identify risk or presence of malnutrition in particular. Examples that are appropriate for older people include the Mini Nutritional Assessment – Short Form (Rubenstein et al., 2001) and the Malnutrition Universal Screening Tool (MUST) (Malnutrition Advisory Group, 2003). These tools list simple questions about aspects of nutritional health such as current weight, recent weight loss or changes in intake, and symptoms or health conditions that might be affecting eating (such as depression or loss of appetite). The person is then ranked according to the degree of actual malnutrition or the risk of becoming malnourished, and recommendations can be made with respect to whether further assessment and intervention by an accredited practising dietitian is required.

Accredited practising dietitians work with individuals to deeply understand their nutritional status and needs, and to achieve their dietary goals (Dietitians Australia, 2020a). People who may benefit from talking to a dietitian include:

- those living with chronic illnesses, such as diabetes, cardiovascular disease, cancer or gastrointestinal problems such as diverticulitis
- those requiring advice regarding weight loss or gain
- those requiring practical advice regarding access to food, preparation or storage of food, and eating food
- those requiring advice regarding poor overall intake (and whether supplements might be of use)
- those experiencing symptoms that might affect their nutritional status, including nausea, loss of appetite, diarrhoea or constipation, taste changes, and difficulty chewing or swallowing (Dietitians Australia, 2020b, 2020c).

15.8 Getting to know the person: Dulcie's story

Dulcie has settled into her family's home and is enjoying working to establish a new vegetable and herb garden with her grandchildren. Spending time with them helps Dulcie feel like she has some autonomy and purpose in her day-to-day life, as well as the joy of watching them learn about food and gardening.

- Think about Dulcie and John's journey over this chapter. At what stage/s would you refer them to see a dietitian?

FOCUS QUESTION

Nutritional benefits of intergenerational programs

Intergenerational programs that provide older people with the opportunity to interact and engage with younger people have been shown to have a positive impact on well-being and quality of life for all involved (Giraudeau & Bailly, 2019). Activities often included in these programs can be varied in nature, but might include art, music or educational activities, and can be conducted in a variety of settings including child-care facilities, schools, aged care facilities and the home. A systematic review conducted by Galbraith and colleagues (2015) specifically focusing on dementia, found that there were benefits for individuals to engaging in these sorts of programs, including improved sense of self. The key finding was that it doesn't matter what sort of activity is undertaken by people in these programs. What is most important is that the activity is meaningful and helps to build relationships between participants. While there appears to be little evidence in the literature exploring whether these programs directly influence nutritional status, Shlisky and colleagues (2017) argue that intergenerational interactions can address the nutritional and mental well-being of older adults by increasing dietary resilience. Consideration of what would specifically benefit participants (both older and young people) based on their own needs, values and beliefs would be important in determining whether such a program should be implemented.

Learn more
Access additional resources – such as weblinks, further readings and podcasts – to broaden your understanding of this chapter. See the Guided Tour for access details.

Conclusion

While the question of what is 'the best' diet to follow to age well is still unanswered, it is most likely that eating a wide variety of mostly plant-based, nutrient-dense wholefoods on a daily basis and minimising the intake of processed foods, where possible, is an effective approach to ensuring good health and well-being for all age groups. Nutrition needs depend on a multitude of factors that extend beyond just the biomedical and physical aspects of health, to include the social, cultural, environmental and personal circumstances of the individual. Achieving optimal nutritional status at any stage of life depends on consideration of all of these factors to determine meaningful, personally acceptable and sustainable eating patterns. Health professionals such as dietitians, general practitioners and pharmacists are all well positioned to assist people to make the best choices for their circumstances.

We must employ a person-centred approach when trying to assist and support people to eat a healthy diet as they age. We must respect their usual dietary habits and include them in decision making. Getting people to keep following their usual routine and continuing to complete daily tasks such as food preparation will help maintain knowledge and skills as well as esteem and quality of life.

REVISION QUESTIONS

1 Examine your daily food and fluid intake. What aspects fit with and diverge from the healthy diet recommendations?
2 What strategies would you suggest a health professional use to help you improve your diet? What are the lessons for you as an agent of change?
3 What is the potential impact of loneliness, depression and antidepressant medications on an 85-year-old's nutrition and hydration?

REFERENCES

Alisi, L., Cao, R., De Angelis, C., Cafolla, A., Caramia, F., Cartocci, G., Librando, A. & Fiorelli M. (2019). The relationships between Vitamin K and cognition: A review of current evidence. *Frontiers in Neurology, 10*, 239. https://doi:10.3389/fneur.2019.00239

Armstrong, L. E. (2005). Hydration assessment techniques. *Nutrition Reviews, 63*(6 Pt 2), S40–S54. https://doi:10.1111/j.1753-4887.2005.tb00153.x

Baldwin, C. & Weekes, C. E. (2011). Dietary advice with or without oral nutritional supplements for disease-related malnutrition in adults (Review). *Cochrane Database Systematic Reviews, 9*, CD002008. https://doi:10.1002/14651858.CD002008.pub4

Barbagallo, M., Veronese, N. & Dominguez, L. J. (2021). Magnesium in aging, health and diseases. *Nutrients, 13*(2), 463. https://doi.org/10.3390/nu13020463

Bartl, R. & Bunney, C. (2015). *Best Practice Food and Nutrition Manual for Aged Homes* (2nd edn). https://x2x8z3r3.stackpathcdn.com/wp-content/uploads/BestPracticeFoodandNutritionManualforAgedCare.pdf

Bernoth, M. A., Dietsch, E. & Davies, C. (2013). 'Two dead frankfurts and a blob of sauce': The serendipity of receiving nutrition and hydration in Australian residential aged care. *Collegian, 21*(3), 171–2. http://dx.doi.org/10.1016/j.colegn.2013.02.001

Bernstein, M. & Munoz, N. (2012). Position of the Academy of Nutrition and Dietetics: Food and nutrition for older adults: Promoting health and wellness. *Journal of the Academy of Nutrition and Dietetics, 112*(8), 1255–77. http://doi:10.1016/j.jand.2012.06.015

Calder, P. C., Carr, A.C., Gombart, A. F. & Eggersdorfer, M. (2020). Optimal nutritional status for a well-functioning immune system is an important factor to protect against viral infections, *Nutrients, 12*, 1181; http://doi:10.3390/nu12041181

Chaffee, B. W. & Weston, S. J. (2010). Association between chronic periodontal disease and obesity: A systematic review and meta-analysis. *Journal of Periodontology, 81*(12), 1708–24.

Chapman, N. A., Jacobs, R.J. & Braakhuis, A. J. (2019). Role of diet and food intake in age-related macular degeneration: A systematic review. *Clinical and Experimental Ophthalmology, 47*, 106–127 http://doi:10.1111/ceo.13343

Charlton, K. E. (2015). Mental health: New horizons in nutrition research and dietetic practice. *Nutrition & Dietetics, 72*(1), 2–7. https://doi.org/10.1111/1747-0080.12178

Cheng, F. W., Gao, X., Mitchell, D. C., Wood, C., Rolston, D. D. K., Still, C. D. & Jensen, G. L. (2016). Metabolic health status and the obesity paradox in older adults, *Journal of Nutrition in Gerontology and Geriatrics, 35*(3), 161–76. http://doi:10.1080/21551197.2016.1199004

Clinton, S. K., Giovannucci, E. L. & Hursting, S. D. (2020). The World Cancer Research Fund/American Institute for Cancer Research third expert report on diet, nutrition, physical activity, and cancer: Impact and future directions, *The Journal of Nutrition*, https://doi.org/10.1093/jn/nxz268

Commonwealth of Australia (2019). Royal Commission into Aged Care Quality and Safety. Interim report: Vol. 1. Information gathered and some conclusions. https://agedcare.royalcommission.gov.au/publications/interim-report-volume-1

Commonwealth of Australia (2021a). Royal Commission into Aged Care Quality and Safety Final report: Vol. 1. Summary and recommendations. https://agedcare.royalcommission.gov.au/publications/final-report-volume-1

Commonwealth of Australia (2021b). Royal Commission into Aged Care Quality and Safety. Final report: Vol. 4A. Hearing overviews and case studies. https://agedcare.royalcommission.gov.au/publications/final-report-volume-4a

Craenen, K., Verslegers, M., Baatout, S. & Abderrafi Benotmane, M. (2020). An appraisal of folates as key factors in cognition and ageing-related diseases. *Critical Reviews in Food Science and Nutrition, 60*(5), 722–39. http://doi:10.1080/10408398.2018.1549017

Cruz-Jentoft, A. J., Dawson Hughes, B., Scott, D., Sanders, K. M. & Rizzoli, R. (2020). Nutritional strategies for maintaining muscle mass and strength from middle age to later life: A narrative review. *Maturitas, 132*, 57–64. https://doi.org/10.1016/j.maturitas.2019.11.007

Das, A., Hsu, M. S. H., Rangan, A. & Hirani, V. (2020). Dietary or supplemental intake of antioxidants and the risk of mortality in older people: A systematic review. *Nutrition & Dietetics.* https://doi:10.1111/1747-0080.12611

Department of Social Services (DSS) (2014). Charter of Care Recipients Rights and Responsibilities – Residential Care. https://www.dss.gov.au/sites/default/files/documents/04_2015/charter_of_care_recipients_rights_responsibilities_-_residential_care.pdf

Desbrow, B. & Irwin, C. (2019). Hydration. In R. Belski, A. Forsyth & E. Mantzioris (eds). *Nutrition for Sport, Exercise and Performance: A Practical Guide for Students, Sports Enthusiasts and Professionals*. Allen & Unwin.

Dietitians Australia (2020a). Definition of a Dietitian. https://dietitiansaustralia. org.au/what-dietitans-do/ definition-of-a-dietitian/

Dietitians Australia (2020b). Improving Patient Outcomes through Medical Nutrition Therapy. https://member. dietitiansaustralia.org.au/ Common/Uploaded%20 files/DAA/Resource_ Library/2020/Improving_ Patient_Outcomes- Updated2020.pdf

Dietitians Australia (2020c). Why Choose an Accredited Practising Dietitian? https:// dietitiansaustralia.org.au/ what-dietitans-do/choosing- your-nutrition-expert/

Dietitians of Canada. (2015). Gerontology – Hydration: Summary of Recommendations and Evidence. Practice-based Evidence in Nutrition [PEN]. www.pennutrition. com/KnowledgePathway. aspx?kpid-7997

Dinu, M., Pagliai, G., Casini, A. & Sofi, F. (2018). Mediterranean diet and multiple health outcomes: An umbrella review of meta- analyses of observational studies and randomised trials. *European Journal of Clinical Nutrition, 72*, 30–43. https://doi:10.1038/ ejcn.2017.58

Dolan, E. & Sale, C. (2019). Protein and bone health across the lifespan. *Proceedings of the Nutrition Society, 78*, 45–55. https://doi:10.1017/ S0029665118001180

Donaldson, A. I. C., Johnstone, A. M., de Roos, B. & Myint, P. K. (2018). Role of protein in healthy ageing. *European Journal of Integrative Medicine, 23*, 32–6. https://doi.org/10.1016/j. eujim.2018.09.002

Dorrington, N., Fallaize, R., Hobbs, D. A., Weech, M. & Lovegrove, J. A. (2020). A review of nutritional requirements of adults aged ≥65 years in the UK. *The Journal of Nutrition, 150*, 2245–56. https://doi. org/10.1093/jn/nxaa153

Elizabeth, L., Machado, P., Zinöcker, M., Baker, P. & Lawrence, M. (2020). Ultra- processed foods and health outcomes: A narrative review. *Nutrients, 12*(7), 1955. https://doi.org/10.3390/ nu12071955

Fardet, A. & Boirie, Y. (2014). Associations between food and beverage groups and major diet-related chronic diseases: An exhaustive review of pooled/meta- analyses and systematic reviews. *Nutrition Reviews, 72*(12), 741–62. https:// doi:10.1111/nure.12153

Fatahi, S., Namazi, N., Larijani, B. & Azadbakht, L. (2018). The association of dietary and urinary sodium with bone mineral density and risk of osteoporosis: A systematic review and meta-analysis. *Journal of the American College of Nutrition, 37*(6), 522–32. https://doi:10.1080/073157 24.2018.1431161

Faulkner, J. A., Larkin, L. M., Claflin, D. R. & Brooks, S. V. (2007). Age-related changes in the structure and function of skeletal muscles. *Clinical and Experimental Pharmacology and Physiology, 34*(11), 1091–6. https:// doi: 10.1111/j.1440- 1681.2007.04752.x

Fávaro-Moreira, N. C., Krausch- Hofmann, S., Matthys, C., Vereecken, C., Vanhauwaert, E., Declercq, A., Bekkering, G. E. & Duyck, J. (2016). Risk factors for malnutrition in older adults: A systematic review of the literature based on longitudinal data. *Advances in Nutrition, 7*, 507–22. https:// doi:10.3945/an.115.011254

Ferreira, A., Silva, N., Furtado, M. J., Carneiro, A., Lume, M. & Andrade, J. P. (2020).

Serum vitamin D and age- related macular degeneration: Systematic review and meta-analysis. *Survey of Ophthalmology.* 1–15. https://doi.org/10.1016/j. survophthal.2020.07.003

Flanagan, E., Lamport, D., Brennan, L., Burnet, P., Calabrese, V., Cunnane, S. C., de Wilde, M. C., Dye, L., Farrimond, J. A., Lombardo, N., Hartmann, T., Hartung, T., Kalliomäki, M., Kuhnle, G. G., La Fata, G., Sala-Vila, A., Samieri, C., Smith, A. D., Spencer, J. P. E., Thuret, S., Tuohy, K., Turroni, S., Vanden Berghe, W., Verkuijl, M., Verzijden, K., Yannakoulia, M., Geurts, L. & Vauzour, D. (2020). Nutrition and the ageing brain: Moving toward clinical applications. *Ageing Research Reviews, 62*, 101079. https://doi.org/10.1016/j. arr.2020.101079

Galbraith, B., Larkin, H., Moorhouse, A. & Oomen, T. (2015). Intergenerational Programs for Persons with Dementia: A scoping review. *Journal of Gerontological Social Work, 58*(4), 357–78. https://doi.org/10.1080/016 34372.2015.1008166

Ganapathy, A. & Nieves, J. W. (2020). Nutrition and sarcopenia – What do we know? *Nutrients, 12*, 1755; https://doi:10.3390/ nu12061755

Giraudeau, C. & Bailly, N. (2019). Intergenerational programs: What can school- age children and older people expect from them? A systematic review. *European Journal of Ageing, 16*, 363– 76. https://doi.org/10.1007/ s10433-018-00497-4

Holland, T. M., Agarwal, P., Wang, Y., Leurgans, S. E., Bennett, D. A., Booth, S. L. & Morris, M. C. (2020). Dietary flavonols and risk of Alzheimer dementia. *Neurology, 94*, E1749– E1756. https://doi:10.1212/ WNL.0000000000008981

Hugo, C., Isenring, E., Sinclair, D. & Agarwal,

E. (2018). What does it cost to feed aged care residents in Australia?. *Nutrition & Dietetics, 75*(1), 6–10. https://doi.org/10.1111/1747-0080.12368

Iuliano, S., Poon, S., Wang, X., Bui, M. & Seeman, E. (2017). Dairy food supplementation may reduce malnutrition risk in institutionalised elderly. *British Journal of Nutrition, 117*(1), 142–7. https://doi:10.1017/S000711451600461X

Johnson, S., Nasser, R., Banow, T., Cockburn, T., Voegeli, L., Wilson, O. & Coleman, J. (2009). Use of oral nutrition supplements in long-term care facilities. *Canadian Journal of Dietetic Practice and Research, 70*(4), 194–8. https://doi:10.3148/70.4.2009.194

Kalache, A., de Hoogh, A. I., Howlett, S. E., Kennedy, B., Eggersdorfer, M., Marsman, D. S., Shao, A. & Griffiths, J. C. (2019). Nutrition interventions for healthy ageing across the lifespan: A conference report. *European Journal of Nutrition, 58*(Suppl 1), S1 S11. https://doi.org/10.1007/s00394-019-02027-z

Klimova, B., Novotny, M. & Valis, M. (2020). The impact of nutrition and intestinal microbiome on elderly depression: A systematic review. *Nutrients, 12*, 710. https://doi:10.3390/nu12030710

Kumar, M., Babaei, P., Ji, B. & Nielsen, J. (2016). Human gut microbiota and healthy aging: Recent developments and future prospective. *Nutrition and Healthy Aging, 4*, 3–16, https://doi:10.3233/NHA-150002

Magkos, F. (2019). Metabolically healthy obesity: What's in a name? *American Journal of Clinical Nutrition, 110*, 533–9. https://doi.org/10.1093/ajcn/nqz133

Malnutrition Advisory Group (MAG) (2003). The 'MUST' Explanatory Booklet. A

Guide to the 'Malnutrition Universal Screening Tool' ('MUST') for Adults. http://www.bapen.org.uk/pdfs/must/must_explan.pdf

Mariño, R., Hopcraft, M., Ghanim, A., Tham, R., Khew, C. W. & Stevenson, C. (2015). Oral health-related knowledge, attitudes and self-efficacy of Australian rural older adults. *Gerodontology*. https://doi:10.1111/ger.12202

Martens, P-J., Gysemans, C., Verstuyf, A. & Mathieu, C. (2020). Vitamin D's effect on immune function. *Nutrients, 12*, 1248. https://doi:10.3390/nu12051248

Martinez Leo, E. E. & Segura Campos, M. R. (2020). Effect of ultra-processed diet on gut microbiota and thus its role in neurodegenerative diseases. *Nutrition. 71*, 110609, https://doi.org/10.1016/j.nut.2019.110609

McCance, T., McCormack, B. & Dewing, J., (2011). An exploration of person-centredness in practice. *OJIN: The Online Journal of Issues in Nursing, 16*(2), Manuscript 1. https://doi:10.3912/OJIN.Vol16No02Man01

Miller, V., Webb, P., Micha, R. & Mozaffarian, D. (2020). Defining diet quality: A synthesis of dietary quality metrics and their validity for the double burden of malnutrition. *The Lancet Planetary Health, 4*(8), E352–E370. Global Dietary Database. https://doi.org/10.1016/S2542-5196(20)30162-5

Monteiro, C. A., Cannon, G., Levy, R. B., Moubarac, J-C., Louzada, M. L. C., Rauber, F., Khandpur, N., Cediel, G., Neri, D., Martinez-Steele, E., Baraldi, L. G. & Jaime, P. C. (2019). Ultra-processed foods: What they are and how to identify them. *Public Health Nutrition, 22*(5), 936–41. https://doi:10.1017/S1368980018003762

Mossavagh, E. Z. & Vatanparast, H. (2017).

Current evidence on the association of dietary patterns and bone health: A scoping review. *Advances in Nutrition, 8*, 1–16. https://doi:10.3945/an.116.013326

Mueller, C. M. (2015). Nutrition assessment and older adults. *Topics in Clinical Nutrition, 30*(1), 94–102. https://doi: 10.1097/TIN.0000000000000022

Naja, F. & Hamadeh, R. (2020). Nutrition amid the COVID-19 pandemic: A multi-level framework for action. *European Journal of Clinical Nutrition.* https://doi.org/10.1038/s41430-020-0634-3

National Health and Medical Research Council (NHMRC) (2013). Australian Dietary Guidelines. www.nhmrc.gov.au/adg

National Health and Medical Research Council, Department of Health and Ageing & New Zealand Ministry of Health (2006). Nutrient Reference Values for Australia and New Zealand Including Recommended Dietary Intakes. Commonwealth of Australia.

National Institute on Aging (2006). *Encouraging Eating: Advice for At-home Dementia Caregivers.* www.nia.nih.gov/alzheimers/features/encouraging-eating-advice-home-dementia-caregivers

O'Connell, M. L., Coppinger, T. & McCarthy, A. L. (2020). The role of nutrition and physical activity in frailty: A review. *Clinical Nutrition ESPEN, 35*, 1–11.

O'Connor, J. P., Milledge, K. L., O'Leary, F., Cumming, R., Eberhard, J. & Hirani, V. (2020). Poor dietary intake of nutrients and food groups are associated with increased risk of periodontal disease among community dwelling older adults: A systematic literature review. *Nutrition Reviews, 78*(2), 175–88. https://doi:10.1093/nutrit/nuz035

Pagliai, G., Dinu, M., Madarena, M.P., Bonaccio, M., Iacoviello, L. & Sofi, F. (2021). Consumption of ultra-processed foods and health status: a systematic review and meta-analysis. *British Journal of Nutrition, 125*, 308–18. https://doi:10.1017/S0007114520002688

Perrier, E. T., Armstrong, L. E., Bottin, J. H., Clark, W. F., Dolci, A., Guelinckx, I., ... & Péronnet, F. (2021). Hydration for health hypothesis: A narrative review of supporting evidence. *European Journal of Nutrition, 60*(3), 1167–80. https://doi.org/10.1007/s00394-020-02296-z

Piggott, D. A. & Tuddenheim, S. (2020). The gut microbiome and frailty. *Translational Research, 221,* 23–43.

Popkin, B. M., D'Anci, K. E. & Rosenberg, I. H. (2010). Water, hydration and health. *Nutrition Reviews, 68*(8), 439–58. https://doi:10.1111/j.1753-4887.2010.00304.x

Renehan, E., Dow, B., Lin, X., Blackberry, I., Haapala, I., Gaffy, E., Cyarto, E., Brasher, K. & Hendy, S. (2012). Healthy Ageing Literature Review. Victorian Department of Health. www2.health.vic.gov.au/Api/downloadmedia/%7BAC003F9D-5C1C-4FFB-9F34-199E20EDEED2%7D

Rubenstein, L. Z., Harker, J. O., Salva, A., Guigoz, Y. & Vellas, B. (2001). Screening for undernutrition in geriatric practice: Developing the short-form Mini-Nutritional Assessment (MNA-SF). *Journal of Gerontology, 56*(6), M366–M372.

Samnieng, P., Ueno, M., Shinada, K., Zaitsu, T., Wright, F. A. C. & Kawaguchi, Y. (2011). Oral health status and chewing ability is related to mini-nutritional assessment results in an older adult population in Thailand. *Journal of Nutrition in Gerontology and Geriatrics,* *30*(3), 291–304. https://doi:10.1080/21551197.2011.591271

Sampson, G. (2009). Weight loss and malnutrition in the elderly – the shared role of GPs and ADPs. *Australian Family Physician, 38*, 507–10. www.racgp.org.au/download/Documents/AFP/2009/July/200907sampson.pdf

Samuelson, M. (2013). *Collaborative Decision Making in Early Career Dietetic Practice*. Lambert Academic Publishing.

Scott, A. M., Clark, J., Del Mar, C. & Glasziou, P. (2020). Increased Fluid Intake to Prevent Urinary Tract Infections: Systematic review and meta-analysis. *British Journal of General Practice, 70*(692), e200–e207. https://doi.org/10.3399/bjgp20X708125

Shlisky, J., Bloom, D. E., Beaudreault, A. R., Tucker, K. L., Keller, H. H., Freund-Levi, Y., Fielding, R. A., Cheng, F. W., Jensen, G. L., Wu, D. & Meydani, S. N. (2017). Nutritional considerations for healthy aging and reduction in age-related chronic disease. *Advances in Nutrition, 8,* 17–26. https://doi:10.3945/an.116.013474

Tylka, T. L., Annunziato, R. A., Burgard, D., Danielsdottir, S., Shuman. E., Davis, C. & Calogero, R. M. (2014). The weight-inclusive versus weight-normative approach to health: Evaluating the evidence for prioritizing well-being over weight loss. *Journal of Obesity*. https://dx.doi.org/10.1155/2014/983495

Valdés-Ramos, R., Martínez-Carrillo, B. E., Aranda-González, I. I., Guadarrama, A. L., Pardo-Morales, R. V., Tlatempa, P. & Jarillo-Luna, R. A. (2010). Diet, exercise and gut mucosal immunity. *Proceedings of the Nutrition Society, 69*(4), 644–50.

Vesnaver, E., Keller, H. H., Payette, H. & Shatenstein, B. (2012). Dietary resilience as described by older community-dwelling adults from the NuAge study 'if there is a will—there is a way!'. *Appetite, 58*, 730–8. https://doi:10.1016/j.appet.2011.12.008

Wellman, N. S. & Kamp, B. J. (2012). Nutrition in aging. In L. K. Mahan, S. Escott-Stump & J. L. Raymond (eds.) *Krause's Food and the Nutrition Care Process*. Elsevier, pp. 442–59.

Whitney, E., Rady Rolfes, S., Crowe, T., Cameron-Smith, D. & Walsh, A. (2017). *Understanding Nutrition* (3rd edn). Cengage Learning Australia.

Wilkes, E. A. & Rennie, M. J. (2009). Healthy ageing: Skeletal muscle. In S. Stanner, R. Thompson & J. L. Buttriss (eds). *Healthy Ageing: The Role of Nutrition and Lifestyle*. Wiley-Blackwell, pp. 88–106.

Willis, H. J. & Slavin, J. L. (2020). The influence of diet interventions using whole, plant food on the gut microbiome: A narrative review. *Journal of the Academy of Nutrition and Dietetics, 120*(4), 608–23. https://doi.org/10.1016/j.jand.2019.09.017

World Health Organization (WHO) (2019). Essential Nutrition Actions: Mainstreaming Nutrition through the Life-course. WHO.

Wu, D., Lewis, E. D., Pae, M. & Meydani, S. N. (2019). Nutritional modulation of immune function: Analysis of evidence, mechanisms, and clinical relevance. *Frontiers in Immunology, 9*(3160). https://doi:10.3389/fimmu.2018.03160

Zeng, G., Zhu, W., Lam, W. & Bayramgil, A. (2020). Treatment of urinary tract infections in the old and fragile. *World Journal of Urology, 38*, 2709–20. https://doi.org/10.1007/s00345-020-03159-2

16 Oral Health

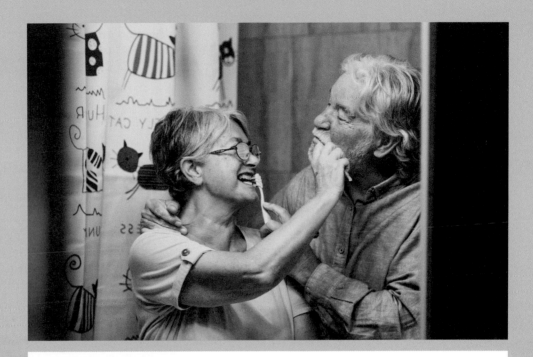

LEARNING OBJECTIVES

After reading this chapter, you will:

» understand age-related changes of the mouth

» explore a basic oral health assessment tool

» become familiar with a basic soft tissue examination

» focus on the more common pathologies that can occur inside and outside of the mouth

» determine when to refer an older person and some referral pathway options.

Introduction

Having a basic understanding of oral health is as important as any other consideration in your journey of lifelong learning as a health-care professional. Why? Because checking someone's mouth, teeth, lips and tongue is as important as checking their general skin integrity and doing their overall health assessment … *it's the same thing!* In fact, studies have concluded that oral health will significantly determine the quality of a person's life (Lewis et al., 2015, p. 96). Oral health care should be considered as important as any other aspect of healthcare. It is everyone's human right to have access to healthcare, including dental care.

The aim of this chapter is to provide health-care professionals with information to do a basic dental exam so they can provide help and support to someone like Anna, who is the person in the case study for this chapter. The goal is to help health professionals know the key indicators to look for, and when, and how to refer the older person for dental care. The aim is to help avoid or reduce the impact that poor oral health can have on an individual, families and the health-care system.

By progressing through Anna's story, significant aspects of oral hygiene will be highlighted to enhance the knowledge and practice of health professionals in this often-neglected aspect of assessing older people.

16.1 Getting to know the person: Anna's story

Anna is 85 years old. She has lived in an aged care facility for three years and has settled in, but misses her home-cooked meals and her independence. Anna was moved into the facility because she has mobility issues related to advanced arthritis and is now in a wheelchair.

Anna used to see her dentist regularly. Since she has had some mobility issues and moved into the nursing home, it has been hard for her and her family to get her out for her yearly dental check-ups. It has been three years since a dental professional has looked at her teeth and gums and undertaken a full dental examination.

Anna still has some of her natural teeth but also wears a partial denture. She finds it hard to use her hands because of the advanced arthritis and loss of strength in her hands and arms. So, it is hard for her to take her denture out to clean it and to brush her natural teeth. She needs help to brush her teeth and clean her denture but feels silly because she can't do it herself. Anna sees the staff are too busy and she hates to ask anyone for help as she doesn't want to be a bother.

Over the past month Anna has had a lot of pain in her mouth, and she finds it hard to eat anything because of the pain. Again, she doesn't say anything because she doesn't want to be a bother and thinks the pain will go away on its own. Staff have noticed that Anna has lost weight and that she isn't eating very much. When they ask her why she isn't eating, she just says that she doesn't like the food and misses her home cooking.

Staff document that Anna has lost her appetite and isn't eating much.

We will explore Anna's story throughout this chapter as just one example of how poor oral health can have a flow-on effect on many other aspects of a person's life. We will explore the impact of treating or neglecting a person's dental symptoms. What if they have no symptoms? What do we look for?

Impacts of oral disease

Figure 16.1, from the NSW Government Department of Health (2014), is a valuable visual representation of the impact and flow-on effect that poor oral health has on the quality of life and health of an older person.

FIGURE 16.1 The impact and flow-on effect of poor oral health on the quality of life of an older person

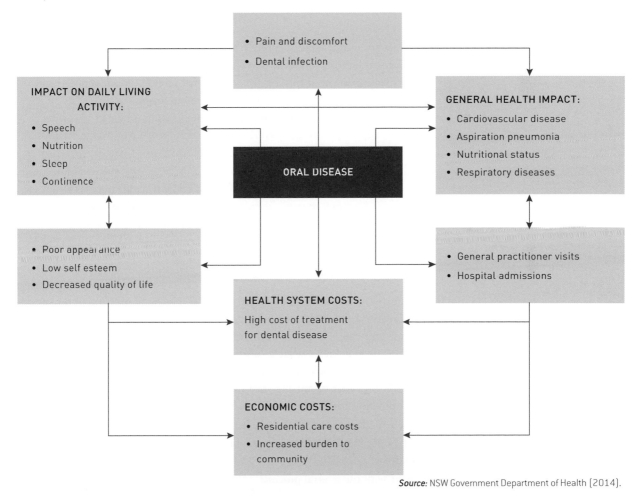

Source: NSW Government Department of Health (2014).

As Anna's story progresses, keep referring to this diagram.
- What is the potential link between Anna's symptoms and her oral health challenges?

FOCUS QUESTION

16.2 Getting to know the person: Anna's story

Family members come to visit Anna and they are worried that she is losing weight and is not her usual happy self. She seems a little withdrawn.

Anna's daughter, Gwen, decides to help her mum brush her teeth and her denture. As she starts to take Anna's denture out, Anna cries out in pain. Gwen goes to get one of the staff members and tells them that her mum appears to be in pain.

The staff member, Hyuk, comes into Anna's room and helps take her denture out. When she looks into Anna's mouth, she reacts with shock and disgust at what she sees. Hyuk doesn't know what she is looking at, but she knows that Anna's mouth does not look right.

Hyuk goes to get another staff member named Yvonne and they find a large, red, swollen area inside Anna's mouth. Gwen asks, 'Has anyone looked in Mum's mouth before? Has anyone been helping her to clean her teeth?' Yvonne replied that it was documented that Anna was not eating well and losing weight. There was nothing documented about Anna's mouth as Anna had not told staff that there was an issue. Yvonne said it was assumed that Anna could brush her own teeth and denture because Anna had never asked for help before.

Anna told her family and the staff that there wasn't an issue and she would be OK: 'It's just a small ulcer'. She states that she doesn't know what all the fuss is about; she has had ulcers before, and they all go away. She says she just wants to spend time with her family and does not want precious time with her family be taken up by talking about something so trivial.

From personal experience working as a dental hygienist in general practice, at university and in residential aged care facilities, the most common situation that I have come across is that nursing staff and carers are not comfortable looking in someone's mouth. Health professionals usually do not know what a 'normal', healthy mouth looks like compared to what an unhealthy mouth looks like. As research has shown, there is limited, if any, oral health education provided to nursing staff in their initial training and their continual professional development (Norrie et al., 2020, p. 537).

The process or procedure of referral can also be very confusing for carers and health professionals if they are concerned about a dental issue. Common questions that health professionals ask are:

• Where do I start with the referral process?

• Who do I refer to?

• Is there even a dental service in town?

16.3 Getting to know the person: Anna's story

Gwen asks the staff what can be done about Anna's mouth and the pain she appears to be in. The staff say they will document the issue and assess the area again soon to see if it goes away. Gwen then asks if she should take her mum to see a dentist. Staff say that it would be very difficult to take Anna out of the facility due to her mobility issues and the nearest dentist is two hours away. It could only really be done if it were urgent, as arranging transport would be difficult. For now, staff will monitor Anna.

Considerations in accessing oral healthcare

Many older people have other complications that affect the possible treatment for oral health care. The following questions may also be pertinent to older people when other issues arise:

- What about cost to the person or family?
- Does that person have a mobility issue?
- Is there travel involved?
- Can that person travel?
- Is there a long waiting list at the public dental clinic?

The aim of this chapter is not to overload or bore you with lots of dental terminology but to give you some visual aids on doing a soft tissue examination and simple explanations about the most common oral pathologies you may come across. This information is just a guide to help make it easier and less daunting to do an oral health assessment. The resources in this chapter will help make the referral pathway look a little clearer and easier even though there is still a fair way to go to making dental care accessible to everyone, including older people and disadvantaged people.

16.4 Getting to know the person: Anna's story

Over the next week, Anna is eating even less and she has lost more weight. She stays in her room more and doesn't want to go to activities.

She isn't socialising with other people and isn't as talkative as usual. Staff find it hard to get her out of bed and her incontinence has gotten worse. She doesn't appear to be her usual happy self; in fact, she has been getting angry and irritable at staff.

The night staff have noted that she is not sleeping well and is often calling out at night. When family come to see her, she stays in bed and doesn't even acknowledge they are there.

Her family have brought in the grandchildren and lots of her favourite foods thinking that this may help. This doesn't appear to work. The family talk to staff members and Anna's doctor. Medications are adjusted and staff members tell Anna's family they will closely monitor her.

Linking oral health with quality of life

Anna's story offers a glimpse of the effect on her quality of life from just one oral health issue. Empowering health professionals to be able to recognise oral health issues and then doing something about them is the focus of the next section. The best way to counteract the flow-on effect of oral health issues is to build your understanding of the changes that occur in the mouth as people age.

FOCUS QUESTIONS

Review Figure 16.1 and link Anna's symptoms with issues identified in the diagram.

- What may have been the outcome for Anna if an oral health and functional assessment had been undertaken when Anna was admitted to the residential aged care facility?

- What oral health services are available, accessible and affordable for older people where you live and work?

Caring for dentures

A full denture is exactly that: the person has none of their own natural teeth and therefore the denture is a complete denture. Figure 16.2a shows an example of a full denture. Even though they do not have their own natural teeth, it is still important to take the dentures out regularly and look under their dentures and around their mouth for any abnormalities or irritations.

A partial denture means that the person still has some of their natural teeth, but not enough, so they need a partial denture. Figure 16.2b shows an example of a lower partial denture. People can also have a partial denture on their top teeth. Again, it's important these are taken out regularly to give the mouth a rest. It's important to check under the denture for any oral tissue abnormalities or irritations.

It's important that appliances like these are cleaned well, twice a day, just like natural teeth as they can harbour plaque (bacteria) and food debris. When cleaning these appliances, it's important to look for any broken or rough areas as these can be a source of irritation in the mouth and a sign of an ill-fitting denture.

FIGURE 16.2 Types of dentures

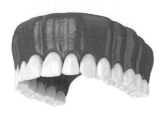

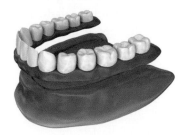

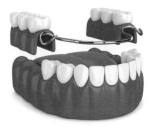

a Full dentures   **b** Partial denture

Age-related changes to the mouth

Does age matter in oral health assessment? Is the issue the age of the individual or other factors that put people at risk of poor oral hygiene?

As skilled clinicians, we look at the individual person, not the number of years lived. For example, the authors of an evidence-based oral health-care assessment called the Seattle Pathway have developed a way to easily recognise an individual's increased risk of oral health conditions based on their dependency, not their age (Pretty et al., 2013).

The Seattle Pathway assesses individuals based on the following:

- no dependency
- pre-dependency
- low dependency
- medium dependency
- high dependency (Pretty et al., 2013).

For example, a 75-year-old man who is fit and well and has good access to dental and medical care could be considered as having no dependency or pre-dependency when it comes to his oral health and general health. He is mobile, can look after himself and would possibly be considered as having a low-to-medium oral health risk.

Compare this with a 50-year-old who has comorbidities, mobility issues and limited access to dental care. This person would be medium-to-high dependency and would therefore have more of a moderate-to-high risk of oral health issues.

The point being, we must treat people as individuals, and the more dependent and frailer individuals become, the more at risk they are of comorbidities, including dental morbidities (Pretty et al., 2013).

As we continue to use the case study of Anna, we can understand the relationship between well-being and oral health. So why is Anna's mouth in the state that it's in?

No matter what age we are, it's important to have our mouths and teeth checked regularly for better oral health, general health and well-being. As we become frailer and have more comorbidities, we become more at risk of dental issues and oral health issues.

In Anna's case she hasn't seen a dental professional for over three years. She is frail and struggles to look after herself.

No one is helping her with cleaning her teeth and denture, so her oral hygiene is poor, and no one is checking her mouth regularly. She leaves her denture in her mouth all the time and no one is checking the denture integrity.

Dentures need to come out of the mouth:

- at night to give the mouth a rest
- for a thorough clean
- to do a check of the mouth
- to check the integrity of the denture.

Anna wears a partial denture that has broken and is rough on her gums and cheek. She also has a broken tooth that the denture sits around, which also stops the denture fitting well.

A couple of things are happening here. If a *denture* does not fit properly, it will rub on gums, teeth and the tissue in the mouth. If there is constant trauma, it can lead to pain and discomfort. It will be less likely to heal in this area because of the constant rubbing due to the ill-fitting denture and the broken tooth. There is a higher risk that the oral cavity can become infected and there is a risk of tissue becoming pre-cancerous with continued trauma.

A *broken tooth* can lead to:

- oral tissue trauma
- a tooth infection or abscess
- serious gum disease
- a major impact on eating, chewing and other general health issues.

If *eating* is compromised, the results include:

- weight loss
- malnutrition and dehydration
- delirium.

Further, the flow-on continues to many other areas of the body.

Anna is not eating because of the pain she is in; her incontinence is worse because of the infection that has started in her mouth, which is impacting on other bodily functions and general health issues. She is getting irritated and less social because of the pain and discomfort she is in, and is isolating herself because of the embarrassment and discomfort she is feeling. She is tired due to lack of sleep and due to being malnourished, dehydrated and having constant pain and an infection in her mouth.

Broken teeth and broken dentures happen, but if found early they can be fixed. If fixed, Anna would be less likely to have all these other health issues.

Anna is not getting help with her oral hygiene routine and therefore no one is regularly checking her mouth for abnormalities. Even if Anna could brush her own teeth and denture, it would still be important for staff members to check her mouth regularly for abnormalities, just as you would check other areas of the body.

Structures of the mouth

Figure 16.3 identifies the major structures of the mouth. It will assist you to understand the names of structures related to oral health and the following sections of the chapter.

FIGURE 16.3 Anatomy of the oral cavity

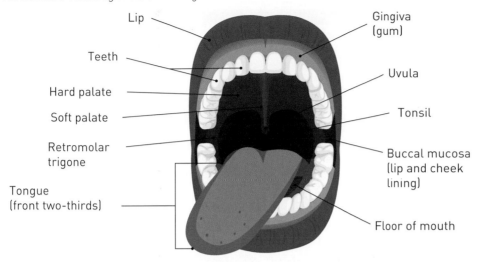

The age-related changes listed in Table 16.1 put older people at a higher risk of many different dental conditions.

TABLE 16.1 Age-related changes to the mouth

AGE-RELATED CHANGE	CAUSE	ISSUES
Xerostomia (dry mouth)	» Polypharmacy » Certain medical conditions (e.g. **Sjogren's syndrome**, diabetes) » Changes to salivary glands – less saliva production	» Increased risk of tooth decay » Increased risk of gum disease » Trouble swallowing » Trouble eating » Discomfort in mouth and throat	**Sjogren's syndrome** An autoimmune condition that can cause a dry mouth.
Tooth decay	» Dry mouth » Increased sugar intake and poor diet » Poor oral hygiene » Gum recession » Poor access to dental care	» Pain » Discomfort » Trouble eating » Gum disease » Broken teeth » Abscess (tooth infection)	
Gum disease **(periodontitis)**	» Dry mouth » Poor oral hygiene » Reduced bone density » Poor access to dental care » Comorbidities	» Pain » Discomfort » Trouble eating » Tooth loss » Bleeding gums » Bad breath » Bad taste in the mouth » General health issues » Gingivitis (red, inflamed gums)	**periodontitis** A bacterial infection that can cause inflammation and bleeding of the gums. In more serious cases it can also lead to bone loss of the jaw.
Gum recession	» Thinner gums » Brushing too hard » Constant rubbing from a denture or other device » Gum disease » Reduced jawbone levels	» Tooth sensitivity » Increased risk of tooth decay » Teeth becoming loose » Wear and tooth erosion	

(Continued)

TABLE 16.1 Continued

AGE-RELATED CHANGE	CAUSE	ISSUES
Missing teeth (**edentulism**)	» Dental caries » Gum disease » Dental abscess and other dental complications	» Trouble eating » Trouble talking » Self-esteem issues » Functional issues in the mouth (how other teeth come together) » More complex dental work (e.g. dentures)
Oral pre-cancer/cancer	» Denture wearing » Bite and chewing changes » Other comorbidities » Smoking	» Ill-fitting dentures -constant rubbing in the mouth » Constantly biting the tongue or cheek

edentulism
No natural teeth.

While Table 16.1 outlines the physiological changes that can happen over time, it does not convey the impacts of oral health on the quality of life of the older person. 'Research has also indicated that tooth loss over time is an ongoing issue for … older people, and there is an association between missing teeth and age as well as missing teeth and oral health-related quality of life' (AIHW, 2018). The pleasure of biting into a crisp apple or chewing a perfectly cooked roast would be lessened by any of these changes. Imagine enjoying life to its fullest if you could only eat soup. These are just some examples, but the point is that all lesions and abnormalities in the mouth should be taken seriously. Any abnormality in the mouth can be a source of:

See Chapter 10 for more detail on age-related changes to all body systems.

- pain
- weight loss (because they cannot eat due to the pain)
- irritability
- being unwell or not seeming like themselves
- reduction in quality of life.

Any abnormality in the mouth, whether it is tooth decay, gum disease, soft tissue lesions or anything else mentioned above, can substantially reduce a person's quality of life if left untreated.

16.5 Getting to know the person: Anna's story

Anna's condition is getting worse. She has had lots of tests done and her medication dose has been increased. No one is sure why her condition has deteriorated. The condition of her mouth has long been forgotten.

Julie, a new staff member, joins the team. The aged care facility that she previously worked at was very thorough in its examinations and assessments on all residents. Oral health assessments were completed on all residents before living at the facility and on a regular basis during their stay.

Julie was helping Anna shower and dress and wanted to help her brush her teeth and denture. When Julie went to remove the denture, Anna cried out in pain. Julie then noticed the large **traumatic ulcer** in Anna's mouth and the broken tooth and denture.

traumatic ulcer
An ulcer that develops through some form of trauma to the mouth.

Julie asked Anna about her pain and discomfort and asked if she had permission to look at her mouth to assess what was going on. Anna gave her verbal consent.

Then Julie decided to do an oral health assessment to document Anna's oral condition.

Julie took notes on what Anna's gums looked like. She noted that Anna's gums looked red and swollen in general, but more so on the top right (patient's right) back area and there was puss and bleeding present here as well.

Julie noted where the denture was broken on the right-hand side. She documented where the ulcer was (top right-hand side on the cheek), how big she thought it was (approximately 1 cm) and that it was red, swollen and raised.

Then Julie noted that Anna's mouth appeared very dry (xerostomia) and her mouth in general did not appear clean, with lots of food debris and plaque everywhere.

She also noted that Anna appeared to be in pain and described how it hurt her to take her denture out. She documented Anna's behavioural changes over the past month. Anna's weight loss and loss of appetite were also added to the assessment.

This oral health assessment was documented and discussed with other staff members and, most importantly, family members were notified. A management plan had to be developed in consultation with Anna and her family. Julie knew it was important to advise Anna's general practitioner (GP) and other staff members involved in Anna's care.

Oral health assessments

An oral health assessment is important for all the reasons mentioned at the beginning of this chapter. It should be a part of your overall health assessment of a person.

A full oral health assessment should be done under the following circumstances:

- Ideally, before someone starts living in an aged care facility and should include an **orthopantomogram (OPG)** x-ray.

- If an oral health assessment has not been completed before entering an aged care facility, then it should be carried out by the nursing staff.

- If someone is receiving home care services and access to a dentist is limited.

Daily assessments should be carried out when helping people brush their teeth and any changes or concerns noted. *Regular assessments are vital for the overall health and well-being of each person.*

orthopantomogram (OPG)
An x-ray of the mouth.

WHAT TO LOOK FOR AND DOCUMENT

When performing an oral health assessment, ensure you consider:

- the individual's health: are other assessments or referrals needed, depending on the pathophysiology?

- any changes to the mouth, cheeks, jaw or lips: you may need to refer the person or keep an eye on this.

Table 16.2 summarises the age-related changes to the mouth, and identifies what is healthy and conditions that raise concerns.

TABLE 16.2 Comparison of a healthy mouth, possible changes and an unhealthy mouth

EXAMINATION	HEALTHY	CHANGES	UNHEALTHY
Lips	Smooth, pink, moist	Dry, chapped or red at corners	Swelling or lumps, red/white/ulcerated/bleeding
Tongue	Moist, pink	Patchy, deep grooves, red, coated	Patch that is red and/or white/ulcerated, swollen
Gums	Moist, pink, no signs of bleeding	Dry, red, swollen, sore, ulcers/sores under dentures	Swollen, bleeding, ulcers, white/red patches, generalised redness under dentures
Saliva	Watery and free flowing	Dry, sticky tissues, person reports a dry mouth	Tissues dry, red, little or no saliva, person reports a dry mouth and difficulty swallowing
Natural teeth	No appearance of decay, no broken teeth	Areas that look like decay or teeth are broken or worn	Areas that look like decay, lots of areas broken or only roots remaining very worn teeth
Dentures	No broken areas, worn regularly with the person's name on them	Broken areas and no name on denture	Lots of broken areas, not fitting well, person doesn't wear them, no name on dentures
Oral cleanliness	Clean, no food particles or plaque in the mouth or on the denture	Food, plaque in small areas of the mouth and denture	Food particles, plaque on most areas of the mouth and denture
Dental pain	No behavioural, verbal or physical signs of dental pain	Verbal or behavioural signs of pain: pulling at the face, chewing lips, not eating, changed behaviour	Physical signs of pain (swelling of cheek, gum, broken teeth, ulcers), as well as verbal and/or behavioural (pulling at the face, not eating, changes in behaviour)

Source: NSW Government Department of Health, 2014.

A BASIC ORAL EXAMINATION

buccal cavity
Structures of the mouth, including lips, cheeks, salivary glands and tongue.

Table 16.3 outlines the steps for a basic oral examination. When doing a soft tissue exam on a person, you can use their toothbrush as a retraction tool. In these photos, a dental mirror is being used, but the handle of a toothbrush will work just as well. These pictures represent a healthy mouth.

TABLE 16.3 Steps in a basic oral examination

EXAMINATION AREA	WHAT TO LOOK FOR IN YOUR ASSESSMENT OF THE BUCCAL CAVITY	IMAGE OF A HEALTHY MOUTH
In the **buccal cavity**, look for all of the following: *Cheeks*	» Note the colour: normal pink appearance » This is a healthy mouth » There are no lesions, the tissue looks intact	

TABLE 16.3 Continued

EXAMINATION AREA	WHAT TO LOOK FOR IN YOUR ASSESSMENT OF THE BUCCAL CAVITY	IMAGE OF A HEALTHY MOUTH
Upper lip and top front teeth	» Note the colour: normal pink appearance » The tissue appears intact » Note the teeth: there appears to be no discoloration and the tooth surface appears intact; there are no breakages or holes	
Upper corners of the mouth and upper posterior teeth	» Note the colour of the tissue: there are no breakages in the tissue integrity » Note the teeth: there are no discoloured areas and the tooth surfaces appear intact	
Lower lip and lower front teeth	» Note the healthy pink colour and intact tissue » You may sometimes see blood vessels closer to the surface. » Note the teeth: no holes or discolouration; the surfaces are intact	
Lower corners of the mouth, lips and teeth	» Tissue is pink and intact » Note the saliva and moist appearance of the surrounding tissue » The tooth surfaces appear intact	
Floor of the mouth, under tongue and bottom teeth	» Tissue is pink and intact » Note the saliva flow » Teeth appear intact » There are no unusual lumps or discolouration » Note the raised area on the floor of the mouth: this forms the salivary duct under the tongue » Some people have more pronounced veins in this area	
Roof of the mouth and upper teeth	» Note the colour » The colour may change slightly towards the back of the mouth as in this photo » There can also be grooves and ridges towards the front of the mouth (this is normal) » It is *not* normal if any areas are discoloured, swollen or there are any breaks in the tissue	
Top of the tongue	» If possible, try to get the person to stick out their tongue » If this is not possible, you can get a good view of the tongue when you are looking at other areas of the mouth » An unhealthy tongue is dry, may be coated and the tissue isn't intact	

(Continued)

SIMONE ALEXANDER

TABLE 16.3 Continued

EXAMINATION AREA	WHAT TO LOOK FOR IN YOUR ASSESSMENT OF THE BUCCAL CAVITY	IMAGE OF A HEALTHY MOUTH
Side of the tongue	» Note the intact tissue » There are no signs of lesions or inflammation	
Under the tongue	» This is a good example of the blood vessels that can be pronounced under the tongue	

Photos courtesy of Dr Sue-Ching Yeoh.

16.6 Getting to know the person: Anna's story

When Gwen was notified about the decline in Anna's mouth, and her general health, she stated she wanted the best treatment for her mum. However, a few concerns were raised.

Gwen lives several hundred kilometres from the facility. The only dental surgery is a few hours away and there is the issue of Anna's mobility. Her general health has declined so much over the past month, due to her mouth condition, that getting her out of bed would be a major issue.

They also didn't know if the local dentist would be able to see someone so frail and with mobility issues. Would the local dental surgery be able to fit her and her wheelchair in the surgery? How long would they need to make the appointment for as a two-hour trip to see the dentist would be hard enough, let alone doing it several times.

In addition, Anna tells Gwen that she doesn't want to go and that everyone is making a fuss about nothing.

How were they going to transport her there?

Family members would have to take time off work to be with her and although they wanted to be there to help her, taking time off work wasn't always easy for them.

Referral to a dentist

A referral to a dentist is needed:

- *any time* there are unhealthy-looking areas in someone's mouth or damage to dentures
- if there is any doubt as to what you see in and around someone's mouth and/or if there is a general change in behaviour. For example, loss of appetite, loss of weight, insomnia or a change in mood. Be alert for oral health issues for the person who is unable to report dental issues such as a person with a neurological disfunction like dementia.

The referral process is:

- First document the concerns/findings.
- Notify or refer your concerns to their GP.
- Notify family members if the person cannot give consent to treatment and/or the family has power of attorney.
- Find out whether the person has a dentist you can refer them to. If not, contact the local area health dental service.
- Decide whether the person can be moved. If not, are there dental services in the local area that can come to the facility? You can find this out through the local area health service. If there are no dental services available and the person cannot be moved, your referral will rely totally on their GP.

16.7 Getting to know the person: Anna's story

Anna's condition is getting worse. Her incontinence is more frequent, and she has become frailer and lost more weight. She has started to get other medical complications like pressure injuries and infections.

The family and facility know they must do something about her mouth immediately. They must manage her pain so she can eat and drink to get her strength back.

They make an appointment with a dental surgery a few hours away. The dentist is very accommodating and is able to treat someone with such complex medical and mobility issues.

Patient transport is arranged and Julie is allocated to accompany Anna. All medical documentation is taken so the dentist can see Anna's medical history. Julie is also able to discuss any issues with the dentist. Gwen has arranged time off work to be there for Anna's dental appointment.

After getting all of Anna's medical history and discussing the chief concerns with Anna, Gwen and Julie, the dentist starts an oral health assessment. Julie observes the oral examination.

For the oral examination, the dentist:

- removes Anna's denture, noting the broken area on the right-hand side of the denture

- looks around the external structures of the mouth – the lips, outer cheek and jaw – noting that Anna's lips are dry and chapped
- examines Anna's mouth, beginning with her tongue. Gently, with some gauze, the dentist holds the tip of Anna's tongue, moving it left and right to see the sides of the tongue. Her tongue is coated white and is dry
- gently pulls out her top and bottom lips to look and feel right around the inside of her lips. The dentist makes a note of a traumatic ulcer measuring 2 cm × 2 cm on the upper right-hand side of Anna's mouth

denture stomatitis
Red appearance where the denture sits.

- looks under Anna's tongue and on the roof of her mouth noting **denture stomatitis** (redness where the denture sits) on the roof of Anna's mouth
- undertakes a full gum and tooth assessment, makes notes and takes photographs of Anna's teeth, gums and the traumatic ulcer.

After a thorough examination, the dentist discusses their findings with Anna, Gwen and Julie. The dentist concludes that Anna's pain and discomfort has come from a severe traumatic ulcer resulting from a broken denture that is not fitting well. Because it is broken and not fitting well, it is rubbing Anna's cheek and gums constantly; therefore, the tissue has no chance of healing. Anna also has a broken tooth that has become infected.

The dentist also had concerns about Anna's poor oral hygiene. The dentist says her gums are red and swollen from lots of plaque (bacteria) in her mouth and she has food debris between her teeth and under and on her denture. Her poor oral hygiene is contributing to her red and swollen gums and would not be helping her general health or the other dental issues in her mouth.

Anna manages the four-hour round trip but is exhausted after her very long day.

FOCUS QUESTIONS

- What are the challenges in ensuring that older people receive the oral assessment and dental care they need?
- What are the implications of not assessing Anna's oral health?
- What strategies can we use as health professionals to promote oral health care for older people?

Common pathologies

angular cheilitis
A condition causing dry, sometimes moist, cracked corners of the mouth.

Although you may think that you will never need the following information, it may make the difference in the quality of life of an older person. The visual recognition of something you see in an older person and the terminology may be helpful in documenting your observations. Table 16.4 offers vocabulary, definitions and photographs of common pathologies in oral health.

TABLE 16.4 Common pathologies in oral health

VOCABULARY AND DEFINITION	WHAT TO LOOK FOR IN YOUR ASSESSMENT OF THE BUCCAL CAVITY	PHOTOGRAPH
Angular cheilitis Dry, sometimes moist, cracked corners of the mouth	Note the corners of the mouth. See how they appear cracked and irritated. They can appear dry like this photo or moist. **Angular cheilitis** is usually associated with a candida infection/thrush (fungal infection). Antifungal creams are usually recommended. If in doubt, refer the person to their GP or a dental professional. Document what you see so changes over time can be noted.	
Denture stomatitis A red appearance where the denture sits; almost takes the shape of the denture	As the name suggests, this type of fungal infection can be found on the roof of the mouth where the denture sits. Most of the time you can see the fungal infection follows the outline of the denture. This can be common in ill-fitting dentures, poor oral hygiene, not taking dentures out regularly and either a general or localised candida infection. This can be in association with angular cheilitis or a stand-alone infection. Sometimes it can appear red as in the photo and sometimes it can appear red and have a white film on top. Please refer to the person's GP or a dental professional. Document what you see so changes over time can be noted.	
Traumatic ulcer An ulcer that develops through some form of trauma to the mouth tissue	Note how the tissue looks red and swollen. Also see how the tissue looks ulcerated and not intact. Refer to the healthy-looking tissue in Table 16.3 and note the difference. This will give you a better understanding of what healthy looks like and what unhealthy looks like. Traumatic ulcers can occur due to: » bite trauma » ill-fitting dentures » sharp, broken teeth » other objects (for example, but not limited to, nail biting, pen chewing, foreign objects) **These lesions should be documented, and referral is important as it can be a chronic, painful area of trauma, and it could become a pre-cancerous/cancerous lesion.**	

Photos courtesy of Dr Sue-Ching Yeoh.

16.8 Getting to know the person: Anna's story

In the following month, Anna goes back to the dentist and has her broken tooth extracted and her denture fixed so that it fits comfortably.

The dentist treats her gum disease and works with family and staff to show them the best way to look after Anna's oral health. The dentist shows them ways they can help Anna brush her teeth and look after her denture and her mouth.

As a consequence, her ulcer heals with help from the dentist and regular monitoring from staff members at the facility. A well-fitting denture, removal of the broken tooth and better oral hygiene will ensure that healing continues, there is no further deterioration in her oral health and her overall health continues to improve.

About a month after her dental work, Gwen and Julie notice that Anna is eating well and socialising more. Her incontinence has reduced, and she is starting to regain quality of life. Anna interacts more and appears happier. She states that her pain has gone.

FOCUS QUESTIONS

- According to Anna's story, what impact can a dental issue have on an older person's physical, social and emotional well-being?
- What about the impact it has on the family, the facility and the health system? If we go back to the start of the chapter, can you see how Anna's story fits into Figure 16.1?
- Consider the outcomes of oral pain on a person with later stage dementia:
  - Could it be a cause of behaviours of concern?
  - What are the outcomes for that person if poor oral health is not assessed and addressed?

Learn more
Access additional resources – such as weblinks, further readings and podcasts – to broaden your understanding of this chapter. See the Guided Tour for access details.

Conclusion

The most important thing to remember with regard to oral health is that we want to aim for the best quality of life for everyone we care for. Try not to be too concerned about looking into someone's mouth; it is just like doing any other assessment. It might feel slightly strange because you are not yet familiar with it, but like anything, the more you do it the less daunting it becomes and the more skilled you become at assessing oral health.

Given what you have learnt in this chapter, and the understanding you have on the impact oral disease can have on someone's overall health and quality of life, hopefully you will feel confident to incorporate an oral health assessment in the care you give.

This chapter has shown through pictures and Anna's story that '[m]outh pain can be devastating for the elderly, compound psychosocial problems, frustrate carers and nursing home staff and disrupt family dynamics' (Foltyn, 2015, p. 86). Through your astute assessment and appropriate referral, you can prevent the devastating impacts of poor oral hygiene on older people.

Anna's story is just one example of the impact that poor oral health can have on anyone. As a health professional working with older people, you have the capacity to assess, intervene and make a significant difference in the individual's quality of life.

1   What are the challenges to accessing oral health care for older people? What are some ways to overcomes these?

2   What are the consequences of poor oral health for older people?

3   List three signs that would alert you to the possibility an older person has an oral health pathology. How will you remember to notice these signs when working with older people?

4   Consider the current Australian dental health system in relation to financial and access issues. How do these contribute to and detract from oral health for people as they age?

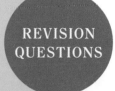

REVISION QUESTIONS

ACKNOWLEDGMENT

The author would like to thank Dr Sue-Ching Yeoh, Oral Medicine Specialist, for her permission to use all the photographs shown in this chapter.

REFERENCES

Australian Institute of Health and Welfare (AIHW) (2018). Older Australia at a Glance. AIHW. www.aihw.gov.au/reports/older-people/older-australia-at-a-glance/contents/health-functioning/oral-health-disease

Foltyn, P. (2015). Ageing, dementia and oral health. *Australian Dental Journal*, *60*(S1), pp. 86–94. https://doi.org/10.1111/adj.12287

Lewis, A., Wallace, J., Deutsch, A. & King, P. (2015). Improving the oral health of frail and functionally dependent elderly. *Australian Dental Journal*, *60*(S1), pp. 95–105. https://doi.org/10.1111/adj.12288

Norrie, T. P., Villarosa, A. R., Kong, A. C., Clark, S., Macdonald, S., Srinivas, R., Anlezark, J. & George, A. (2020). Oral health in residential aged care: Perceptions of nurses and management staff. *Nursing Open, 7*, 536–46. https://doi.org/10.1022/nop2.418

NSW Government Department of Health (2014). Oral Health Care for Older People in NSW: A Toolkit for Oral Health and Health Service Providers. www.health.nsw.gov.au/oralhealth/prevention/Pages/oral-health-older-people-toolkit.aspx

Pretty, I. A., Ellwood, R. P., Lo, E. C. M., MacEntee, M. I., Muller, F., Thomson, W. M., Putten, G. V., Ghezzi, E. M., Walls, A. & Wolff, M. S. (2013). The Seattle Care Pathway for securing oral health in older patients. *Gerodontology, 31*(S1), pp. 77–87.

17 Mobility and Falls Prevention

KRISTY ROBSON

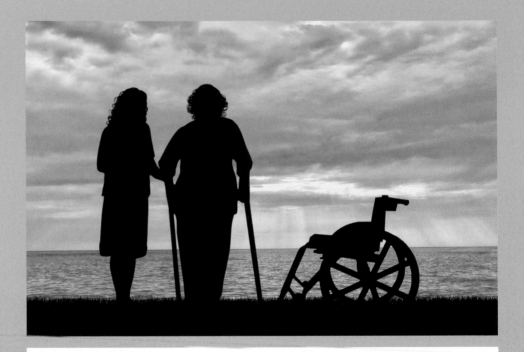

LEARNING OBJECTIVES

After reading this chapter, you will:

» understand the importance of mobility in the older person

» appreciate the impact of mobility issues and falling on the older person and the wider community

» describe the factors that can affect mobility and the potential to fall as we age

» identify the common causes of falls in the older population and describe how to assess an older person's risk of falls

» appreciate the complexity associated with identifying, managing and preventing the risk of falling in older people

» value the importance of empowering older people to keep active but remain safe.

Introduction

This chapter explores the importance of mobility in ensuring independence and autonomy through healthy ageing and discusses the complexity of managing mobility issues and falls risk in the older population. The chapter also provides context to challenges and benefits associated with empowering older people to safely remain active.

17.1 Getting to know the couple: Trish and Robert's story

Trish and Robert are both in their late 70s and are very independent. They live in the family home in a regional community. They have four adult children and eight grandchildren, who all live away from the area, except for their youngest daughter who still lives close by with her three small children and works part time.

Trish's medical history includes hypertension, Type 2 diabetes, which is diet controlled, and osteoarthritis in her right knee, for which she takes regular pain medication. Her doctor is now testing her for osteoporosis. In addition to the antihypertensive and pain medication, Trish takes aspirin and a cholesterol tablet daily. Trish also wears glasses as she is short-sighted. She walks daily with her small dog, Louie, to keep active and keep her knee moving; otherwise it becomes very stiff. On recommendation from her doctor, she has just started a weekly gentle exercise class with her friends to help her lose a bit of weight.

Robert does not have any significant medical history other than he had a mild stroke five years ago, which left his left leg a bit weak. He now takes aspirin and is on antihypertension medication for mildly elevated blood pressure.

Trish and Robert are keen gardeners and are known around the district for their roses. They have a large yard that includes a number of fruit trees, which Robert still prunes every year, although this is becoming harder since the stroke. Both Trish and Robert are active members of the local Probus Club, which meets monthly. They enjoy the social engagement and volunteer to assist in local community projects.

Their house is an older style house with multiple smaller rooms. It is single storey, but there are steps leading up to the front door and to the large backyard. Trish has a number of rugs over the polished floorboards throughout the house. They are both very independent and are still able to do all the jobs around the house. Robert usually looks after the outside jobs such as mowing the lawns and cleaning the gutters while Trish focuses on the inside chores, regularly using a small, sturdy stepladder to reach up to the high cupboards in the kitchen and bedrooms and to do the dusting.

Last month, Trish went to hang the washing out. Louie came racing up to her and she didn't see him as she was carrying the washing basket and tripped over him. Robert was out volunteering at a Probus event and when he came home, he heard Louie barking in the backyard and went to investigate. He found Trish lying on the ground in a lot of pain, especially around her right hip. Trish had tried to get up from the ground after falling, but she struggled to move because of the pain. She had no way of contacting anyone as she had left her mobile phone in the house and she tried to call out but the next-door neighbours weren't home. Robert immediately called an ambulance, which transported Trish to the local hospital where she was diagnosed with a hip fracture. There were complications associated with Trish's surgery because of the now diagnosed osteoporosis, so she had to stay in hospital for more than three weeks.

WHAT CAN AFFECT MOBILITY AS WE AGE?

Mobility is key to healthy ageing and is intimately linked to overall health status and quality of life (Webber et al., 2010). The importance of ensuring improved quality of life for people as they age is gaining momentum and the call to action has been assisted by the World Health Organization (WHO) declaring a decade of healthy ageing from 2021 to 2030, in order to shine a light on the importance of ensuring all older people have an opportunity to age well (WHO, 2021). The overarching goal of this decade is to improve or maintain older people's functional ability, as it is functional ability and mobility that enable well-being and are closely linked to quality of life. Optimal mobility can be defined as the ability to safely and reliably move from one area to another (Franke et al., 2020), where reduced mobility can be defined as a limitation in an older person's physical ability to navigate their environment (Sundar et al., 2016). Mobility limitations in older people are common (Musich et al., 2018). It has been reported that up to one-third of older people have difficulty in walking three street blocks (Centers for Disease Control and Prevention, 2009). Reduced mobility has been shown to cause a decrease in social participation, leading to isolation and loneliness and loss of independence (Terrill et al., 2016) as well as significantly increasing the risk of falls and fall-related injuries (Musich et al., 2018). Functional decline, including reduced mobility, is also one of the main contributors to entering into residential aged care (Chyr et al., 2020).

A number of risk factors can affect an older person's mobility, but a combination of risk factors is likely to cause the greatest threat to mobility (Musich et al., 2018). The key areas to think about when considering risk factors associated with limited mobility are illustrated in Figure 17.1. **Chronic disease** can include conditions such as arthritis, diabetes, obesity, musculoskeletal impairments, and the neurological and balance issues seen in Parkinson's disease or stroke; all have an impact on mobility (Fasano et al., 2017; Stubbs et al., 2016). Psychosocial conditions such as fear of falling, depression or cognitive impairment can also result in reduced mobility (Lavedán et al., 2018; Sakurai & Okubo, 2020). Injury such as falling can result in significant impacts on an older person's mobility, not only directly after the injury, but also in the longer term if ongoing physical and psychological restrictions occur as a result of the injury.

chronic disease
A pathological condition that interrupts the normal functions of the body and tends to be slow in progression and prolonged in duration.

FIGURE 17.1 Key areas that can affect mobility in older people

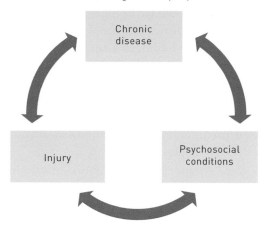

Issues arising in one of these areas, whether it is initially chronic disease, psychosocial conditions or injury, increases the risk of developing issues in the other two areas; that is, they are often interrelated and it is important to address all key areas when working with older people to maintain or improve their mobility. Alongside the consequences that reduced mobility has for the individual older person, it is important to consider its impact on their family, the wider community and the health sector at large, especially considering the ageing Australian population. At least four public health burdens have been shown to be associated with limited or restricted mobility in older populations (Satariano et al., 2012). These burdens and associated consequences are presented in Table 17.1.

morbidity
The burden of disease/ pathophysiology experienced by a person.

mortality
Contributing to death.

TABLE 17.1 Public health burdens associated with mobility issues in the older person

PUBLIC HEALTH BURDEN	CONSEQUENCES FOR OLDER PEOPLE	CITED BY
Restrictions in walking and driving limit access to goods and services	» Challenging to navigate shops and supermarkets, resulting in decreased nutritional options and compromising health » May not be able to attend medical or health services in a timely manner, reducing the capacity to provide preventative services » Living in rural areas may add further challenges to access goods and services	Viljanen et al. (2016) Satariano et al. (2012) Camarero & Oliva (2019)
Reduced mobility is linked to health problems and injury	» Increased sedentary behaviour as a result of mobility limitations is associated with obesity, cardiovascular disease, diabetes, poor cognition and depression » Increased risk of falls is strongly linked to mobility issues	Musich et al. (2018) Satariano et al. (2012) Vinik et al. (2017) Burton et al. (2018)
Decreased mobility may result in social isolation and limited engagement in the community	» Less likely to engage in regular social interactions » Social isolation can be associated with **morbidity** and **mortality** in older people » This can be especially problematic in rural areas » Mobility restrictions limit opportunities to be active members of the community	Peterson & Molina (2021) Petersen et al. (2020) Inder et al. (2012) Gardiner et al. (2018) Bu et al. (2020)

The Royal Commission into Aged Care Quality and Safety (Commonwealth of Australia, 2021) has specifically highlighted the important role health professionals can play in facilitating enhanced quality of life for older people, specifically around mobility. While the focus of the Royal Commission into Aged Care Quality and Safety (Commonwealth of Australia, 2021) was on the current challenges associated with caring for older people who require additional support and assistance, it is important to highlight the role health professionals can play in optimising mobility and independence proactively before older people become reliant on aged care services so that we can delay functional decline and reduce the risk of early dependence on an aged care system that is clearly struggling and likely to take significant time to improve.

A number of key recommendations of the Royal Commission into Aged Care Quality and Safety (Commonwealth of Australia, 2021) have highlighted the need to provide greater enhanced care to support older people living within their own home for longer, including the need for older people to have their mobility within their home environment assessed by health professionals to identify when interventions, assistive technology and home modifications may be warranted to enable older people to live more safely and maintain their independence, particularly if there are concerns about their functional mobility. While undertaking these types of assessments for individuals who may be accessing aged care services, health professionals should also be mindful of the current or potential mobility challenges that may exist in spouses as the role of informal care is seen as critical to facilitating the ability for older people to remain in their own home. Rapid functional decline in a spouse or carer as a result of a fall-related injury, for example, can also often result in an early transition to a residential aged care facility.

17.2 Getting to know the couple: Trish and Robert's story

It has been two months since Trish's fall and the subsequent surgical repair of her hip fracture. As a result, her mobility has significantly declined. She is now reliant on a walking aid to get around her home and community, and she continues to have difficulty sitting for long periods, especially in the car, due to restrictions in the range of motion in her hip. Her surgeon and physiotherapist are hopeful they will be able to gain more range of motion in her hip, but it will take time and continual rehabilitation. She cannot drive at the moment and is reliant on Robert to assist her in a range of daily activities and to do most of the household duties.

FOCUS QUESTIONS

- Reflecting on Table 17.1 and Trish's story, what impact have her fall injury and subsequent decline in mobility had on Trish and Robert?
- Given Trish's current level of mobility, how and why is she at risk of further mobility decline or injury?
- As an informal carer for Trish, how can Robert be supported to maintain his own mobility and independence?

WHY ADDRESS MOBILITY AND FALLS RISK IN OLDER PEOPLE?

Given that mobility issues are common in the older population, addressing these issues can lead to improved function, safety, community participation and quality of life (Musich et al., 2018). Falls in older people is one of the greatest contributors to mobility issues in this population group and can result in significant morbidity, early admission to residential aged care and even mortality. Older people have increased susceptibility for injury given the increase prevalence of:

- age-related physiological changes
- comorbidities and chronic disease
- delayed functional recovery.

These can all lead to musculoskeletal deconditioning, which further increases the risk of subsequent falling (Tsai, 2017).

Falling has a significant impact not only on the individual, but also on family and friends, the community and the health sector at large. In Australia, falls are one of the leading causes of unintentional non-fatal injuries – with fall-related hospital admission rates being the highest in older people – and are the leading cause of injury-related hospitalisation (Pointer, 2013).

Evidence suggests that mobility issues, including falls, are complex to address in the older population. The demographic, physiological, psychological and health status of the individual, as well as the health behaviours and living environment, need to be considered in order to successfully manage these issues (Stenholm et al., 2015).

> You can find more information on age-related changes in Chapter 10 and on multimorbidity in Chapter 18.

COMMON CAUSES OF FALLS IN THE OLDER POPULATION

The definition of a fall is a challenging one as there is little universal consensus. Older people will often describe a fall as a loss of balance or unsteadiness (Huang et al., 2012), whereas health-care providers commonly talk about the consequences of falling, such as injury, the health of the person and the anatomical landing point (Zecevic et al., 2006). The World Health Organization defines a fall as 'inadvertently coming to rest on the ground, floor or other lower level, excluding intentional change in position to rest in furniture, wall or other objects' (WHO, 2007, p. 1). However, the more commonly cited original definition, which is still widely used today, is from the Kellogg international working group on the prevention of falls in the elderly, which defines a fall as 'unintentionally coming to ground, or some lower level not as a consequence of sustaining a violent blow, loss of consciousness, sudden onset of paralysis as on stroke or an epileptic seizure' (Gibson et al., 1987).

Risk factors

There are many specific causes of falling in the older population. The literature commonly talks about three broad falls risk categories or domains: intrinsic risk factors, extrinsic risk factors and behavioural risk factors.

Intrinsic risk factors are defined as relating to the human body and incorporate a range of different areas including chronic disease, muscle and balance limitations, multiple medications and types of medications, age, cognitive impairment and incontinence (Gale et al., 2018; Ganz & Latham, 2020; Sharif et al., 2018).

Extrinsic risk factors are defined as external or environmental factors that interact with us. These types of risk factors include cracked footpaths or pavers, steps, vegetation such as leaves or seed pods on the ground, hoses, rugs, pets, slippery floor surfaces, poor lighting and bad footwear or long clothing (Gale et al., 2018; Moncada & Mire, 2017; Sharif et al., 2018).

The *behavioural risk factors* cited in the literature include reduced physical activity and fear of falling (Painter et al., 2012), individual personality traits leading to risk-taking behaviour (Hallgren & Aslan, 2018; Zhang et al., 2019) and hurrying when walking (Clemson et al., 2019). More current research has found that the value that older people place on independence can strongly influence their risk-taking behaviour (Robson et al., 2018). If older people valued independence more highly than keeping safe, they may often knowingly undertake high-risk activities, such as climbing ladders to clean the gutters, which pose a risk to falling (Robson et al., 2018). Robson et al. (2018) also found that older people continued to undertake high-risk activities unknowingly because they didn't perceive they could result in a fall. Previous experience of a fall also plays a role in risk-taking decisions. That is, even if an older person fell doing a high-risk activity, they were still likely to continue to undertake that task if they sustained only minor or no injury, compared to if they sustained a more severe injury as a result of the fall (Robson et al., 2018).

The concept of the interplay between the falls risk domains is illustrated by Alice's story.

17.3 Getting to know the person: Alice's story

Alice fell off her small stepladder in the backyard while she was pruning a bush that had some overhanging branches. These branches were overhanging her main path to the clothesline, which irritated Alice every time she went to hang the washing out. She was planning on getting her son to do it for her, but he hadn't had a chance to come around. She chose to use the stepladder that she uses in the house and do this task herself. Alice hurt her knee in the fall, but she felt it was not bad enough to see anyone about it. Both her son and her doctor were unaware that she had fallen.

The risk factors associated with this incident are shown in Table 17.2.

TABLE 17.2 Interplay between the different falls risk domains in Alice's case study

EXTRINSIC RISK FACTORS	INTRINSIC RISK FACTORS	BEHAVIOURAL RISK FACTORS
» The ladder placed on uneven ground » The bush and branches at an obscure angle, making them hard to reach » Wearing unsupportive shoes » Time of day influences the amount of light in the area	» Alice's muscle strength – her ability to get up and down the ladder successfully » Alice's balance on the ladder and ability to reach outside her centre of gravity to prune the branch » Any vision issues may lead Alice not to be able to see the steps on the ladder	» Alice's decision that she can successfully complete the task herself rather than wait for her son without considering all the risks » Believing she has made the risk safer by using a stepladder that she often uses inside the house, but fails to recognise that the ground surface is different from inside the house » Concealing the fall from her family and health professionals limits the opportunities to put in place preventative interventions to manage her risk

As you can see, there are a lot of interplaying risks that could have contributed to Alice's fall. The underpinning issue is that Alice chooses not to disclose her fall to her family and health practitioner. This is a missed opportunity to openly discuss the issues Alice may be facing in her day-to-day activities and limits the ability to implement strategies to assist her. When managing falls risk, it is important not to just focus on one or two of the obvious risk factors, but rather to consider all factors that may have contributed to the fall. For example, focusing on improving her muscle strength and balance is a common, evidence-based intervention that may provide her with some protective mechanisms to reduce her falls risk. However, there are two issues with this:

1 This approach does not provide Alice with a contextual understanding of all of the risk factors that may have contributed to her fall, and simple adjustments such as wearing more appropriate footwear, making sure the stepladder is on an even surface and undertaking the task at the brightest time of the day, alongside ongoing strength and balance exercises, may provide Alice with greater protective value than strength and balance training alone.

2 If we as health professionals just focus on referring her to strength and balance training, once Alice has completed this training she may believe that she is safer than she really is because she has done what the health professional has recommended without considering of all the potential risk factors within each of the three domains.

RISK FACTORS FOR OLDER PEOPLE IN HOSPITALS AND RESIDENTIAL FACILITIES

Falls in a hospital or residential setting add further considerations as older people in these settings tend to be less independent and have a greater incidence of chronic and acute conditions compared to older people living in the community (Morris & O'Riordan, 2017) all of which can increase their risk of falling. Evidence suggests that in residential aged care one in every two older people will fall within 12 months of admission, and 3 to 5 per cent of these will fracture their hips as a result (Burland et al., 2013; Vlaeyen et al., 2015). Within hospitals, in-patient falls can result in severe injury, long-term disability and even death (Lerdal et al., 2018). They also increase health-care costs, lengthen hospital stays and use additional hospital resources (Francis-Coad et al., 2018; Morello et al., 2015). Morello et al. (2015) found in a multisite prospective cohort study that a fall within the inpatient setting can contribute up to eight additional days to a hospital stay and an average of $6669 to the health-care cost incurred by the health service.

Early identification of older people admitted to hospital or residential aged care who are at risk of falling is essential to manage the risk of injury and further functional decline (Francis-Coad, 2018; Hayakawa et al., 2014).

Key risk factors specifically related to falls within hospital settings and residential facilities include:

- *intrinsic factors* – age, reduced strength and balance, illness leading to functional deterioration, chronic disease, visual or hearing impairment, cognitive impairment or confusion, hypotension, urinary incontinence, fear of falling and polypharmacy (more than five medications), as well as specific medications (psychotropic and hypnotic medications, antidepressants, antiarrhythmic medications and diuretics) and a previous fall history (Cameron et al., 2018; Morris & O'Riordan, 2017; Najafpour et al., 2019)

- *extrinsic factors* – room design, type of floor surfaces, bed height, bed railings, unfamiliar environment or disorientation and poor lighting (Morris & O'Riordan, 2017; Pati et al., 2021)
- *organisational factors* – the hospital's or residential aged care facility's overall safety culture and philosophy, as well as staff resourcing, can also impact falls risks (Cameron et al., 2018; Morris & O'Riordan, 2017).

17.4 Getting to know the couple: Trish and Robert's story

Trish has started to get more movement in her hip, but is still reliant on a walking stick when walking outside. Robert is struggling to keep on top of all the housework and their garden. Trish is frustrated that she can't help Robert more around the house, but she is too afraid she will fall again and break a bone, especially with the osteoporosis. Robert is worried about Trish's mental state as she now spends most of her time sitting in front of the television and no longer wants to go out and spend time with her friends. Trish and Robert's children have promised to come for a visit and help Robert complete some of the major tasks around the home such as cleaning the windows, but as yet they haven't been able to take time off work. Robert is reluctant to ask for help from their youngest daughter, who lives close by, because she is so busy with her three small children and Robert doesn't want to add to her stress.

FOCUS QUESTIONS

- What factors put Trish and Robert at risk of falling? Consider the different risk factors in all three domains as seen in Figure 17.2.
- In what specific areas might Trish and Robert require additional support to assist with their functional mobility and to undertake activities of daily living safely?

FIGURE 17.2 Interplay between different domains of falls risk factors

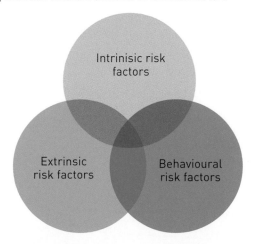

How to assess falls risks in older people

Gaining an early understanding of the difficulties older people have with their functional mobility is the best way to identify older people who may be at risk of falling so that appropriate and proactive interventions can be implemented before serious injury occurs (WHO, 2021). The Australian Commission on Safety and Quality in Health Care (2009) recommends that all older people with a history of two or more falls in the previous year should be referred for a more detailed assessment. International guidelines also recommend that health professionals interacting with older people regularly ask them and/or their carers about their falls history (Moncada & Mire, 2017), regardless of whether the fall resulted in an injury.

As estimates indicate that one-third of older people experience a fall in the community each year (Kenny et al., 2017), it should be every health professional's responsibility to actively engage with older people about their falls history. This is important as the evidence suggests that older people can be reluctant to self-report falls, especially if it resulted in only a minor or no injury (Robson et al., 2018). Health professionals need to ensure that there are no missed opportunities to put in place prevention strategies to reduce an individual's falls risk.

FALLS RISK SCREENING VERSUS FALLS RISK ASSESSMENT

In addition to regularly asking older people about their falls history, screening tools are useful to guide the decision of whether a more detailed assessment needs to be undertaken. Exceeding the threshold score for the specific screening tool should prompt a more thorough falls risk assessment as soon as practicable (Australian Commission on Safety and Quality in Health Care, 2009). The purpose of falls risk assessment is to develop an individualised plan for preventing falls by identifying the key factors contributing to the older person's increased risk of falling.

Table 17.3 shows validated assessments tools for screening of falls risk commonly used in Australia.

TABLE 17.3 Validated screening and assessment tools to determine the falls risk in older people

CLINICAL SETTING	ASSESSMENT TOOL	DESCRIPTION	OUTCOME MEASURE	EQUIPMENT NEEDED	REFERENCES
Community-based screening	Timed Up and Go Test (TUG)	Measures the time taken for a person to rise from a chair and walk 3 metres at a normal pace with their usual assistive device, turn, return to the chair, and sit down	A time of 12 seconds or greater indicates an increased risk of falling.	» Chair » Measured point of 3 metres » A watch with a minute hand or stopwatch	Close & Lord (2011) Alexandre et al. (2012)

(Continued)

TABLE 17.3 Continued

CLINICAL SETTING	ASSESSMENT TOOL	DESCRIPTION	OUTCOME MEASURE	EQUIPMENT NEEDED	REFERENCES
Community-based screening	Sit to Stand (STS)	Measures lower limb strength, speed and coordination through recording the time taken to complete five STS sequences as fast as possible from a chair	A time of 12 seconds or greater indicates an increased risk of falling.	Chair of standard height (43 cm)	Tiedemann et al. (2008)
Community-based assessment	Quickscreen	A multifactorial assessment tool designed for use in clinical settings. Involves measuring a range of fall-related factors – previous falls, medication use, vision, peripheral sensation, lower-limb strength, balance and coordination – in order to determine whether an individual is at risk of a fall and which particular factors contribute to the specific risk	A score of 4 or more indicates there is an increased risk of falling.	» A low-contrast eye chart » Monofilament for measuring touch sensation » A small step	Close & Lord (2011) Tiedemann et al. (2012).
Emergency-department screening	Prevention of Falls in the Elderly Trial (PROFIT)	Used on older people presenting to an emergency department as a result of a fall. Patients are screened using three questions: » Have you had any other falls in the past 12 months? » Have you fallen indoors? » Have you been unable to get up after your fall?	If the answer is 'yes' to any of these questions, further assessment is required.	Questionnaire	Close et al. (2003) Close & Lord (2011)
Emergency-department screening	FROP-Com screening tool	Patients are screened using three factors: » steadiness during walking and turning » history of falls in the past 12 months » the need for assistance with activities of daily living.	A score of 4 or more indicates a high risk.	Questionnaire	Russell et al. (2009)
In-hospital screening	Ontario Modified STRATIFY	A weighted questionnaire with six questions asked relating to falls, cognition, transfer and mobility skills, vision and toileting	A score of 9 or more indicates a high risk of falls.	Questionnaire	Barker et al. (2011) Close & Lord (2011)

TABLE 17.3 Continued

CLINICAL SETTING	ASSESSMENT TOOL	DESCRIPTION	OUTCOME MEASURE	EQUIPMENT NEEDED	REFERENCES
In-hospital and residential assessment tool	Peninsula Health Falls Risk Assessment Tool (FRAT)	Patients are assessed in three areas: » falls risk status » risk factor checklist » action plan. (Part 1 can also be used for fall screening.)	A score of 12 or more indicates an increased risk of falls.	Questionnaire	Stapleton et al. (2009)
In-hospital assessment tool	Falls risk for hospitalised older people (FRHOP)	Comprehensive assessment tool that includes a range of falls risk factors, which are graded from nil (0) to high (3) risk	An overall score of 23 or more, or more than four items rated in the high category, indicates an increased risk of falling.	Questionnaire	Hill et al. (2004)
In-hospital and residential care assessment tool	Falls Risk Assessment and Management Plan (FRAMP)	A comprehensive assessment that includes screening, and specific interventions targeted to the individual with multidisciplinary input	If the answer is 'yes' to any of the initial screening questions, further assessment is required.	Questionnaire	Western Australian Department of Health (2015)
Residential care facilities	Care Home Falls Screen (CaHFRiS)	A weighted questionnaire with seven items asked related to cognitive function, behaviour, standing balance, use of walking aids, falls history and use of certain medications	The number of risk factors identified relates to the likelihood of a fall in the next 6 months represented as a percentage.	Questionnaire	Whitney et al. (2012)

OTHER KEY AREAS TO CONSIDER WHEN ASSESSING FALLS RISK

If you do not have access to specific screening tools in the community setting, you still have an important role to play in identifying older people who may be at risk of falling and could benefit from further assessment.

Examples of key questions that could be asked of an older person or their carer that would prompt further evaluation of the level of falls risk are:

- Do you have difficulty walking?
- Do you have difficulty getting up from furniture, such as a chair, lounge or the bed?
- Do you have joint stiffness or pain?
- Do you have leg or foot pain?
- Do you have problems with your balance?
- Do you have vision problems?
- Do you have a chronic disease – such as diabetes, hypertension, arthritis, osteoporosis, Parkinson's disease or multiple sclerosis – or have you been diagnosed with cognition difficulties?
- Are you on more than five medications?

- Are you afraid of falling?
- Have you had a fall in the past 12 months?

If the older person or their carer answers 'yes' to any of these questions, you should refer them for further falls risk assessment.

Health professionals and falls prevention

Managing falls risk in our older populations is complex and challenging. To achieve effective outcomes, a comprehensive approach that may include a range of different health professionals (depending on the older person's identified risk factors) is needed. Figure 17.3 outlines the types of health professionals who may be involved in managing falls risk in older people.

FIGURE 17.3 Key health professionals involved in the assessment and management of falls risk in older people

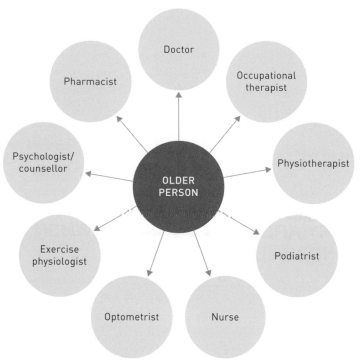

17.5 Getting to know the person: Jim's story

Jim is a 72-year-old man who has had three falls in the past 12 months. His last fall resulted in him badly spraining his right shoulder; this has limited his ability to play golf and undertake some of his regular daily activities and tasks. When presenting to his local doctor about his shoulder injury, he comments that he has noticed his eyesight and balance isn't that good and he sometimes feels dizzy when getting out of bed in the morning, and is worried it might have something do with his new blood-pressure medication. Jim also indicates he has been having a bit of trouble walking because of the pain in his ankles. Jim's last fall has really had a significant impact on him because he can't get out and play golf with his friends, he doesn't have many other interests and he feels he is starting to get a bit weaker. He also had to cancel his last optometry appointment because he could not drive himself due to shoulder pain.

- What is the role of each of the professionals identified in Figure 17.3 in keeping Jim safe from falls?

FOCUS QUESTION

Intervention strategies

With the support of a multi-professional approach to falls prevention, several intervention strategies have been shown to be effective in reducing or managing falls risk in older populations. Intervention strategies can be classified into three categories:

- single interventions, such as vitamin D supplements, home modifications, exercise programs, vision review, medication review, and strength and balance programs
- multiple interventions, such as the Stepping On program, strength and balance with patient education, and exercise groups with home modification
- multifactorial interventions. These are interventions that have three or more components (e.g. exercise with vision assessment and home assessment, or medication review with patient education and strength and balance classes).

EXERCISE INTERVENTIONS

Evidence suggests that several exercise programs – either home-based or group-based programs such as tai chi and strength and balance training – can reduce the rate of falls, but only if older people continue with this type of exercise over the long term (Langhammer et al., 2018; Sherrington et al., 2017; Robson et al., 2021).

HOME MODIFICATIONS

Home risk assessment and modifications have been seen to be effective in older people who are at high risk of falls (Clemson et al., 2019; Stark et al., 2017). Occupational therapists can review potential hazards in the home such as slippery floors, mats or poor lighting, and unsafe behaviour like leaving clutter in high traffic areas or wearing loose shoes or clothes that are too long. Discussion with the older person about their daily mobility issues or challenges can lead to modifications to reduce the risk. However, the fact that there is a home hazard isn't enough to cause a fall; rather, it is the interaction between the physical limitations of the older person and their exposure to a home hazard that creates the greatest risk (Mackenzie & Byles,

2018). Therefore, home assessment and modification should always be considered as part of a multifactorial approach for managing falls risk (Clemson et al., 2019).

MEDICATION REVIEWS

Older people use more medications due to the increased presence of chronic disease (Andersen et al., 2020). Polypharmacy, defined as the use of five or more medications, has been seen to increase the risk of falls (Morin et al., 2019). Older people who visit multiple medical practitioners or fill their prescriptions at different pharmacies may also increase their risk of negative consequences associated with polypharmacy (Kim & Parish, 2017). There is also a range of medications that specifically increase the risk of falling: psychotropic drugs, benzodiazepines, atypical antipsychotics, antidepressants, opioids and antihypertensive and cardiovascular medications (Ie et al., 2021). Regular medication reviews with a pharmacist and/or medical practitioner are important to reduce the risk of falls.

VITAMIN D SUPPLEMENTATION

There has been mixed evidence for the support of vitamin D supplementation and its effectiveness in reducing the risk of falls (Chakhtoura et al., 2020), except in older people with low levels of vitamin D (Remelli et al., 2019). However, there is clear evidence that vitamin D supplementation can prevent fractures (Chakhtoura et al., 2020), which may reduce the risk of a more injurious fall. Vitamin D deficiency has also been linked to reduced neuromuscular function (Machaj et al., 2020), which may also increase the risk of falls. Therefore, the use of vitamin D may be a useful fall-related intervention (Australian Commission on Safety and Quality in Health Care, 2009).

IMPROVING VISION

Impaired vision is an independent risk factor for older people (Australian Commission on Safety and Quality in Health Care, 2009). A decrease in vision has been seen to increase the incidence in falls and other injuries (Saftari & Kwon, 2018). Eye diseases such as cataracts, glaucoma, macular degeneration or conditions that affect contrast sensitivity or visual acuity have all been shown to increase the risk of falls (Ehrlich et al., 2019; Nguyen et al., 2021).

Regular vision screening and eye examinations should be included as part of a multifactorial approach to reducing fall rates (Moncada & Mire, 2017). In addition, older people are likely to benefit from regular assessment of their glasses prescriptions (Delbaere et al., 2021). The use of bifocal or multifocal lenses has also been shown to increase the risk of falling when walking outside (Chang, 2021). Avoiding these types of lens when walking is preferable for people who are at high risk of falls.

Evidence also suggests that performing cataract surgery on the first affected eye can successfully reduce the rate of falls (Boyd et al., 2020). Early identification and management of cataracts is also useful (Nguyen et al., 2021).

MANAGING LOWER LIMB ISSUES AND FOOTWEAR

Foot pain and deformity are significant problems, with one study showing one in five older people report foot pain, arching or stiffness on most days (Awale et al., 2017).

Foot pathology is likely to result in older people having difficulty performing daily tasks such as walking (Menz et al., 2018; Spink et al., 2011). Foot deformity such as reduced ankle flexibility, muscle weakness, joint deformity and pain changes the body's weight distribution over the feet, impairing the abilities to walk and maintain balance (Menz et al., 2018) and resulting in increased risk of falls. Assessment and management by a podiatrist for gait and lower limb pathology has shown to be effective in reducing this risk (Spink et al., 2011).

Appropriate footwear is also important. Older people who wear shoes that are slip on and not adequately secured to the foot, and which have low or no heels and minimal sole contact with the ground have been shown to suffer more falls (Hatton & Rome, 2019). Wearing slippers or socks regularly has also been associated with falls (Davis et al., 2019). Showing older people the appropriate footwear to wear both inside and outside the home is important in managing the risk of falls. Specific features that older people should consider when choosing footwear include soles that are firm with a tread, low heels and a supportive heel counter around the ankle (Hatton & Rome, 2019).

INCONTINENCE MANAGEMENT

Urinary and faecal incontinence have been seen to increase the risk of older people falling in the community (Schluter et al., 2018). If incontinence issues are identified, the person should be referred to establish the underlying cause and so appropriate management can be instigated.

SYNCOPE MANAGEMENT

Any older person who reports an unexplained fall should be appropriately assessed to identify the underlying cause. Older people are more likely to have syncope events due to the ageing process linked to reduced **cerebral perfusion** (Australian Commission on Safety and Quality in Health Care, 2009). The more common causes of syncope include vasovagal syncope (fainting), **postural hypertension**, **carotid sinus hypersensitivity**, **cardiac arrhythmias**, **aortic stenosis** and **transient ischaemic attacks** (Australian Commission on Safety and Quality in Health Care, 2009).

FEAR OF FALLING

Fear of falling is a significant issue that older people can face regardless of whether they have fallen previously or not (Lavedán et al., 2018). Older people who fear they will fall commonly avoid activity, which can lead to negative consequences such as decreased quality of life, functional decline and potential institutionalisation (van Haastregt et al., 2013).

Cognitive behaviour therapy has been shown to be successful in reducing the fear of falling, which may reduce the risk of falls in this group of older people (Whipple et al., 2018). Strategies such as home-based exercise, fall prevention programs and community-based tai chi also assist with developing confidence in older people navigating their home and community (Whipple et al., 2018).

MULTIPLE INTERVENTIONS

Multifactorial interventions involve more than one form of intervention clustered together and older people may receive different combinations of interventions based on their

cerebral perfusion
The flow of blood to and around the brain.

postural hypertension
Decrease in blood pressure on standing.

carotid sinus hypersensitivity
A condition that causes slowing of the heart and reduced blood pressure making a person vulnerable to falls.

cardiac arrhythmias
Irregular heartbeats.

aortic stenosis
Loss of elasticity of the artery taking blood from the heart.

transient ischaemic attack
A disruption to the circulation in the brain causing temporary loss of awareness; can be a precursor to a major cerebral disruption or stroke.

individual needs and identified risks (Hopewell et al., 2018). Falls prevention programs that include a combination of targeted strength and balance exercise and education sessions is an example of a multifactorial intervention as it involves both exercise and education (Robson et al., 2021) and has proven to be successful in reducing the risk of falls

FALLS PREVENTION EDUCATION

Currently it is inconclusive whether falls prevention education alone reduces falls in older people (Hopewell et al., 2018).

Management of falls risk in hospital and residential facilities

Falls in hospital or residential facilitates are common events (LeLaurin & Shorr, 2019) and can result in injuries and sometimes death (Cameron et al., 2018). The incidence of falls in residential care facilities is reported to be three times that seen in the community (Cameron et al., 2018). All staff who work within a hospital or residential care setting have a role to play in reducing or preventing falls in older people.

Older people presenting to a hospital or living in a residential aged care facility should be appropriately screened and assessed for falls risk during the admission phase. Reassessment should be undertaken if their condition changes or every six months. Due to the frailty and complexity of the types of conditions that older people have in both hospital and residential aged care, effective falls prevention is challenging in this space and there has been limited evidence to support a universal approach to managing this issue in these settings. However, systematic reviews have indicated that instigating a multifactorial approach to assessment may reduce 20 to 30 per cent of falls in these types of environments (Cameron et al., 2018).

Within these settings, a broad range of interventions are in use, from regular mobility and exercise, medication reviews, environmental or assistive technologies to the social environment, including targeting staff culture and organisational change (Cameron et al., 2018). In addition to commonly used strategies to manage the risk of falls in the community, the following may be of use for frailer older people:

- If mobility issues are identified, assessment for walking aids may be useful (Burton et al., 2018).
- Older people identified with cognitive impairments need to have falls risk factors addressed and may benefit from the use of hip protectors to reduce the risk of hip fractures (Korall et al., 2019). Electronic alarm systems have also been found to be effective in managing the risk of falls in people with cognitive impairment (Melin, 2018).
- Any incontinence issues should be appropriately identified, and strategies put in place to manage these, including toileting protocols (Schluter et al., 2018).
- Visual problems should be assessed and strategies implemented to assist with vision impairment, such as the use of luminous commode seats and toilet signs as well as night sensors (Palmer, 2018).
- Low beds have demonstrated a reduction in fall rates within the hospital setting (Palmer, 2018).

- Ensuring the physical environment is safe for older patients is also important, so personal belongings and equipment should be in easy reach; and furniture, lighting, floor surfaces, clutter and spills should all be managed appropriately (Australian Commission on Safety and Quality in Health Care, 2009; Palmer, 2018).

- Other useful strategies include flagging high-risk patients with alert bracelets or symbols (Zanker & Duque, 2020), individual observation (Shekelle et al., 2019) and volunteer sitter programs (Saunders et al., 2019).

Reflect on Trish and Robert's story.

- Think about the fall-related risk factors that you identified for Trish and Robert in all three domains (extrinsic, intrinsic and behavioural). What types of interventions could you facilitate with them to reduce their risk of falling?

- Think about the types of referral pathways that may be useful in assisting in their safety. Are there any other strategies outside health referrals that you think may be helpful for Trish and Robert?

FOCUS QUESTIONS

Identifying and managing falls risk in the community

In the following section we will discuss the complex nature of assessing and supporting older people living in the community who are vulnerable to having a fall.

EARLY IDENTIFICATION

Early identification of older people who may be at high risk of falling is important so that effective intervention strategies can be implemented. However, the challenge becomes being able to appropriately identify 'at risk' individuals, as many older people are reluctant to admit to health professionals that they have fallen (Dollard et al., 2014; Robson et al., 2018). This reluctance can be because they don't perceive their fall experience to be an issue, especially if there was little or no injury, or they may be worried that health professionals will think they are not coping, resulting in loss of independence (Robson et al., 2018).

ACTIVELY ENGAGING IN COMMUNICATION

It is important that all health professionals actively engage in communication with older people about their falls history. If they assume that the older person will inform them, then a considerable number of falls that health professionals are unaware of are likely to be occurring (Robson et al., 2018). This reduces the ability to address key risk factors before more significant injury occurs. This also poses significant challenges from an injury risk management perspective because, without a systematic approach towards identifying 'at risk' older people, appropriate and timely falls interventions are unlikely to be implemented in this vulnerable population.

OTHER CHALLENGES

Even if older people are successfully identified and referred to fall-related interventions, there are still challenges associated with managing the falls risks. Several factors can influence the uptake of fall-related interventions, such as:

- the value older people place on independence
- the level of understanding older people have about risk
- the willingness to accept support.

All of the above influence behavioural decisions by the older person to undertake a risky activity or task. If the older person doesn't perceive they are at risk, even if they have previously fallen, they may not engage with interventions they have been referred to (Gardiner et al., 2017; Robson et al., 2018). Even if they do attend intervention strategies such as falls risk education programs, they may not take on board the advice they are given to reduce their risk (Robson et al., 2018). *It is important that health professionals don't assume that because they have referred an older person to a service that deals with falls intervention, they have done their part.* Adequate follow-up and ongoing communication with the older person are key. If the older person is reluctant to take recommendations on board, a dialogue should be opened as to why it is important, during which alternative options could be offered.

CONTINUAL REASSESSMENT

Continual reassessment of older people's falls risk is important due to comorbidities and the ageing process itself. The consequences of a lack of routine follow-up may mean that any falls intervention that was previously instigated may no longer be the most appropriate one or may not address all of the current risk factors, leaving older people vulnerable to subsequent falls with more severe outcomes.

REGIONAL AND RURAL AREAS

Access and availability to falls-related assessment and interventions in regional or rural areas also provides unique challenges. Lack of specific health professionals and resources means that available staff need to be flexible to undertake transdisciplinary practice in key areas such as falls assessment and the implementation of interventions. That is, most common falls risk assessments can be undertaken by any health professional. Interventions such as strength and balance programs, home assessments and footwear advice that would be traditionally done by allied health staff (exercise physiology, occupational therapy, physiotherapy or podiatry) with up-skilling, could be undertaken by other local health professionals such as community nurses. Engaging community members in rural townships to run exercise programs that incorporate strength and balance components, for example, or tai chi, can also be a useful strategy when there is limited resourcing.

EMPOWERING OLDER PEOPLE TO REMAIN ACTIVE BUT KEEP SAFE

Falls-related injury in older populations is a significant issue not only for the older person, but also for their family, the health sector and the wider community. Our role as health professionals is:

- not to limit independence for older people
- to enable them to remain active while keeping safe
- to reduce their risk of injurious falls.

Given that the home environment is the most common location for falls, education on potential risk factors is an important aspect of allowing older people to make decisions on how to undertake necessary tasks safely or assisting them to decide whether a task poses too great a risk and external support is needed. Empowering older people to make appropriate decisions on risks using a person-centred approach is likely to have the greatest impact on managing the burden of falls-related injuries.

Evidence suggests that traditional health messages focusing on falls prevention are less effective than those on healthy ageing and maintaining safe independence (Gardiner et al., 2017). Alongside positive health messages, there needs to be greater involvement of the community in raising awareness of the risk factors linked to falls and to reduce the stigma associated with falling (Robson et al., 2018). By enhancing the general awareness within the community, there is likely to be a better understanding by both older people and health professionals of the need to manage risk early, before injury occurs.

Person-centred approaches to injury risk management also have a number of benefits, including enabling greater discussion about the individual goals or activities of the person; providing common alignment with the most appropriate interventions that will enable the person to achieve their individual goals or activities; and prompting older people to articulate what is important to them through shared decision making, rather than the health professional informing them about what they need to do (Reuben & Tinetti, 2012). A person-centred approach also enables the development of behavioural change through a greater understanding of the perspective and psychosocial context of the older person (Yardley et al., 2015). Ensuring older people are active participants rather than passive recipients in the management of falls-related risks (Child et al., 2012) may go some way towards increasing our ability to successfully reduce fall rates within the community as our population ages.

Conclusion

Falls injuries in older people is a significant health issue not only in Australia, but also across the globe. If we are going to curb the increasing trend of falls-related injuries, effective models of care are needed to both identify those individuals at greatest risk of falls and to allow for person-centred interventions to be successfully implemented. Every health professional who interacts with older people has a role to play in discussing mobility concerns and falls risk. Continued open dialogue between health professionals and older people is needed so that a greater understanding of the range of individual risks that contribute to falling are identified and managed before significant injury occurs. Ongoing conversations on the everyday functional challenges that older people face will enable more proactive and early interventions to be instigated to mitigate against mobility decline while empowering older people to maintain their independence and autotomy through safe and active engagement. Given that by 2051 it is estimated that 24 per cent of the Australian population will be over the age of 64, a holistic and collaborative approach that promotes safe independence is critical; otherwise, we are unlikely to be able to curb the increasing trend of falls-related injuries and hospitalisation.

Learn more
Access additional resources – such as weblinks, further readings and podcasts – to broaden your understanding of this chapter. See the Guided Tour for access details.

KRISTY ROBSON

REVISION QUESTIONS

1 How can issues with mobility affect healthy ageing?

2 What factors contribute to falls in older age?

3 How would you assess an older person for falls risk?

4 What strategies can you implement to assist in managing falls risks in older people?

5 As a health professional, how can you actively contribute to the narrative of improving functional mobility to enhance independence and autonomy for older people, as advocated by the Royal Commission into Aged Care Quality and Safety and the WHO's Decade of Healthy Ageing?

REFERENCES

Alexandre, T. S., Meira, D. M., Rico, N. C. & Mizuta, S. K. (2012). Accuracy of timed up and go test for screening risk of falls among community-dwelling elderly. *Brazilian Journal of Physical Therapy, 16*(5), 381–8. https://doi.org/10.1590/s1413-35552012005000041

Andersen, C. U., Lassen, P. O., Usman, H. Q., Albertsen, N., Nielsen, L. P. & Andersen, S. (2020). Prevalence of medication-related falls in 200 consecutive elderly patients with hip fractures: A cross-sectional study. *BMC Geriatrics, 20*(1), 1–9. https://doi.org/10.1186/s12877-020-01532-9

Australian Commission on Safety and Quality in Health Care (ACSQHC) (2009). Preventing Falls and Harm from Falls in Older People: Best Practice Guidelines for Australian Community Care. ACSQHC. www.safetyandquality.gov.au/publications-and-resources/resource-library/preventing-falls-and-harm-falls-older-people-best-practice-guidelines-australian-community-care

Awale, A., Hagedorn, T. J., Dufour, A. B., Menz, H. B., Casey, V. A. & Hannan, M. T. (2017). Foot function, foot pain, and falls in older adults: The Framingham foot study. *Gerontology, 63*(4), 318–24. https://doi.org/10.1159/000475710

Barker, A., Kamar, J., Graco, M., Lawlor, V., & Hill, K. (2011). Adding value to the STRATIFY falls risk assessment in acute hospitals. *Journal of Advanced Nursing, 67*(2), 450–7. https://doi.org/10.1111/j.1365-2648.2010.05503.x

Boyd, M., Kvizhinadze, G., Kho, A., Wilson, G. & Wilson, N. (2020). Cataract surgery for falls prevention and improving vision: Modelling the health gain, health system costs and cost-effectiveness in a high-income country. *Injury Prevention, 26*(4), 302–9. http://dx.doi.org/10.1136/injuryprev-2019-043184

Bu, F., Abell, J., Zaninotto, P. & Fancourt, D. (2020). A longitudinal analysis of loneliness, social isolation and falls amongst older people in England. *Scientific Reports, 10*(1), 1–8. https://doi.org/10.1038/s41598-020-77104-z

Burland, E., Martens, P., Brownell, M., Doupe, M. & Fuchs, D. (2013). The evaluation of a fall management program in a nursing home population. *The Gerontologist, 53*(5), 828–38. https://doi.org/10.1093/geront/gns197

Burton, E., Lewin, G., O'Connell, H. & Hill, K. D. (2018). Falls prevention in community care: 10 years on. *Clinical Interventions in Aging, 13*, 261–9. https://doi.org/10.2147/CIA.S153687

Camarero, L. & Oliva, J. (2019). Thinking in rural gap: Mobility and social inequalities. *Palgrave Communications, 5*(1), 1–7. https://doi.org/10.1057/s41599-019-0306-x

Cameron, I. D., Dyer, S. M., Panagoda, C. E., Murray, G. R., Hill, K. D., Cumming, R. G. & Kerse, N. (2018). Interventions for preventing falls in older people in care facilities and hospitals. *Cochrane Database of Systematic Reviews, 9*. https://doi.org/10.1002/14651858.CD005465.pub4

Centers for Disease Control and Prevention (2009). Prevalence and most common causes of disability among adults – United States, 2005. *Morbidity and Mortality Weekly Report, 58*(16), 421–6.

Chakhtoura, M., Chamoun, N., Rahme, M. & Fuleihan, G. E.-H. (2020). Impact of vitamin D supplementation on falls and fractures – A critical appraisal of the quality of the evidence and an overview of the available guidelines, *Bone, 131*, 115112. https://doi.org/10.1016/j.bone.2019.115112

Chang, D. H. (2021). Multifocal spectacle and monovision treatment of presbyopia and falls in the elderly. *Journal of Refractive Surgery, 37*(S1), S12–S16. https://doi.org/10.3928/1081597X-20210408-02

Child, S., Goodwin, V., Garside, R., Jones-Hughes, T., Boddy, K. & Stein, K. (2012). Factors influencing the implementation of fall-prevention programmes: A systematic review and synthesis of qualitative studies. *Implementation Science, 7*(91), 1–14. https://doi.org/10.1186/1748-5908-7-91

Chyr, L. C., Drabo, E. F. & Fabius, C. D. (2020). Patterns and predictors of transitions across residential care settings and nursing homes among community-dwelling older adults in the United States. *The Gerontologist, 60*(8), 1495–503. https://doi.org/10.1093/geront/gnaa070

Clemson, L., Stark, S., Pighills, A. C., Torgerson, D. J., Sherrington, C. & Lamb, S. E. (2019). Environmental interventions for preventing falls in older people living in the community. *Cochrane Database of Systematic Reviews, 2019*(2). https://doi.org/10.1002/14651858.CD013258

Close, J. C. T., Hooper, R., Glucksman, E., Jackson, S. H. & Swift, C. G. (2003). Predictors of falls in a high risk population: Results from the prevention of falls in the elderly trial (PROFET). *Emergency Medicine Journal, 20*(5), 421–5. https//doi.org/10.1136/emj.20.5.421

Close, J. C. T. & Lord, S. R. (2011). Fall assessment in older people. *British Medical Journal, 343*(d5153), 579–82. https://doi.org/10.1136/bmj.d5153

Commonwealth of Australia (2021). Royal Commission into Aged Care Quality and Safety. Final report: Care, dignity and respect. Vol. 1, Summary and recommendations. https://agedcare.royalcommission.gov.au/sites/default/files/2021-03/final-report-volume-1_0.pdf

Davis, A., Haines, T. & Williams, C. (2019). Do footwear styles cause falls or increase falls risk in healthy older adults? A systematic review. *Footwear Science, 11*(1), 13–23. https://doi.org/10.1080/19424280.2018.1555861

Delbaere, K., Sherrington, C. & Lord, S. R. (2021). Fall prevention interventions. In D. W. Dempster, J. A. Cauley, M. L. Bouxsein & F. Cosman (eds), *Marcus and Feldman's Osteoporosis* (5th edn), pp. 1627–47 (Ch. 68). https://doi.org/10.1016/B978-0-12-813073-5.00068-X

Dollard, J., Braunack-Mayer, A., Horton, K. & Vanlint, S. (2014). Why older women do or do not seek help from the GP after a fall: A qualitative study. *Family Practice, 31*(2), 222–8. http://dx.doi.org/10.1093/fampra/cmt083

Ehrlich, J. R., Hassan, S. E. & Stagg, B. C. (2019). Prevalence of falls and fall-related outcomes in older adults with self-reported vision impairment. *Journal of the American Geriatrics Society, 67*(2), 239–45. https://doi.org/10.1111/jgs.15628

Fasano, A., Canning, C. G., Hausdorff, J. M., Lord, S. & Rochester, L. (2017). Falls in Parkinson's disease: A complex and evolving picture. *Movement Disorders, 32*(11), 1524–36. https://doi.org/10.1002/mds.27195

Francis-Coad, J., Etherton-Beer, C., Burton, E., Naseri, C. & Hill, A. M. (2018). Effectiveness of complex falls prevention interventions in residential aged care settings: A systematic review. *JBI Evidence Synthesis, 16*(4), 973–1002. https://doi.org/10.11124/JBISRIR-2017-003485

Franke, T., Sims-Gould, J., Chaudhury, H., Winters, M. & McKay, H. (2020). Re-framing mobility in older adults: An adapted comprehensive conceptual framework. *Qualitative Research in Sport, Exercise and Health, 12*(3), 336–49. https://doi.org/10.1080/2159676X.2019.1575269

Gale, C. R., Westbury, L. D., Cooper, C. & Dennison, E. M. (2018). Risk factors for incident falls in older men and women: The English longitudinal study of ageing. *BMC Geriatrics, 18*(1), 1–9. https://doi.org/10.1186/s12877-018-0806-3

Ganz, D. A. & Latham, N. K. (2020). Prevention of falls in community-dwelling older adults. *New England Journal of Medicine, 382*(8), 734–43. https://doi.org/10.1056/NEJMcp1903252

Gardiner, C., Geldenhuys, G. & Gott, M. (2018). Interventions to reduce social isolation and loneliness among older people: An integrative review. *Health & Social Care in the Community, 26*(2), 147–57. https://doi.org/10.1111/hsc.12367

Gardiner, S., Glogowska, M., Stoddart, C., Pendlebury, S., Lasserson, D. & Jackson, D. (2017). Older people's experiences of falling and perceived risk of falls in the community: A narrative synthesis of qualitative research. *International Journal of Older People Nursing, 12*(4), E12151. https://doi.org/10.1111/opn.12151

Gibson, M. J., Andres, R. O., Isaacs, B., Radebaugh, T. & Worm-Petersen, J. (1987). The prevention of falls in later life: A report of the Kellogg International Work Group on the prevention of falls by the elderly. *Danish Medical Bulletin, 43*(S4), 1–24.

Hallgren, J. & Aslan, A. K. D. (2018). Risk factors for hospital readmission among Swedish older adults. *European Geriatric Medicine, 9*(5), 603–11. https://doi.org/10.1007/s41999-018-0101-z

Hatton, A. L. & Rome, K. (2019). Falls, footwear, and podiatric interventions in older adults. *Clinics in Geriatric Medicine, 35*(2), 161–71. https://doi.org/10.1016/j.cger.2018.12.001

Hayakawa, T., Hashimoto, S., Kanda, H., Hirano, N., Kurihara, Y., Kawashima, T. & Fukushima, T. (2014). Risk factors of falls in inpatients and their practical use in identifying high-risk persons at admission: Fukushima Medical University

Hospital cohort study. *BMJ Open, 4*(8), E005385. https://doi.org/10.1136/bmjopen-2014-005385

Hill, K., Vrantsidis, F., Jessup, R., McGann, A., Pearce, J. & Collins, T. (2004). Validation of a falls risk assessment tool in the sub-acute hospital setting: A pilot study. *Australasian Journal of Podiatric Medicine, 38*(4), 99–108.

Hopewell, S., Adedire, O., Copsey, B. J., Boniface, G. J., Sherrington, C., Clemson, L., Close, J. & Lamb, S. E. (2018). Multifactorial and multiple component interventions for preventing falls in older people living in the community. *Cochrane Database of Systematic Reviews, 7*. https://doi.org/10.1002/14651858.CD012221.pub2

Huang, A. R., Mallet, L., Rochefort, C. M., Eguale, T., Buckeridge, D. L. & Tamblyn, R. (2012). Medication-related falls in the elderly: Causative factors and preventive strategies. *Drugs Aging, 29*(5), 359–76. https://doi.org/10.2165/11599460-000000000-00000

Ie, K., Chou, E., Boyce, R. D. & Albert, S. M. (2021). Fall risk-increasing drugs, polypharmacy, and falls among low-income community-dwelling older adults. *Innovation in Aging, 5*(1), igab001. https://doi.org/10.1093/geroni/igab001

Inder, K. J., Lewin, T. J. & Kelly, B. J. (2012). Factors impacting on the well-being of older residents in rural communities. *Perspectives in Public Health, 132*(4), 182–91. https://doi.org/10.1177/1757913912447018

Kenny, R. A., Romero-Ortuno, R. & Kumar, P. (2017). Falls in older adults. *Medicine, 45*(1), 28–33. https://doi.org/10.1016/j.mpmed.2016.10.007

Kim, J. & Parish, A. L. (2017). Polypharmacy and medication management in older adults. *Nursing Clinics of North America, 52*(3), 457–

68. https://doi.org/10.1016/j.cnur.2017.04.007

Korall, A. M., Feldman, F., Yang, Y., Cameron, I. D., Leung, P.-M., Sims-Gould, J. & Robinovitch, S. N. (2019). Effectiveness of hip protectors to reduce risk for hip fracture from falls in long-term care. *Journal of the American Medical Directors Association, 20*(11), 1397–403. https://doi.org/10.1016/j.jamda.2019.07.010

Langhammer, B., Bergland, A. & Rydwik, E. (2018). The importance of physical activity exercise among older people. *BioMed Research International.* https://doi.org/10.1155/2018/7856823

Lavedán, A., Viladrosa, M., Jürschik, P., Botigué, T., Nuín, C., Masot, O. & Lavedán, R. (2018). Fear of falling in community-dwelling older adults: A cause of falls, a consequence, or both? *PLoS ONE, 13*(3), e0194967. http://doi.org/10.1371/journal.pone.0194967

LeLaurin, J. H. & Shorr, R. I. (2019). Preventing falls in hospitalized patients: State of the Science. *Clinics in Geriatric Medicine, 35*(2), 273–83. https://doi.org/10.1016%2Fj.cger.2019.01.007

Lerdal, A., Sigurdsen, L. W., Hammerstad, H., Granheim, T. I., Risk Study Research Group & Gay, C. L. (2018). Associations between patient symptoms and falls in an acute care hospital: A cross-sectional study. *Journal of Clinical Nursing, 27*(9–10), 1826–35. https://doi.org/10.1111/jocn.14364

Machaj, D., Cyboran, K., Płaczek, A., Baran, M. & Wojnowski, M. (2020). The importance of vitamin D3 supplementation in orthopedics – literature review. *Journal of Education, Health and Sport, 10*(5), 118–22. https://doi.org/10.12775/JEHS.2020.10.05.011

Mackenzie, L. & Byles, J. (2018). Scoring the home falls and accidents screening tool for health professionals (HOME FAST-HP): Evidence from

one epidemiological study. *Australian Occupational Therapy Journal, 65*(5), 346–53. https://doi.org/10.1111/1440-1630.12467

Melin, C. M. (2018). Reducing falls in the inpatient hospital setting. *International Journal of Evidence-Based Healthcare, 16*(1), 25–31. https://doi.org/10.1097/XEB.0000000000000115

Menz, H. B., Auhl, M. & Spink, M. J. (2018). Foot problems as a risk factor for falls in community-dwelling older people: A systematic review and meta-analysis. *Maturitas, 118*, 7–14. https://doi.org/10.1016/j.maturitas.2018.10.001

Moncada, L. V. V. & Mire, L. G. (2017). Preventing falls in older persons. *American Family Physician, 96*(4), 240–7. https://www.aafp.org/afp/2017/0815/p240.html

Morello, R. T., Barker, A. L., Watts, J. J., Haines, T., Zavarsek, S. S., Hill, K. D., Brand, C., Sherrington, C., Wolfe, R., Bohensky, M. A. & Stoelwinder, J. U. (2015). The extra resource burden of in-hospital falls: A cost of falls study. *Medical Journal of Australia, 203*(9), 367. https://doi.org/10.5694/mja15.00296

Morin, L., Larrañaga, A. C., Welmer, A.-K., Rizzuto, D., Wastesson, J. W. & Johnell, K. (2019). Polypharmacy and injurious falls in older adults: A nationwide nested case-control study. *Clinical Epidemiology, 11*, 483–93. https://doi.org/10.2147/CLEP.S201614

Morris, R. & O'Riordan, S. (2017). Prevention of falls in hospital. *Clinical Medicine, 17*(4), 360–62. https://doi.org/10.7861/clinmedicine.17-4-360

Musich, S., Wang, S. S., Ruiz, J., Hawkins, K. & Wicker, E. (2018). The impact of mobility limitations on health outcomes among older adults. *Geriatric Nursing, 39*(2), 162–9. https://doi.org/10.1016/j.gerinurse.2017.08.002

Najafpour, Z., Godarzi, Z., Arab, M. & Yaseri, M. (2019). Risk factors for falls in hospital in-patients: A prospective nested case control study. *International Journal of Health Policy and Management*, 8(5), 300–6. https://doi.org/10.15171/ijhpm.2019.11

Nguyen, T., Combs, E. M., Wright, P. J. & Corbett, C. F. (2021). Reducing fall risks among visually impaired older adults. *Home Healthcare Now*, 39(4), 186–93. https://doi.org/10.1097/NHH.0000000000000995

Painter, J. A., Allison, L., Dhingra, P., Daughtery, J., Cogdill, K. & Trujillo, L. G. (2012). Fear of falling and its relationship with anxiety, depression, and activity engagement among community-dwelling older adults. *American Journal of Occupational Therapy*, 66(2), 169–76. https://doi.org/10.5014/ajot.2012.002535

Palmer, R. M. (2018). The acute care for elders unit model of care. *Geriatrics*, 3(3), 59. https://doi.org/10.3390/geriatrics3030059

Pati, D., Valipoor, S., Lorusso, L., Mihandoust, S., Jamshidi, S., Rane, A. & Kazem-Zadeh, M. (2021). The impact of the built environment on patient falls in hospital rooms: An integrative review. *Journal of Patient Safety*, 17(4), 273–81. https://doi.org/10.1097/PTS.0000000000000613

Petersen, N., König, H.-H. & Hajek, A. (2020). The link between falls, social isolation and loneliness: A systematic review. *Archives of Gerontology and Geriatrics*, 88, 104020. https://doi.org/10.1016/j.archger.2020.104020

Peterson, D. & Molina, A. (2021). An Analysis of the Costs and Benefits of Providing Increased Mobility to Reduce Social Isolation Among America's Aging Population. U.S. Department of Transportation. www.ugpti.org/resources/reports/downloads/surtcom21-06.pdf

Pointer, S. (2013). *Trends in hospitalised injury, Australia: 1999-00 to 2010–11.*

Australian Institute of Health and Welfare. https://apo.org.au/node/35340

Remelli, F., Vitali, A., Zurlo, A. & Volpato, S. (2019). Vitamin D deficiency and sarcopenia in older persons. *Nutrients*, 11(12), 2861. https://doi.org/10.3390/nu11122861

Reuben, D. B. & Tinetti, M. E. (2012). Goal-oriented patient care – An alternative health outcomes paradigm. *New England Journal of Medicine*, 366(9), 777–9. https://doi.org/10.1056/NEJMp1113631

Robson, K., Ahasan, N., Barnes, C., Murphy, K. & Pope, R. (2021). Increasing physical activity in older Australians to reduce falls: A program evaluation. *Internet Journal of Allied Health Sciences and Practice*, 19(3), 3.

Robson, K., Coyle, J. & Pope, R. (2018). Exploration of older people's perceptions of behavioural factors associated with falls. *Age and Ageing*, 47(5), 734–40. https://doi.org/10.1093/ageing/afy051

Russell, M. A., Hill, K. D., Day, L. M., Blackberry, I., Gurrin, L. C. & Dharmage, S. C. (2009). Development of the falls risk for older people in the community (FROP-Com) screening tool. *Age and Ageing*, 38(1), 40–6. https://doi.org/10.1093/ageing/afn196

Saftari, L. N. & Kwon, O.-S. (2018). Ageing vision and falls: A review. *Journal of Physiological Anthropology*, 37(1), 1–14. https://doi.org/10.1186/s40101-018-0170-1

Sakurai, R. & Okubo, Y. (2020). Depression, fear of falling, cognition and falls. In M. Montero-Odasso & R. Camicioli, (eds). *Falls and Cognition in Older Persons* (pp. 49–66). Springer. https://doi.org/10.1007/978-3-030-24233-6_4

Satariano, W. A., Guralnik, J. M., Jackson, R. J., Marottoli, R. A., Phelan, E. A. & Prohaska, T. R. (2012). Mobility and aging: New directions for public health action. *American Journal of Public*

Health, 102(8), 1508–15. https://doi.org/10.2105/AJPH.2011.300631

Saunders, R., Seaman, K., Graham, R. & Christiansen, A. (2019). The effect of volunteers' care and support on the health outcomes of older adults in acute care: A systematic scoping review. *Journal of Clinical Nursing*, 28(23–24), 4236–49. https://doi.org/10.1111/jocn.15041

Schluter, P. J., Arnold, E. P. & Jamieson, H. A. (2018). Falls and hip fractures associated with urinary incontinence among older men and women with complex needs: A national population study. *Neurourology and Urodynamics*, 37(4), 1336–43. https://doi.org/10.1002/nau.23442

Sharif, S. I., Al-Harbi, A. B., Al-Shihabi, A. M., Al-Daour, D. S. & Sharif, R. S. (2018). Falls in the elderly: Assessment of prevalence and risk factors. *Pharmacy Practice*, 16(3), 1–7. https://doi.org/10.18549/pharmpract.2018.03.1206

Shekelle, P. G., Greeley, A. M., Tanner, E. P., Mak, S. S., Begashaw, M. M., Miake-Lye, I. M., & Beroes-Severin, J. M. (2019). *One-to-one observation: A systematic review.* Evidence Synthesis Program, Health Services Research and Development Service, Office of Research and Development, Department of Veterans Affairs. https://www.hsrd.research.va.gov/publications/esp/one-to-one-obsv-REPORT.pdf

Sherrington, C., Michaleff, Z. A., Fairhall, N., Paul, S. S., Tiedemann, A., Whitney, J., Cumming, R. G., Herbert, R. D., Close, J. C. & Lord, S. R. (2017). Exercise to prevent falls in older adults: An updated systematic review and meta-analysis. *British Journal of Sports Medicine*, 51(24), 1750–8. https://doi.org/10.1136/bjsports-2016-096547

Spink, M. J., Menz, H. B., Fotoohabadi, M. R., Wee, E., Landorf, K. B., Hill, K.

D. & Lord, S. R. (2011). Effectiveness of a multifaceted podiatry intervention to prevent falls in community dwelling older people with disabling foot pain: Randomised controlled trial. *British Medical Journal, 342*(online), d3411. https://dx.doi.org/10.1136/bmj.d3411

Stapleton, C., Hough, P., Oldmeadow, L., Bull, K., Hill, K. & Greenwood, K. (2009). Four-item fall risk screening tool for subacute and residential aged care: The first step in fall prevention. *Australasian Journal on Ageing, 28*(3), 139–43. https://doi.org/10.1111/j.1741-6612.2009.00375.x

Stark, S., Keglovits, M., Arbesman, M. & Lieberman, D. (2017). Effect of home modification interventions on the participation of community-dwelling adults with health conditions: A systematic review. *American Journal of Occupational Therapy, 71*(2), 7102290010p1–7102290010p11. https://doi.org/10.5014/ajot.2017.018887

Stenholm, S., Shardell, M., Bandinelli, S., Guralnik, J. M. & Ferrucci, L. (2015). Physiological factors contributing to mobility loss over 9 years of follow-up – Results from the InCHIANTI study. *Journals of Gerontology. Series A, Biological Sciences & Medical Sciences, 70*(5), 591–7. https://doi.org/10.1093/Gerona/glv004

Stubbs, B., Schofield, P. & Patchay, S. (2016). Mobility limitations and fall-related factors contribute to the reduced health-related quality of life in older adults with chronic musculoskeletal pain. *Pain Practice, 16*(1), 80–9. https://doi.org/10.1111/papr.12264

Sundar, V., Brucker, D. L., Pollack, M. A. & Chang, H. (2016). Community and social participation among adults with mobility

impairments: A mixed methods study. *Disability and Health Journal, 9*(4), 682–91. https://doi.org/10.1016/j.dhjo.2016.05.006

Terrill, A. L., Molton, I. R., Ehde, D. M., Amtmann, D., Bombardier, C. H., Smith, A. E. & Jensen, M. P. (2016). Resilience, age, and perceived symptoms in persons with long-term physical disabilities. *Journal of Health Psychology, 21*(5), 640–9. https://doi.org/10.1177/1359105314532973

Tiedemann, A., Lord. S. & Sherrington, C. (2012). The Quickscreen tool – A validated falls risk assessment, development and implemented in Australia for use in primary care. *Injury Prevention, 18*(S1), A1–A246. https://doi.org/10.1136/injuryprev-2012-040580e.16

Tiedemann, A., Shimada, H., Sherrington, C., Murray, S. & Lord, S. (2008). The comparative ability of eight functional mobility tests for predicting falls in community dwelling older people. *Age and Ageing, 37*(4), 430–5. https://doi.org/10.1093/ageing/afn100

Tsai, L.-T. (2017). Walking, physical activity and life-space mobility among older people. *Studies in Sport, Physical Education and Health, 254.* https://jyx.jyu.fi/bitstream/handle/123456789/52956/978-951-39-6965-3_vaitos17022017.pdf?sequence=1&isAllowed=y

van Haastregt, J., Zijlstra, G., Hendriks, M., Goosens, M., van Eijk, J. & Kempen, G. (2013). Cost-effectiveness of an intervention to reduce fear of falling. *International Journal of Technology Assessment in Health Care, 29*(3), 219–26. https://doi.org/10.1017/S0266462313000275

Viljanen, A., Mikkola, T. M., Rantakokko, M., Portegijs, E. & Rantanen, T. (2016). The association between transportation and life-space mobility in community-dwelling older people with or

without walking difficulties. *Journal of Aging and Health, 28*(6), 1038–54. https://doi.org/10.1177/0898264315618919

Vinik, A. I., Camacho, P., Reddy, S., Valencia, W. M., Trence, D., Matsumoto, A. M., & Morley, J. E. (2017). Aging, diabetes, and falls. *Endocrine Practice, 23*(9), 1120–42. https://doi.org/10.4158/EP171794.RA

Vlaeyen, E., Coussement, J., Leysens, G., Van der Elst, E., Delbaere, K., Cambier, D., Denhaerynck, K., Goemaere, S., Wertelaers, A., Dobbels, F., Dejaeger, E. & Milisen, K. & Center of Expertise for Fall and Fracture Prevention Flanders. (2015). Characteristics and effectiveness of fall prevention programs in nursing homes: A systematic review and meta-analysis of randomized controlled trials. *Journal of the American Geriatrics Society, 63*(2), 211–1. https://doi.org/10.1111/jgs.13254

Webber, S. C., Porter, M. M. & Menec, V. H. (2010). Mobility in older adults: A comprehensive framework. *The Gerontologist, 50*(4), 443–50. https://doi.org/10.1093/geront/gnq013

Western Australian Department of Health (2015). Development of the Falls Risk Assessment and Management Plan. Health Strategy and Networks Branch, Western Australian Department of Health. https://ww2.health.wa.gov.au/-/media/Files/Corporate/general%20documents/falls/PDF/Dev-of-FRAMP.pdf

Whipple, M. O., Hamel, A. V. & Talley, K. M. (2018). Fear of falling among community-dwelling older adults: A scoping review to identify effective evidence-based interventions. *Geriatric Nursing, 39*(2), 170–7. https://doi.org/10.1016/j.gerinurse.2017.08.005

Whitney, J., Close, J. C. T., Lord, S. R. & Jackson, S. H. D. (2012). Identification of high risk fallers among older people living in residential care facilities: A simple screen based on easily collectable measures. *Archives of Gerontology and Geriatrics, 55*(3), 690–5. https://doi.org/10.1016/j.archger.2012.05.010

World Health Organization (WHO) (2007). WHO Global Report on Falls Prevention in Older Age. WHO. https://apps.who.int/iris/handle/10665/43811

World Health Organization (WHO) (2020). UN Decade of Healthy Ageing (2021–2030). WHO. https://www.who.int/initiatives/decade-of-healthy-ageing

World Health Organization (WHO) (2021). Step safely: Strategies for preventing and managing falls across the life-course. https://apps.who.int/iris/bitstream/handle/10665/340962/9789240021914-eng.pdf

Yardley, L., Morrison, L., Bradbury, K. & Muller, I. (2015). The person-based approach to intervention development: Application to digital health-related behavior change interventions. *Journal of Medical Internet Research, 17*(1), E30. https://doi.org/10.2196/jmir.4055

Zanker, J. & Duque, G. (2020). Approaches for falls prevention in hospitals and nursing home settings. In M. Montero-Odasso & R. Camicioli, (eds). *Falls and Cognition in Older Persons.* Springer, pp. 245–59. https://doi.org/10.1007/978-3-030-24233-6_14

Zecevic, A. A., Salmoni, A. W., Speechley, M. & Vandervoort, A. A. (2006). Defining a fall and reasons for falling: Comparisons among the views of seniors, health care providers, and the research literature. *The Gerontologist, 46*(3), 367–76. https://doi.org/10.1093/geront/46.3.367

Zhang, W., Low, L. F., Schwenk, M., Mills, N., Gwynn, J. D. & Clemson, L. (2019). Review of gait, cognition, and fall risks with implications for fall prevention in older adults with dementia. *Dementia and Geriatric Cognitive Disorders, 48*(1–2), 17–29. https://doi.org/10.1159/000504340

18 Managing Multiple Chronic Conditions (Multimorbidity)

ALISON DEVITT

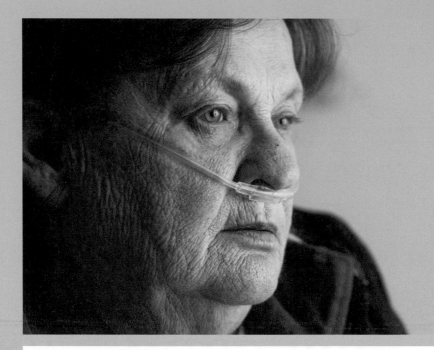

LEARNING OBJECTIVES

After reading this chapter, you will:

» describe the multifaceted impact of multiple chronic conditions on the older person and the ways this influences their experience of illness

» compare various evidenced-based models of care that have common elements proven to be successful in chronic disease management

» differentiate prevention, early detection and early treatment across the chronic disease continuum and how they are key population health strategies

» implement collaborative, person-centred care, which makes up the principles that underpin chronic disease management

» describe the role of the multidisciplinary team for the management of chronic and complex conditions

» integrate the health and social services at administrative and service delivery levels that are needed to facilitate continuity of care and timely access to services.

Introduction

Many older people are managing **multiple chronic conditions (MCCs)**. Successful management impacts an older person's functional independence and quality of life significantly (Commonwealth of Australia, 2020). This chapter explores the unique challenges of people living with MCCs and outlines approaches to healthcare that have proven to better cater for **multimorbidity**.

multiple chronic conditions (MCCs)
The coexistence of two or more long-term or permanent health conditions in a person.

multimorbidity
The presence of multiple chronic conditions that collectively have an adverse effect on the health and well-being of the person living with them.

18.1 Getting to know the person: Jack's story

Jack has been living with diabetes since he was 39 years old. At first, he controlled his blood sugar levels by taking hypoglycaemic medications. He had no other major health complications and considered himself to be generally healthy. Jack had an active social life and played golf with his work colleagues on a regular basis. He enjoyed his career, where he indulged in his love of cars by working as a manager at a motor dealership. On the weekend he would drive his three sons to their football games in the newest car, to the envy of all their friends. His wife, Jean, managed the household affairs, and prepared Jack's meals every day. This typically included two pieces of white toast with jam for breakfast, a piece of cake for morning tea, a meat and salad sandwich on white bread for lunch, biscuits or fruit with a cup of tea in the afternoon, meat and three vegetables for dinner and a piece of toast before going to bed. Jack's family and career were his pride and joy.

Jack, his wife and family will be the focus of the chapter in order to engage you with a situation that will stimulate your thinking, illustrate concepts and introduce models of care for older people with MCC.

18.2 Getting to know the person: Jack's story

When Jack retired, he moved with Jean to a rural town to be close to their grown-up children and young grandchildren. They planned to travel around Australia when they were no longer required to babysit their grandchildren. During their early years of retirement, Jack's diabetes progressed and he required insulin to manage his blood sugar levels. Some days he found it difficult to self-administer the injection because osteoarthritis was affecting his hands. He also developed peripheral neuropathy, which caused burning pain in his legs; this prevented him from sleeping at night. Mobilising became increasingly difficult, and he no longer wanted to play golf because at times he would lose his balance. His vision was affected by bilateral glaucoma and he did not feel safe driving. His GP prescribed regular tramadol (a pain killer) and suggested that he purchase a walking aid. He also suggested that Jack ask his children to drive him the long distances to his specialist medical appointments, but Jack refused to be seen using a walking aid in public, and he did not want to bother his children to drive him to his increasingly frequent appointments.

chronic disease
A pathological condition that interrupts the normal functions of the body and tends to be slow in progression and prolonged in duration.

chronic condition
Any ongoing or recurring health issue that has a significant impact on the person and/or family or other carers, and requiring a long period of supervision, monitoring and care.

The rates of **chronic disease** are rising in Australia and so is multimorbidity (the coexistence of two or more **chronic conditions** in a person that collectively have an adverse effect on their health and well-being). It is estimated that one in four Australians have two or more of the eight selected chronic conditions measured in the 'Australia's Health 2018' report (AIHW, 2018). The prevalence of multimorbidity increases with age, with almost one in three Australians aged 65 years or older reported as having at least three or more chronic conditions (AHMAC, 2017). These individuals often require complex disease management and experience worse health outcomes, which are associated with increased health costs (AHMAC, 2017). The growing burden of multimorbidity in our ageing population will place more importance on the care and treatment of people who require complex disease management, including the need for a skilled aged care workforce who are able to effectively care for older people, who are often among the most complex to manage (Commonwealth of Australia, 2019b).

Impact of multimorbidity

A growing number of older Australians are required to manage MCCs. This has a significant impact on their lives, their families and/or their carers and on the health-care system. In the experience of people living with MCCs, it is more complex than having a single chronic disease (Duguay et al., 2014, p. 15). This perception is supported by the fact that multimorbidity is associated with suboptimal health outcomes, including:

quality of life
An individual's subjective perception of their life based on an evaluation of the positive and negative aspects.

- reduced **quality of life**
- declines in physical, mental and social functionality
- higher rates of unplanned hospitalisation
- psychological distress
- increased risk of mortality.

All of these place a heavy demand on health-care resources (Cheng et al., 2019; Shad et al., 2017).

The presence of several health problems in a system as complex as the human body results in a variety of interactions (illness–illness, treatment–treatment, treatment–illness) that adversely affect one another. There are interactions between the health conditions themselves that can have physical, psychological and social impacts (Coventry et al., 2015; Duguay et al., 2014). For example, Jack has insomnia because of peripheral neuropathy pain. Because his sleep quality is poor, his body is unable to recover from the pain. These factors contribute to daytime fatigue and can heighten psychological distress and depression, which may lead to social withdrawal. This can become a vicious cycle as social disconnectedness has been identified as a risk factor for depression (Santini et al., 2020). Other causes of harm in people with MCCs are treatment-related interactions and conflicts (see Table 18.1 for impacts of multimorbidity, common issues and intervention). For example, the management of osteoarthritis with non-steroidal anti-inflammatory agents when peptic ulcer disease is a coexisting condition is problematic because these medications can cause upper gastric bleeding and may cause an ulcer. Because of these complex interactions, each person living with MCCs presents with their own unique set of issues, symptoms, challenges and attitudes towards illness. This requires person-centred approaches to management of multimorbidity and individually tailored interventions (Pert et al., 2020).

Several studies have also revealed common themes in the experience of people living with MCCs, most prominently that it is disruptive to everyday life and impacts the quality of life due to:

- time-consuming treatments
- required **self-care**
- travelling to various medical appointments
- managing symptoms
- polypharmacy (Duguay et al., 2014; O'Brien et al., 2014).

It is important that health-care providers understand that multimorbidity creates a cascade of medical and emotional crises that adversely affect one another. These inevitably have implications for various dimensions of personhood, including physical, psychosocial and emotional well-being. This requires a collaborative and holistic approach to assessment and interventions, which are managed and prioritised in conjunction with the patient and their family (Duguay et al., 2014). Table 18.1 outlines the multifaceted impact of multimorbidity with examples of common issues and interventions.

self-care
Individuals taking the actions required to care for their own health and well-being; in the context of multimorbidity this includes actions to effectively manage their chronic conditions and to prevent further illness.

TABLE 18.1 Impacts of multimorbidity: common issues and interventions

IMPACTS	ISSUES	INTERVENTIONS
Physical	Symptoms produced by the health condition and/or treatment can be debilitating. Some common symptoms include: » pain » dyspnoea » nausea » constipation » diarrhoea » fatigue » muscle weakness » cognitive dysfunction (Coventry et al., 2015; Larsen, 2019).	» Assess for common symptoms. » Partner with the patient to establish a care plan to control and prevent exacerbation of their symptoms. This will often require the use of multiple techniques, tailored to suit the unique needs and preferences of the individual (Larsen, 2019).
	Physical loss may cause disability and functional impairment. This may affect activity levels and independence (Coventry et al., 2015; Duguay et al., 2014).	» Perform activities of daily living assessment. » Perform a falls risks assessment. » Make referrals to support services as required to enable independence and self-care.

(Continues)

TABLE 18.1 Continued

Psychological	The illness experience is associated with a variety of negative emotions including powerlessness, anger, despair, distress, discouragement, chronic sorrow, devaluation of self, anxiety and fear of losing independence (Coventry et al., 2015; Larsen, 2019; Porter et al., 2020).	» Chronic health conditions often have no cure and affect everyday life to varying degrees. The long-term nature of **chronic illness** requires health-care professionals to listen to and understand the patient's experience with illness (Larsen, 2019). » Encourage, but do not force, the verbalisation of feelings. » The Trajectory Framework, a nursing model for chronic illness management developed by Corbin and Strauss (1991), assists nurses to identify and understand the phases of the chronic illness experience (Corbin, 1998).
	» Mental health issues are more common in people with chronic disease (Coventry et al., 2015). » The greater number of chronic conditions an individual has, the more vulnerable they become to depression (Spangenberg et al., 2011). » People who experience chronic pain are at high risk of depression (Sheng et al., 2017). » Depression is also common in spouses and carers of people with MCCs (Pierce & Lutz, 2019).	» Recognise the risk factors for depression. » Ask patients about their mental and emotional health in a sensitive manner. Listen and provide a validating and empathetic response. » Assess for depression using a screening tool such as the DMI-10 or DMI-18, specifically for measuring depression in people with medical health conditions. » Make a referral to a mental health practitioner. » Share information with the patient about mental health and well-being. » Encourage activities that promote mental health such as social reconnection and exercise. » Assess the caregiver for stress and fatigue and the need for respite (Pierce & Lutz, 2019).
Social	Disease management regimens, decreased activity levels, disability and financial burdens can place limitations on an individual's social engagement or prevent them from fulfilling their valued social roles. This can lead to social isolation (Nicholas & Nicholson, 2019).	» Assess for social isolation. » Help patients to adapt/adjust to changes using problem-solving techniques. » Help patients set realistic goals and expectations. » Make environmental modifications to enable people to maintain independence, self-care and social roles.
	Many people living with disability report experiencing stigma. Stigmatisation excludes individuals from full social interaction and alters social relationships (Mauk, 2019). In healthcare it can be associated with inequitable treatment.	» Health professionals need to examine their own biases, attitudes, perceptions and actions carefully. » Encouraging a patient's participation in health-care decision making is an outward demonstration of respect and regard for that person. » Support groups can offer moral support and a source of acceptance. However, this approach may not be helpful for all people as some stigmatised individuals do not feel comfortable with other stigmatised individuals because it can heighten the issues they face.

chronic illness
The human experience of prolonged symptoms and suffering. It refers to how the disease or condition is perceived by the person experiencing it, as well as their caregiver/s.

Review Chapter 5 on family relationships and informal carers to assist your understanding.

CHALLENGES FOR THE HEALTH SYSTEM, THE PATIENT AND THEIR FAMILY

The multifaceted impact of multimorbidity translates into complex and costly care needs associated with increased demands on health-care resources, including GPs, medical specialists, psychologists and other allied health consultations, pharmaceutical prescriptions, acute and community care services and other medical expenditures (AIHW, 2018). More concerning is the impact of the health-care system on individuals living with MCCs and their families and/or carers who are required to navigate and respond to myriad health services and information sources (AHMAC, 2017).

Barriers to optimal health

The Royal Commission into Aged Care Quality and Safety (Commonwealth of Australia, 2021) reported several factors within the current health system that are contributing to incomplete care and suboptimal health outcomes for aged care consumers requiring healthcare for MCCs. They include:

- failure to coordinate care
- poor communication between health-care providers, particularly during hospitalisation events
- administration requirements of clinicians resulting in insufficient time for adequate health provider and patient interactions
- lack of integration between health and community sectors
- patients receiving conflicting treatment advice from different health professionals (see Table 18.2).

TABLE 18.2 Barriers to optimal health outcomes and their impact on the patient and health system

BARRIER TO OPTIMAL HEALTH OUTCOMES	IMPACT ON THE PATIENT – EXAMPLES FROM JACK'S STORY	IMPACT ON THE HEALTH SYSTEM
Failure to coordinate care	Jack sees multiple health professionals (endocrinologist, podiatrist, dietician, diabetes educator, vascular surgeon, ophthalmologist) and is asked to retell his story each time.	» Cost of time of each specialist, conflicting treatment regimens, unnecessarily repeating diagnostic tests and screening. » Assumptions can be made about who is taking responsibility for certain aspects of care and as a result patients can 'fall through gaps' in care.
Poor communication between health providers	Communication between Jack's GP and his medical specialists is one-way.	This hinders shared decision making.
Administration requirements of clinicians resulting in lack of time for health provider and patient interactions	When Jack is admitted to hospital for intravenous antibiotics to treat an infected leg ulcer, he wants to talk to the medical registrar about his concern that his wife, who is becoming more forgetful, is at home alone. He does not get the chance because all the doctors seem to be in a rush and are focused on his wound and medications and documenting notes on their computer.	» Health professionals address the presenting or immediate problem, and do not provide comprehensive and holistic care. » Health professional job dissatisfaction. » A reactive approach to healthcare is less cost-effective than preventative and comprehensive care across the continuum of chronic disease.
Lack of integration of health services with social services	During a health assessment, the practice nurse identifies that Jack is not coping at home and needs home care support. She emails a referral form to the age care assessment team and advises Jack that he will go on their waiting list for a home visit to assess his eligibility for a home-care package.	Support services are not provided in a timely manner.
Patients receiving conflicting treatment advice	Jack's GP advised him that he needs to take his prescribed non-steroidal anti-inflammatories to control his pain. Another specialist advised him to stop taking them because he is prone to peptic ulcers. Jack stops taking his anti-inflammatories without an alternative analgesic to replace it and his pain flares up.	» It is difficult for patients to know what advice to follow so they may not follow any advice or may follow inappropriate advice. This may cause harm to the patient and consequently burden the acute care sector with higher rates of unplanned hospital admissions. » Patient distrust of health-care providers and the health system.

Chapter 2 provides an overview of policies in Australia that affect healthcare and older people.

The illness experience is 'the lived experience of individuals and families with chronic disease' (Larsen, 2019, p. 67). It refers to how the disease or condition is subjectively perceived and responded to physically, psychologically, socially and emotionally, including actions people take that affect their health for better or worse (Larsen, 2019; Porter et al., 2020). For example, hypertension may have little impact on the day-to-day life of a person, so if a person believes that illness is a debilitating condition, they may not perceive hypertension as an illness. In contrast, conditions such as rheumatoid arthritis may significantly restrict an individual's physical functioning and social responsibilities because of obvious symptoms such as pain, and therefore the person living with this condition may perceive it as an illness.

FOCUS QUESTIONS

- Reflect on your own experiences with health and illness. What influences your health behaviours and perceptions of chronic illness?
- How has Jack's illness experience evolved as the impact of his conditions progressed?
- Using Jack's story as an example, how does a person's values, interests and self-perception affect their illness experience?
- What 'self-care' activities will be required of Jack to maintain his health? How may this impact on his illness experience?

Models of care

patient-centred approach
A respectful relationship between health-care professionals, the health system and patients and their families that involves patients in shared decisions about their own health to develop a personalised care plan.

collaboration
Health-care professionals working together to achieve greater impacts on patient health outcomes than they could in isolation.

relationship-centred care
A reciprocal relationship between health-care professionals and patients that promotes a sense of belonging and security.

In Australia, the National Strategic Framework for Chronic Conditions provides approaches to healthcare that cater for multimorbidity (AHMAC, 2017). It embraces a **patient-centred approach**, which includes **collaboration** and partnership (AHMAC, 2017). Together, these principles encourage health-care providers to work with their patients in compassionate and respectful ways, acknowledging their unique and holistic health needs as fellow human beings, and reinforcing their power to make important contributions to their own health-care decisions (Larsen, 2019). Considering this knowledge, the Australian Royal Commission into Aged Care Quality and Safety (Commonwealth of Australia, 2019b, p. 2) found that the current aged care system is more focused on the funding relationship between providers and government than the choices of older people seeking care. Therefore, for older people and their families to receive real choices in their care, the aged care system requires a systemic overhaul, moving away from funding models that promote one-off transactions between health providers and 'consumers' to a system that facilitates patient-centred and **relationship-centred care** (Commonwealth of Australia, 2019b, p. 3). The Royal Commission into Aged Care Quality and Safety (Commonwealth of Australia, 2019b, p. 4) recommends that:

> Aged care must be designed for the people it is intended to help, and based on their dignity, rights, choices, quality of life, involvement and feedback. Aged care should be delivered in the context of trusting, respectful and collaborative relationships between the person receiving care, their family, staff and management (Commonwealth of Australia, 2019b, p. 4).

A new aged care system that has these qualities is urgently needed to better cater for the complex health needs of older people living with MCCs and to ensure their active participation in their own health-care decision making (Commonwealth of Australia, 2019a).

There are often similar approaches for the prevention and management of many chronic conditions. In Australia, the following approaches have been emphasised by the health-care system as they reduce the impact of chronic diseases and better cater for multimorbidity:

- focus on prevention or delay of chronic disease
- timely detection and intervention
- integration and **continuity of care** coordination
- empowering the individual to self-manage their health challenges (AHMAC, 2017; AIHW, 2016).

These approaches will be discussed in more detail as they apply to the role of health-care professionals working in multidisciplinary teams.

continuity of care
Using a care coordination health-care model to provide consistency of care and continuity of information to improve patient outcomes.

PREVENTION OR DELAY OF CHRONIC DISEASE

Health promotion is an important element in preventing or delaying the onset of chronic disease in older people (AHMAC, 2017). It is most effective when implemented during the early years of an individual's life, which are formative for their health in older life. However, that is not to say that it is too late for older people with chronic disease to change their lifestyles and improve their health. In 2001, the World Health Organization (WHO) publicised that a healthy lifestyle is important for every stage of life (as cited in Golinowska et al., 2017). Evidence has shown that limiting alcohol consumption, exercising, quitting smoking and participating in social activities can help to inhibit the progression of many diseases and prevent the loss of functional capacity (Golinowska et al., 2017). Health promotion targeted to older people with MCCs requires health professionals to take an individualised approach that aims to maintain and increase the older person's functional capacity and improve self-care. Older people living with MCC also tend to have unique health issues such as social isolation and suffering from loneliness. Health promotion activities that encourage community involvement and social connectedness can contribute to improved quality of life (Golinowska et al., 2017).

health promotion
The process of enabling people to increase control over and to improve their health.

TIMELY DETECTION AND INTERVENTION

Timely and appropriate detection and intervention involves recognising the risk factors for chronic conditions and taking appropriate action to monitor for signs and symptoms commonly associated with them. In the context of multimorbidity, it also involves monitoring for the emergence of complications associated with existing conditions (AHMAC, 2017). In Australia, one approach to early detection and intervention of health issues in older people is an annual **health assessment**. These are funded by Medicare and are often performed by a registered nurses in collaboration with a GP in a primary health setting. Assessment of older people requires strong assessment skills, particularly since multimorbidity creates challenges for the assessment process because of:

- multiple interactions between chronic conditions, medications and other treatment, which often result in complex and competing health needs. The cause of presenting symptoms can be difficult to differentiate between primary conditions, an exacerbation of symptoms, the predicted progression of the disease or new pathology unrelated to the known conditions
- atypical presentations. Older people may present with subtle, ill-defined or unexplained deterioration in function rather than 'textbook' signs and symptoms of disease.

health assessment
An Australian Government initiated program where older people undergo a full health check each year to prevent and/or address any changes that have occurred.

For example, an asymptomatic urinary tract infection may be the possible cause of unexplained, acute change in cognition

- polypharmacy, which makes older people at risk of adverse drug events and medication errors. This adds to the complexity of the patient assessment

- ageism and stigmatisation of older people and the ageing process, which can reduce the awareness of health practitioners and contribute to mistreatment and misdiagnosis

- communication barriers such as low health literacy, cognitive impairment and changes in sensory capacity (e.g. vision and hearing), which may make history taking and assessment difficult (Smith, 2017; Commonwealth of Australia, 2021).

Polypharmacy is explained in detail in Chapter 14.

COMPREHENSIVE ASSESSMENT

In response to these challenges, the person-centred 'comprehensive assessment' was developed. Unlike traditional health assessments, which are typically focused on presenting health symptoms, a comprehensive assessment focuses on individuals with complex health problems and involves input and findings from a team of professionals from different health disciplines who collectively assess all domains of an individual's life relevant to overall health and well-being (Welsh et al., 2014). This allows them to better understand the unique risk factors and holistic health needs of patients to form appropriate assessment, care planning, goal setting, monitoring and other relevant decision making such as treatment and referrals (ACSQHC, 2020). Areas typically assessed include:

- clinical assessment and diagnosis
- medications
- functionality (medical, physical and social)
- psychological assessment (mental health and cognition)
- nutritional status and needs
- social support and carer strain
- living environment
- people involved in care
- planned or ongoing interventions, including preventative interventions such as vaccinations
- monitoring plans such as escalation plans and review dates (ACSQHC, 2020; Smith, 2017).

care plan
A plan of action, agreed between a patient and their health-care providers, that identifies their health-care needs, services that are needed, and a list of health goals and specific actions that are required to meet them.

Screening tools can be used to identify common conditions associated with ageing, including dementia, depression, vision impairment and skin integrity. Referrals can be made for additional screening services such as bone density scans, hearing tests, mammograms, oral health check, bowel cancer screening and other pathology tests. This opportunistic approach to prevention and early detection serves the purpose of identifying actual and potential health risks that will guide the development of interventions to promote and protect health.

You can find more information on carer strain in Chapters 5 and 7.

A person-centred approach to the assessment should establish or update the patient's goals of care, including clinical and personal goals, advanced **care plans** and preferences for end-of-life care or treatment-limiting orders (ACSQHC, 2020). Overall, this comprehensive approach ensures that the person is at the centre of their healthcare and improves diagnostic accuracy and the effectiveness of timely interventions (ACSQHC, 2020; Smith, 2017).

Communication is incredibly important during the assessment. Barriers to communication may result in inaccurate findings, misdiagnosis and mistreatment (Smith, 2017). In older people communication may be hindered by:

- hearing impairment
- vision impairment
- changes in cognition
- depression
- health literacy status
- culturally and linguistically diverse background.

These aspects should be assessed at the beginning of the process to ensure that interventions can be put in place to enhance the communication – for example, ask the older person to put in their hearing device (Smith, 2017). It is also essential that the health professional continues to check the patient's understanding throughout the assessment and ensures that any information given to them is suited to their health literacy needs.

> You can find information on assessing people with culturally and linguistically diverse backgrounds in Chapters 3 and 5.

18.3 Getting to know the person: Jack's story

During a routine health assessment, the nurse discovered that Jack's pain, along with insomnia at night, fatigue during the day and constipation, was continuing to worsen and was affecting his activities of daily living and overall quality of life. The nurse shared this information with the GP, who prescribed Coloxyl for Jack's constipation, Normison to help him sleep at night and non-steroidal anti-inflammatory agents for osteoarthritis pain. This new medication regimen did help with his symptoms, but he developed a new symptom: epigastric pain and nausea after eating. An endoscopy revealed a stomach ulcer. The gastroenterologist told him to stop taking the non-steroidal anti-inflammatories. His pain was now more severe than before. Jack returned to his GP and expressed that he felt frustrated and hopeless about his situation, and that he saw no point in living if his condition was only going to get worse as he got older. The only thing keeping him around was Jean, who had been diagnosed with early-stage dementia. Jean had been his carer for many years. Now he was caring for her. His GP prescribed him opioids for pain and amoxapine for depression.

- In a system as complex as the human body, the presence of several health problems results in multiple interactions: disease–disease, disease–treatment and treatment–treatment. Identify and discuss Jack's multiple medication interactions and their implications.
- How has Jack's illness experience continued to evolve with the deterioration of his health?
- What screening tools could the clinicians have used during their assessments to identify some of Jack's risk factors earlier?

FOCUS QUESTIONS

- coordinating multidisciplinary teamwork
- continuity of care by engaging directly with the patient and their family and/or carers across the continuum of care in collaboration with other health providers
- providing ongoing support and advocating on behalf of the patient and their family/or carer within the system
- allocating health-related system resources
- facilitating optimal transition of the patient between health-care settings, including acute, rehabilitation and palliative care
- providing ongoing assessments and evaluation of the plan of care.

> The registered nurse's role on multidisciplinary teams is an important aspect of professional practice. See Chapters 13 and 19 for more on this.

The services offered by care coordinators have demonstrated significant improvements in self-management and reduced potentially preventable hospitalisation. However, the most significant characteristic and benefit of the care coordinator role is the development of a trusting relationship that empowers the patient on their journey with chronic illness and makes them feel safe, cared for and respected (Porter et al., 2020). Based on these significant benefits, the development of the care coordinator or case manager role in aged care services is a key recommendation of the Australian Royal Commission into Aged Care Quality and Safety (Commonwealth of Australia, 2021).

PATIENT SELF-MANAGEMENT

Patient self-management is a patient's knowledge, skills and confidence to take on the role of managing their health and healthcare (Hibbard et al., 2005 in Consumers Health Forum of Australia, 2019, p. 5). There is a strong evidence base around self-management as a core component of chronic disease management, with studies demonstrating decreased presentations to hospital, improved adherence to agreed treatment plans and goals, improved clinical indicators (such as HBA1c), beneficial effects on a person's ability to manage activities of daily living, increased self efficacy and well-being, and a sense of control over their own health situation (Contant et al., 2019; CHFA, 2019; Duguay et al., 2014). However, it must be noted that the complex nature of multimorbidity makes self-management more difficult for people living with MCCs compared to people living with a single chronic disease. In several studies of the experiences of adults living with multimorbidity, participants expressed that self-management was a challenge but that support, encouragement and regular follow-up from their health providers had a positive influence on them engaging in self-management practices (Duguay et al., 2014).

Active engagement through advanced care planning

Although self-management support can be highly effective, we need to recognise that there are older people with complex care needs who have limited capacity for self-management. However, this does not mean they are expected to play a passive role in their health decision making. The National Strategic Framework for Chronic Conditions emphasises that 'wherever possible, individuals should be actively engaged in shared decision-making processes, with care partnerships created between individuals and their health care providers, carers, families and communities as appropriate' (AHMAC, 2017, p. 31). In many cases, multimorbidity is often accompanied by periods of decline and in its advanced stages can lead to disability and impaired decision making. **Advanced care planning** in the early stages of chronic conditions is important as it ensures active engagement of individuals to make informed decisions about end-of-life care and to plan appropriately for the future when they may lose capacity to speak for themselves (AHMAC, 2017). This involves having a sensitive conversation with individuals and their significant others where they are prompted to think about, reflect, discuss and communicate their wishes for care and treatment should the time come when they are unable to speak for themselves.

advanced care planning
The process of developing a plan for an individual's health and personal care in accordance with their own personal values, belief systems and care preferences.

18.4 Getting to know the person: Jack's story

As time went by, Jack's daily struggle with pain was having a bigger impact on his sleep and mobility. He voiced his concern to his GP, who asked Jack if he had been taking his analgesics on a regular basis, as had been prescribed. Jack confessed that he often missed doses and he only took the analgesia when the pain was extreme. The GP told Jack that he needed to take the medications in the way that they were prescribed or they would not have the desired effect. Jack left the clinic feeling like the appointment had been a waste of time because there had been no resolution to his problems.

- In what context has the term 'non-compliance' traditionally been used in healthcare?

- Does the use of this word support the principles of person-centred care and partnership?

- If a patient is not adhering to the recommended medication or treatment plan, what could be a potential reason for this? Give an example from Jack's situation.

- You are the nurse sharing the care coordination of Jack with his GP. How would you advocate for Jack in this situation?

FOCUS QUESTIONS

Health coaching

Health coaching is an intervention that supports patient self-management. The technique applies psychological principles to motivate and support health behaviour change to improve self-management and health outcomes. It is more than just education, which is not enough to provoke significant changes in health behaviour because it does not focus on patient psychological motivators for change (Gale, 2012; Huffman, 2014; Kubina & Kelly, 2007). There are many and varied social and emotional reasons why people do not change their health behaviour, including:

- a lack of readiness to change

- a conflict of values

health coaching
An evidenced-based technique that applies psychological principles to motivate and support health behaviour change to improve health outcomes.

- inadequate support from their family, workplace or community
- lack of financial resources
- lack of access to services
- the belief that their health is unimportant.

Often, health professionals' recommendations simply 'do not match the needs or desires of the person' (Kubina & Kelly, 2007, p. 60). Health professionals who shift their role from clinical expert to that of coach show that self-management support can be effective, enabling 'the expert patient' to play an active role in their care and to discover their motivation to change (Kubina & Kelly, 2007).

Lacking confidence to alter and self-manage their conditions is one of the biggest barriers to health behaviour change (Huffman, 2014). There is evidence to show that building self-efficacy (gaining confidence in one's own ability to change) is a key component of chronic disease self-management (Gale, 2012). Health coaching utilises psychological and behavioural interventions to enhance self-efficacy, which involves:

- assessing the person's health needs, values and understanding of healthy behaviour
- providing treatment recommendations in a way that increases the person's acceptance of the information
- identifying barriers to health behaviour change
- building the patient's skills in problem solving
- changing unhelpful thinking patterns
- encouraging self-regulation and self-management of treatment regimens associated with their chronic diseases
- setting achievable goals that reduce their lifestyle risk factors (including smoking, binge drinking, sedentary lifestyle and poor dietary habits)
- providing regular follow-up for support and accountability (Kubina & Kelly, 2007).

Health coaching is most effective when the health professional applies the principles of motivational interviewing. Motivational interviewing is a conversational skill that aims to identify a person's stage of change, exploring and resolving their ambivalence to change, tapping into their intrinsic motivations to change and assessing their readiness to change (Huffman, 2014; Kubina & Kelly, 2007). Motivational interviewing principles include:

- open-ended questions
- empathy in listening
- reflective listening
- eliciting what the patient already knows about their health and condition(s)
- asking permission to provide them with helpful information when needed (Huffman, 2014).

Table 18.4, adapted from Huffman (2014), summarises and compares the key elements of traditional health education with health coaching to support self-management.

As health professionals transition from being solely educators to health coaches who recognise the social construct of health behaviours and implement patient-centred interventions that enhance self-efficacy, we are more likely to see patients alter their health behaviour to promote their own health.

TABLE 18.4 Traditional health education versus health coaching

TRADITIONAL HEALTH EDUCATION	HEALTH COACHING
Diagnosis driven	Collaborates to understand the social context of patients' lives and their health behaviours
Creates dependency	Empowers patient and their family/carer
Providers do the talking	Provider actively listens, checks the patient's understanding and asks for permission to give information when required
Follows provider's agenda	Addresses patient's concerns and needs

18.5 Getting to know the person: Jack's story

When Jack commenced on the amoxapine, he found that his blood sugar level readings were becoming higher than usual, so his endocrinologist changed his type of insulin. One day, soon after the change to Jack's insulin, his son became concerned when no one answered the home phone. He went to his parents' house and found Jack on the floor. He was sweating and could not talk or move. His son called the ambulance and Jack was taken to hospital, where he was treated for hypoglycaemia. While he was in the emergency department, the nurses discovered he also had an infected ulcer on his heel. He needed to stay in hospital for IV antibiotics. When Jack's son said he would take the week off work to stay with Jean, Jack agreed to be admitted to hospital. Secretly he was grateful to have a rest from Jean. They had been arguing constantly because of her forgetfulness. During his time in hospital, he felt anxious about going home and sad about the prospect of moving into a nursing home where he believed he would lose his independence and dignity. Although there were nurses constantly around him in hospital taking his blood sugar levels, administering his medications and treating his wounds, he felt alone and could not talk to anyone about his fears.

- How has hospitalisation contributed to Jack's sense of powerlessness?
- What strategies can health professionals use to empower patients in hospital?
- How can self-management techniques be adapted and used by nurses to support people with chronic conditions while they are in hospital?
- Create an open-ended question that a nurse could use to encourage Jack to talk about his concerns and needs.
- Imagine that you are the hospital diabetic nurse educator and you have been asked to see Jack to talk to him about his elevated blood sugar levels. When you ask him about his diet you discover that, although he believes he has a healthy diet, many of his food choices have a high glycaemic index. Using Table 18.4 as a guide, how would you use health coaching to help Jack change his dietary habits, compared to the traditional method of health education?

FOCUS QUESTIONS

18.6 Getting to know the person: Jack's story

One day in hospital, a new nurse called Sonya came in to see Jack. She warmly extended her hand to greet him as she introduced herself as a nurse care coordinator. She explained her role to Jack and asked if he had any questions or concerns he would like to discuss with her. The nurse appeared to have a lot of clinical expertise and she seemed genuinely interested in more than his infected ulcer and high blood sugar readings. Jack felt he could trust this nurse and he voiced his fears and concerns to her. The nurse care coordinator asked Jack's permission to invite his family to sit down together with them to talk about his health and how he is managing at home with Jean so that they could develop a plan to support him. Jack agreed to this and felt peace of mind in knowing that his health providers and family would now understand his struggles and that he could have a voice in how his care would progress.

FOCUS QUESTIONS

- How has this nurse shown person-centred care?
- How has this empowered Jack?
- Identify barriers that prevent health-care professionals from offering person-centred care in acute care settings. What actions could you take to remove or work around these barriers?

Issues with hospitalisation, innovative responses and future directions

primary care
The first point of contact and closest health service for consumers to access in the community that offers a range of health services to prevent disease and support people managing their health at home.

This chapter has provided evidence for the preference of managing multimorbidity in **primary care** settings. However, there will most likely come a time when an older person with MCCs will require hospitalisation for acute or emergency care. Hospitalisation is a point of vulnerability for older people with MCCs, with increased risk of:

- physical and cognitive functional decline related to prolonged hospital stays
- adverse events when starting new therapies
- inappropriate treatment
- conflicts between interventions
- medication errors
- complications post-discharge (Elliott & O'Callaghan, 2011; Commonwealth of Australia, 2021).

These poor health outcomes are generally associated with breakdowns in care during hospitalisation, including:

- clinicians' lack of clarity about their role in the multidisciplinary health-care team
- failure to manage comorbidities

- inadequate engagement of patients in care planning and communication
- lack of communication at transitions of care
- inadequate discharge planning
- poor medication reconciliation on discharge (ACSQHC, 2017).

Poor medication reconciliation on discharge is a major concern for people managing complex medication regimens. When their medications are changed in hospital, it can result in medication errors post-discharge, which accounts for two-thirds of the people being readmitted to hospital (Elliott & O'Callaghan, 2011; Commonwealth of Australia, 2021).

Promisingly, a number of nurse-led models of care have been successful at preventing unplanned hospitalisation of older people living with MCCs and reducing post-discharge complications. The Aged Care Emergency (ACE) program supports the staff of residential aged care facilities (RACFs) to care for residents with acute, non-life-threatening conditions within the facility, and potentially avoid unnecessary transfer to the hospital. When transfer to the emergency department is required, the ACE program has demonstrated improved emergency care for people living in RACFs as a result of the direct collaboration with an experienced acute aged care nurse (Agency for Clinical Innovation, 2019).

Nurse-led **in-home telemonitoring** is emerging as another approach that is improving patient outcomes in community aged care (Devitt, 2018). Trials in Australia have demonstrated reduced unplanned hospitalisations of older people with MCCs because of improved chronic disease self-management and as a result of clinicians receiving early warning of deterioration, enabling early intervention (Devitt, 2017). In this model, the nurse is vital to its success, acting as a care coordinator who is the central point of contact for the patient and health team. Important interventions undertaken by the nurse in this role include monitoring and assessment, health coaching, sharing of information between health providers, making referrals and developing relationship-based partnerships with patients and their families. The Royal Commission into Aged Care Quality and Safety (Commonwealth of Australia, 2021) recognised that assistive technology has significant potential to support older people to remain living in their own homes, rather than moving to residential aged care. It recommended that technology is included in aged care strategies and government funding is allocated towards it.

in-home telemonitoring
Remotely monitoring a patient in their home using technology that tracks their vital signs and electronically transmits the information to health professionals for assessment.

18.7 Getting to know the person: Jack's story

When Jack no longer required intravenous antibiotics, he was discharged home with a community nurse organised to provide wound care. Sonya, the nurse care coordinator, arranged a time to meet with Jack and Jean and one of their sons at their house to discuss their needs. Jack shared that his top priority was that Jean was well looked after and that they could remain living together in their home for as long as possible. Together, they identified and prioritised several issues and needs that were important to them:

1   Jean's dementia was getting worse. Jack needed to constantly keep his eye on her, and this was stressful for him.

2   Jean could no longer cook so they were ordering take-away food for most meals and this was contributing to his poor blood sugar control.

3   Their son was worried that if Jack had another hypoglycaemic event, Jean would not know how to call for an ambulance.

4   Jack is confused about what medications he can take for his pain control.

5   Jack is seeing several different doctors and specialists and he feels like he is spending most of his time going to medical appointments.

6   They want to go to the services club to have a drink with their friends, but Jack's poor mobility is a barrier and this upsets him.

FOCUS QUESTION

- After reading this chapter, how would you as Jack's care coordinator work with Jack and his family to address these issues and needs?

Learn more
Access additional resources – such as weblinks, further readings and podcasts – to broaden your understanding of this chapter. See the Guided Tour for access details.

Conclusion

At a time when Australia's population is ageing and the need to care for people with MCCs is becoming commonplace, there is a critical need to restructure both the health-care and aged care systems to focus on the prevention and better management of chronic health conditions. This will require the development of new strategies that enable health care and aged care services to provide integrated, multidisciplinary and coordinated care. This is an exciting time for health-care professionals, with new roles in care coordination, case management and health coaching approaches to chronic disease management. This requires health-care professionals to change the way they perceive their roles, from focusing on clinical tasks and patient compliance to partnering with patients in their communities and homes to establish what is important to them for their health. In recent years, the aged care system has been critically reviewed to ensure it meets the health needs and challenges of our ageing population. What it has taught us is that there is a need for a revival of the basic principles of caring and connecting in compassionate and respectful ways with fellow human beings across the lifespan. This is the essence of excellent care from the viewpoint of patients and their families living with illness. Individuals and families living with and managing the daily impact of multimorbidity require trusted health professionals to walk alongside and support them on their illness journey, partnering with 'expert patients' to help them find meaning in their experience and their own motivation to change and adapt in ways that are necessary for them to promote their health and well-being.

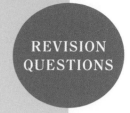

1   Based on the barriers to optimal health outcomes in Table 18.2, what are some strategies that health-care professionals could employ to lessen their personal involvement in adding to the barrier?

2   When you are expected to provide health education, how could you utilise strategies of health coaching? Create a plan for using techniques to effectively engage older people in self-management for a common health problem.

REVISION QUESTIONS

REFERENCES

Agency for Clinical Innovation. (2019). Aged Care Emergency. https://aci.health.nsw.gov.au/networks/eci/administration/models-of-care/ace

Australian Commission on Safety and Quality in Health Care (ACSQHC) (2017). Safety Issues at Transitions of Care: Consultation Report on Pain Points Relating to Clinical Information Systems. ACSQHC.

Australian Commission on Safety and Quality in Health Care (ACSQHC) (2020). Implementing the Comprehensive Care Standard: Clinical assessment and diagnosis. ACSQHC. http://www.safetyandquality.gov.au

Australian Health Ministers' Advisory Council (AHMAC) (2017). National Strategic Framework for Chronic Conditions. Australian Government. www.health.gov.au/resources/publications/national-strategic-framework-for-chronic-conditions

Australian Institute of Health and Welfare (AIHW) (2016). Australia's Health 2016 Series no. AUS 199. AIHW.

Australian Institute of Health and Welfare (AIHW) (2018). Australia's Health Series no. 16. AUS 221. AIHW.

Australian Institute of Health and Welfare (AIHW) (2020). Experiences in Health Care of People with Chronic Conditions: How GPs and Other Specialists Communicate with Their Patients 2017–18. AIHW.

Cheng, C., Bai, J., Yang, C. Y., Li, M., Inder, K. & Chan, W. C. (2019). Patients' experience of coping with multiple chronic conditions: A qualitative descriptive study. *Journal of Clinical Nursing, 28*(24), 4400–11.

Commonwealth of Australia (2019a). Royal Commission into Aged Care Quality and Safety (RCACQS). Interim report: Neglect. Vol. 2. Hearing Overviews and Case Studies. https://agedcare.royalcommission.gov.au/sites/default/files/2019-12/interim-report-volume-2_0.pdf

Commonwealth of Australia (2019b). Royal Commission into Aged Care Quality and Safety (RCACQS). Aged Care Program Redesign: Services for the Future. Consultation Paper 1. https://agedcare.royalcommission.gov.au/sites/default/files/2019-12/consultation-paper-1.pdf

Commonwealth of Australia (2020). Royal Commission into Aged Care Quality and Safety (RCACQS). Review of Innovative Models of Aged Care. Research Paper 3. https://agedcare.royalcommission.gov.au/sites/default/files/2020-01/research-paper-3-review-innovative-models-of-aged-care.pdf

Commonwealth of Australia (2021). Royal Commission into Aged Care Quality and Safety (RCACQS). Final report: Care, dignity and respect. Vol. 1, Summary and recommendations. https://agedcare.royalcommission.gov.au/sites/default/files/2021-03/final-report-volume-1_0.pdf

Consumers Health Forum of Australia (CHFA) (2019). Patient Activation in Australian with Chronic Illness – Survey Results. https://chf.org.au/publications/patient-activation-australians-chronic-illness-survey-results

Contant, E., Loignon, C., Bouhali, T., Almirall, J. & Fortin, M. (2019). A multidisciplinary self-management intervention among patients with multimorbidity and the impact of socioeconomic factors on results. *BMC Family Practice, 20*(53).

Corbin, J. (1998). The Corbin & Strauss chronic illness trajectory model: An update. *Scholarly Inquiry for Nursing Practice, 12*(1), 33–41.

Corbin, J. & Strauss, A. (1991). A nursing model for chronic illness management based upon the trajectory framework. *Scholarly Inquiry for Nursing Practice, 5*(3), 155–74.

Coventry, P.A., Small, N., Panagioti, M., Adeyemi, I. & Bee, P. (2015). Living with complexity; marshalling resources: A systematic review and qualitative meta-synthesis of lived experience of mental and physical multimorbidity. *BMC Family Practice, 16,* 171–83. https://doi:10.1186/s12875-015-0345-3

Department of Health & Ageing (2012). Indigenous Chronic Disease Package: Care Coordination and Supplementary Services. Program Guidelines.

www.mdas.org.au/
getattachment/HEALTH-
SERVICES/Chronic-
Disease-Management/
Care-Coordination-and-
Supplementary-Services-
Progr/Nov-2012-CCSS-
guidelines.pdf.aspx

Devitt, A. (2017). Nursing reflections on a pilot project: Improving outcomes in chronic disease management using nurse-led home monitoring. *The Hive, 19,* 28–9.

Devitt, A. (2018). Improving the lives of rural residents using nurse-led telemonitoring in community aged care. *Australian Nursing and Midwifery Journal, 25*(7), 32.

Duguay, C., Gallagher, F. & Fortin, M. (2014). The experience of adults with multimorbidity: A qualitative study. *Journal of Comorbidity, 4,* 11–21.

Elliott, R. A. & O'Callaghan, C. J. (2011). Impact of hospitalisation on the complexity of older patient's medication regimens and potential for regimen simplification. *Journal of Pharmacy Practice and Research, 41*(1), 21–5.

Gale, J. (2012). *A Practical Guide to Health Behaviour Change Using the HCA Approach.* Health Change Australia.

Golinowska, S. & Sowa, A. (2017). Quality and Cost-Effectiveness in Long-Term Care and Dependency Prevention: The Polish Policy Landscape. CASE Research Paper, (489).

Hancock, N., Scanlan, J. N., Gillespie, J. A., Smith-Merry, J. & Yen, I. (2017). Partners in Recovery Program Evaluation: Changes in unmet needs and recovery. *Australian Health Review, 42*(4), 445–52.

Hibbard, J. H., Mahoney, E. R., Stockard, J. & Tusler, M. (2005). Development and testing of a short form of the patient activation measure. *Health Services Research, 40*(6p1), 1918–30.

Huffman, M. (2014). Using motivational interviewing through evidence-based health coaching. *Home Healthcare Nurse, 32*(9), 543–8.

Kubina, N. & Kelly, J. (2007). *Navigating Self-Management: A Practical Approach to Implementation for Australian Health Care Agencies.* Whitehorse Division of General Practice.

Larsen, P. D. (2019). The illness experience. In P. D. Larsen (ed.). *Lubkin's Chronic Illness: Impact and Intervention* (10th edn). Jones and Bartlett Learning.

Mauk, K. L. (2019). Rehabilitation. In P. D. Larsen (ed.). *Lubkin's Chronic Illness: Impact and Intervention.* Jones and Bartlett Learning.

Miller, E., Stanley, J., Gurney, J., Stairmand, J., Davies, C., Semper, K., Dowell, A., Lawrenson., Mangin, D. & Sarfati, D. (2018). Effect of multimorbidity on health service utilisation and health care experiences. *Journal of Primary Health Care, 10*(1), 44–53.

Nicholas, R. & Nicholson Jr. (2019). Social isolation. In P. D. Larsen, (ed.). *Lubkin's Chronic Illness: Impact and Intervention.* Jones and Bartlett Learning.

O'Brien, R., Wyke, S., Watt, G., Guthrie, B, & Mercer, S. (2014). The 'everyday work' of living with multimorbidity living in socioeconomically deprived areas of Scotland. *Journal of Comorbidity, 4*(1), 1–10. https://doi:10.15256/joc.2014.4.32

Pert, A., Barton, C., Lewis, V. & Russell, G. (2020). A state-of-the-art review of the experience of care coordination interventions for people living with multimorbidity. *Journal of Clinical Nursing, 29,* 1445–56. https://doi:10.1111/jocn.15206

Pierce, L. L. & Lutz, B. J. (2019). Family caregiving. In P. D. Larsen, (ed.). *Lubkin's Chronic Illness: Impact and Intervention.* Jones and Bartlett Learning.

Porter, T., Ong, B. B. & Sanders, T. (2020). Living with multimorbidity? The lived experience of multiple chronic conditions in later life. *Health, 24*(6), 701–18. https://doi:10.1177/1363459319834997

Santini, Z. I., Cornwell, E.Y., Koyanagi, A., Nielsen, L., Hinrichsen, C., Meilstrup, C., Madsen, K. & Kouchede (2020). Social disconnectedness, perceived isolation, and symptoms of depression and anxiety among older Americans (NSHAP): A longitudinal mediation analysis. *Lancet Public Health, 5,* E63–E70.

Shad, B., Ashouri, A., Hasandokht, T., Rajati, F., Salari, A., Naghshbandi, M. & Mirbolouk, F. (2017). Effects of multimorbidity on quality of life in adult with cardiovascular disease: A cross-sectional study. *Health and Quality of Life Outcomes, 15*(1), 240.

Sheng, J., Liu, S., Wang, Y. & Zhang, X. (2017). The link between depression and chronic pain: Neural mechanisms in the brain. *Neural Plasticity, 9724371.* https://doi:10.1155/2017/9724371

Smith, B. (2017). Care of the person in the emergency department. In A. Johnson & E. Chang (eds), *Caring for Older People in Australia: Principles for Nursing Practice* (2nd edn). John Wiley & Sons.

South Australian Department of Health (2009). *Health Service Framework for Older People 2009–2016: Improving Health and Wellbeing Together.* Author.

Spangenberg, L., Forkmann, T., Brahler, E. & Glaesmer, H. (2011). The association of depression and multimorbidity in the elderly: Implications for the assessment of depression. *Psychogeriatrics, 11*(4), 227–34.

Welsh, T. J., Gordon, A. L. & Gladman, J. R. (2014). Comprehensive geriatric assessment – A guide for the nonspecialist. *International Journal Clinical Practice, 68*(3), 290– 3.

19 End-of-life Care

JENNY MCKENZIE AND MELISSA BRODIE

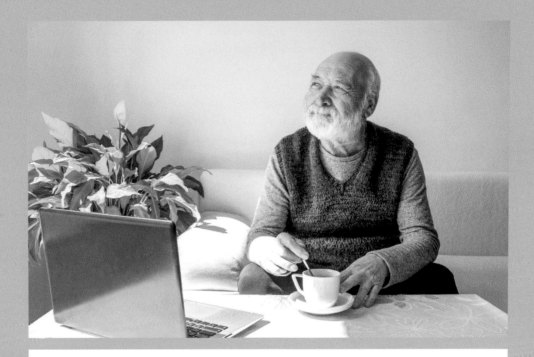

LEARNING OBJECTIVES

After reading this chapter, you will:

» anticipate the possibility of facilitating a good death when the person and their family are setting their own goals for end-of-life care

» demonstrate sophisticated communication and assessment skills to identify pain and manage symptoms

» validate that palliative care continues after death for the family and loved ones

» develop self-care strategies and recognise managing compassion fatigue as necessary for a sustainable career.

Introduction

end of life
The last few weeks of life, in which a patient with a life-limiting illness is rapidly approaching death.

Caring for people at the end of their lives will be a part of every registered nurse's career, no matter their specialty. Care at the **end of life** is directed towards easing physical symptoms caused by illness and allaying the emotional concerns of the dying person, carers and family. How carers and families perceive the quality of their loved one's care at the end of life will affect their progression through bereavement and ultimately their responses when facing their own death. By their actions and words, registered nurses can have an impact on the trauma of loss and grief for the family and are remembered for the presence or absence of compassionate care.

It is estimated that 70 per cent of deaths in Australia are expected deaths (Swerrisen & Duckett, 2014). These deaths are caused by chronic illnesses such as cancer, cardiovascular disease and respiratory disease. However, causes of death in Australia are changing and the following points indicate the reason for this change:

- Over the past century, the rate of death per 1000 people has gone down by one-third (ABS, 2020).
- People are less likely to die young.
- People are more likely to die from chronic diseases as opposed to sudden, traumatic deaths.
- In 1900, 23 per cent of the population died before the age of five years and less than 5 per cent lived past their 85th birthday. The figures are now reversed.
- In 2019, less than 1 per cent of the population died before the age of five and nearly 40 per cent lived past the age of 85 years (ABS, 2020).
- Most of these people died from chronic disease.
- Death is becoming more predictable (Swerrisen & Duckett, 2014).

Dying in modern Australia is very much the domain of the aged. Two-thirds of Australians who die each year are in the 75–95-year-old age bracket. The advent of chronic disease as the major cause of death and the likelihood that people will know they are going to die means that many people expect to be able to have a say in how and where they die, what death should like and the direction of their journey.

This chapter aims to provide registered nurses and health-care professionals with information about how to assist dying people, their carers and their families to plan for the end of life and provide a 'good death' as envisioned by the person.

Palliative care

palliative care
The person- and family-centred care provided for a person with an active, progressive, advanced disease, who has little or no prospect of cure and who is expected to die, and for whom the primary goal is to optimise the quality of life.

pain
An unpleasant sensory and emotional experience associated with actual or potential tissue damage.

Palliative care is care that is given when there is no possibility of a cure for an illness. According to the World Health Organization (2020), palliative care:

> … is an approach that improves the quality of life of patients (adults and children) and their families who are facing problems associated with life-threatening illness. It prevents and relieves suffering through the early identification, correct assessment and treatment of **pain** and other problems, whether physical, psychosocial or spiritual.

Addressing suffering involves taking care of issues beyond physical symptoms.
Palliative care uses a team approach to support patients and their caregivers. This
includes addressing practical needs and providing bereavement counselling. It
offers a support system to help patients live as actively as possible until death …

The process of dying is an individual one. For the dying person, it is a solo journey
without the benefit of a map or directions from those who have travelled there before them.
For health professionals, carers' families and loved ones of the dying person, feelings about
death are unique and individual to their life experiences and beliefs. For many, a good
death may be considered an extension of the concept of ageing and living well. Despite the
individual nature of death, the concept of having a good death resonates. A review of the
literature reveals recurring themes as to what is considered a good or bad death. Table 19.1
summarises the themes related to these concepts.

TABLE 19.1 Characteristics of a good and a bad death

GOOD DEATH	BAD DEATH	REFERENCES
» Death free from pain » Sense of a life well lived » Sense of community » Death within bounds of acceptable clinical and ethical standards » Sense of privacy and dignity » Dying in the chosen environment » Having time to say goodbye and complete life tasks » Access to spiritual and emotional supports » Respect for cultural traditions	» Painful death » Uncontrolled symptoms » Loss of control (decision making, who is present at death) » Loss of independence » Lack of information about disease and dying process » Not being able to choose where they die » Poor communication of treatment and care options » Failure to establish the dying person's wishes	Swerrisen & Duckett (2014) Rainsford et al. (2018) Cottrell & Duggleby (2016)

Registered nurses spend more time with patients than any other health professional
in the caring team. This relationship enables registered nurses to strongly advocate for
their patients, placing registered nurses in a unique position to play an advocate role for
dying people (Evenblij et al., 2019). Registered nurses are perceived as key facilitators
for a good death. The following personal story illustrates how a registered nurse can
facilitate a good death.

19.1 Getting to know the person: Josie's story

Josie was a much-loved 72-year-old mother, grandmother and friend to all who
were privileged to know her. She had lived independently since the death of her
husband five years earlier and enjoyed her active life with family and friends. After
many months of vague symptoms and frustrating unsuccessful visits to doctors,
Josie presented to hospital deeply jaundiced. Josie was diagnosed with inoperable
advanced metastatic pancreatic cancer and was referred to palliative care.

The first meeting with Josie was memorable. She was bright yellow due to her jaundiced skin, sitting high up in bed, holding court and basking in the love of the many family members crowded around her bed. The love and support for Josie was tangible. The palliative care nurse introduced herself to Josie and her family and asked if it was a convenient time to talk. Invited to join the group, the nurse was very quickly told that Josie had an advance care plan. She wanted to be kept comfortable: 'Whatever Josie wants or needs she will get it'.

The nurse informed the group of the role of palliative care and the range of services available to support Josie's care at the end of her life. It was soon established that Josie was experiencing very little symptom discomfort. She proudly informed the nurse that she had only cried twice. That was when she had telephoned her sister to tell her that she had cancer and said goodbye to her, because she knew she would never see her again. When asked why it would not be possible to see her sister, the nurse was told that Josie's sister lived in Perth and could not travel. Again, the palliative care nurse asked why seeing each other was not possible. Josie was not actively dying and had minimal discomfort from symptoms. Physically, there was no reason why Josie could not travel to Perth if that was what she wanted to do, the caveats being that she needed to travel imminently, not plan an extended stay, and for them all to discuss a plan for what to do if Josie's health deteriorated or if she died while she was away.

The suggestion was greeted with silence, which was broken by a now smiling Josie asking, 'Can I really?' After answering more questions and supporting the concept of flying first class, the palliative care nurse organised a time to visit the next day and informed the surgeon of the result of the palliative care consultation with Josie and her family and the developing plan for Josie to travel to Perth.

The next day, the palliative care nurse returned to be greeted by an ecstatic Josie. First-class flights had been booked for Josie and three family members. She was flying out the next morning and would return five days later. Her adult children, although very supportive of Josie, had some reservations. The reservations were openly discussed, and attempts made to trouble-shoot solutions; their main focus was assisting their beloved Josie to achieve her last wish.

On her return home from Perth, the family reported that Josie was experiencing a marked increase in fatigue. The family contacted the palliative care team, who made arrangements to admit Josie directly to the inpatient palliative care unit.

Josie died five days later, elated and at peace that she had seen her much-loved sister. Her family were overjoyed to have her home, safe in their arms. They labelled her death as perfect because she left the world without the appearance of suffering and having achieved her dying wish.

INTEGRATED CARE AND MULTIDISCIPLINARY TEAMS IN PALLIATIVE CARE

Integrated care encompasses a range of steps to support a holistic approach to palliative and end-of-life care. It is the underlying foundation for all the required services to provide seamless, quality care for the older person at the centre of care.

Palliative and end-of-life care can be complex and requires multiple levels of holistic care from a range of diverse services and support systems. Many services are needed throughout the trajectory of palliative care, especially towards the end of life. Integrated care is the underlying foundation for providing seamless quality care between all health services to provide the best possible care with the older person at the centre of care. It is a model of care that focuses on bringing a holistic approach to meet all the needs of the older person – not a one-size-fits-all model – and empowers and supports the seamless care needed and provided (Gilbert et al., 2020).

To assist in facilitating an integrated care approach, a **multidisciplinary team** (MDT) is formed as the foundation of the collaborative team. Depending on who is needed, an MDT may consist of services such as allied health, social work, specialist palliative care, general practitioners and any other service that may assist in collaborative care (NSW Ministry of Health, 2019). The MDT works alongside the older person and focuses on how best to create a coordinated approach as a team to encompass current and anticipated care needs. Utilising an MDT approach provides clear, seamless care, reducing the anxiety and stress of coordinating care for the individual, their carer and their family.

integrated care
Provision of well-connected, effective and efficient care that takes account of and is organised around a person's health and social needs.

multidisciplinary team
A team that includes professionals from a range of disciplines consisting of a group of experts whose goal is comprehensive patient-centred care.

Legal issues related to the end of life

For registered nurses working with patients coming to the end of their life, it is important to know about the legal concepts and how to apply them in their jurisdiction. By having this knowledge, you are able to discuss advance care planning and end-of-life goal-setting with confidence and sensitivity with a patient and their family. You should try to find out who is the individual's enduring guardian and enduring power of attorney to ensure that the correct decision makers are in place. Where possible, the individual should be given the opportunity to validate the goals for their care and what care they wish to receive when they are dying. Such conversations can be difficult, and clinicians may be fearful of introducing the topic of mortality for fear of upsetting people or removing hope. In reality, advance care plans may need to be revisited many times over the course of an individual's illness and should be viewed as an opportunity to check that you are working as a team with your patients and their families towards a shared goal as nominated by the individual. Resources to support conversations about advance care planning and end-of-life goal setting can be found at Advance Care Planning Australia (n.d.), Palliative Care Australia (n.d.) and ELDAC (End of Life Direction for Aged Care, n.d.).

VOLUNTARY ASSISTED DYING

voluntary assisted dying (VAD)
A process of self-administering a medication for the purpose of causing death in accordance with the steps and processes set out in law. It is only for those who face an inevitable, imminent death as a result of an incurable disease, illness or medical condition.

euthanasia
The merciful killing of a patient suffering from a terminal disease or in an irreversible coma.

Voluntary assisted dying (VAD), assisted dying or **euthanasia** is gradually becoming legal in jurisdictions in Australia. At the time of writing, laws have been passed in Victoria, South Australia, Western Australia, Queensland and Tasmania. It would be realistic to assume that other jurisdictions in Australia will follow suit in time. This is an emerging area in healthcare in Australia, and we urge you as health-care professionals to access up-to-date information at End of Life Law in Australia (n.d.).

VAD is a divisive topic for many health-care professionals. Being aware of the divisions this may cause; being aware of your own stance on VAD and the self-education requirements around VAD; knowing how to communicate effectively with patients and families about VAD; and understanding how VAD laws may be applied in your jurisdiction are integral to health-care workers' ability to provide care in this space. Individuals seeking information on or access to VAD should be supported. Palliative care and end-of-life principles of equity, respect and non-abandonment apply for individuals seeking VAD (Palliative Care Australia, 2019).

19.2 Getting to know the person: Roger's story

Roger was a 66-year-old businessman. He had been married to Jan for 44 years and they had two adult children. Roger had begun to transition to retirement from his successful business two years ago, but still worked part time 'to keep his hand in'. Six months earlier, Roger had been playing golf. A couple of times that day he had stumbled 'over nothing' and disturbingly could not pick up his golf club at the end of the day. On returning home, Jan called an ambulance, fearing that Roger had had a stroke. It was not a 'stroke', but the commencement of the journey to being diagnosed with **motor neurone disease**.

motor neurone disease
A neurodegenerative disease that causes rapidly progressive muscle weakness. It is a life-limiting disease.

On his first meeting with palliative care, Roger was quick to point out his well-organised status. He had revised his will, made his funeral arrangements and developed his advance care plan (ACP) with his GP. The registered nurse allowed Roger and Jan to discuss what was important to them and answered questions about the role of palliative care and symptom control. The closeness and ease between Roger and Jan was palpable; it was very clear that they had a very close relationship and had discussed his goals of care. Roger firmly stated a number of times his desire not to prolong his life; quality was important to him and 'if I can't wipe my bum, then I want to be dead'. At the time of the first meeting, Roger was still able to walk, with effort and the occasional use of a walker, when tired. When shaking the nurse's hand on greeting he had a notable weakness.

Over a series of visits, it was reiterated that Roger did not wish to prolong his life, did not want artificial feeding via percutaneous endoscopic gastrostomy (PEG) or airway assistance via continuous positive airway pressure (CPAP), and this was all documented in his ACP. Roger formed a strong therapeutic relationship with all members of his caring team.

Over the following eight months, Roger's mobility and upper limb motor function progressively declined. He could no longer 'wipe [his] own bum', an indicator of good quality of life for him, and he was requiring increasing assistance. On one visit, he surprised the palliative care nurse by telling her that he was booked in to have a PEG inserted and had an appointment to see the respiratory physician about CPAP. When asked what had changed for him, he stated that life was better than he thought it would be when he lost his ability to self-care. He found happiness in his time with Jan, his grandchildren and other family and friends. He wasn't ready to die. The nurse supported his decision and reassured him that his journey with the palliative care team would continue, with him in charge.

Six weeks after this, Roger developed a chest infection. This was a catalyst for another discussion about palliation versus active treatment. Again, at odds with his previously written ACP, Roger opted to be admitted to hospital for intravenous antibiotics. The first-line antibiotics did not have the desired effect. It was evident that Roger's health was deteriorating. In accordance with Roger's wishes, Jan informed the palliative care nurse that they did not wish to continue antibiotics. The nurse advocated on their behalf for aggressive pursuit of palliative measures and cessation of antibiotics. Roger's family and all stakeholders in his care had a meeting. Roger's treatment goals were renegotiated, and palliative management of his symptoms prioritised. He died in hospital 24 hours later. Unfortunately, due to his rapidly progressing respiratory failure, Roger did not have the opportunity to die at home, but he did die surrounded by the family he loved.

- How were Roger's life goals respected?
- What were the types of support offered by the palliative care nurse?
- What legal considerations were in place to support Roger and his family?

FOCUS QUESTIONS

Communication

The key skill for registered nurses to provide quality care for people at the end of their life is skilled, sensitive communication. Without the ability to communicate effectively, astute assessment and symptom management and the principles of good end-of-life/palliative care such as advance care planning, establishing goals of care and planning a good death are not

JENNY MCKENZIE AND MELISSA BRODIE

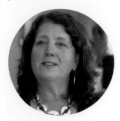

achievable. The ability to communicate effectively enables the registered nurse to develop strong therapeutic relationships with the person, their family and carers (Clayton et al., 2019; Hernandez-Marrero et al., 2019).

Communication skills is an area of study that is often neglected in health education. Many registered nurses do not feel they are adequately skilled to initiate or guide a conversation about end-of-life care issues, so they avoid them. For patients, their families and carers, encountering the health system or being admitted to hospital is an intimidating experience. It can be confronting, cold and demeaning sharing their most intimate details with strangers. It can feel like an invasion of their person, especially if they are being touched without so much as an introduction. Add to this being told they have a life-limiting illness, or have to be admitted to hospital due to a deterioration in their chronic or life-limiting illness, and it is little wonder that people and families often rate their dealings with health-care professionals poorly.

Allowing individuals to raise concerns about and discuss their greatest fears – such as loss of independence, becoming a burden and having an uncertain future – is central to providing good palliative and end-of-life care (Murray et al., 2017).

CONVERSATION STARTERS

The health professional often feels confronted and even fearful of talking to a person and their family about death and palliative care. Research has shown that people and their families expect health professionals to introduce the conversation around death and dying (Clayton et al., 2005; Olsson et al., 2020). Many health professionals feel uncomfortable about this conversation and do not know how to start.

Communication skills are developed over time, but to assist you in your professional practice here are some strategies to guide you. Ensure you deliver the information in the correct cultural context for each person.

1   Preparation:
    »   Familiarise yourself with the person's history and current health issues.
    »   Allow yourself to mentally prepare (emotional intelligence).

2   Environment:
    »   Ensure privacy.
    »   Ensure it is quiet, and there will be no interruptions.
    »   Include a support person if that is the wish of the patient.
    »   Try to seat all parties: do not stand over the person.

3   How to begin:
    »   Clarify what the person and support people present already know.
    »   Acknowledge the difficult time that the person and family may have had to get to this point.

4   Starting points:
    »   'How do you think you are going?'
    »   'What do you expect?'
    »   (To the family) 'Have you noticed any changes to [name of person's] health?'
    »   'Since I saw you last, I can see that things have changed for you.'
    »   Acknowledge the fear and uncertainty of their poor health status and their future.

» Avoid jargon and health-related technical terms. Tumour, metastasis, neoplasm, spot and cancer are often used interchangeably and cause misunderstanding and confusion (Omori et al., 2020).

» Avoid being blunt. Telling a patient and/or their family to 'get your affairs in order' or 'Betty's dying' and walking out of the room is an insensitive way to inform patients and/or family.

» Provide information at the person's/family's pace, and check for understanding by asking the person to repeat what you have said in their own words. Written material may be helpful so the person can have certainty and refresh their memory after you have left them (Clayton et al., 2007; Anderson et al., 2019).

> Building rapport is an important skill. Chapters 3, 12, 13 and 14 include more information about this skill.

ACTIVE LISTENING

Active listening is an extension of everyday communication skills. It involves the listener giving their full and undivided attention to the person who is talking. While listening, body language and facial expression may also be noted; these may emphasise what is truly important for the person being listened to. When building a therapeutic relationship, active listening builds trust. Show a genuine interest by not interrupting and by allowing the person to tell their story and direct you to their biggest concerns (Robertson, 2005; Widera et al., 2020; Wittenberg et al., 2015).

Here are some strategies to facilitate your development of active listening skills. According to Denise Winkler, a co-editor of this book, 'this is the most important gift a health professional can extend to a dying person and their family. During the weeks my beloved husband was in palliative care, the active listening of a few registered nurses made the experience and the subsequent grief less traumatic'.

Learn more
Watch Video 11.2: Denise talks about the importance of active listening.

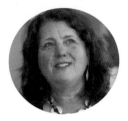

Attentive body language

* Employ posture and gestures that show involvement and engagement.
* Use body movement that demonstrates interest and engagement; avoid larger-than-life gestures.
* Use facial expressions that reflect the emotions being expressed by the person and family.
* Make sensitive eye contact (remember cultural considerations).

'Following' skills (giving the speaker space to tell their story their way)

* Show interest.
* Offer minimal verbal encouragements.
* Ask infrequent, timely and considered questions.
* Employ attentive silences.

'Reflecting' skills (checking that the listener has the story correct and is showing acceptance)

* Paraphrase by putting the information in another way (watch their facial expressions, which demonstrate comprehension).

- Reflect back feelings and content to ensure you understand what is being said.
- Summarise major issues and be prepared to put these in writing (Robertson, 2005; Wittenberg et al., 2015; Widera et al., 2020).

Active listening takes time and practice. It is a valuable tool in end-of-life care when establishing goals of care with a person, clarifying what is important at the end of life and determining what a good death may look like for that individual. However, in a health situation where rapid clinical decision making is required, active listening is not the correct communication tool.

Person-centred approach

The cornerstone of quality palliative and end-of-life care is placing the individual at the front of decision making, and establishing what is important to that individual and their goals. This is especially true when interacting with individuals who are identified as having greater health needs, including First Nations peoples; care leavers – that is, individuals who were in institutional or out-of-home care, including foster care in the twentieth century (Australian Healthcare Associates, 2019) – individuals with a disability; individuals who are experiencing homelessness; lesbian, gay, bisexual, transgender, gender diverse, intersex, queer, asexual and questioning (LGBTIQ+); and those from culturally and linguistically diverse backgrounds (AIHW, 2019). Caring for these groups can also be challenging for health-care staff; and, as a registered nurse, being aware of your own prejudices and belief system (McGee & Johnson, 2014) is essential when providing care in a person-centred approach. A registered nurse can display acceptance by reviewing advance care plans and, if possible, allowing individuals and their family/family member of choice (as subject-matter experts on their loved one) a voice to be heard; using interpreters; involving community decision makers as decided by the individual; accessing Aboriginal health workers (AHWs); and involving religious/spiritual guides. This list is not exhaustive, but by considering promoting a person-centred approach and allowing for collateral information-gathering, an individualised care plan can be formulated.

....

EXAMPLE DIALOGUE

Conversation starters you can use to display acceptance may include:

- How can we best help you?
- What do I need to know to provide the best care for you and your family?
- What would you like us to call you?
- What is your preferred pronoun: he, she or they?
- Who is your best support person or persons? (This might not be a blood relative.)
- Is there anything I can read, or person I can talk to, to assist us to care for you?

Allow time and privacy for these conversations, understanding that there can be fear of judgment, persecution and distrust of health-care providers, which can make rapport-building difficult.

....

19.3 Getting to know the person: Essie's story

Essie grew up in a very remote area of New South Wales. As a young woman, she moved to Sydney and worked for the Education Department to promote education opportunities for First Nations children. In her early seventies, she was diagnosed with advanced lung cancer. She felt guilty towards herself and her family because she blamed the cancer on smoking 'as a youngster'. Initially, she was accompanied to palliative care appointments by an AHW, with no goal except to yarn and answer any questions. As a rapport was established, she started going alone. Essie's goal was to live with her daughter for as long possible, then – when it was time (and not before!) – to return to Country to die. Knowing this was Essie's ultimate goal, the palliative care nurse worked with Essie's GP and the AHW teams locally and at her health service on Country to ensure continuity of care.

Essie's health started to deteriorate rapidly and she made the call to go back to Country. Essie's family drove her home, taking with them a pre-organised portable oxygen concentrator. The convoy left at 4 am. According to Essie's daughter, the trip home was harrowing and they doubted Essie would make it. However, as Essie approached Country, she regained some strength. She arrived home, acknowledged being home and expressed joy at being there and seeing her people. Her health quickly worsened and she died later that night.

- How was a rapport built with Essie?
- Were Essie's wishes for end-of-life care supported? How?

FOCUS QUESTIONS

Caring for our diverse community requires a patient-centred approach for individuals who are approaching the end of their life and the families who support them. See Table 19.2 for examples of diversity and hints for providing care.

TABLE 19.2 Examples of diversity and strategies for providing care

GETTING TO KNOW THE PERSON	STRATEGIES
Terry was in her late sixties. She had spent most of her life in jail after killing the man who raped her. Her family by choice were Pauline (a former brothel madam whom she met in jail) and Bazza (an active IV drug user and loyal long-time friend). Terry wanted to be looked after at home by the only people she felt ever loved her. They were concerned about legalities and that they would get raided by the police. Bazza was keen to prove that he would not steal and use Terry's S8 medication. Terry was well cared for and died at home with her family of choice. At the time of death they called the palliative care team, who were able to guide proceedings post death.	» Long, respectful conversation about end-of-life goals » Expressed admiration for the love and support they have as their family unit and their determination to overcome barriers » Educating Pauline about legalities of home death and cautioning against calling an ambulance or police, and making palliative care or Terry's GP the first contact for assistance » Encouraging Bazza to reconnect with his drug and alcohol worker » Discussing the risk mitigation of having S8s in a home with an active IV drug user. (Pauline took ownership of this problem. She procured a safe for storage and initiated a highly detailed diary of Terry's symptoms and medications.)

(Continued)

TABLE 19.2 Continued

GETTING TO KNOW THE PERSON	STRATEGIES
Bob and Serg were in their late eighties. They had been a couple for seventy years, since meeting as teenagers at boarding school. Bob had been living with dementia and his care needs had exceeded the care that Serg could provide at home. Transition to living separately has been difficult. Serg was pining the lack of physical touch and no longer sharing a bed. He felt self-conscious visiting the facility and scared to touch or get close to Bob in case he was reported. Serg had lived through decades of persecution from when homosexuality was considered a crime, then the 1980s to 1990s when HIV/AIDS was labelled the 'gay disease'. Today, same-sex marriage is legal and HIV a chronic disease, but many in this community live with a trauma-laden past.	» Bob's palliative care team had known the couple for many months and had built a strong rapport. Serg felt comfortable discussing his fears with them, but was not sure how his desire to get into bed and cuddle Bob would be interpreted by staff at the facility. » With Serg's consent, the palliative care nurse discussed his concerns with the facility manager. » The manager was embarrassed on hearing about Serg's concerns because no one had thought to enquire about Bob's relationship status (the next of kin was Bob's nephew). » Once informed, the facility was quick to respond to Serg's needs. Bob's nephew brought a bed in and the nursing staff assisted to position it next to Bob's high/low bed at the appropriate height. The facility was very clear that when Serg was staying the night they would keep overnight cares to a minimum, limiting interruption to the couple's time together. » Three months after entering the facility, Bob died peacefully, with Serg cuddled up next to him in bed.
Tiges had lived a nomadic existence for most of his life. At time he was diagnosed with a terminal illness, he was living in his car. Post diagnosis, he decided to remain there. When living in the car was no longer physically possible, Tiges moved into a homeless shelter. Once his care needs exceeded what the shelter could provide, he moved into a palliative care unit. In that unit, the nurses were respectful of Tiges' goal to stay outside and placed him in a room with a courtyard. They moved the bed close to the open door just before he died. After Tiges died, his sister was called and informed. She was grateful to hear how well Tiges was cared for at the end of his life, and that he did not die alone in an unknown place as she had always feared he might.	» Palliative care caught up with Tiges around town, in parks, by the river – wherever the weather and Tiges' sense of adventure took him. » A rapport was built after a series of non-judgmental visits. He consented to being referred to the local homeless outreach worker, with whom palliative care collaborated to plan what Tiges' end-of-life care might look like. » Tiges' goal was to stay outside for as long as possible. » Tiges disclosed he made a yearly phone call to his sister on his mum's birthday. He did not want her to know about his illness (she'd make a fuss and want to look after him) but consented to her being told of his death so she wouldn't worry about him.
Johnno was born with a severe intellectual disability, diagnosed as being severely autistic and thought to have an unnamed syndrome that affected his hearing. He had spent his life in institutionalised care, where he liked to be outside playing with toys in the sandpit. In his late sixties, Johnno was diagnosed with very advanced metastatic melanoma. Johnno was visited at regular intervals by palliative care at his group home. Group home staff had access to palliative care's on-call system for support out of hours. When it became clear that Johnno's health was deteriorating, he was moved into the palliative care unit for end-of-life care. The disability support workers continued to be with him and supported him until he died.	» Initial palliative care visits took place in hospital, with palliative care engaging Johnno's disability support workers to learn his behaviours if he had pain or was upset. » Johnno was involved in conversations about his care even though he was non verbal. » Meetings including his sister, GP, oncologist and disability workers were organised to plan care for Johnno, including end of life. Johnno's sister expressed her wish for Johnno to die in the inpatient palliative care unit. » Palliative care held an education session with Johnno's disability workers at his group home. Education was provided on palliative care, Johnno's disease, what may happen next, pain and symptom management. An open question and answer session was facilitated. » Palliative care viewed the disability support workers as family for Johnno and experts on his comfort. Palliative care's role was to take the information provided and adjust Johnno's pain medications accordingly. The goal was to make Johnno as comfortable as possible so he could be outside and play with his tractors.

Caring for people of diverse cultures and backgrounds is challenging. No one expects registered nurses to be experts on all vulnerable groups, but it is not unreasonable to expect nurses to educate themselves. By informing yourself and providing culturally safe, sensitive care, the patient-centred approach to care becomes the norm.

OXFORD UNIVERSITY PRESS

You can expect that, due to life experiences, persecution, government policy, societal expectations and the ages of the individuals being cared for, any individual may have been exposed to (multiple) traumas during their lifetime. As such, a trauma-informed approach to care should be considered. **Trauma-informed care** is an approach to care provision that assumes that all individuals potentially have a history of trauma or lived experience that may impact how they respond to the care you provide (NSW Health, 2020; ACI, 2019; Blue Knot Foundation, n.d.).

Tenets of trauma-informed care include being open minded and compassionate; empowering individuals and providing choice; providing a culturally safe environment; and working collaboratively in partnership with the individual and their carers (Kezelman, 2016).

Assessment

Identification and treatment of problematic symptoms are key in palliative and end-of-life care. Impeccable assessment is required to achieve optimal symptom control at the end of life. Assessment of symptoms needs to be performed regularly and repeated as needed to monitor the success of the interventions employed and to allay symptom distress. Developing a strong therapeutic relationship grounded in good communication skills improves the quality of information assessed.

People with life-limiting illnesses often experience a common suite of symptoms:

* pain
* **nausea** and **vomiting**
* **dyspnoea**
* **constipation**
* **fatigue**
* **anorexia**.

Common psychological symptoms experienced include anxiety, depression and general emotional distress. Personal distress may also stem from the person's spiritual beliefs, culture or deficits in social support. The Palliative Care Outcomes Collaborative (PCOC) is a voluntary framework that guides routine clinical assessment and response aimed at measuring and improving quality of care at the end of life (Masso et al., 2015). The individual's physical, social, spiritual and cultural needs are assessed using common assessment tools, which helps to create a common language for planning and delivering palliative care (PCOC, n.d.)

Here are descriptions of some standardised assessment tools:

* The palliative care phase uses the descriptors 'stable', 'unstable', 'deteriorating' and 'terminal' to assist with identifying the person's location on their illness trajectory.
* The System Assessment Score is a score, ideally rated by the person, of common palliative care symptoms (pain, dyspnoea, nausea, bowels, anorexia and **insomnia**) from 0 (no distress) to 10 (extreme distress). Repetition of scoring can map the effect of treatment interventions.
* Resource Utilisation Groups – Activities of Daily Living (RUG/ADL) is a measure of loss of ability to self-care (it scores bed mobility, toileting and the ability to transfer and eat). The scores vary from being independent to requiring extensive assistance.

trauma-informed care
Care that is aware of trauma symptoms and accepts the role it plays in a person's life.

nausea
A feeling of sickness with an inclination to vomit.

vomiting
Expulsion of stomach contents through the mouth.

dyspnoea
A subjective experience of difficulty in breathing.

constipation
Difficulty passing stools; incomplete or infrequent passing of hard stools.

fatigue
A subjective experience defined as a persistent and distressing sense of tiredness that is not proportional to activity, not relieved by sleep or rest, and which interferes with normal functioning.

anorexia
A lack of appetite and weight loss in advanced life-limiting illness.

See Chapters 10 and 11 for more on assessing the older person's physiological changes.

insomnia
A long period of time when a person is unable to fall asleep or stay asleep.

- The Australian Modified Karnofsky Score is a measure of health status. A score of 100 is indicative of full health and no signs of disease; 0 indicates a person is dead.
- The Palliative Care Problem Severity Score is a clinician screening tool that monitors overall consideration of pain, other symptoms, psychological/spiritual distress and family/carer distress.

Tools such as these enable an overall picture of the person with a life-limiting illness, and may be used to trigger referral to specialist palliative care services (Murray et al., 2017). To achieve relief from symptom distress, a comprehensive assessment is required. At the end of life, it is unlikely you will be able to complete a full, comprehensive assessment in one session with the person. Allowing the person to direct the flow of information with sensitive direction from you, the registered nurse, helps to build a therapeutic relationship and improve the quality of information offered. A series of visits will enable you to achieve a thorough assessment and more easily develop goals of care. A general health assessment and listing the person's medications (including over-the-counter and natural therapies) is the starting point for achieving a comprehensive assessment.

Pain and symptom management

Good symptom management relies on impeccable assessment and evaluation of each symptom. Decisions made about treatment of symptoms are often evaluated on a benefit-versus-burden approach, with consideration given to overall health and well-being, and where the person is on their health trajectory in relation to death (Palliative Care Expert Group, 2016). Life goals of the person and family wishes may also be considered before embarking on extensive investigations or aggressive treatment.

PHARMACOLOGICAL TREATMENTS

Medication management of symptoms in palliative and end-of-life care should be evidence based and tailored to suit the individual person. When prescribing for people experiencing symptoms at the end of life, frequent assessment for efficacy of treatment and ongoing adjustment to the pharmacological regimen is needed for maximum benefit with minimal side effects. In palliative and end-of-life care, registered nurses – with their ongoing, closer relationships with people and their families – are in the ideal position to assess patients, document their findings and communicate findings with other members of the multidisciplinary team (PalliAged, 2019).

You can find more information on pharmacology in Chapter 14.

non-pharmacological treatments
Strategies to relieve pain and/or promote comfort that do not rely on medications.

Non-pharmacological treatments are often used alongside pharmacological therapies. Many patients and their families may already be using some of these; it is useful to establish what they are using or have used when completing a comprehensive assessment of symptoms and to document any strategies the person and family have used. Referral to occupational therapists, physiotherapists, dieticians, social workers and support services for help with personal care or housekeeping may also assist with symptom management. Once the registered nurse has direction from the person or their proxy, a comprehensive assessment can be pursued. Individual symptoms may be assessed, as shown in Table 19.3.

TABLE 19.3 Non-pharmacological treatment strategies for symptoms

SYMPTOM	POINTS TO CONSIDER	NON-PHARMACOLOGICAL TREATMENT STRATEGIES
Delirium	» If an older person is confused, *always* assume delirium. » Any symptoms in this table can manifest themselves as confusion and delirium.	» Assess and intervene according to the assessed need.
Pain	» Severity, score out of 10 (0 = no pain, 10 = extreme pain) is the most common method. Visual analogue scales may also be used. Standardised scoring across the health setting is paramount. » Location of pains (the person may have more than one pain) » Duration of pain » What does the pain feel like? Descriptors are a useful tool for attributing the origin of pain. » What makes the pain better or worse? » Is the pain new? How long has the pain been there? » Current medications for pain and what has previously been tried » Impact of pain on life » Physical examination	» Hot or cold packs » Positioning » Relaxation » Distraction therapy » Referral for support services to assist with activities of daily living » Listening to the person's story can itself be a therapeutic intervention.
Nausea	» Severity (can the person keep down water? If not, urgency of symptom resolution increases) » Consider possible causes (environment, non-compliance with medications, recent treatment disease status) » Frequency » Onset/duration » What makes nausea better or worse? » Medication use » Ease of vomiting (no warning and effortless vomiting or nausea, retching and heaving) » Description of vomit, undigested food, offensiveness, bile » Bowel (last bowel motion and description, nausea is often a sign of constipation) » Oral cavity, signs of candidiasis, ill-fitting dentures, ulcers, dry mouth » Physical examination (look, feel and listen)	» Small, frequent meals » Consider environment, odour and visual » Consider positioning when trying to eat » Check oral cavity; utilise mouthwashes; refer to dental services » Check bowels; consider constipation management » Review diet: avoid spicy fatty foods and foods that may be arduous to eat » Review medication regimen; administer anti-emetic half an hour prior to attempting to eat
Dyspnoea	» Severity (ability to talk, ability to self-care, at rest) » Occurrence, on exertion or at rest » What makes it better or worse? » Complications, febrile, overall health, underlying condition/comorbidities » Physical examination » Related cough	» Position upright or semi-upright » Open window for air circulation » Use a fan. Recent research has unequivocally proven that use of fans and room air provides as much relief to people as providing oxygen (Swan et al., 2019) » Ease the activity burden » Communicate in a calm manner » Remain with the person » Refer to occupational therapy for equipment » Use low-dose opioids and benzodiazepine » Use of oxygen unnecessarily medicalises natural dying. Oxygen via a mask or nasal prongs can cause extra discomfort by drying out oral and nasal mucosa.

(Continued)

TABLE 19.3 Continued

SYMPTOM	POINTS TO CONSIDER	NON-PHARMACOLOGICAL TREATMENT STRATEGIES
Constipation	» Date of last bowel motion » Pre-illness bowel habit » Description of bowel motion, size, consistency, feeling of emptiness post bowel motion » Medication and aperient use (include long-term aperient use, natural therapies, lifelong use of Epsom salts) » Physical examination (consider rectal examination)	» Prevention is better than cure: educate people and families on how to prevent constipation » Encourage drinking of fluids » Monitor bowel habit » Gentle exercise » Gentle abdominal massage
Insomnia	» Physical symptoms to prevent sleep » Sleep patterns » Sleep hygiene » Emotional concerns » Depression	» Good sleep hygiene » Counselling for improved emotional well-being » Refer to social worker for financial assistance if concerns over this are keeping the person awake at night
Anorexia	» Assess meaning (poor intake from early satiety, nausea preventing sufficient oral intake) » Establish quantities of food and/or liquid intake » Consider causes (ill-fitting dentures, oral candidiasis, ulcers, pain, nausea, fatigue) » Assess impact on loved ones	» Small, appetising meals » Refer to a dietician » Educate on the natural dying process: loss of interest in food and drinking are part of the dying process » Counsel and support family about their loved one's lack of interest in food » Mouth care

Source: adapted from Ferrell & Paice, 2019; Matzo & Witt Sherman, 2018; Palliative Care Expert Group, 2016.

19.4 Getting to know the person: Samira's story

Samira is a 72-year-old woman who was diagnosed with metastatic pancreatic cancer six months ago. The referral stated that the reason for referral was that Samira wished to know more about end-of-life care.

The palliative care nurse introduced herself and explained the role of palliative care to Samira. She started the conversation by acknowledging Samira's health journey and allowed Samira to take the lead. It quickly became apparent that, although Samira confirmed that seeking information about end-of-life care was her primary goal, she was clearly having pain issues. The nurse observed that Samira was holding herself in a rigid manner and trying not to move; on movement, she grabbed and splinted her abdomen and her facial expression was frowning and fearful.

Acknowledging Samira's desire for information, the nurse asked about Samira's level of comfort, explaining that she did not appear to be comfortable and asked if she could help.

Samira started crying. She was scared that her worsening pain meant imminent death and had not taken the prescribed morphine as it was the 'death drug'.

The nurse quickly reassured her about the use of morphine in cancer pain and gave her information about pain. Samira scored her pain at 8/10, and said that she wasn't sleeping well and felt teary and emotional all the time. The nurse offered to get Samira's morphine and administer a dose while she was in attendance.

After reassuring Samira again about the safety of morphine and promising Samira that she was not imminently dying, Samira agreed to try the morphine and was given a dose at the rate prescribed by her GP.

The nurse stayed with Samira, chatting about non-threatening topics, and after 15 minutes the nurse observed a change in Samira's posture and body language. Samira appeared more relaxed. She allowed five more minutes to pass before asking Samira to re-score her pain. Samira's pain had settled to 4/10.

Samira again started to cry, this time with relief at having less pain and for the kindness the nurse had shown. The nurse dedicated the rest of the visit to pain education, commencing a pain diary and devising a pain-management plan with Samira. Once Samira appeared less fearful of morphine and committed to the plan, the nurse made a time to return the next day to review her. She indicated to Samira that she would be sharing information of the visit with her GP and oncologist.

- How would you devise a plan of care for Samira to cover the relevant health issues identified in her story?

- How would you manage pain and the side effects of analgesia?

- What other symptoms experienced by Samira would you include in the pain-management plan? How would you work with her to keep her comfortable?

FOCUS QUESTIONS

Nursing care for the imminently dying

All care should be directed at providing comfort to the dying person and their family. Be a compassionate presence. Prior to attending nursing care for your dying patient or patient with reduced consciousness levels, *always* reintroduce yourself and inform them of your intended actions. Show respect. Nursing care should be directed towards the actions in Table 19.5.

Registered nurses often act as guides for families of dying people. Many people have not been exposed to the natural process of dying and it can be frighteningly unfamiliar territory over which they may feel they have no control. Families may require an explanation of the bodily process of dying, reassurance about comfort levels, encouragement to have quality time with the dying person (talking, music, religious rites) and support through a gamut of emotions (sadness, numbness and happiness to anger are all normal emotional responses) (Palliative Care Expert Group, 2016).

Many individuals, as they draw closer to the end of their life or with worsening health, will lose weight and experience a decreased desire to eat (see Table 19.4). The causes of this are multifactorial, and efforts should be made to treat reversible causes. It might be necessary to refer the patient to a speech pathologist or accredited dietitian. The dying individual should be supported to eat or drink if they wish to (Hodgkinson et al., 2016). Goal-setting should gravitate towards allowing food and drink for pleasure and maintaining weight, not towards a relentless pursuit of regaining lost weight (Hashimie et al., 2020; Druml et al., 2016; Arends et al., 2017).

JENNY MCKENZIE AND MELISSA BRODIE

TABLE 19.4 Strategies for addressing a decreased desire to eat

POTENTIAL CAUSES FOR DECREASED APPETITE	STRATEGIES
Medication interaction	» Consider recent medication changes » Request pharmacist review
Ill-fitting dentures	» Request a dental review » Check mouth for oral thrush » Check mouth for ulcers
Failure to respect long-standing food preferences	» Experiment with food textures and temperature » Encourage social habit and atmosphere at meal times » Encourage family to bring in favourite foods » Encourage small snacks often » Offer caloric-rich foods

Providing food to those we love has strong symbolic meaning in all cultures (Hashimie et al., 2020). Families may react emotionally to what they view as starvation during the natural dying process so they may keep attempting to feed their loved one and/or request artificial feeding and hydration. Gentle education about the natural dying process and poor outcomes from artificial feeding and hydration may assist them to process their grief and emotions.

Conversation points for these family members include validating their feelings and providing education.

EXAMPLE DIALOGUE

Yes, I can see how concerned you are for your father. During the dying process, the body does not need the same level of fluid or nutrition as when living an active life. To artificially feed or hydrate your father now may increase his symptoms (oedema, stomach cramps, increased incontinence, moist breathing) and make him feel worse. I can reassure you that research proves that the worst symptom of dehydration is having a dry mouth, which is why we perform regular mouth care on him. Can I show you how to do that?'

Table 19.5 offers some strategies that can be used to assist a dying person to feel more comfortable.

TABLE 19.5 Nursing care for the person who is close to death

ACTION	POINTS TO CONSIDER	STRATEGIES
Eye care	» Dry eye syndrome » As an individual is dying, natural ability to lubricate eyes lessens and they no longer blink. » Family can be taught eye care	» Lubricating eye drops » Maintain individual's regular prescribed eye-drop regime. » Saline eye cleanse to clean away eye discharge » Warm, wet face washer lain across closed eyes
Mouth care	» Assess the condition of the mouth. » Assess for and treat oral thrush. » Teach the family to attend to mouth care. » Keep the patient's lips moist.	» Use solutions to moisten the mouth that are palatable to the patient. » Use regular mouth care with plain water, sodium bicarbonate mouth swabs. » Consider substitute saliva products – but these are not always well tolerated due to 'mouth feel'. » Apply lip balm.

TABLE 19.5 Continued

ACTION	POINTS TO CONSIDER	STRATEGIES
Personal care	» If person is in a domestic setting, consider referral to support services for assistance with personal care.	» Give analgesia prior to washing if pain is an issue. » Give opioid/benzodiazepine prior to washing if the patient has refractory dyspnoea and consider a modified hygiene regimen, such as a bath or 'shampoo in a bag' products. » Keep the patient informed and do not rush the activity.
Pressure area care and maintenance of skin integrity	» Consider pressure-relieving aids for inpatient and domestic settings. » Monitor skin integrity and treat wounds accordingly.	» Position the patient for comfort — never nurse a dyspnoeic patient flat. » Consider analgesia prior to position changes. » Remember that lying in the same position for an extended time can cause discomfort.
Emotional care of the dying person	» Observe the patient for non-verbal indicators of distress. » Enquire about special requests for the patient.	» Involve the patient and family in care-making decisions. » Maintain compassionate care and respect. » Refer the patient to pastoral care, a social worker or other assistance as requested.
Spiritual care	» Not just religious beliefs » Maintain respect for patient and family's unique needs. » Ask them how you can support them or who they may want you to contact. » Older people go through life reviews and revisit regrets and traumas. They may just need someone to listen to their concerns or triumphs.	» Establish religious or spiritual requirements as part of your assessment. » This may include having favourite music playing, having favourite objects nearby or having rituals completed. » Involve religious or spiritual guides as required. » Use technology such as iPads to enable the person to make contact with people at a distance from them. » Provide them with the materials and opportunities to document concerns.
Assessment and management of symptoms	» Be vigilant and observe patient and family non-verbal cues. » If the patient is unable to respond, ask the family about their beliefs on comfort level and respond accordingly.	» Ask the patient if they are able to respond. » Non-verbal indicators of distress may include, but are not restricted to, groaning, grimacing, frowning and appearing to hold tension. » Attune yourself to the tension in the room; it may indicate distress in the patient or family members attending. » Use prn medications as required by the patient. » Consider constipation/urinary retention if there is a sudden increase in distress levels.
Care of family	» Keeping the family informed minimises distress. » Involve the family in decision making.	» Compassionate care of the patient reduces family/carer distress. » Giving information can provide reassurance. » Refer the patient to pastoral care or a religious minister of choice.

Source: adapted from Ferrell & Paice 2019; Matzo & Witt Sherman, 2018; Palliative Care Expert Group, 2016.

COMMUNICATION: 'HOW LONG HAVE I GOT?'

There are many ways to respond to such a question. The following information is based on many years of clinical practice in palliative care and observations of senior medical and nursing staff well practised in having discussions about death and dying.

On occasion, a person may ask for a time frame for when they are likely to die. Alternatively, a family member may ask for an approximate time frame for the death of their loved one. It is important to answer this question in an honest manner. Responding flippantly, as in giving reassurance that death is not going to happen or ignoring the question is unhelpful. Families often seek time frames to death for planning, although at times it is also a cry for reassurance at a difficult time.

Before answering, ask why they wish to know. Often, the desire to know may be driven by relatives or friends living far away and wanting to see them before dying, or a desire to be around for a special occasion (such as a wedding, birth or Christmas).

By giving time frames to approximate time of death such as hours to days, days to weeks, weeks to months, and months to years, the person requesting the information should have enough detail to make relevant decisions without the burden of being given an exact time. Any requests for time frames should be handled with respect and kindness. Honest conversation around time frames enables families to prioritise quality time with their loved one and ultimately improves outcomes for the bereaved (Brighton & Bristowe, 2016).

The will to live is a very strong primal drive; many people will live longer in the dying phase of life than what is expected. Families and loved ones may need reassurance, education and support during this time. As registered nurses, we are privileged to care for exceptional people.

Transformation of hope in end-of-life care

Hope is an emotion experienced through all stages of life. A child may hope for the biggest piece of cake, a teenager's hope may be directed towards being beautiful and famous and, for adults, hope may be about being happy and maintaining good health. By definition, hope is a pleasant feeling linked to a belief that the desired outcome could happen (Harpham, 2017). Hope has long been recognised as an important component of a terminally ill person's existential needs (Olsson et al., 2010; Lohne, 2021). For people and families living with life-limiting illness, hope is the belief that better days or moments can come: it gives a sense of what is possible. Hope can also be considered respite from the reality of their current situation and evolves and changes over the progression of the dying process. As a registered nurse, you can enhance the person's experience of hope by recognising this need and through skilled, therapeutic communication.

THE CHANGING FACE OF HOPE

At diagnosis, there is often:

- hope for a cure
- hope of living a normal life.

   As the disease progresses, there is:

- hope for prolonging life
- hope for good symptom control
- hope for maintaining control of decision making
- hope for gaining pleasure from life (days of good health, sunny days, presence of loved ones).

As death comes closer, there is:

- hope for comfort
- reflection of a life well lived
- hope for a good death (Yun et al., 2018; Bartlett, 2019; Lohne, 2021).

Living with a life-limiting illness is living life with multiple losses including, but not restricted to, altered body image, altered function, loss of employment, loss of social standing or loss of position in one's individual family. In the context of living with a life-limiting illness, hope may have many transformations (Lohne, 2021).

Health professionals have a role in assisting people to balance hope with the reality of living with a life-limiting illness. Australian society values open disclosure and truth telling. When communicating about a life-limiting illness, it is important to have a balance between honesty and being sensitive to maintain hope. Insensitive, tactless delivery of information can cruelly remove a person's hope, making their everyday existence harder to endure.

PRESERVING HOPE

Many health professionals worry that providing realistic information on prognosis may 'take away hope'. Research does not support this fear and suggests that individuals and carers have better outcomes psychologically if they are able to have honest conversations on prognosis (Kelemen et al., 2017).

To safely navigate the balance between honesty and hope, health professionals might want to consider:

- *Communication:*
  - » Before discussing a prognosis, establish how much the person wishes to know, and respect that request.
  - » Respect cultural differences and attitudes about death and dying; employ cultural sensitivity.
  - » Document the set beliefs the person and family may have to share with the rest of the caring team to ensure ongoing, appropriate, respectful communication.
  - » Reassure the person and their family that they will not be abandoned.
- *Physical aspects*:
  - » Refer the person to an occupational therapist for aids and equipment to assist with preservation of physical independence.
  - » Refer them to physiotherapy for a gentle exercise program.
  - » Refer them to support services for personal care or domestic assistance.

Recognising imminent death

Registered nurses are the health professional group most likely to recognise that a person is close to dying. Signs that an individual is likely to die within *weeks* include:

- noticeable functional decline over the past week or two
- increasing fatigue
- increasing **somnolence**
- decreasing interest in food

somnolence
Sleepiness or drowsiness.

- appearance of being unwell
- social withdrawal
- increasing of symptoms from disease (Glare, 2005; Hodgkinson et al., 2016; Palliative Care Expert Group, 2016).

Noticing these changes should trigger conversations within the health-care team and with the person and their family. The person's overall general health should be reviewed to rule out other causes for the changes to health and treat any reversible illness. Common causes for health deterioration in an aged person include:

- urinary tract infection
- mouth ulcers, ill-fitting dentures or oral candidiasis
- peripheral oedema indicative of altered heart or lung function
- chest infection
- pulmonary oedema
- altered blood sugar levels
- constipation
- anaemia.

Depending on the results of the clinical review, consideration should be given to the benefit of diagnostic testing such as blood tests. If the decline in the person's health is deemed to not have a reversible or easily treated cause, it might be appropriate to have a conversation with the person and/or family to check their perception of their and their loved one's current health.

As days or weeks pass, the likelihood that the person is dying may or may not declare itself. Signs of *imminent death* may include:

- altered vital signs (consider negotiating ceasing unnecessary treatment with family)
- increased pallor
- refusal of food or fluids
- reduced ability or inability to swallow (cease unwarranted medications, consider use of **parenteral** medications, through continuous infusion, for symptom control)
- increased somnolence
- difficulty in rousing the person
- an altered breathing pattern
- skin changes
- increased pain/dyspnoea or other symptoms
- reduced urine output (Hodgkinson et al., 2016; Palliative Care Expert Group, 2016).

parenteral
When something is put into the body by a means other than the mouth or rectum (e.g. an injection).

Declaring death

Legal obligations and practices concerning death vary between countries and even from state to state in Australia. It is important that health professionals familiarise themselves with practices in their own health setting. A person is considered deceased when there is an absence of:

- response to external stimuli
- muscular movement

- reflexed
- breathing
- pulse
- eye response (Palliative Care Expert Group, 2016).

EXAMPLE DIALOGUE

Communicating death

What to say when a person has just died:

- 'I am very sorry for your loss … I can see how Joan was loved by you all …'
- 'It's OK to cry …'
- 'Condolences to you all …'
- 'I can see Joan is at peace; she looks so relaxed.'
- 'Please take your time. Would you like to be alone? … I will be outside if you need me.'

Phrases to *avoid*:

- 'Joan would want you to get on with your life …'
- Inferring that the deceased was aged, so it was time they died.
- 'Joan is in a better place now.'
- 'Be strong.'
- 'Don't cry.'
- 'I know how you feel … ' (As observers, even if we have suffered a similar bereavement we are not privy to the intimacy of others' relationships. It is impossible to know just how the recently bereaved person is feeling.)
- Being overly sympathetic; offer empathy instead.

Role of the registered nurse at time of death

The role of the registered nurse at the time of death is often to confirm to the attending family that the person has died or to call family who are not present to inform them of the death. The registered nurse will then contact medical staff to confirm death or follow state/local policy to declare life extinct. Interactions with the family require compassion and kindness. Initially, offer your condolences. Once the family have had a bit of time with their loved one, it may be prudent to offer to reposition and freshen up the appearance of the deceased. This may include removing hospital equipment in line with setting policy and the appropriate Coroners Act (if relevant), repositioning the deceased and washing them. When the family return to the room, reassure them that they may take their time, and offer to answer any questions and to contact any person required to attend to the deceased.

It is then appropriate to be a compassionate presence in the room or, alternatively, to pop in and out of the room, offering support. The family's mood and response will dictate the level of support and presence you, the registered nurse, needs to offer.

Once it becomes clear that the family are ready to leave (this may be minutes after the death or it may be more than an hour), assist them to pack the deceased's belongings and inform them of the next steps they will need to attend to. Providing written information according to the health settings policy will also be beneficial.

As registered nurses, we often develop strong relationships with people we care for and their families. This is particularly true when working in aged care or community-based care, where the therapeutic relationship may be ongoing for many months or years. It is natural for nurses to feel sadness and a level of bereavement when a person they have grown close to dies. Expressing your loss to your colleagues, or how you will miss the deceased to their family, is acceptable. It may assist with your own emotional health and ability to cope, and improve your personal resilience.

Compassion fatigue

As we mentioned earlier in the chapter, registered nurses spend more time in direct contact with patients than any other health professionals. This is particularly true for registered nurses working in palliative and aged care who can care for their cohort for many months or years (Pereira et al., 2021). This can put registered nurses at a higher risk of physical and emotional distress, which may manifest as **compassion fatigue**.

Compassion fatigue has been increasingly researched over recent years and is now a well-recognised challenge for registered nurses working in palliative and aged care. Due to their prolonged contact with individuals with serious illnesses reaching the end of their lives, and the intense emotional connections that these caring relationships can develop, these registered nurses are at higher risk of developing compassion fatigue (Klein et al., 2018). It can be defined as 'a state of exhaustion and dysfunction – biologically, physically and socially – as a result of prolonged exposure to compassion stress and all that it evokes' (Cross, 2019). Compassion fatigue is characterised by an inability to continue being nurturing, by apathy and by cynicism (Boyle, 2015). Table 19.6 indicates the differences between **burnout** and compassion fatigue.

compassion fatigue
A state of biological, physical and social exhaustion and dysfunction resulting from prolonged exposure to compassion stress and everything that comes with it.

burnout
A state of emotional, physical and mental exhaustion caused by excessive and prolonged stress.

TABLE 19.6 Burnout versus compassion fatigue

BURNOUT	COMPASSION FATIGUE
Burnout is commonly associated with workplace stressors: » manager unresponsiveness » lack of camaraderie and team work » working short staffed » conflict » intense workloads.	Compassion fatigue is commonly associated with stress experienced from relationships with people and families: » caring for multiple people with debilitating illness » repeated traumatic events » witnessing tragedies and feeling unable to help.

Source: adapted from Melvin, 2015; Boyle, 2015.

Compassion fatigue can present as physical symptoms such as chronic fatigue, insomnia, gastrointestinal disturbances, headache and muscle tension. Emotionally, nurses may experience feelings of sadness, mood swings, apathy, poor concentration, poor memory, irritation and cynicism (Boyle, 2015). It is being increasingly recognised that compassion fatigue is complex and affects nurses (poor job satisfaction and personal cost), employers (difficulty retaining and attracting staff) and patients (poor satisfaction with care received) (Cross, 2019). Strategies to combat compassion fatigue are layered. Self-awareness, knowledge of work setting supports (formal and informal) and strong self-care strategies are essential. Accessing tools such as the 'Self-Care Matters (Aged Care)' resource (Palliative Care Australia, 2020) and being informed about palliative care (Frey et al., 2018) as well as reflective writing (Tonarelli et al., 2018) may increase resilience and decrease the risk of compassion fatigue for registered nurses. Caring for people and families at the end of life is a rewarding area of nursing. Nurses can gain immense satisfaction from helping people achieve a good death and hearing families say 'thank you for your compassionate care'.

Conclusion

Learn more
Access additional resources – such as weblinks, further readings and podcasts – to broaden your understanding of this chapter. See the Guided Tour for access details.

In spite of advances in medicine to combat disease, death is an inevitable outcome for us all. Registered nurses are uniquely placed in the health-care team to be advocates and guides for their patients and their families as they reach the end of their life and to provide compassionate care.

> Jenny (a chapter co-author) shares the origins of her interest in palliative care: As a second-year student nurse more than 30 years ago, a time when my clinical skills were developing, I was privileged to care for a gracious older woman named Maisie. Caring for Maisie and her family was an educational experience not available in a classroom or by reading a textbook. She and her family's dignified response to care, gratitude for being kept informed, and the significance and comfort felt from well-attended mouth care, pressure area care and personal care all contributed to her ability to preserve hope in the face of death. This experience of providing good-quality care at the end of life and witnessing the benefits of a strong therapeutic relationship formed a passion in me for promoting quality care at the end of life. Now I am passing this passion and knowledge onto you.

1   Consider your previous experiences of death. How have they influenced your ability to care for someone who is dying?

2   What are the significant aspects of communication that must be taken into account when interacting with someone who is dying? And their family?

3   A person who is receiving palliative care complains of breathlessness and abdominal pain. Identify the assessments a registered nurse would undertake. What documentation is required? What other members of the multidisciplinary team need to be involved? Outline the clinical care that a registered nurse could undertake to alleviate the patient's symptoms.

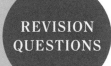

REVISION QUESTIONS

REFERENCES

Advance Care Planning Australia (n.d.). www. advancecareplanning.org.au/

Agency for Clinical Innovation (ACI) (2019). Trauma-informed Care and Mental

Health in NSW. www.aci. health.nsw.gov.au/__data/ assets/pdf_file/0008/561977/ ACI-Mental-Health-Trauma-informed-care-mental-health-NSW.pdf

Anderson, R. J., Bloch, S., Armstrong, M., Stone, P. C. & Low, J. T. S. (2019). Communication between healthcare professionals and relatives of patients

JENNY MCKENZIE AND MELISSA BRODIE

approaching the end of life: A systematic review of qualitative evidence. *Palliative Medicine, 33*(8), 926–41.

Arends, J., Bachmann, P., Baracos, V., Barthelemy, N., Bertz, H. & Bozzetti, F. (2017). ESPEN guidelines on nutrition in cancer patients. *Clinical Nutrition*, 36(1),11–48.

Australian Bureau of Statistics (ABS) (2020). Deaths, Australia. www.abs.gov.au

Australian Healthcare Associates (2019). Exploratory Analysis of Barriers to Palliative Care: Literature Review. www.health.gov.au/resources/publications/exploratory-analysis-of-barriers-to-palliative-care-literature-review

Australian Institute of Health and Welfare (AIHW) (2019). Australia Burden of Disease Study: Impact and Causes of Illness and Death in Australia 2015. www.aihw.gov.au/reports/burden-of-disease/burden-disease-study-illness-death-2015/summary

Bartlett, M. (2019). Finding hope in dying. *BMJ, 366.* https://doi:10.1136/bmj.l2416

Blue Knot Foundation (n.d.) Trauma Informed Care and Practice. www.blueknot.org.au/Resources/Information/Trauma-Informed-Care-and-Practice

Boyle, D. (2015). Compassion fatigue: The cost of caring. *Nursing, 45*(7), 48–51.

Brighton, L. J. & Bristowe, K. (2016). Communication in palliative care: Talking about the end of life, before end of life. *Postgrad Med J., 92,* 466–70.

Clayton, J., Butow, P. & Tattersall, M. (2005). When and how to initiate discussion about prognosis and end of life issues. *Journal of Pain and Symptom Management, 30*(2), 132–44.

Clayton, J., Hancock, K., Butow, P., Tattersall, M. & Currow, D. (2007). Clinical practice guidelines for communicating prognosis and end of life issues with adults in the advanced stages of a life-limiting illness, and their

caregivers. *Medical Journal of Australia, 186*(12), 577–9.

Clayton, J. M., Ritchie, A. J. & Butow, P. N. (2019) Enabling better end of life communication in residential aged care. *Patient Education and Counseling, 102,* 2131–3.

Cottrell, L. & Duggleby, W. (2016). The 'good death': An integrative literature review. *Palliative and Supportive Care, 14,* 686–712.

Cross, L. (2019). Compassion fatigue in palliative care nursing: A concept analysis. *Journal of Hospice & Palliative Care Nursing 21*(1).

Druml, C., Ballmer, P., Druml, W., Oehmichen, F., Shenkin, A., Singer, P., Soeters, P., Weimann, A. & Bischoff, S. (2016). ESPEN guideline on ethical aspects of artificial nutrition and hydration. *Clinical Nutrition 35,* 545–56.

End of Life Direction for Aged Care (ELDAC) (n.d.). www.eldac.com.au

End of Life Law in Australia (n.d.). Euthanasia and Assisted Dying. https://end-of-life.qut.edu.au/euthanasia

Evenblij, K., Koppel, Mt., Smets, T., Widdershoven, G. A. M., Onwuteaka-Philipsen, B. D. & Pasman, H. R. W. (2019). Are care staff equipped for end-of-life communication? A cross-sectional study in long-term care facilities to identify determinants of self-efficacy. *BMC Palliative Care, 18,* 1.

Ferrell, B. R. & Paice, J. (2019). *Oxford Textbook of Palliative Nursing* (5th edn). Oxford University Press.

Frey, R,. Robinson J,. Wong, C. & Gott M (2018). Burnout, compassion fatigue and psychological capital: Findings from a survey of nurses delivering palliative care. *Applied Nursing Research. 43,* 1–9.

Gilbert, A. S., Owusu-Addo, E., Feldman, P., Mackell, P., Garratt, S., M. & Brijnath B. (2020). Models of Integrated Care, Health and Housing: Report prepared for the Royal Commission into Aged Care

Quality and Safety. National Ageing Research Institute.

Glare, P. (2005). Clinical predictors of survival in advanced cancer. *The Journal of Supportive Oncology, 3*(5), 331–9.

Harpham, W. (2017). Healing hope. *Oncology Times,* 25 May.

Hashimie, J., Schultz, S. & Stewart, J. (2020) Palliative care for dementia 2020 update. *Clinical Geriatriatric Medicine 36,* 329–39.

Hernandez-Marrero, P., Fradique, E. & Martins Pereira, S. (2019) Palliative care nursing involvement in end-of-life decision-making: Qualitative secondary analysis. *Nursing Ethics, 26*(6), 1680–95.

Hodgkinson, S., Ruegger, J., Field-Smith, A., Latchem, S. & Ahmedzai, S. (2016) Care of dying adults in the last days of life. *Clinical Medicine 16*(3), 254–8.

Kelemen, A. M., Kearney, G., Pottash, M. & Groninger, H. (2017). Poor prognostication: Hidden meanings in word choices. *BMJ Supportive & Palliative Care 7,* 267–8.

Kezelman, C. (2016). Trauma-informed care and practice in nursing. *Australian Nursing and Midwifery Federation, 24*(2). www.anmf.org.au.

Klein, C. J., Riggenbach-Hays, J. J., Sollenberger, L. M., Harney D. M. & McGarvey J. S. (2018). Quality of life and compassion satisfaction in clinicians: A pilot intervention study for reducing compassion fatigue. *American Journal of Hospice and Palliative Medicine, 35*(6) 882–8.

Lohne, V. (2021). 'Hope as a lighthouse': A meta-synthesis on hope and hoping in different nursing contexts. *Scandinavian Journal of Caring Sciences.* 3 March.

Masso, M., Allingham, S. F., Banfield, M., Johnson, C. E., Pidgeon, T., Yates, P. & Eager, K. (2015). Palliative care phase: Inter-rater reliability and acceptability in national study. *Palliative Medicine, 29,* 22–30.

Matzo, M. & Witt Sherman, D. (2018). *Palliative Care Nursing* (5th edn). Springer Publishing Company.

McGee, P. & Johnson, M. (2014). Developing cultural competence in palliative care. *British Journal of Community Nursing, 19*(2).

Melvin, C. (2015). Historical review in understanding burnout, professional compassion fatigue, and secondary traumatic stress disorder from a hospice and palliative nursing perspective. *Journal of Hospice and Palliative Nursing, 17*(1), 66–72.

Murray, S., Kendall, M., Mitchell, F., Moine, S., Amblas-Novellas, J. & Boyd, K. (2017). Palliative care from diagnosis to death. *BMJ, 356,* j878. https://doi:10.1136/bmj.j878

NSW Health (2020). What is Trauma Informed Care? www.health.nsw.gov.au/mentalhealth/psychosocial/principles/Pages/trauma-informed.aspx

NSW Ministry of Health (2019). NSW Health End of Life and Palliative Care Framework 2019–2024. https://agedcare.royalcommission.gov.au/system/files/2020-06/NDH.0008.0004.0001.pdf

Olsson, L., Ostlund, P. S., Jeppsson Grassman, E. & Friedrichsen, M. (2010). Maintaining hope when close to death: Insight from cancer people in palliative home care. *International Journal of Palliative Nursing, 16*(12), 607–12.

Olsson, M. M., Windsor, C., Chambers, S. & Green, T. (2020) A scoping review of end of life communication in international palliative care guidelines for acute care settings. *Journal of Pain and Symptom Management, 62*(2), 425–37.

Omori, M., Jayasuriya, J., Scherer, S., Dow, B., Vaughan, M. & Savvas, S. (2020) The language of dying: Communication about end-of-life in residential aged care. *Death Studies.* 13 May. https://doi:10.1080/07481187.2020.1762263

PalliAged (2019). Prescribing Guidance. www.palliaged.com.au/Portals/5/Documents/GP_Pharmacological_Management.pdf

Palliative Care Australia (n.d.). https://palliativecare.org.au

Palliative Care Australia (2019). Voluntary Assisted Dying in Australia: Guiding Principles for Those Proving Care to People Living with a Life-Limiting Illness. https://palliativecare.org.au/wp-content/uploads/dlm_uploads/2019/06/PCA-Guiding-Principles-Voluntary-Assisted-Dying.pdf

Palliative Care Australia (2020). Self-Care Matters Aged Care. https://palliativecare.org.au/resources/self-care-matters-aged-care

Palliative Care Expert Group. (2016). Therapeutic Guidelines: Palliative Care. Version 4. Therapeutic Guidelines Limited.

Palliative Care Outcomes Collaborative (PCOC). (n.d.). www.uow.edu.au/ahsri/pcoc

Pereira S. M., Hernandez, P., Pasman, H. R., Capelas, M. L., Larkin, P. & Francke, A. L. (2021). Nursing education on palliative care across Europe: Results and recommendations from the EAPC Taskforce on preparation for practice in palliative care nursing across the EU based on an online-survey and country reports. *Palliative Medicine 35*(1), 130–41.

Rainsford, S., Macleod, R. D., Glasgow, N. J., Wilson, D. M., Phillips, C. B. & Wiles, R. B. (2018). Rural residents' perspectives on the rural 'good death': A scoping review. *Health and Social Care in the Community, 26*(3), 273–94.

Robertson, K. (2005). Active listening: More than just paying attention. *Australian Family Physician, 34*(12), 1053–5.

Swan, F., English, A,. Allgar, V., Hart, S. & Johnson, M. (2019). The hand-held fan and the calming hand for people with chronic breathlessness: A feasibility trial. *Journal of Pain and Symptom Management, 57*(6).

Swerrisen, H. & Duckett, S. (2014). *Dying Well.* Grattan Institute.

Tonarelli, A., Consentino, C., Tomasoni, C., Nelli, L., Damiani, I., Goisis, S., Sarli, L. & Artioli, G. (2018). Expressive writing: A tool to help health workers of palliative care. *ACTA Biomed for Health Professionals, 89*(Suppl. 6) 35–42.

Widera, E., Anderson W. G., Santhosh, L., McKee, K. Y., Smith, A. K. & Frank, J. (2020). Family meetings on behalf of patients with serious illness. *The New England Journal of Medicine, 383*(11).

Wittenberg, E., Ferrell, B. R., Goldsmith, J., Smith, T., Glajchen, M. & Handzo, G. F. (2015). *Textbook of Palliative Care Communication.* Oxford University Press.

World Health Organization (WHO) (2020). Palliative Care.

Yun, Y. H., Kim, K. N., Sim, J. A., Kang, E. K., Lee, J., Choo, J., Yoo, S. H., Kim, M., Kim, A. E., Kang B. D., Shim, H. J., Song, E. K., Kang J. H., Kwon, J. H., Lee, J. L., Lee, S. N., Maeng, C. H., Kang, E. J., Do, Y. R., Choi, Y. S. & Jung K. H. (2018). Priorities of a 'good death' according to cancer patients, their family caregivers, physicians, and the general population: A nationwide survey. *Supportive Care in Cancer. 26,* 3479–88.

GLOSSARY

ableism
Discrimination in favour of able-bodied people.

accord
An official agreement between two or more parties.

acopic
A derogatory term referring to not being able to cope.

active ageing
A program of policies and discourses that generally encourage people to remain physically, socially and mentally active as they age.

acute abdominal emergencies
Sudden, severe abdominal pain that is considered life-threatening.

acute care
Secondary healthcare where a person receives treatment for a sudden, short-term illness or exacerbation of a chronic condition.

advanced care planning
The process of developing a plan for an individual's health and personal care in accordance with their own personal values, belief systems and care preferences.

adverse drug reaction
An untoward drug effect (unintended and occurring at normal dose) that may reflect the drug's action in other body tissues, causing mild to severe side effects, including toxicities, allergic reactions and idiosyncratic side effects.

aetiology
The cause or set of causes, or manner of a disease or condition.

ageing well
The ability to maintain a sense of physical, mental and social health over time.

ageist attitude
An attitude, based on the age of the person, that fails to respect the uniqueness of the individual and instead stereotypes older people as all being the same.

akinetic
The loss of the normal ability to move the muscles.

aldosterone
A hormone that is significant for homeostasis as it regulates sodium, potassium and hydrogen; it has implications for cognition, nervous innervation and hydration for an older person.

amyloidosis
A condition caused by the deposit of abnormal proteins in the muscle of the heart impacting cardiac muscle contraction.

angular cheilitis
A condition causing dry, sometimes moist, cracked corners of the mouth.

anorexia
A lack of appetite and weight loss in advanced life-limiting illness. It may be emotionally troubling for patients and loved ones.

anticholinergic
An agent that causes the loss of water in the body.

anticoagulant
Medication that thins the blood and makes a person vulnerable to bleeding.

aortic stenosis
Loss of elasticity of the artery taking blood from the heart.

apnoea
When someone stops breathing.

arteriosclerotic
Referring to the hardening of the walls of the arteries, causing impeding of blood flow.

auscultate
Listen to the sounds of various body structures, usually with a stethoscope.

authentic partnership
A partnership focusing on the decision-making processes of the older person, family members, health professionals and local community through joint efforts, discussion and regular critical reflection.

baby boomer generation
People born between 1945 and the mid 1960s.

baroreceptor
A bundle of nerve endings in the atria of the heart, the vena cava, aortic arch and carotid sinuses, assisting in the regulation of blood pressure.

behavioural disturbances
Changes in the way a person acts that are generally distressing and puts them or others at risk.

benzodiazepines
A group of drugs that depress the nervous system.

beta-blockers
Drugs that block the effects of the hormone adrenaline.

bioavailability
The percentage of the administered dose of the unchanged drug that reaches the systemic circulation; for intravenous drugs, it is 100 per cent as the drug is administered directly into the circulatory system.

biotransformation
The process by which the body breaks down and converts a drug into an inactive metabolite, a more potent active metabolite or a less active metabolite.

buccal cavity
Structures of the mouth including lips, cheeks, salivary glands and tongue.

burnout
A state of emotional, physical and mental exhaustion caused by excessive and prolonged stress.

calcium channel blockers
Drugs that prevent calcium entering the cells of the heart and arteries.

cardiac arrhythmias
Irregular heartbeats.

care coordinator
A health professional who works collaboratively with patients, general

practice, allied health, First Nation health services, social service providers and other people responsible for part of a patient's care, to organise and facilitate person-centred delivery of care.

care plan

A plan of action, agreed between a patient and their health-care providers, that identifies their health-care needs, services that are needed, and a list of health goals and specific actions that are required to meet them.

carotid sinus hypersensitivity

A condition that causes slowing of the heart and reduced blood pressure making a person vulnerable to falls.

cerebral perfusion

The flow of blood to and around the brain.

cerumen

A substance excreted by the sebaceous glands in the ear canal; accumulation of cerumen retards the sound waves reaching the tympanic membrane and affects hearing.

chemoreceptor

A cell that is sensitive to changes in chemical concentrations and initiates changes to nervous impulses as a result of those changes.

chronic condition

Any ongoing or recurring health issue that has a significant impact on the person and/or family or other carers, and requiring a long period of supervision, monitoring and care. Examples include, but are not limited to, long-term pain, mental health conditions, musculoskeletal conditions, hypertension, disability and syndromes.

chronic disease

A pathological condition that interrupts the normal functions of the body and tends to be slow in progression and prolonged in duration. Examples are cardiovascular disease, cancers, chronic kidney disease, respiratory diseases and diabetes. It is uncommon that it will resolve spontaneously, and it is rarely cured completely.

chronic illness

The human experience of prolonged symptoms and suffering. It refers to how the disease or condition is perceived by the person experiencing it, as well as their caregiver/s.

collaboration

Health-care professionals working together to achieve greater impacts on patient health outcomes than they could in isolation.

compassion fatigue

A state of exhaustion and dysfunction – biologically, physically and socially – as a result of prolonged exposure to compassion stress and everything that comes with it.

constipation

Difficulty passing stools; incomplete or infrequent passing of hard stools.

Consumer Directed Care (CDC)

An approach to service delivery where the individual receiving the service determines the types of services, from whom, when and how these services will be delivered, giving individuals choice and flexibility.

continuity of care

Using a care coordination health-care model to provide consistency of care and continuity of information to improve patient outcomes.

coronary angiogram

A procedure in which pictures of the heart and its arteries are taken.

costal cartilage

Cartilage between the ribs and the sternum.

Council on the Ageing (COTA)

A group claiming to represent seniors having a central role in policy development in NACA.

creatinine

A product of protein metabolism in the muscle; it is excreted in the urine.

cultural awareness

The emotional, social, economic and political context in which people exist. Understanding culture and having an awareness of one's own culture.

cultural diversity

Having a mix of people from different cultural backgrounds. It can include differences in cultural/ethnic identity, language, country of birth, religion, heritage/ancestry, national origin and/or race (Diversity Council of Australia (DCA)).

cultural practice

The traditional and customary practices of a particular ethnic or other cultural group.

cultural safety

An outcome that enables safe service to be determined by those who receive the service. Cultural safety is determined by First Nations individuals, families and communities.

cultural sensitivity

Alerts practitioners to the validity of difference and starts a self-exploration process of their own experience and realities of life and the effect this could have on others. Having an awareness of any cultural issues in health-care delivery and the policies and practices involved.

culturally appropriate care

More than just awareness of cultural differences, this focuses on the capacity of the health system to improve health and well-being by integrating culture into the delivery of health-care services.

culturally safe residential aged care

A concept that aims to ensure service users of a different cultural background from the caregiver/practitioner can feel safe in their experience of care; where there is no assault, challenge or denial of identity of who they are and what they need. It is about shared respect, shared meaning, living and working together with dignity, and truly listening.

delirium

A sudden onset of confusion that can be resolved when the cause is identified and treated.

dementia

A syndrome – usually of a chronic or progressive nature – in which there is deterioration in cognitive function (i.e. the ability to process thought) beyond what might be expected from normal ageing.

denture stomatitis

Red appearance where the denture sits.

despair

To be without hope.

***Diagnostic and Statistical Manual of Mental Disorders* (DSM-5)**

A manual of descriptions, symptoms and other criteria for diagnosing mental disorders.

discourse

Foundational ways of understanding the world and how these influence what we see, what we value and how we act.

discretionary choices

Foods that contain large amounts of fat, sugar, sodium or alcohol, and as a result may also be high in calories and lack important nutrients. Examples are cakes, sweet and savoury biscuits, ice cream, beer, wine, takeaways and chips.

disenfranchisement

The state of being deprived of a right or privilege, often the right to vote.

diverticula

Sacs or pouches that form at weaknesses in the wall of the gastrointestinal system; they can trap food, leading to ulceration and infection.

dyad

A social group that consists of two members – for example, husband and wife – or a caregiver and a care recipient.

dyspnoea

A subjective experience of difficulty in breathing.

edentulism

No natural teeth.

end of life

The last few weeks of life, in which a patient with a life-limiting illness is rapidly approaching death.

euthanasia

The merciful killing of a patient suffering from a terminal disease or in an irreversible coma.

evidence-based practice

An approach to practice that encourages practitioners to combine research evidence with their own growing understanding and the knowledge of the unique context within which they are working. When working with an individual or a family, this means you are adapting the scientific evidence to suit the individual person's circumstances. In this way of practising, you are also giving the knowledge and understanding of all individuals involved in practice equal weighting – that is, the practitioner's knowledge or the scientific evidence is not considered superior to that of the individual receiving care.

familial

Relating to or involving a family.

fatigue

A subjective experience defined as a persistent and distressing sense of tiredness that is not proportional to activity, not relieved by sleep or rest, and which interferes with normal functioning.

filial

Referring to a child's relationship with or feelings towards their parents.

formal care

Services and supports provided by paid health care, aged care and other professionals.

for-profit

An organisation that operates in the private sector with the aim of making a profit for its owners.

Fourth Age

A period towards the end of life, older than 80 years, which is typically characterised by sickness, dependency, frailty and the imminence of death.

frailty

Clinically defined as three or more of the following: weight loss, fatigue, weakness, slow walking speed and less activity.

free market

A situation where supply and demand are free from any form of regulation by government or any other authority.

free will

The ability to act as you choose without being confined by fate.

gastrointestinal

Related to the digestive system.

generativity

Focusing on perpetuating and moulding the next generation.

gerontologist

A scientist who focuses on supporting education about and understanding of ageing.

gerontology

The study of all aspects of ageing: social, spiritual, psychological, physical, cultural and cognitive.

gerotranscendence

Described as not just a continuation of the activity patterns and values of mid life, but rather a transformation characterised by new ways of understanding life, activities, oneself and others.

glomerular filtration rate (GFR)

A measure used to check how well the kidneys are working.

glomerulus

The site where waste is exchanged from the capillaries in the kidneys into the end of nephrons (Bowman's capsule).

half-life

The time the body takes to excrete half of the dose of a drug.

health assessment

An Australian Government initiated program where older people undergo a full health check each year to prevent and/or address any changes that have occurred.

health coaching

An evidenced-based technique that applies psychological principles to motivate and support health behaviour change to improve health outcomes.

health promotion

The process of enabling people to increase control over and to improve their health.

healthy ageing

The development of mental, social and physical well-being across the lifespan.

heterogeneous

Diverse, different, varied, mixed.

heteronormativity

Consciously or subconsciously using heterosexuality as standard human behaviour, thereby leaving non-heterosexual peoples out of the frame of reference.

high care

Care for older people who require almost complete assistance with most daily living activities including meals, laundry, room cleaning and personal care.

holistic concept

A concept that health requires a view of the individual as an integrated system – including physical, cognitive, spiritual and emotional – rather than one or more separate parts.

homeostatic mechanism
A feedback (loop) mechanism involving organs, glands, tissues and cells that respond to changes in the internal and external environment to enable the body to function at an optimum steady state by regulating body temperature, water balance, acid–base balance, blood pressure, blood glucose and gas concentrations.

hospital-acquired infections
When bacteria or viruses get into the body because of medical treatments.

human rights
Individual and collective rights to food and shelter; rights that are inherent to being human, universal and indivisible.

hyperpigmentation
The staining of skin caused by breakdown of the venous system, common in the lower leg.

hypodypsia
Age-related blunting of the thirst response to dehydration.

hypoglycaemia
Low blood sugar level.

hypovolaemia
Low fluid levels in the body.

identity management
The process by which adults negotiate and construct a personal and social sense of self

idiosyncratic
A rare and unpredictable adverse drug reaction that is specific to the individual (e.g. anaphylaxis); such a reaction is not related to the known pharmacological properties of the drug and does not suggest a dose–response relationship.

individual rights-based approach
An approach that privileges the human rights of the individual over the group or community.

individualised values
Values that emphasise independence and personal fulfilment.

informal care
Unpaid care provided by family, friends, neighbours and other community supports

without support from a government agency or service provider.

in-home telemonitoring
Remotely monitoring a patient in their home using technology that tracks their vital signs and electronically transmits the information to health professionals for assessment.

innervation
The excitement of nerves in an area or organ of the body.

insomnia
A long period of time when a person is unable to fall asleep or stay asleep.

integrated care
Provision of well-connected, effective and efficient care that takes account of and is organised around a person's health and social needs.

integrity
Being true to yourself, honest and undivided.

integument
The skin, hair and nails.

intergenerational care
The exchange of care and support across generations.

intervention designers
The people responsible for designing interventions to prevent or respond to elder abuse.

iterative personhood
The practice of building, refining and improving personhood over time

lacrimal
Relating to a tear gland in the corner of the eye and the duct system that extends from the eye into the nasal cavity.

lateral violence
Displaced violence directed against one's peers rather than adversaries.

life event
A major change in a person's status or circumstances that affects interpersonal relationships, leisure and recreation activities, or work duties.

low care
Care for older people who can manage their daily chores with minimal assistance from a nurse or carer.

malnutrition
The intake of too little or too much energy, protein or other nutrients, causing negative changes in body weight, muscle and fat mass, functionality and wellness.

marginalisation
The treatment of a person, group or concept as insignificant or peripheral.

market
An arena where commercial dealings are conducted.

marketplace
A place where goods and services are supplied and purchased.

Masters Games
A multi-sport and entertainment event, such as the Australian Masters Games and World Masters Games, held at local, state, national and/or international levels for mature-aged athletes.

Mediterranean diet
A dietary pattern where plant foods (such as fruit, vegetables, grains, legumes, nuts and seeds) make up the majority of the daily diet, with animal foods (such as dairy, fish, eggs and poultry) consumed in lesser quantities. Wine (consumed at meals in low to moderate amounts) and olive oil are also key components of the diet and fruit is a typical finish to a meal.

melanocyte
A skin cell in which the brown or black pigment, melanin, is produced.

men's and women's business
The separate responsibilities of men and women to families, communities, culture and Country that traditional Australian Indigenous cultures had numerous laws governing and which are sacred and remain secret.

mesenteric ischaemia
When blood flow is cut off from part of the small intestine.

metabolite
The intermediate or end product of the breakdown of chemicals in the body.

metastatic cancer
When cancer cells spread from a primary tumour to another part of the body.

micturition
The process of eliminating urine from the bladder through muscle contraction of that organ.

morbidity
The burden of disease/pathophysiology experienced by a person.

mortality
Contributing to death.

motor neurone disease
A neurodegenerative disease that causes rapidly progressive muscle weakness. It is a life-limiting disease.

multidimensional
Containing a number of different levels, including micro (individual), meso (family, group) and macro levels (community, policy, research).

multidisciplinary team
A team that includes professionals from a range of disciplines consisting of a group of experts whose goal is comprehensive patient-centred care.

multimorbidity
The presence of multiple chronic conditions that collectively have an adverse effect on the health and well-being of the person living with them.

multiple chronic conditions (MCCs)
The coexistence of two or more long-term or permanent health conditions in a person.

Multi-Purpose Services Program
Provides integrated health and aged care services to regional and remote communities in areas that can't support a hospital and a separate aged care home.

National Aged Care Alliance (NACA)
An alliance of a number of providers and other groups involved in aged care formed in 2000 and designed to lobby and work with government. It supported a focus on individual choice and control within government-free market policies.

nausea
A feeling of sickness with an inclination to vomit.

neoliberal
Refers to market-oriented policies with minimal regulation and reduced government interference and influence.

nephron
A functional unit of the kidney.

nerve block
Injecting medication around a specific nerve to stop a person feeling pain.

neurotoxicity
Nervous system problems occurring from exposure to chemicals.

non-pharmacological treatments
Strategies to relieve pain and/or promote comfort that do not rely on medications. These can be a broad range of measures depending on the individual's needs. Comfort may include addressing physical, psychological, spiritual, social and financial needs.

non-profits
Organisations with a social mission and not seeking a profit for any individual.

oedema
Swelling of body tissue caused by the excessive accumulation of fluid.

open market
Refers to economic situations where there is free trade.

organisational viability
An organisation's ability to successfully adapt and manage business practices, finances and challenges over the long term.

orthopantomogram (OPG)
An x-ray of the mouth.

orthostatic hypotension
A drop in blood pressure when standing.

ototoxicity
Damage to the inner ear caused by chemicals.

overservicing
Market weaknesses are exploited to make profits by providing more services than are needed as and to those who don't need them.

over-the-counter
Substances purchased by the person, without requiring a prescription, from pharmacies, supermarkets, health-food shops and herbalists.

pain
An unpleasant sensory and emotional experience associated with actual or potential tissue damage. It is an individual experience that occurs when the person says it does and is as severe as the person says it is.

palliative care
The person- and family-centred care provided for a person with an active, progressive, advanced disease, who has little or no prospect of cure and who is expected to die, and for whom the primary goal is to optimise the quality of life.

parenteral
When something is put into the body by a means other than the mouth or rectum (e.g. an injection).

patient-centred approach
A respectful relationship between health-care professionals, the health system and patients and their families that involves patients in shared decisions about their own health to develop a personalised care plan.

peer workers
People who, through their unique and valuable experiences, harness the lived experience of mental ill-health and recovery to support others and foster hope.

periodontal disease
Inflammation of the gums (gingivae) and damage to the bone that anchors teeth in the jaws; also called 'gum disease'.

periodontitis
A bacterial infection that can cause inflammation and bleeding of the gums. In more serious cases it can also lead to bone loss of the jaw.

person-centred approach
A focus on participant involvement in decision making about leisure activities and nurturing individuals' strengths in leisure contexts through leisure experiences.

person-centred care
Treatment and care provided by health services that places the person at the centre of their own care and considers the needs of the older person's carers.

personal protective equipment
Clothing or accessories worn by a worker to protect them from hazards.

personhood
The standing or status bestowed on a human being.

pharmacodynamics
The study of the way a drug affects the body: a primary (desired) or secondary (desired or undesired) physiological effect, or both.

pharmacokinetics
The process of drug movement to achieve drug action, or how a drug is altered as it travels through the body.

physically active leisure
Leisure activity that involves bodily movement.

pinna
The part of the ear that is external to the skull.

pinocytosis
The process by which a cell carries a drug across its membrane by engulfing the drug particles.

polypharmacy
The use of more than five medications, often with medications prescribed to address the side effects of other pharmaceutical products.

postural hypertension
Decrease in blood pressure on standing.

powerlessness
A lack of influence, ability or power.

pressure sores
Wounds caused by prolonged periods of pressure on a part of the body.

primary care
The first point of contact and closest health service for consumers to access in the community that offers a range of health services to prevent disease and support people managing their health at home.

probity regulators
Authorities who undertake an assessment of an applicant's trustworthiness before licensing them to operate in vulnerable sectors.

protectionism
Refers to government policies that restrict commercial activity with the aim of improving safety and/or quality.

psychoactive drugs
Chemicals that affect a person's mental state.

psychomotor behaviour
Physical movements controlled by the brain.

psychotropic agent
Any drug capable of affecting the mind, emotions and behaviour.

public good
A commodity or service that is provided without profit to all members of a society, either by government or by private individuals or organisations.

Purkinje fibre
A fibre that conducts nervous stimuli, initiated by the sinoatrial node, through the atria and across the ventricles of the heart.

quality of life
An individual's subjective perception of their life based on an evaluation of the positive and negative aspects. An introspective assessment of their holistic well-being including their physical, social, spiritual, mental and economic needs and experiences.

recreation
Activity that contributes to one's health and sense of identity (in contrast to traditional understandings of recreation in health-care settings, such as therapeutic recreation).

regulated
Business activity controlled by means of rules or regulations.

relationship-centred care
A reciprocal relationship between health-care professionals and patients that promotes a sense of belonging and security. The model moves beyond focusing on individual medical needs to valuing the person behind the conditions. Health and healing are promoted through an openness to connect, learn and grow.

respiratory depression
Slow and ineffective breathing.

sarcopenia
Commonly recognised as a loss of muscle mass, and therefore decline in function and strength.

sebum
A substance excreted by sebaceous glands to protect and moisturise the skin.

self-care
Individuals taking the actions required to care for their own health and well-being; in the context of multimorbidity this includes actions to effectively manage their chronic conditions and to prevent further illness.

self-determination
The fulfilment of a person's psychological need for autonomy, competence and relatedness.

septic shock
A dangerously low drop in blood pressure due to an infection.

'shame'
An uncomfortable feeling of humiliation or distress caused by being aware of wrong or reckless behaviour.

sinoatrial node
The area of the heart where nervous stimuli are initiated to induce contractions.

Sjogren's syndrome
An autoimmune condition that can cause a dry mouth.

somnolence
Sleepiness or drowsiness.

spousal
Relating to marital or de facto relationships.

stage of life
A period of human existence that has unique characteristics: infancy, early childhood, childhood, adolescence, adulthood, middle adulthood and advanced years.

stagnation
Lack of progression.

step-down care
Hospitals receiving payment to provide rehabilitation care transferred patients to nursing homes where the payment system allowed more therapy and much larger profits.

stereotyping
The belief that all the members of a particular category of people are the same.

strengths-based approach
A social work theory that focuses on an individual's self-determination and strength.

substrate
The natural environment in which an organism lives.

successful ageing
Ageing where the person perceives themselves as healthy, disability (if any exists) is not impeding their enjoyment of life and they are functioning at a level that enables them to be actively engaged in activities they enjoy or find fulfilling.

System Governor
Refers to the overall management function of the controlling Independent Australian Aged Care Commission in Pagone's model and the Department of Health in Brigg's. An Aged Care Advisory Council appointed by the minister would advise on policy matters concerning the performance of the aged care system and on matters of importance from the perspectives of older people who need and use aged care services, the workforce, providers, educators and professionals involved in the provision of aged care.

Third Age
Approximately between the ages of 65 and 80 years, following retirement, and a time when there are fewer responsibilities, coupled with greater freedom to pursue self-fulfilment.

toxicity
Where the blood drug level exceeds the maximum therapeutic range and a harmful and unintended response to the drug results.

transient ischaemic attack
A disruption to the circulation in the brain causing temporary loss of awareness; can be a precursor to a major cerebral disruption or stroke.

trauma-informed care
Care that is aware of trauma symptoms and accepts the role it plays in a person's life. This includes the life of the carer and health professional. Trauma-informed care can change organisational culture to one that values, respects and appropriately responds to the effects of trauma at all levels of the organisation.

traumatic ulcer
An ulcer that develops through some form of trauma to the mouth.

triage category
A numerical system used to determine how quickly people need to be treated when they attend an emergency department.

unregulated
Not controlled or supervised by government regulations or laws.

voluntary assisted dying (VAD)
A process of self-administering a medication for the purpose of causing death in accordance with the steps and processes set out in law. It is only for those who face an inevitable, imminent death as a result of an incurable disease, illness or medical condition.

volunteering sector
Organisations that are not-for-profit and non-governmental.

vomiting
Expulsion of stomach contents through the mouth.

well-being
The contented feeling people have about their holistic state of health and quality of life at any given moment.

wellness model
A model that focuses on valuing wellness and possibilities in later life, as opposed to a disease model, which focuses on illness, dependency and decline.

INDEX